THE ANTICANCER DRUGS

THE ANTICANCER DRUGS

SECOND EDITION

William B. Pratt

Raymond W. Ruddon

William D. Ensminger

Jonathan Maybaum

New York   Oxford
OXFORD UNIVERSITY PRESS
1994

Oxford University Press

Oxford   New York   Toronto
Delhi   Bombay   Calcutta   Madras   Karachi
Kuala Lumpur   Singapore   Hong Kong   Tokyo
Nairobi   Dar es Salaam   Cape Town
Melbourne   Auckland   Madrid

and associated companies in
Berlin   Ibadan

Published by Oxford University Press, Inc.
200 Madison Avenue, New York, New York 10016

Oxford is a registered trademark of Oxford University Press

Library of Congress Cataloging-in-Publication Data
The Anticancer drugs / William B. Pratt . . . [et al.]. — 2nd ed.
  p. cm.   Rev. ed. of: The anticancer drugs / William B. Pratt, Raymond W.
Ruddon. 1979.
Includes bibliographical references and index.
ISBN 0-19-506738-X — ISBN 0-19-506739-8 (pbk.)
1. Cancer—Chemotherapy.   2. Antineoplastic agents.
3. Antineoplastic agents—Testing.   I. Pratt, William B., 1938–
[DNLM: 1. Antineoplastic Agents.   QV 269 A62954 1994]
RC271.C5P72 1994
616.99'4061—dc20
DNLM/DLC
for Library of Congress   93-5964

1 3 5 7 9 8 6 4 2

Printed in the United States of America
on acid-free paper

Preface to Second Edition

This text offers an up-to-date review of the field of cancer chemotherapy, including some of the new approaches to biological treatments of cancer and potential targets for new drug design. A detailed description of the pharmacology, mechanisms of action, toxicity, resistance mechanisms, and clinical usefulness of each class of drugs is given. We have emphasized the concepts involved in determining the mechanism of action and development of resistance, the determinants of drug responsiveness to chemotherapeutic agents, and a rationale for their clinical use in various types of cancer.

We have organized the text in a way that we think will make it easy for the reader to conceptualize how drugs work and to categorize them by their mechanism of action. The aim is to help the reader understand the rationale for chemotherapy with respect to the biology of the cancer cell and to tumor growth kinetics. Drawing on the fields of medicinal chemistry, pharmacology, biochemistry, cell biology, molecular biology, and clinical medicine, the book is extensively referenced and provides a historical background for the development of each class of drugs.

In the first edition of this text we discussed the anticancer drugs in terms of their effects on biochemical pathways. Since that edition was written in the late 1970s, the tools of molecular biology and cell biology have been widely used to describe the mechanisms of drug action on cells and how these events lead to cell death. The concepts derived from this work have contributed greatly to our understanding of the determinants of tumor cell responses and resistance as well as to our understanding of the pathophysiological basis for the undesirable clinical effects of these drugs. To help condense this considerable body of information into readable form, two new authors have helped write the second edition. Dr. Maybaum is an expert in cancer pharmacology, specializing in mechanisms of antimetabolite drug action and the phenomenon of programmed cell death. Dr. Ensminger is an expert in the clinical pharmacology of anticancer drugs, in particular in innovative methods of drug delivery. When we began writing this edition, all of the authors were members of the faculty of the Department of Pharmacology and members of the Cancer Pharmacology Program at the University of Michigan. Dr. Ruddon subsequently moved to the University of Nebraska, where he is currently director of the Eppley Institute for Research in Cancer and Allied Diseases.

Ann Arbor, Michigan   W.B.P.
Omaha, Nebraska   R.W.R.

Contents

PART 3

CLINICAL CANCER CHEMOTHERAPY

PART 4

NEW DIRECTIONS IN CANCER CHEMOTHERAPY

Principles of Cancer Chemotherapy

The Cancer Problem

Cancer is a dread disease. Indeed, it is many diseases. That's one of the problems. There are several initiating causes, several cofactors and promoters, and several kinds of cellular damage inflicted on the body's own cells. Cancer arises from cells in the body that were once normal cells. These "transformed" cells grow and divide and keep dividing in an uncontrolled manner. Yet they differ only subtly at first from the cells in the normal tissue from which they arise. Thus, the biochemistry and molecular regulatory mechanisms of cancer cells are similar to the body's own cells. In the words of Walt Kelly: "We have met the enemy and they are us."

Cancer is not like a bacterial infection that the body recognizes as foreign in the way, for example, that the body recognizes an invading staphylococcus as foreign to itself. It is true that the body can mount a partial immune reaction against cancer cells, but as a cancer grows, these immune mechanisms are overwhelmed and only weakly effective.

A question about finding a cure for cancer might be posed in the following way: "When will cures be found for the many different types of cancer?" As will be pointed out later in this book, there are many success stories in cancer treatment. These include acute lymphocytic leukemia of childhood, Hodgkin's disease, Burkitt's lymphoma, Ewing's sarcoma (a form of bone cancer), Wilm's tumor (a kidney cancer in children), rhabdomyosarcoma (a cancer of the muscle tissue), choriocarcinoma (a malignancy of placental trophoblast), testicular can-

cer, certain ovarian cancers, and osteogenic sarcoma. In all of these examples, therapy with anticancer drugs has played a major role. Unfortunately, these cancers are of relatively low incidence compared to breast, lung, colon, and prostate cancer, the most common types of cancer in adults. In these latter forms of cancer, early diagnosis and prompt treatment with surgery, often in combination with radiotherapy and chemotherapy, still hold out the best hope of long-term survival. The reasons why some cancers are harder to treat than others will be discussed in some detail in Chapter 3. Suffice it to say here that some cancers are more susceptible than others to anticancer drugs. Moreover, some cancers metastasize early and become much harder to eradicate in body sites distant from the primary locus of the tumor.

Everyone wants to know when there will be cures for the major forms of cancer. We now understand much more about the cellular and molecular biology of cancer, about the kinds of cell-surface antigens that tumor cells produce and about how the body's immune system reacts to them, about the growth factors that tumor cells make, about the "tumor suppressor genes" that they are lacking, and about the "oncogenes" that are activated in cancer cells. These new findings in cancer biology are being translated slowly but surely into clinically viable treatment strategies, and one can predict that in the next five to ten years gene replacement therapy, antisense gene therapy, adoptive immunotherapy, and growth factor antagonists will take their place in standard medical practice along with surgery, radiation, and chemotherapy.

Why is it all taking so long? Part of the reason is that cancer researchers have had to unlock a lot of the deep secrets of life itself—how normal cells grow, divide, and differentiate—in order to understand how a cancer cell is abnormal. This has taken time and has had to await advances in molecular biology and fundamental cell biology that in some ways are still only beginning to illuminate these areas. As Alexander Fleming, the discoverer of penicillin, said: "The spores didn't just stand up on the agar and say, 'I produce an antibiotic, you know.'"

Cancer Epidemiology

Each year in the United States more than one million people are diagnosed with cancer, and this number does not include the 600,000 cases of nonmelanoma skin cancer (mostly due to sun overexposure) diagnosed annually.[1] About 500,000 people die from cancer each year in the United States. One person dies from cancer every 62 seconds. About 76,000 children between the ages of 3 and 14 die of cancer each year. Most of the 157,000 people diagnosed yearly with lung cancer will die of their disease. Almost all of the patients diagnosed with pancreatic, liver, or esophageal cancer will die within five years of diagnosis.

About 76 million Americans, or 30% of the population, now living will eventually get cancer. The disease will strike three out of four families. In addition to the individual physical and emotional burden, there is a huge financial burden—both to the family involved and to the nation. It is estimated that the total cost of cancer in the United States is about $72 billion a year, $22 billion in direct medical costs and $50 billion in lost wages and productivity.[2]

Not all the news is bad, however. There are over six million Americans alive today who have had cancer. Over half of them can be considered "cured" in that they have had no evidence of disease for at least five years past the time of treatment. Since the average age of onset of cancer is about 67 years of age[3] (averaged for both sexes and all forms of cancer),

most people surviving past five years are expected to have a normal life span.

Much progress has been made in the early diagnosis and treatment of cancer. At the turn of the twentieth century, few cancer patients survived. By the 1930s, less than one in five was alive five years after diagnosis. In the 1940s, this figure reached one in four, in the 1960s one in three, and by 1990 it was close to 50%.

Cancer Incidence and Mortality Rates

The current incidence and mortality rates for cancer in the U.S. are shown in Figure 1–1. For men, the most commonly diagnosed cancers are prostate, lung, colon, and urinary bladder. For women, the most common are cancer of the breast, colon, lung, and uterus. The highest mortality rates for men are from lung, prostate, and colon cancer, whereas for women the highest death rates are from lung, breast, and colon cancer, in that order. The death rates for individual cancers differ from the incidence rates because of the better "curability" of some cancers compared with others. The remarkable increase in female lung cancer mortality in recent years, to the point where it surpasses breast cancer deaths, is almost certainly due to the increased amount of cigarette smoking among women (Fig. 1–2).[4]

The trends in cancer mortality in the United States are depicted in Figure 1–3. There are some encouraging and some troubling signs. Although the mortality rate for lung cancer in men is leveling off, the sharp rise of lung cancer deaths in women continues to drive the trendline upward. Although the mortality rate for breast cancer has been relatively constant, there has been a disturbing rise in the incidence rate. This incidence of breast cancer increased about 1% a year from the early 1970s to the late 1980s, and has gone from 85 cases to 105 cases per 100,000 women during that time. Some of this increased incidence is likely due to more active screening programs, including mammography, but this cannot be the complete answer. The risk factors for breast cancer include early menarche and late menopause, childlessness, first childbirth after age 30, and family history of breast cancer. The larger number of women delaying having children may contribute to this increase, but that isn't clear yet.

Cancer incidence by site and sex*

Prostate 132,000	Breast 180,000
Lung 102,000	Colon & rectum 77,000
Colon & rectum 79,000	Lung 66,000
Bladder 38,500	Uterus 45,500
Lymphoma 27,200	Lymphoma 21,200
Oral 20,600	Ovary 21,000
Melanoma of the skin 17,000	Melanoma of the skin 15,000
Kidney 16,200	Pancreas 14,400
Leukemia 16,000	Bladder 13,100
Stomach 15,000	Leukemia 12,200
Pancreas 13,900	Kidney 10,300
Larynx 10,000	Oral 9,700
All sites 565,000	All sites 565,000

Cancer deaths by site and sex

Lung 93,000	Lung 53,000
Prostate 43,000	Breast 46,000
Colon & rectum 28,900	Colon & rectum 29,400
Pancreas 12,000	Pancreas 13,000
Lymphoma 10,900	Ovary 13,000
Leukemia 9,900	Uterus 10,000
Stomach 8,000	Lymphoma 10,000
Esophagus 7,500	Leukemia 8,300
Liver 6,600	Liver 5,700
Brain 6,500	Brain 5,300
Kidney 6,400	Stomach 5,300
Bladder 6,300	Multiple myeloma 4,500
All sites 275,000	All sites 245,000

*Excluding nonmelanoma skin cancer and carcinoma in situ.

Figure 1-1 (From *Cancer Facts and Figures—1992*)[1]

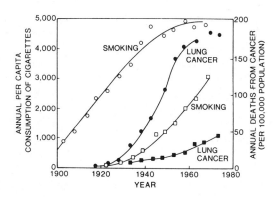

Figure 1-2 Trends in smoking prevalence and lung cancer in British males and females. The data for this chart are from England and Wales. In men, smoking (O) began to increase at the beginning of the 20th century, but the corresponding trend in deaths from lung cancer (●) did not begin until after 1920. In women, smoking (□) began later, and the increase in lung cancer deaths in women (■) has appeared only recently. (From Loeb *et al.*)[4]

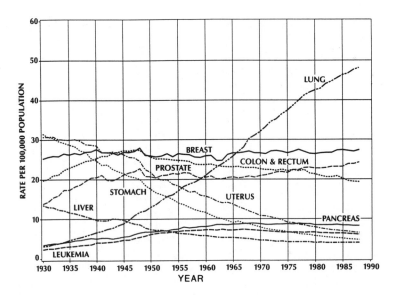

Figure 1-3 Cancer death rates by site, United States, 1930–88. Rates are adjusted to the age distribution of the 1970 census population. Sources of Data: National Center for Health Statistics and Bureau of the Census, United States. Note: Rates are for both sexes combined except breast and uterus (female population only) and prostate (male population only). (From *Cancer Facts and Figures—1992*).[1]

Other risk factors, including dietary ones, may also be involved. The fact that the mortality rates for breast cancer have not changed significantly (Fig. 1–3) even though the incidence has risen indicates that improved diagnosis and treatment have had some impact.

Mortality rates for uterine cancer have been going down since the late 1940s, due primarily to earlier diagnosis and treatment of endometrial and cervical cancer. The Papanicolaou (Pap) test for cervical cancer has clearly had an important role in the earlier diagnosis of cervical cancer.

Among the gastrointestinal tract cancers, stomach cancer mortality has been decreasing since the early 1900s, presumably due to better storage of foods and less use of nitrates and other food-curing agents; deaths due to colorectal cancer have decreased slightly; and a disturbing increase in deaths due to pancreatic cancer has been noted.

Five-Year Survival Rates

Figure 1–4 emphasizes the importance of early diagnosis in the survival of cancer. In every case, survival is better when the disease is localized to a primary site. Once regional spread has occurred, survival rates go down, and they decrease dramatically once distant metastasis has occurred.

Cancer by Age and Race

Cancer is a disease of aging. As noted above, the average age of diagnosis of cancer is 67 years. Thus, as a higher proportion of the population reaches age 60 and beyond, the incidence of cancer would be expected to rise due to that factor alone. When the death rates for cancer are corrected for age, however, some trends are evident that cannot be explained by aging of the population. Death rates from several kinds of cancer have increased in people over age 54 in the last two decades in the United States and five other industrial countries.[5] Mortality from brain tumors, multiple myeloma, breast cancer, and malignant melanoma increased in this age group in the United States, England and Wales, France, West Germany, Italy, and Japan. The greatest overall increase occurred in men between the ages of 75 and 84. Excluding mortality from lung and stomach cancer (which varied in trends among the countries studied), cancer death rates increased by at least 15% between 1968 and

1987 in all six countries. Since most adult malignant tumors require about 20 years to appear after an initiating carcinogenic insult, these data suggest that some environmental exposures or lifestyle changes have occurred in the past 20 or more years that affect susceptibility to certain cancers.[5] Interestingly, death rates for certain cancers in the United States, such as lung (males only), colon and rectum (whites only), ovary, uterus, urinary bladder (both sexes), and Hodgkin's disease (both sexes) appear to be going down, primarily in individuals under age 55. For all cancer sites combined, cancer mortality has decreased for age groups under age 45 and increased for age groups over age 55 from 1950 to 1989.[3]

Table 1–1 shows the trends in five-year survival by site of cancer and by race. One thing is immediately clear: five-year survival rates for most cancers are lower for African-Americans than for Caucasians. Over the past 30 years, overall cancer death rates rose by almost 50% for blacks and about 10% for whites.[1] Blacks had significantly higher cancer mortality rates

for lung, colon-rectum, prostate, and esophagus cancers. The reasons for this lower survival rate aren't entirely clear, but they include less access to and utilization of diagnostic tests that could detect cancer earlier. For example, a poll sponsored by the American Cancer Society in 1987 indicated that 88% of white women as opposed to 79% of black women had had a Pap test performed at some time.[1] Proctoscopic exams had been done on 29% of whites and 22% of blacks. As a reflection of this, data show that significantly more whites than blacks are diagnosed in the early, localized stages of cancer.

Similar surveys have shown that Hispanic Americans are not adequately aware of many of the warning signals of cancer or of ways to reduce cancer risk. Nor do they tend to seek early detection or treatment.[1]

Access to medical care, due to its perceived high cost and the feeling that the health care system may not respond to their needs, may also contribute to the discrepancies in survival rates among various ethnic groups.

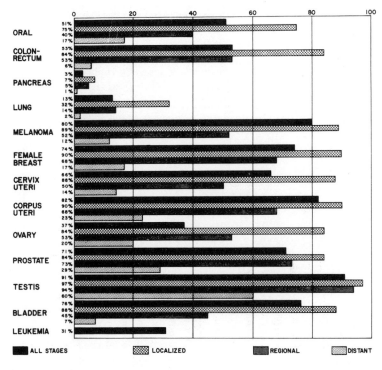

Figure 1–4 Five-year cancer survival rates (adjusted for normal life expectancy) for selected sites. This chart is based on cases diagnosed in 1974–1985. Source: Cancer Statistics Branch, National Cancer Institute.

Table 1-1 Trends in Survival by Site of Cancer, by Race. Cases Diagnosed in 1960–63, 1970–73, 1974–76, 1977–80, 1981–87

Site	White					Black				
	Relative 5-Year Survival					Relative 5-Year Survival				
	1960–63[1]	1970–73[1]	1974–76[2]	1977–80[2]	1981–87[2]	1960–63[1]	1970–73[1]	1974–76[2]	1977–80[2]	1981–87[2]
All sites	39	43	50	51	53*	27	31	39	39	38
Oral cavity and pharynx	45	43	55	54	54	—	—	35	34	31
Esophagus	4	4	5	6	9*	1	4	4	4	6*
Stomach	11	13	14	16	16*	8	13	16	16	17
Colon	43	49	50	53	58*	34	37	46	48	47
Rectum	38	45	49	51	55*	27	30	41	37	44
Liver	2	3	4	3	5	—	—	1	3	5
Pancreas	1	2	3	2	3*	1	2	2	5	4
Larynx	53	62	66	67	68	—	—	59	58	54
Lung and bronchus	8	10	12	13	13*	5	7	11	12	11
Melanoma of skin	60	68	80	82	82*	—	—	69†	51‡	70
Breast (female)	63	68	75	75	78*	46	51	63	63	63
Cervix uteri	58	64	69	68	68	47	61	63	62	57
Corpus uteri	73	81	89	86	84*	31	44	62	56	56
Ovary	32	36	36	38	39*	32	32	41	40	36
Prostate gland	50	63	67	72	76*	35	55	58	62	63*
Testis	63	72	79	88	93*	—	—	77†	73†	94
Urinary bladder	53	61	74	76	79*	24	36	48	55	59*
Kidney and renal pelvis	37	46	52	51	53	38	44	49	57	52
Brain and nervous system	18	20	22	24	24*	19	19	27	28	33
Thyroid gland	83	86	92	92	94	—	—	87	92	94
Hodgkin's disease	40	67	71	73	77*	—	—	68	73	74
Non-Hodgkin's lymphoma	31	41	47	49	51*	—	—	48	49	45
Multiple myeloma	12	19	24	25	26*	—	—	27	32	28
Leukemia	14	22	34	36	36*	—	—	31	30	29

Source: Cancer Statistics Branch, National Cancer Institute.

[1] Rates are based on End Results Group data from a series of hospital registries and one population-based registry.

[2] Rates are from the SEER Program. They are based on data from population-based registries in Connecticut, New Mexico, Utah, Iowa, Hawaii, Atlanta, Detroit, Seattle–Puget Sound and San Francisco–Oakland. Rates are based on follow-up of patients through 1988.

*The difference in rates between 1974–76 and 1981–87 is statistically significant (p < 0.05).

†The standard error of the survival rate is between 5 and 10 percentage points.

‡The standard error of the survival rate is greater than 10 percentage points.

—Valid survival rate could not be calculated.

(From *Cancer Facts and Figures—1992.*)[1]

Factors in Cancer Causation

Table 1–2 lists the risk factors for cancer deaths and their relative significance according to various cancer epidemiologists.[6] Most cancer epidemiologists agree that tobacco smoking is a key factor in causing about 30% of all cancers. Smoking is a risk factor not only for lung cancer but also for cancers of the mouth, pharynx, larynx, esophagus, urinary bladder, pancreas, and kidney.[6]

"Lifestyle" is the next most commonly agreed-upon cause of cancer. Risk factors here include diet, alcohol use, reproductive and sexual behavior, and exposure to sunlight. Risk for colon, breast, and uterine cancers is higher in obese people. A lot of circumstantial evidence indicates that high-fat diets contribute to the development of breast, colon, prostate, ovarian, and endometrial uterine cancers.[7] Several studies suggest that diets high in grain fiber, fruits and vegetables, and foods rich in vitamins A and C reduce the risk of breast and of colorectal cancers.[7-13] Hence, the American Cancer Society and the National Cancer Institute have recommended diets low in fat and high in grains, fruits and vegetables, and certain vitamins.

Heavy alcohol use, particularly when accompanied by cigarette smoking, has been linked to the cause of liver, mouth, larynx, pharynx, and esophagus cancers. Sexual contact with a variety of partners has been linked to a higher incidence of cervical carcinoma, and in the recent past to AIDS, which is associated with Kaposi's sarcoma and non-Hodgkin's lymphoma. As noted above, early menarche, late menopause, delaying childbirth, and childlessness are risk factors in breast cancer. High exposure to the ultraviolet irradiation of sunlight is associated with increased risk for squamous cell carcinoma of the skin and melanoma.[6,14]

Interestingly, pollution and industrial exposure to carcinogens are thought by some cancer epidemiologists to be relatively low on the risk factor scale.[6,15] However, this conclusion is controversial. Clearly, high workplace exposures to aromatic amines, polycyclic aromatic hydrocarbons, pesticides, radon, asbestos, and certain

Table 1–2 *Proportions of Cancer Deaths Attributed to Various Different Factors.* (From Doll and Peto[6])

Factor or Class of Factors	Percent of All Cancer Deaths	
	Best Estimate	Range of Acceptable Estimates
Tobacco	30	25–40
Alcohol	3	2–4
Diet	35	10–70
Food additives	<1	−5[a]–2
Reproductive and sexual behavior	7	1–13
Occupation	4	2–8
Pollution	2	<1–5
Industrial products	<1	<1–2
Medicines and medical procedures	1	0.5–3
Geophysical factors[b]	3	2–4
Infection	10?	1–?
Unknown	?	?

[a]Allowing for a possibly protective effect of antioxidants and other preservatives.
[b]Geophysical factors also cause a much greater proportion of nonfatal cancers (up to 30% of all cancers, depending on ethnic mix and latitude) because of the importance of UV light in causing the relatively nonfatal basal cell and squamous cell carcinoma of sunlight-exposed skin.

other chemical or physical agents have been linked to human cancers (Table 1–3).

Relative Role of Environmental and Genetic Factors in Cancer Causation

There is now little doubt that cancers are caused by factors related to the environment (up to 85%, by some estimates). There is compelling evidence to support this. If one looks, for example, at the range in the incidence of common cancers in different areas of the world, variations up to 300-fold for certain cancers can be seen (Table 1–4). What it is in local environments that affects the susceptibility of specific organs to cancer is not always

Table 1–3   *Established Human Carcinogenic Agents and Circumstances.* (From Doll and Peto[6])

Agent or Circumstance	Type of Exposure[a]			Site of Cancer
	Occupation	Medical	Social	
Aflatoxin			+	Liver
Alcoholic drinks			+	Mouth, pharynx, larynx, esophagus, liver
Alkylating agents:				
Cyclophosphamide		+		Bladder
Melphalan		+		Marrow
Aromatic amines:				
4-Aminodiphenyl	+			Bladder
Benzidine	+			Bladder
2-Naphthylamine	+			Bladder
Arsenic[b]	+	+		Skin, lung
Asbestos	+			Lung, pleura, peritoneum
Benzene	+			Marrow
Bis(chloromethyl) ether	+			Lung
Busulphan		+		Marrow
Cadmium[b]	+			Prostate
Chewing (betel, tobacco, lime)			+	Mouth
Chromium[b]	+			Lung
Chlornaphazine		+		Bladder
Furniture manufacture (hardwood)	+			Nasal sinuses
Immunosuppressive drugs		+		Recticuloendothelial system
Ionizing radiations[c]	+	+		Marrow and probably all other sites
Isopropyl alcohol manufacture	+			Nasal sinuses
Leather goods manufacture	+			Nasal sinuses
Mustard gas	+			Larynx, lung
Nickel[b]	+			Nasal sinuses, lung
Estrogens:				
Unopposed		+		Endometrium
Transplacental (DES)		+		Vagina
Overnutrition (causing obesity)			+	Endometrium, gallbladder
Phenacetin		+		Kidney (pelvis)
Polycyclic hydrocarbons	+	+		Skin, scrotum, lung
Reproductive history:				
Late age at 1st pregnancy			+	Breast
Zero or low parity			+	Ovary

Agent or Circumstance	Type of Exposure[a]			Site of Cancer
	Occupation	Medical	Social	
Parasites:				
Schistosoma haematobium			+	Bladder
Chlonorchis sinensis			+	Liver (cholangioma)
Sexual promiscuity			+	Cervix uteri
Steroids:				
Anabolic (oxymetholone)		+		Liver
Contraceptives		+		Liver (hamartoma)
Tobacco smoking			+	Mouth, pharynx, larynx, lung, esophagus, bladder
UV light	+		+	Skin, lip
Vinyl chloride	+			Liver (angiosarcoma)
Virus (hepatitis B)			+	Liver (hepatoma)

[a]A plus sign indicates that evidence of carcinogenicity was obtained.
[b]Certain compounds or oxidation states only.
[c]For example, from X rays, thorium, Thorotrast, some underground mining, and other occupations.

Table 1–4   *Worldwide Variation in the Incidence of Common Cancers. Range of Variations is Expressed for Ages 35–64.* (Data from Doll[16])

Type of Cancer	High-incidence Area	Low-incidence Area	Range of Variation
Skin	Australia (Queensland)	India (Bombay)	>200
Buccal cavity	India	Denmark	>25
Nasopharynx	Singapore*	England	40
Bronchus	England	Nigeria	35
Esophagus	Iran	Nigeria	300
Stomach	Japan	Uganda	25
Liver	Mozambique	Norway	70
Colon	U.S. (Connecticut)	Nigeria	10
Rectum	Denmark	Nigeria	20
Pancreas	New Zealand†	Uganda	5
Breast	U.S. (Connecticut)	Uganda	5
Cervix uteri	Columbia	Israel	15
Corpus uteri	U.S. (Connecticut)	Japan	10
Ovary	Denmark	Japan	8
Bladder	U.S. (Connecticut)	Japan	4
Prostate	U.S.‡	Japan	30
Penis	Uganda	Israel	300

The U.S. data are taken from the Connecticut Tumor Registry, because it is the oldest cancer registry based upon a defined population in this country.
*Chinese.
†Maori.
‡Blacks.

clear. In some cases, it appears to be due to certain behavioral factors—e.g., the high incidence or oral cancers in some areas of Asia where betel nut chewing is common and the increased incidence of cancer of the palate in areas of Asia, Africa, and South America where smoking with the lighted end of a cigar in the mouth was practiced. Carcinogens in the diet most likely play a large role. In Thailand, Singapore, Swaziland, and Mozambique, for example, the incidence of liver cancers is proportional to the amount of aflatoxin contamination of foods,[16] although some studies in China indicate that liver cancer rates are more related to infection with hepatitis B virus and to consumption of alcohol and daily intake of cadmium from foods of plant origin than to aflatoxin in the diet.[17] It appears that hepatitis B virus infection and aflatoxin exposure act as co-carcinogens for the liver. The decreasing incidence of stomach cancer in the United States has been attributed to a decrease in the consumption of smoked foods, whereas the cause of colon cancer is attributed, at least in part, to an increased intake of fat and relative lack of fiber in the typical United States diet.

The argument that the incidence of many cancers is related to the environment is greatly strengthened by the observation that when populations emigrate, the incidence of cancer in the offspring of the same ethnic group more closely approaches that of their country of residence than that of the country of their ancestry. An example is seen in the mortality rates for various cancers among native Japanese, the children of Japanese immigrants to the United States (Nisei), and the general U.S. population (Table 1–5).[18] In the Nisei population, mortality rates have decreased for stomach cancer and

increased for cancer of the colon, lung, and breast; these rates are approaching the rates in the United States. It is interesting that in areas of Japan where Western dietary habits are becoming widespread, the trends in incidence of various cancers resemble those in the United States.[19]

Nevertheless, genetic factors play an important role in cancer causation. A few cancers have a definite inheritance, whereas others may arise in individuals with a genetic defect that makes them more susceptible to potentially carcinogenic agents.

Inherited cancers represent a small fraction, perhaps 1–2%, of total cancers.[20] A high percentage of certain tumors, however, are genetically determined. For example, dominant genetic inheritance accounts for about 40% of retinoblastomas and 20–40% of Wilm's tumors (embryonal renal tumors) and neuroblastomas. Familial multiple polyposis of the large bowel is another example of a disease that is transmitted as a Mendelian-dominant trait, with about an 80% penetrance rate. Cancer of the large bowel will eventually occur in nearly 100% of untreated patients with familial multiple polyposis. There is also a predisposition to develop a variety of other neoplasms, particularly subcutaneous tumors and osteomas, in these latter patients.

For some hereditary cancers, a specific chromosomal alteration has been identified that presumably predisposes to the cancer. For example, in some patients with Wilm's tumor, a renal cancer seen in children, the short arm of chromosome 11 has a deletion in band 13,[21] and in some children with retinoblastoma the long arm of chromosome 13 has a deletion in band 14.[22] In the latter example, the finding that in some cases a deletion in the long arm of chromosome 13 is present in the tumor cells and not in peripheral lymphocytes of the same patients suggests that this alteration is related to a second mutagenic event. It is now known that the deleted portion of chromosome 13 in retinoblastoma contains a tumor suppressor gene called RB.[23] Similar deletions in other forms of human cancer may also represent the loss of tumor suppressor genes[24] (see Chapter 14).

Other genetically inherited conditions carry a predisposition to cancer involving the inter-

Table 1–5 *Standardized Mortality Ratios for Selected Cancer Sites.* Data for Stomach, Colon, and Lung, Males Only; Data for Breast, Females Only. (Data from Haenzel and Kurihara[18])

Cancer Site	Native Japanese	Nisei	General U.S. Population
Stomach	100	38	17
Colon	100	288	489
Lung	100	166	316
Breast	100	136	591

action of genetic and environmental factors. These include xeroderma pigmentosum (characterized by extreme sensitivity to sunlight, an incidence of skin cancer approaching 100%, and, frequently, neurologic deficiencies), ataxia telangiectasia (progressive cerebellar ataxia, dilated blood vessels, immune deficiencies), and Fanconi's anemia (hematologic deficiency leading to anemia and hemorrhage with an increased risk for leukemia). These rare, autosomal recessive genetic disorders have in common an inability to repair DNA damaged by such potentially carcinogenic substances as ultraviolet radiation, ionizing radiation, or chemical carcinogens.

A number of familial "clusters" of various cancers have been reported. The implication of this is that there is some familial, but as yet genetically undefined predisposition to develop certain cancers. For example, breast cancer has for many years been considered to have a familial association,[25] although as yet there is no clearly defined genetic mechanism to explain it. Similar associations have been noted for ovarian cancer.[26] Some genetic studies have also associated occurrence of breast cancer with a variety of other tumors in the same families.[27] These include associations between breast cancer and ovarian cancer, gastrointestinal tract cancer, soft tissue sarcoma, brain tumors, or leukemia.

Biology of the Cancer Cell

The hallmarks of malignant neoplastic tissue are unregulated cell proliferation, invasiveness, and metastasis to distant sites in the body. The histopathologic characteristics include increased numbers of mitotic cells in a tissue field, evidence of cells breaking tissue barriers (e.g., the basal lamina of epithelial tissues), presence of incompletely differentiated or undifferentiated cell types, and cells with large nuclei and prominent nucleoli.

Some of the biochemical characteristics of malignant cells are shown in Figure 1–5. "Transformed" malignant cells in culture, as well as cancer cells isolated directly from malignant tumors, display several alterations in

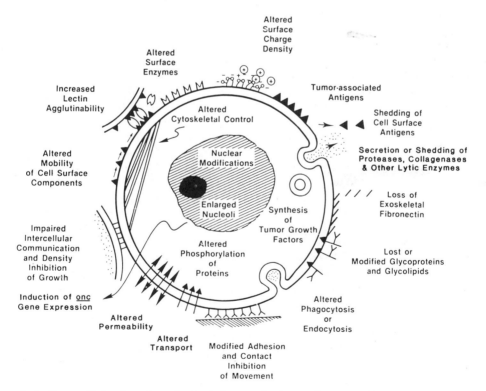

Figure 1–5 Some cellular alterations observed after neoplastic transformation. (Modified from Nicolson.[28])

cell-surface biochemistry, including altered cell-surface glycoproteins and glycolipids that may be recognized by the body as foreign, tumor-associated antigens. In addition, these cells secrete tissue-digesting lytic enzymes such as proteases, collagenases, and glycosidases. They also produce altered extracellular matrix components (i.e., laminin, fibronectin) and/or receptors for these (integrins). Cancer cells may secrete a variety of growth factors, some of which may stimulate their own growth ("autocrine" stimulation). Cancer cells tend to have high rates of nucleic acid biosynthesis and higher levels of the enzymes involved in these pathways. Cancer cells have a variety of genetic alterations, some evident only at the gene level and some more global changes in chromosomal structure, such as chromosomal deletions, rearrangements, or duplications. Activation or mutation of cellular oncogenes is also a common phenomenon in cancer cells. As noted above, loss of so-called tumor suppressor genes is now being recognized as a common occurrence in human cancer.[24]

All of these alterations in cancer cells are potential targets for anticancer drugs to attack. The trick is to design agents that selectively kill cancer cells and leave the normal cells in the body unharmed. That has proved extremely difficult to do for the reason noted above—i.e., that cancer cells arise from normal tissue. In the succeeding chapters of this book, the mechanisms of action and the toxic side effects of the various classes of anticancer drugs will be described in detail. In Chapters 13 and 14, we will describe some of the newer strategies for improving the selective toxicity and therapeutic index of anticancer therapies.

To understand the difficulties in cancer treatment, it is important to note why cancer kills patients. The factors involved in the invasion and spread of cancer are the ones most devastating to the patient and the ones leading to fatality. If the invasion and metastatic spread of cancer could be controlled, many patients, perhaps most patients, could survive the disease. Thus, defining the biochemical mechanisms for invasion and metastasis is a key step in designing agents that will block the killing effects of cancer.

Cancerous growths affect patient function in the following ways:[28]

1. They may grow and expand in confined space and destroy normal tissue by crowding out normal cells (e.g., certain brain tumors).
2. They have a high metabolic rate and produce nutritional deficits out of proportion to their tissue mass.
3. They decrease host defense mechanisms against infections.
4. They often produce hormonelike substances that have peripheral effects in the body, the so-called paraneoplastic syndromes. These include hypercalcemia, ectopic production of hormones such as ACTH, calitonin, ADH, and chorionic gonadotropin, and release of "toxohormones" that inhibit metabolic functions in normal tissues.
5. They invade through tissues and cause hemorrhage and infection.
6. They metastasize to distant organs (e.g., liver, brain, lungs, bone) and destroy these tissues.

Role of Drugs in Cancer Treatment

The ultimate clinical effectiveness of any anticancer drug requires that it kill malignant tumor cells *in vivo* at doses that allow enough cells in the patient's critical tissues (e.g., bone marrow, gastrointestinal tract) to survive so that recovery can occur. This is difficult to accomplish because, in general, anticancer drugs are most useful against malignant tumors with a high proportion of dividing cells, and some normal tissues such as the bone marrow and GI tract also have a high cell-proliferation rate. Anticancer drugs used by themselves are primarily effective against high-growth-fraction tumors such as the leukemias and lymphomas. The most common malignant tumors, however, are "solid" tumors, including those of the colon, rectum, lung, and breast. These tumors usually have a low proportion of dividing cells and therefore are less susceptible to treatment by drugs alone.

It is apparent from the data in Table 1–1 that significant, though relatively small increases, in five-year survival rates for the major solid tumors have occurred since the 1960s. Nevertheless, there have been striking improvements in the survival rates for certain of the less common tumors. A significant number of patients with gestational choriocarcinoma, childhood ALL, Hodgkin's disease, Burkitt's lymphoma, and testicular cancer as well as Wilm's tumor, osteogenic sarcoma, and rhabdomyosarcoma are now being cured by chemotherapy (Table 1–6).[29]

Surgery, radiotherapy, and chemotherapy are all effective treatments for cancer and have been used alone and in combination. Surgery and radiotherapy can often eradicate primary or localized disease but may ultimately fail because the cancer has metastasized to other areas of the body. In such instances, chemotherapy, if used properly, may control or eliminate metastatic disease and reduce mortality. Chemotherapy combined with surgery or radiotherapy or both, so-called adjuvant therapy, has increased survival rates for a number of solid tumors that were formerly treated by only one therapeutic modality. Medical oncologists, surgeons, and radiotherapists now work closely together in order to maximize the effectiveness of combined treatment modalities by monitoring the sequence and timing of their use.

In many multimodality treatment protocols, the first treatment is often local control, either by surgery or irradiation, followed by chemotherapy to treat metastatic tumor foci. More recently, an approach utilizing chemotherapy as the first-line treatment followed by surgery or radiation therapy has been employed. The rationale for this so-called neoadjuvant chemotherapy, a term coined by Emil Frei,[30] is that the primary tumor can be shrunk before local eradication is attempted, and micrometastatic foci can be attacked initially, without waiting until local treatment is completed.

New drugs and new therapeutic approaches continue to be discovered and put into clinical practice. Some of the newer immunologic and genetic approaches will be discussed in Chapter 14. The discovery of new anticancer drugs and the more efficacious use of available ones depend to a large extent on a thorough knowledge of the chemistry and pharmacology of the drugs that have already proven to be effective. The purpose of this book is to provide a fundamental approach to understanding the treatment of cancer with drugs by presenting in a simplified, yet sufficiently detailed, manner the chemistry and pharmacology of current drugs as well as of drugs in the "pipeline" from laboratory to clinic. In addition, some insights into new anticancer drug design are given. It is conceded at the outset that cancer chemotherapy is often more empirical than rational, a fact that does not detract from the intelligence or dedication of the clinicians and scientists involved; rather, it speaks to the complexity of the issues they face.

REFERENCES

1. *Cancer Facts and Figures—1992*, American Cancer Society, Inc., Atlanta, 1992.

Table 1–6   *Cures in Advanced Cancer.* (From Krakoff[29])

Type of Cancer	Cure Rate	
	1955	1986
Gestational trophoblastic tumors	0	>90% (moderate tumor burden) >60% (high tumor burden)
Acute lymphoblastic leukemia (children)	0	75%
Acute lymphoblastic leukemia (adults)	0	40%
Acute myeloblastic leukemia	0	15%
Hodgkin's disease	0	80%
Non-Hodgkin's lymphoma (children)	0	60%
Diffuse histiocytic lymphoma	0	50%
Burkitt's lymphoma	0	50%
Testicular tumors	0	90%

2. *Cancer Facts and Figures—1989,* American Cancer Society, Inc., Atlanta, 1989

3. B. F. Hankey, L. A. Gloeckler Ries, B. A. Miller, and C. L. Kosary: "Overview" in *Cancer Statistics Review 1973–1989,* ed. by B. A. Miller, L. A. Gloeckler Ries, B. F. Hankey, C. L. Kosary, and B. K. Edwards, National Cancer Institute. NIH Pub. No. 92-2789, 1992, pp. I.1–I.55.

4. L. A. Loeb, V. L. Ernster, K. E. Warner, J. Abbotts, and J. Laszlo: Smoking and lung cancer: An overview. *Cancer Res. 44:*5940 (1984).

5. D. L. Davis, D. Hoel, J. Fox, and A. Lopez: International trends in cancer mortality in France, West Germany, Italy, Japan, England and Wales, and the USA. *Lancet 336:*474 (1990).

6. R. Doll and R. Peto: The causes of cancer. *J. Natl. Cancer Inst. 66:*1191 (1981).

7. R. L. Prentice, M. Pepe, and S. G. Self: Dietary fat and breast cancer: A quantitative assessment of the epidemiological literature and a discussion of methodological issues. *Cancer Res. 49:*3147 (1989).

8. M. L. Slattery, A. W. Sorenson, A. W. Mahoney, T. K. French, D. Kritchevsky, and J. C. Street: Diet and colon cancer: Assessment of risk by fiber type and food source. *J. Natl. Cancer Inst. 80:*1474 (1988).

9. J. L. Freudenheim, S. Graham, P. J. Horvath, J. R. Marshall, B. P. Haughey, and G. Wilkinson: Risks associated with source of fiber and fiber components in cancer of the colon and rectum. *Cancer Res. 50:*3295 (1990).

10. A. S. Whittemore, A. H. Wu-Williams, M. Lee, Z. Shu, R. P. Gallagher, J. Deng-ao, Z. Lun, W. Xianghui, C. Kun, D. Jung, C.-Z. Teh, L. Chengde, X. J. Yao, R. S. Paffenbarger, Jr., and B. E. Henderson: Diet, physical activity, and colorectal cancer among Chinese in North America and China. *J. Natl. Cancer Inst. 82:*915 (1990).

11. B. Trock, E. Lanza, and P. Greenwald: Dietary fiber, vegetables, and colon cancer: critical review of the meta-analyses of the epidemiologic evidence. *J. Natl. Cancer Inst. 82:*650 (1990).

12. G. R. Howe, T. Hirohata, T. G. Hislop, J. M. Iscovich, J.-M. Yuan, K. Katsouyanni, F. Lubin, E. Marubini, B. Modan, T. Rohan, P. Toniolo, and Y. Shunzhang: Dietary factors and risk of breast cancer: Combined analysis of 12 case-control studies. *J. Natl. Cancer Inst. 82:*561 (1990).

13. J. J. DeCosse, H. H. Miller, and M. L. Lesser: Effect of wheat fiber and vitamins C and E on rectal polyps in patients with familial adenomatous polyposis. *J. Natl. Cancer Inst. 81:*1290 (1989).

14. P. T. Strickland, B. C. Vitasa, S. K. West, F. S. Rosenthal, E. A. Emmett, and H. R. Taylor: Quantitative carcinogenesis in man: solar ultraviolet B dose dependence of skin cancer in Maryland watermen. *J. Natl. Cancer Inst. 81:*1910 (1989).

15. B. N. Ames and L. S. Gold: Too many rodent carcinogens: Mitogenesis increases mutagenesis. *Science 249:*970 (1990).

16. R. Doll: "Introduction," in *Origins of Human Cancer,* ed. by H. H. Hiatt, J. D. Watson, and J. A. Winsten. Cold Spring Harbor Laboratory, N.Y., 1977, pp. 1–12.

17. T. C. Campbell, J. Chen, C. Liu, J. Li, and P. Parpia: Nonassociation of aflatoxin with primary liver cancer of a cross-sectional ecological survey in the People's Republic of China. *Cancer Res. 50:*6882 (1990).

18. W. Haenszel and M. Kurihara: Studies of Japanese migrants. I. Mortality from cancer and other diseases among Japanese in the United States. *J. Natl. Cancer Inst. 40:*43 (1968).

19. T. Hirayama: "Changing patterns of cancer in Japan with special reference to the decrease in stomach cancer mortality," in *Origins of Human Cancer,* ed. by H. H. Hiatt, J. D. Watson, and J. A. Winsten. Cold Spring Harbor Laboratory, N.Y., 1977, pp. 55–75.

20. A. G. Knudson, Jr.: "Genetic predispositions to cancer," in *Origins of Human Cancer,* ed. by H. H. Hiatt, J. D. Watson, and J. A. Winsten. Cold Spring Harbor Laboratory, N.Y., 1977, pp. 45–52.

21. U. Francke, L. G. Holmes, L. Atkins, and V. M. Riccardi: Aniridia—Wilm's tumor association: Evidence for specific deletion of 11p 13. *Cytogenet. Cell Genet. 24:*185 (1979).

22. J. J. Yunis and N. Ramsey: Retinoblastoma and subband deletion of chromosome 13. *Amer. J. Dis. Child. 132:*161 (1978).

23. S. H. Friend, H. R. Bernards, S. Rogelj, R. A. Weinberg, J. M. Rapaport, D. M. Abert, and T. P. Dryja: A human DNA segment with properties of the gene that predisposes to retinoblastoma and osteosarcoma. *Nature 323:*643 (1986).

24. R. Sager: Tumor suppressor genes: The puzzle and the promise. *Science 246:*1406 (1989).

25. M. T. Macklin: Comparison of the number of breast cancer deaths observed in relatives of breast cancer patients, and the number expected in the basis of mortality rates. *J. Natl. Cancer Inst. 22:*927 (1959).

26. J. F. Fraumeni, Jr., G. W. Grundy, E. T. Creagan, and R. B. Everson: Six families prone to ovarian cancer. *Cancer 36:*364 (1975).

27. H. T. Lynch, R. E. Harris, H. A. Guirgis, K. Maloney, L. L. Carmody, J. F. Lynch: Familial association of breast/ovarian carcinoma. *Cancer 41:*1543 (1978).

28. R. W. Ruddon: *Cancer Biology,* 2nd ed., New York: Oxford University Press, 1987, pp. 190–296.

29. I. Krakoff: Cancer chemotherapeutic agents. *Ca—A Cancer Journal for Clinicians 37:*93 (1987).

30. E. Frei III: What's in a name—neoadjuvant. *J. Natl. Cancer Inst. 80:*1088 (1988).

CHAPTER TWO

Some Milestones in the Development of Cancer Chemotherapy

Although the concept of treating cancer with drugs goes back at least 500 years when preparations of silver, zinc, and mercury were used, the usefulness of drugs in the systemic treatment of cancer was first documented in 1865 when Lissauer gave potassium arsenite (Fowler's solution) to a patient with leukemia and noted a positive effect.[1] Successful systemic cancer chemotherapy, however, was not really developed until almost 80 years later. It is ironic that the first effective anticancer drug was developed as a war gas, not a medicine. This drug was nitrogen mustard, whose precursor, sulfur mustard (H-gas), had been used on the battlefield in 1917. Sulfur mustard was known to be an extremely irritating vesicant that burns the eyes, skin, and respiratory tract. It was not until later in the war, however, that it was recognized that sulfur mustard had other toxic effects.[2] The gas also produced leukopenia, aplasia of the bone marrow, dissolution of lymphoid tissue, and ulceration of the gastrointestinal tract in military personnel exposed to high concentrations. Another instance of exposure further demonstrated the systemic toxic effects of sulfur mustard. Although it was never used in combat during World War II, an unfortunate wartime incident exposed naval personnel and an unknown number of civilians to mustard gas.[3] General Eisenhower had ordered that a stockpile of mustard gas be kept near the front for possible use in a reprisal if the Nazis resorted to chemical warfare. Such a stockpile was on board the Liberty Ship S.S. *John Harvey* in Bari Harbor (Italy) in December 1943 when a German air strike destroyed the ship, releasing mustard gas and a mustard-containing oil slick into the harbor. Survivors in the sea and those on land who were exposed to the fumes developed severe, unusual burns to the eyes, skin, and respiratory tract. The nature of these burns went undiagnosed for several days because the Allied port authority, presumably out of fear of enemy reprisals and the negative effect of any publicity, refused to reveal the nature of the cargo of the *John Harvey*. By a careful and painstaking investigation, Lieutenant Colonel Stewart F. Alexander, a U.S. Army physician with training in chemical warfare, determined the nature of the poison but by then it was too late to help a number of the victims. The fatality rate was over 13% of those exposed,[3] with many fatalities due to infection and internal bleeding.

In 1931, Adair and Bagg[4] applied sulfur mustard to squamous carcinomas and also injected it directly into tumors in humans, but it was considered too toxic for systemic use. As the engines of war were again set in motion during the 1930s, another mustard, nitrogen mustard, was developed for possible combat use. A few years later, the known lymphocytolytic effects of the mustards prompted Alfred Gilman and his colleagues to examine the antitumor effect of a nitrogen mustard in lymphosarcoma-bearing mice. It was found to have an effect, and in

17

November 1942, Gilman, Goodman, Lindskog, and Dougherty began the first clinical trial of nitrogen mustard in a patient with lymphosarcoma. Since it was wartime and all the information obtained on this compound was classified, its usefulness in the treatment of cancer did not become generally known until 1946 when a review by Gilman and Philips was published.[5] That review marks the beginning of modern cancer chemotherapy. One of the first nitrogen mustards shown to be clinically effective (HN_2 or mechlorethamine) is still used as an anticancer drug, and a host of more recently synthesized alkylating drugs, based to a large extent on the original "parent compound," are now widely used in the treatment of cancer.

It is of some interest (and a cause for consternation) that the clinical course of the first patient treated with nitrogen mustard is still reflected in the use of anticancer drugs today.[6] A patient in the terminal stages of lymphosarcoma was selected as a suitable subject. The patient had large tumor masses in the mediastinum and axilla and at other sites. Breathing, chewing, and swallowing were very difficult, and the patient was cyanotic. Based on the earlier animal studies, it was decided to administer a daily dose of 0.1 mg/kg of the nitrogen mustard intravenously for 10 days, unless the total granulocyte count dropped below 5000/cubic millimeter. Within 48 hours of treatment, softening of the tumor masses was detected. By day 4, the patient's obstructive difficulties were relieved, and a few days after therapy was terminated, the cervical and axillary tumor masses had receded. Unfortunately, although the antitumor effect of the drug was very pronounced, about 3½ weeks after initiation of therapy the total white blood cell count was down to 200 cells/cubic millimeter. Subsequently, the bone marrow gradually recovered, but so did the tumor. A second, shorter course of treatment produced a transient improvement, and a third course had virtually no effect. Thus, the therapy-limiting effect of marrow toxicity and the development of drug resistance, both of which are still problems in cancer chemotherapy, were observed in this very first patient.

The second successful anticancer drug to be used clinically belongs to the so-called antimetabolite class. Antimetabolites structurally resemble a natural metabolite necessary for cellular function and interfere with its normal utilization. They are basically of three types: antifolates, antipurines, and antipyrimidines. The first antifolate to be employed clinically was aminopterin. Following a report that a "folic acid concentrate" inhibited sarcoma growth in mice, Sidney Farber investigated the effects of folic acid conjugates and antagonists in leukemic children. He found that the conjugates accelerated the leukemic process in bone marrow but that certain antagonists were cytotoxic in that they induced a marked hypocellularity in the marrow. In November 1947, when a sufficient amount of pure aminopterin, the most potent antifolate then known, became available, Farber gave the drug to a series of 16 children with acute leukemia.[7] Dramatic, albeit temporary, remissions were noted in 10 of the 16. This spurred a search for more powerful and less toxic antagonists to folic acid. In 1949, Seeger and his colleagues[8] synthesized amethopterin (methotrexate) and shortly thereafter it was used clinically. Although the search for the "more powerful and less toxic" drug of Farber's dream continued, no antifolate significantly better than methotrexate has been developed, and this drug is still the member of its class that is most widely used clinically. It should be noted that the use of methotrexate to treat women with gestational choriocarcinoma provided the first example of a drug-induced cure of a cancer.[9]

The development of antipurines as anticancer and antiviral drugs has a long history, dating back to the pioneering work of George Hitchings and Gertrude Elion in the early 1940s at the Wellcome Research Laboratories.[10] At that time knowledge about the synthesis and structure of nucleic acids was primitive. The theory was that purine and pyrimidine nucleotides were strung together in some manner, but neither the nature of the internucleotide linkage nor the helical structure of DNA had been established. It wasn't until 1953 that Watson and Crick published the structure of DNA.[11]

Nevertheless, in the early 1940s Hitchings postulated, based on the antimetabolite theory of the action of sulfonamides interfering with the utilization of the nutrient paraaminoben-zoic acid in bacteria, that it might be possible to stop a cell's nucleic acid synthesis with a nucleic acid base analog.

In 1944, when Gertrude Elion joined the lab, she was given the assignment of synthesizing some purine and pyrimidine analogs. For this she had to go back to the manuscripts of Emil Fischer in the old German chemical literature to ad some of the methods, since so few chemists were interested in the synthesis of nucleic acid bases at the time she started her work.

By 1948, Elion and Hitchings had some good leads. They found that 2,6-diaminopurine inhibited the growth of the microorganism *Lactobacillus casei* and that this inhibition could be reversed by adenine. They deduced that adenine and 2,6-diaminopurine were anabolized by the same enzyme and that the product of diaminopurine anabolism interfered with purine interconversion. That was a big conceptual breakthrough. They went on to show that diaminopurine inhibited the growth of AKR mouse leukemia *in vivo* and of tumor cells in culture, but its toxicity was such that it was not considered a good drug for clinical use.

By 1951, they had synthesized and tested over 100 purine analogs in the antimicrobial screen. By then it had become clear that the substitution of sulfur for oxygen at position 6 of guanine and hypoxanthine produced compounds with significant activity against rodent tumors and leukemia.[12] 6-Mercaptopurine and 6-thioguanine were among the most active, and these findings led to clinical trials in 1953 of 6-MP in children with acute leukemia.[13] 6-MP was found to induce complete remission in these children, although most of them eventually relapsed. Today, the use of 6-MP in combination with other drugs for induction and maintenance therapy can cure almost 80% of children with acute lymphocytic leukemia—quite an accomplishment when you consider that, before the development of 6-MP, the average survival time of children with ALL was 3 to 4 months.

6-Thioguanine, although it was actually synthesized earlier than 6-MP, was found to be more active versus some rodent tumors, but also more toxic. Nevertheless, 6-TG has been a useful drug for the treatment of acute myelo-cytic leukemia, together with a pyrimidine-type antimetabolite, cytosine arabinoside.

Experiments with purine analogs led Elion and Hitchings and their coworkers to the discovery of several other clinically useful drugs. Among them are azathioprine, an immunosuppressive drug useful in kidney transplantation; allopurinol, a xanthine oxidase inhibitor effective in the treatment of gout; and acyclovir, an acyclic guanine analog that is a potent inhibitor of herpes viruses. For their seminal and continued contributions to the development of effective drugs for the treatment of cancer and other diseases, George Hitchings and Gertrude Elion were awarded the Nobel Prize in 1988.

Antipyrimidines were developed during attempts to synthesize analogs that could inhibit uracil utilization by tumors. Heidelberger *et al.*[14] reasoned that since a number of experimental tumors had been reported to use more uracil than orotic acid for nucleic acid synthesis (the reverse is true for many normal tissues), an antimetabolite resembling uracil might be utilized preferentially by tumors and therefore might inhibit tumor growth specifically. He thought that, since "acetic acid is vinegar and fluoroacetic acid is a rat poison," a fluorine-substituted compound might be active. Such a substitution is possible on the 5 and 6 positions of the uracil ring, but the 5-substituted derivative is both easier to make and more stable. In addition, Heidelberger predicted that a substituent in the 5 position would block the formation of thymine nucleotides from uracil nucleotides. This prediction turned out to be correct and the result was a new anticancer drug, 5-fluorouracil. This was the first clinically effective antipyrimidine, but others have followed. The most prominent of these analogs is cytosine arabinoside, which was first used in patients in the early 1960s and is a mainstay of antileukemic therapy today.[15]

Sidney Farber also introduced another class of drugs into the clinic. In 1954, he used actinomycin D, one of a series of cytotoxic antibiotics isolated from a *Streptomyces* species[16] to treat metastatic Wilm's tumor in children. The demonstrated effectiveness of actinomycin D led to the development of a large number of antibiotics with activity against rodent and human malignancies. The antitumor antibiotics differ from antibiotics used as antibacterial drugs in that the former are markedly cytotoxic to mammalian cells. The clinically effective antitumor antibiotics include mitomycin,[17] active against chronic myelogenous leukemia and gastrointestinal tumors; mithramycin, testicular tumors;[18] bleomycin,[19] testicular cancer, lymphomas, and some squamous cell carcinomas; daunorubicin,[20,21] acute leukemias; and doxorubicin (Adriamycin)[22], leukemias and a wide spectrum of solid tumors including both carcinomas and sarcomas. Doxorubicin was found to be effective against a wider variety of solid tumors than any other drug in clinical use at the time. Doxorubicin, one of the anthracyiline class of antitumor antibiotics, was discovered in soil samples in Italy. Other anthracylines of this class include the poetically named marcellomycin, musettamycin, and rudolfomycin, after characters in Puccini's opera *La Boheme*.

Serendipity played a role in the introduction of the vinca alkaloids, antimitotic agents that are extracted from periwinkle plants. Periwinkle has been used in folk medicine for centuries, and more recently, a claim that an extract of these plants could produce hypoglycemia led to testing for this effect. Noble *et al.*[23] could not substantiate this claim, but they found granulocytopenia and bone marrow suppression in their experimental rats. Johnson *et al.*[24] later demonstrated that alkaloid fractions of the periwinkle plant had antileukemic activity in mice. Of the four alkaloids that showed such activity, only vincristine and vinblastine have been used to treat cancer in humans. They have proven effective in the treatment of leukemias, lymphomas, and some carcinomas.

Serendipity also played a major role in the discovery of another useful clinical anticancer drug, cisplatin. In 1965, Barnett Rosenberg and his colleagues were studying the effects of electric current on cell division in cultures of *Escherichia coli*. When *E. coli* were placed in an electrolysis chamber equipped with platinum electrodes and aerated with air or oxygen, the proliferation of the microorganism was inhibited.[25] They found that oxygen and platinum electrodes were required for the effect. When nitrogen or helium was bubbled through the chamber, no effect of the electric field was detected on bacterial growth. After ruling out several possible causes of the inhibitory effect, such as changes in temperature, pH, magnesium ion concentration, or exposure to ultraviolet light, they reasoned that some chemical change produced in the culture medium by electrolysis was responsible for the observed effect. To test this, they took "conditioned" medium from the electrolysis chamber and inoculated it with *E. coli*. The bacteria didn't divide. Next they tested the requirement for various salts in the medium and found that chloride salts seemed to be the most effective.

It was known that solutions of acidified chloride salts could attack platinum electrodes during electrolysis. They therefore suspected that a platinum salt was the active ingredient. Eureka. When they added to an *E. coli* culture a solution of $(NH_4)_2 PtCl_6$, maintaining a concentration of the Pt (IV) oxidation state of the metal at 10 ppm, they got the same effect as in the electrolysis chamber. This verified that a platinum salt was the active agent. Further experiments showed that other group VIIIb transition metals such as rhodium could have similar effects, but the platinum compounds were more potent. Various platinum salts were subsequently synthesized and *cis*-diamminetetrachloroplatinum (IV), but not the *trans* isomer, was shown to be the most effective,[26] and later to be a potent inhibitor of sarcoma 180 and L1210 leukemia in mice.[27]

These results led to clinical trials of the drug in 1972, and it was found to be effective against a number of human cancers. However, it was nearly discarded in the early 1970s because of its marked gastrointestinal and renal toxicities. When it became known that these negative side effects could be alleviated by antiemetic drugs and aggressive hydration of the patient, cisplatin became a mainstay of anticancer therapy. It is an integral part of a curative drug combination regimen for testicular cancer and is an important drug in the treatment of ovarian, head and neck, bladder, lung, and cervical cancers.[28]

Most anticancer drugs act by inhibiting nucleic acid synthesis or function. Very few inhibit tumor-cell proliferation by blocking protein synthesis. One of those that does is the enzyme L-asparaginase. It was discovered to affect tumor cell proliferation by Kidd, who was attempting to grow transplanted mouse lymphoma cells in vivo.[29] For mammalian cells to grow in culture, it usually requires the addition of animal serum. Kidd had added various sera to the cultures to see which would provide an appropriate growth stimulus. What he found was that the lymphoma cells would grow perfectly well in the presence of horse or rabbit serum, but not in guinea pig serum. To make a long story short, he determined that guinea pig serum contained an enzyme that degraded asparagine. The lymphoma cells required an exogenous source of asparagine for their growth, since they lacked the enzyme for synthesis of the amino acid. It was later found that human acute lymphocytic leukemia cells also require exogenous asparagine, and that their growth is inhibited by L-asparaginase. This drug has been used successfully in childhood ALL in combination with other drugs, particularly in patients refractory to other first-line therapeutic regimens.

The development of antiestrogens for the treatment of breast cancer is another interesting chapter in the history of anticancer drug therapy. It stems back to an observation made about 100 years ago by Beatson that removal of the ovaries was beneficial to patients with mammary cancer.[30] Later it was found by Dao and Huggins that oblation of the adrenal gland[31] and by Pearson and Ray that hypophysectomy[32] were also beneficial for some women with breast cancer. As the chemistry and biology of estrogens and gonadotropins became better known, it became clearer that hormones play a key role in the growth of mammary cancer as well as in mammary gland growth and development. The development of sensitive bioassays in rodents[33] and of methods to study specific binding of estrogenic compounds to their receptor[34] provided a way to develop compounds with estrogenic and antiestrogenic activity.

It soon became apparent that the typical phenanthrene steroid hormone nucleus was not necessary for estrogenic activity. This led in the 1930s to the synthesis of a large number of phenolic and triphenolic compounds, such as diethylstilbestrol, with potent estrogenic activity.[35] Somewhat later it was found that a number of triphenylethylene derivatives could also bind to estrogen receptors, and in this case produce antiestrogenic effects (for review, see ref. 36). Among the best studied of the latter are ethamoxytriphetol (MER-25) and tamoxifen (ICI 46,474).

Roy Hertz at NIH and Robert Kistner at Harvard were the first to study the effects of MER-25 in women with breast cancer, and both reported favorable results.[36] Unfortunately, the drug also produced hallucinations and psychotic episodes, and so it was abandoned for use in cancer patients. Further use of antiestrogens in breast cancer was abandoned for more than a decade. Then along came tamoxifen, which proved to be a potent antiestrogen in animal bioassays and inhibitor of estrogen binding to its receptor. It also inhibited the growth of human breast cancer cells in culture. Tamoxifen has now been studied in a wide range of breast cancer patients in a number of countries. The drug has been shown to provide a survival advantage as an adjuvant with surgery and other chemotherapeutic agents and also when used as a long-term adjuvant prophylactic therapy to delay disease recurrence.[36] It is now also being tested as a chemopreventive agent in women at risk to develop breast cancer.

One of the recently approved anticancer drugs for clinical use is etoposide (VP16), a semisynthetic derivative of podophyllotoxin, which is extracted from the May apple plant (*Podophyllum peltatum*). This plant was used as a cathartic for centuries. The history of its use can be traced back to an early English book of folk remedies, the *Leech Book of Bald* (A.D. 900–950). The plant was also used by American Indians and early colonists for its emetic, cathartic, and deworming properties. It was in the U.S. Pharmacopoeia until 1942, when it was finally dropped because of its reported toxicity. As part of a National Cancer Institute screen of natural products for anticancer activity, extracts of the plant were found to have antitumor effects. Two semisynthetic glycosides of the active components have been made, etoposide and teniposide. Both have significant anticancer activity. Etoposide has shown important therapeutic activity against lung and testicular cancer as well as against Hodgkin's and diffuse histiocytic lymphomas.

So-called biological-response modifiers are among the newest therapeutic approaches to cancer therapy. These are natural compounds, usually small polypeptides, produced by cells in the body that modulate the production and function of immune system cells. Many of these are called cytokines or lymphokines because they are often produced by blood forming cells and affect the proliferation and differentiation of blood cell elements. The first one of these used in cancer chemotherapy was interferon.

Interferon was discovered in 1957 by two virologists, A. Isaacs and J. Lindemann, who were looking for a substance that blocks viral infection of cells.[37] Their research was prompted by the clinical observation that patients seldom come down with two viral infections at the same time. We now know that this isn't necessarily true, especially in immunosuppressed patients, who may have an opportunistic infection with a second virus, e.g., patients with HIV-induced AIDS who become co-infected with herpes viruses or cytomegalovirus. They found that conditioned medium removed from influenza-virus-infected chicken cells grown in culture prevented infection of other cultures of chicken cells challenged with a different virus. They named this interfering substance "interferon."

Since the early studies, interferons have been purified and the genes cloned. There are three general groups: IFN-α, -β, and -γ. They are produced by lymphoid-type cells primarily, and their function appears to result from stimulation of natural killer cells and macrophages to improve their ability to attack tumor cells in the body. IFN-α has received the most use clinically, but IFN-γ is also being evaluated. The most obvious clinical success has been against a rare leukemia called "hairy cell" leukemia.

Interleukin-2 (IL-2) was originally called T-cell growth factor (TCGF), because it was first found in conditioned medium of mitogen-stimulated lymphocytes and observed to be a factor necessary for T-lymphocytes to grow in culture.[38] Because of its ability to promote proliferation of lymphocytes that can kill tumor cells, it is being used to stimulate lymphokine-activated killer (LAK) cells or tumor infiltrative lymphocytes (TIL cells) in culture prior to and after their administration to cancer patients. This so-called "adoptive immunotherapy," developed by Steven Rosenberg and his colleagues

at the National Cancer Institute, has shown promise in the treatment of renal cell tumors and melanoma.[39]

Tumor necrosis factor (TNF) is another naturally produced peptide that can affect tumor cell growth. In the late 1800s, it was noted that a few cancer patients had a regression of their tumors after a severe systemic bacterial infection. This prompted William Coley in 1893 to try injecting a mixture of killed bacteria (*Streptococcus pyogenes* and *Serratia marescens*) into cancer patients. In a few cases, this concoction (called "Coley's toxins") produced some remarkable remissions when injected directly into tumors. This experimental approach was continued somewhat sporadically over a number of years until the 1930s, and then was abandoned.

The use of bacterial filtrates underwent a resurgence in the 1970s when the mycobacterium BCG, an organism similar to the tuberculosis-causing organism, and the corynebacterium *C. parvum* were found to induce tumor necrosis when injected into tumor-bearing mice. These agents were also found to induce a heightened immune response in patients and were used clinically in a number of experimental therapeutic protocols. Additional data indicated that an extract of gram-negative bacteria containing a lipopolysaccharide (LPS) called endotoxin could induce tumor necrosis when injected with BCG into sarcoma-bearing mice, but not when these agents were added directly to cultures of murine tumor cells. When the serum of the BCG-LPS-injected mice was added to the cultures, however, the cells were killed. These results, obtained by Lloyd Old and his colleagues, led to the conclusion that BCG and LPS were eliciting the release of some cytotoxic factor into the serum of the tumor-bearing animals.[40] This factor, dubbed tumor necrosis factor (TNF), has been purified from mouse and rabbit serum and also from cultures of human lymphoblastoid cells.[41] It is a protein of about 45,000 molecular weight. The TNF gene has been cloned and recombinant TNF has been tested in clinical trials, with some mixed results (see Chapter 14).

Interestingly, the use of TNF is the first approach to gene therapy for cancer patients. Rosenberg and Anderson and their colleagues at NCI have transfected the TNF gene into patients' TIL cells and placed them back into the same patients from whom the cells were derived. The concept here is that the TIL cells will localize in the tumor and release TNF to kill the tumor cells.

Another recently developed approach to direct therapeutic agents selectively to tumors is the use of monoclonal antibodies. Köhler and Milstein showed that fusion of an antigenically stimulated lymphocyte with a malignant myeloma cell, whose protein synthetic machinery is primarily geared to producing immunoglobulins, results in formation of a hybrid cell (hybridoma) that secretes large amounts of highly specific antibodies.[42] Each hybridoma clone makes an antibody with exquisite specificity to a particular epitope of the antibody-eliciting molecule. In 1984, Drs. Köhler and Milstein were awarded the Nobel Prize in Physiology and Medicine for this work. Such monoclonal antibodies have been made against human tumor antigens and are being used clinically to detect tumor cells in the body as well as to tar-

get anticancer drugs and radionuclides directly to tumors (see Chapter 14).

New drugs and new therapeutic approaches continue to be developed for the treatment of cancer. Some of the promising new ideas, such as tumor suppressor gene replacement therapy, antisense genes that inhibit the expression of oncogenes, growth factor antagonists, and monoclonal antibodies will be discussed in Chapter 14. Nevertheless, "classical" anticancer drugs are, and will remain, a mainstay of cancer treatment. The rate of approval of anticancer drugs is shown in Figure 2–1.[43] There was a rapid acquisition of new drugs from 1955 through the 1970s. Most of these were based on parent compounds developed as a result of the pioneering work described in this chapter.

Many of the promising recent advances in cancer chemotherapy have come about from the more effective application of drugs already available. These advances include: (1) the use of more effective drug combinations to maximize tumor cell kill and minimize toxicity, (2) cir-

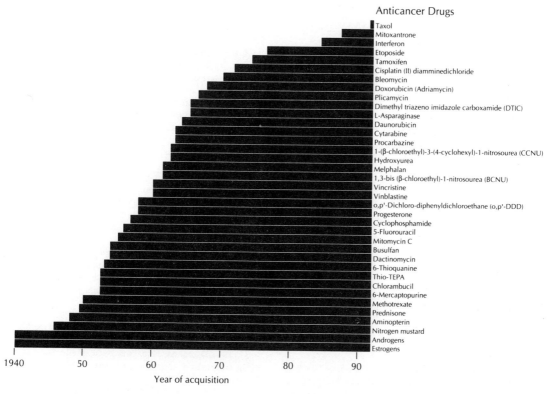

Anticancer Drugs

Taxol
Mitoxantrone
Interferon
Etoposide
Tamoxifen
Cisplatin (II) diamminedichloride
Bleomycin
Doxorubicin (Adriamycin)
Plicamycin
Dimethyl triazeno imidazole carboxamide (DTIC)
L-Asparaginase
Daunorubicin
Cytarabine
Procarbazine
1-(β-chloroethyl)-3-(4-cyclohexyl)-1-nitrosourea (CCNU)
Hydroxyurea
Melphalan
1,3-bis (β-chloroethyl)-1-nitrosourea (BCNU)
Vincristine
Vinblastine
o,p'-Dichloro-diphenyldichloroethane (o,p'-DDD)
Progesterone
Cyclophosphamide
5-Fluorouracil
Mitomycin C
Busulfan
Dactinomycin
6-Thioquanine
Thio-TEPA
Chlorambucil
6-Mercaptopurine
Methotrexate
Prednisone
Aminopterin
Nitrogen mustard
Androgens
Estrogens

1940   50   60   70   80   90

Year of acquisition

Figure 2–1   Acquisition of new anticancer drugs since 1940. (Modified from Krakoff.[43])

cumventing toxic effects by improving the timing of drug delivery, better hydration of patients, and the use of better antiemetic drugs, and (3) autologous bone marrow transplantation, which allows the use of much higher doses of marrow-toxic anticancer drugs by reconstituting a patient's bone marrow. These advances will be discussed in later chapters.

REFERENCES

1. Lissauer: II. Zwei Fälle von Leucaemie. *Berl. Klin. Wochenschr.* 40:403 (1865).

2. E. B. Krumbhaar and H. D. Krumbhaar: The blood and bone marrow in yellow cross gas (mustard gas) poisoning: Changes produced in the bone marrow of fatal cases. *J. Med. Res.* 40:497 (1919).

3. G. B. Infield: *Disaster at Bari.* New York: The Macmillan Co., 1971.

4. F. E. Adair and H. J. Bagg: Experimental and clinical studies on the treatment of cancer by dichloroethyl sulfide (mustard gas). *Ann. Surgery* 93:190 (1931).

5. A. Gilman and F. S. Philips: The biological actions and therapeutic applications of β-chloroethyl amines and sulfides. *Science* 103:409 (1946).

6. A. Gilman: The initial clinical trial of nitrogen mustard. *Am. J. Surgery* 105:574 (1963).

7. S. Farber, L. K. Diamond, R. D. Mercer, R. F. Sylvester, and J. A. Wolff: Temporary remissions in acute leukemia in children produced by folic acid antagonist, 4-aminopteroyl-glutamic acid (aminopterin): *New Engl. J. Med.* 238:787 (1948).

8. D. R. Seeger, D. B. Cosulich, J. M. Smith, and M. E. Hultquist: Analogs of pteroylglutamic acid. III. 4-amino derivatives. *J. Am. Chem. Soc.* 71:1753 (1949).

9. R. Hertz, J. Lewis, Jr., and M. B. Lippsett: Five years' experience with the chemotherapy of metastatic choriocarcinoma and related trophoblastic tumors in women. *Am. J. Obstet. Gynec.* 82:631 (1961).

10. G. B. Elion: The purine path to chemotherapy. *Science* 144:41 (1989).

11. J. D. Watson and F. H. C. Crick: Molecular structure of nucleic acids. A structure for deoxyribose nucleic acid. *Nature* 171:737 (1953).

12. G. B. Elion, E. Burgi, and G. H. Hitchings: Studies on condensed pyrimidine synthesis: IX. The synthesis of some 6-substituted purines. *J. Am. Chem. Soc.* 74:411 (1952).

13. J. H. Burchenal, M. L. Murphy, R. R. Ellison, D. A. Karnofsky, M. P. Sykes, T. C. Tan, L. A. Leone, L. F. Craver, H. W. Dargeon, and C. P. Rhoads: Clinical evaluation of a new antimetabolite, 6-mercaptopurine, in the treatment of leukemia and allied diseases. *Blood* 8:965 (1953).

14. C. Heidelberger: "Fluorinated pyrimidines," in *Progress in Nucleic Acid Research and Molecular Biology*, ed. by J. N. Davidson and W. E. Cohn. New York: Academic Press, 1965, pp. 1–50.

15. R. R. Ellison, J. F. Holland, M. Weil, C. Jacquillat, M. Boiron, J. Bernard, A. Sawitsky, F. Rosner, B. Gussof, R. T. Silver, A. Karanas, J. Cuttner, C. L. Spurr, D. M. Hayes, J. Blom, L. A. Leone, F. Haurani, R. Kyle, J. L. Hutchinson, R. J. Forcier, and J. H. Moon: Arabinosyl cytosine: A useful agent in the treatment of acute leukemia in adults. *Blood* 32:507 (1968).

16. S. A. Waksman and H. B. Woodruff: Bacteriostatic and bacteriocidal substances produced by a soil actinomycetes. *Proc. Soc. Exptl. Biol.* 45:609 (1940).

17. S. Shiba and T. Taguchi: Experimental and clinical studies on mitomycin C. Study on Mitomycin C, No. 101, June 1959.

18. J. H. Brown and B. J. Kennedy: Mithramycin in the treatment of disseminated testicular neoplasms. *N. Engl. J. Med.* 272:111 (1965).

19. H. Umezawa, K. Maeda, T. Takeuchi, and Y. Okami: New antibiotics, bleomycin A and B. *J. Antibiot.* (Tokyo) 19:200 (1966).

20. A. Di Marco, M. Soldati, A. Fioretti, and T. Dasdia: Richerche sull'attiva' della daunomicina ser cellule normali e neoplastiche coltivate *in vitro*. *Tumori* 49:235 (1963).

21. M. Dubost, P. Gantner, R. Maral, L. Ninet, S. Pinner, J. Preud Homme, and G. H. Werner: Un nouvel antibiotique à proprietes antitumorales. *C. R. Acad. Sc. Paris,* Série D 257:1813 (1963).

22. F. Arcamone, G. Cassinelli, G. Fantini, A. Grein, P. Orezzi, C. Poli, and C. Spalla: Adriamycin, 14-hydroxy-daunomycin, a new antitumor antibiotic from *S. peucetius var. caecius*. *Biotechnol. Bioeng.* 11:1101 (1969).

23. R. L. Noble, C. T. Beer, and J. H. Cutts. Further biological activities of vincaleukoblastine—an alkaloid isolated from *Vinca rosea* (L). *Biochem. Pharmacol.* 1:347 (1958).

24. I. S. Johnson, J. G. Armstrong, M. Gorman, and J. P. Burnett, Jr.: The *Vinca* alkaloids: A new class of oncolytic agents. *Cancer Res.* 23:1390 (1963).

25. B. Rosenberg, L. Van Camp, and T. Krigas: Inhibition of cell division in *Escherichia coli* by electrolysis products from a platinum electrode. *Nature* 205:698 (1965).

26. B. Rosenberg, L. Van Camp, E. B. Grimley, and A. J. Tomson: The inhibition of growth and cell division in *Escherichia coli* by different ionic species of platinum (IV) complexes. *J. Biol. Chem.* 242:1347 (1967).

27. B. Rosenberg, L. Van Camp, J. E. Trosko, and V. H. Mansour: Platinum compounds: A new class of potent antitumor agents. *Nature* 222:385 (1969).

28. P. J. Loehrer and L. H. Einhorn: Diagnosis and treatment; drugs five years later: Cisplatin. *Ann. Int. Med.* 100:704 (1984).

29. J. G. Kidd: Regression of transplanted lymphoma induced in vivo by means of normal guinea pig serum. I. Course of transplanted cancers of various kinds in mice and rats given guinea pig serum, horse serum, or rabbit serum. *J. Exp. Med.* 98:565 (1953).

30. G. T. Beatson: On the treatment of inoperable cases of carcinoma of the mamma: Suggestions for a new method of treatment with illustrative cases. *Lancet* 2:104 (1896).

31. T. L. Dao and C. Huggins: Bilateral adrenalectomy in the treatment of cancer of the breast. *AMA Arch. Surg.* 71:645 (1955).

32. O. H. Pearson and B. S. Ray: Results of treatment of metastatic mammary carcinoma. *Cancer* 12:85 (1959).

33. E. Allen and E. A. Doisy: The induction of a sexual mature condition in immature females by injection of ovarian follicular hormone. *Am. J. Physiol. 69:*577 (1924).

34. E. V. Jensen, M. Numata, S. Smith, T. Suuki, P. I. Brecker, and E. R. De Sombre: Estrogen-receptor interaction in target tissues. *Dev. Biol. Suppl. 3:*151 (1969).

35. E. C. Dodds, L. Golberg, W. Lawson, and R. Robinson: Oestrogenic activity of alkylated stilboestrols. *Nature 142:*34 (1938).

36. L. J. Lerner and V. C. Jordan: Development of antiestrogens and their use in breast cancer: Eighth Cain Memorial Award Lecture. *Cancer Res. 50:*4177 (1990).

37. A. Isaacs and J. Lindemann: Virus interference. I. The interferon. *Proc. Roy. Soc. Ser. B 147:*258 (1957).

38. J. W. Mier and R. C. Gallo: Purification and some characteristics of human T-cell growth factor from phytohemagglutinin-stimulated lymphocyte-conditioned media. *Proc. Natl. Acad. Sci. USA 77:*6134 (1980).

39. S. A. Rosenberg, M. T. Lotze, L. M. Muril, S. Leitman, A. E. Chang, S. E. Ettinghausen, Y. L. Matory, J. M. Skibber, E. Shiloni, J. T. Vetto, C. A. Seipp, C. Simpson, and C. M. Reichert: Observations on the systemic administration of autologous lymphokine-activated killer cells and recombinant interleukin-2 to patients with metastatic cancer. *New Engl. J. Med. 313:*1485 (1985).

40. L. J. Old: Tumor necrosis factor (TNF). *Science 230:*630 (1985).

41. B. Y. Rubin, S. L. Anderson, S. A. Sullivan, B. D. Williamson, E. A. Carswell, and L. J. Old: Purification and characterization of a human tumor necrosis factor from the LUKII cell line. *Proc. Natl. Acad. Sci. USA 82:*6637 (1985).

42. G. Köhler and C. Milstein: Continuous cultures of fused cells secreting antibody of predefined specificity. *Nature 256:*495 (1975).

43. I. H. Krakoff: Cancer chemotherapeutic agents. *Ca— A Journal for Clinicians 37:*93 (1987).

Determinants of Drug Responsiveness

Cancer chemotherapy can be curative for about twelve kinds of human cancer. These include childhood leukemia, pediatric solid tumors such as Wilm's, rhabdomyosarcoma, Ewing's sarcoma, osteosarcoma, testicular cancer, choriocarcinoma in women, Hodgkin's disease and certain other lymphomas, and, if diagnosed and treated early, some breast cancers. Many malignant solid tumors are extremely difficult to cure with chemotherapy. These include colon, lung and breast (later stage), and pancreatic carcinomas. Why the difference? Why are some tumors responsive to drugs and others not? Can anything be done to improve the responsiveness of tumors that are not sensitive to drugs? These questions will be approached in this chapter and in Chapter 4.

The responsiveness of tumors to drugs depends on several factors. These can be categorized as determinants relating to the nature of the cancer itself; to the pharmacology, timing and combination of the drugs used; and to the patient—e.g., the state of health, location and blood supply of the tumor, and ability to mount an immune response.

Tumor Determinants

Growth Fraction and Mass Doubling Time

To understand how anticancer drugs work and why certain tumors are sensitive to such drugs, it is helpful to visualize how tumors originate. Malignant tumors arise from the induction of a heritable change in a cell, resulting in the pro-duction of daughter cells which escape the quality control that limits the growth of differentiated adult tissues. During growth and development, the liver, the spleen, and the kidney, for example, attain a predetermined size. A feedback control system, the nature of which is only vaguely understood, signals the tissue when it is time to stop growing. Something like 350 billion cells divide each day in a normal adult, and, potentially, all it takes to initiate a malignant tumor is for one of these divisions to produce a cell that does not respond to the growth-stopping signals. In a tissue exposed to oncogenic (cancer-causing) agents, malignant transformation probably involves stem cells that are responsible for the replacement of cells being lost by normal cell death. These stem cells are "committed" in the sense that normally they will progress only along a certain pathway of differentiation. In other words, a liver stem cell will not become a kidney cell or vice versa. Stem cells have the capacity for proliferation as well as for differentiation, but after a carcinogenic insult, they may lose their ability to differentiate.[1] Once a cell is thus transformed, it may continue to divide *ad infinitum,* limited only by the availability of nutrients and possibly by the host's ability to mount an immunological defense. The transformed cell, then, may be visualized as one that does not progress to a fully differentiated state with limited capacity for cell division. The genes coding for differentiation are either repressed or function imperfectly in the transformed cell, whereas the genes coding for cell proliferation are left "on" instead of being "switched off."

Depending on the type of cancer, the time it takes for the initial transformed cell to produce a clinically detectable tumor may be months or years.[2] One indication that it is often years is the time lag between exposure to a specific carcinogen and the appearance of a diagnosable cancer. Such a lag is observed in people who may smoke an average of one pack of cigarettes or more a day for 20 years before lung cancer appears. Some human tumors grow very rapidly and others very slowly. The mass doubling time of Burkitt's lymphoma, for example, is about 1 day while that of a typical breast cancer mass is about 100 days (Table 3–1).[3] The growth of solid tumors is limited to some extent by the availability of nutrients. Small tumors depend on diffusion for oxygen and other nutrients[4] and for the removal of wastes as long as the cells are within approximately 150 μ of a capillary. Because of this diffusion-limited growth, a steady state is eventually reached in which newly generated cells are balanced by older dying cells. For a spheroidal tumor, the steady state diameter is usually a few millimeters or less. Tumors may remain in this dormant state for years. Usually a neoplasm must be at least 1 cm in diameter ($\simeq 10^9$ cells) to be clinically detectable.

The critical events that initiate the progression of small, avascular neoplasms into large, clinically detectable ones are not yet clear, but Judah Folkman and his colleagues[5] have obtained evidence that tumors, possibly stimulated by anoxia, can release diffusable substances, called tumor angiogenesis factors, that induce the growth of capillaries from the surrounding host tissues into the tumor. Once this occurs, the neoplasm initiates new growth that may continue until the host dies. As the vascularized tumor grows, amino acids, carbohydrates, and other essential nutrients may be consumed at a rapid rate, leading to one of the most common signs of malignant disease, weight loss. Not all parts of a solid tumor become equally well vascularized, however, and a tumor may become too large for capillary growth to keep up. The end result is often a tumor with a necrotic center of dead or dying cells surrounded by a layer of dormant cells and an outer "rim" of dividing cells.

What does this imply for chemotherapy? In Chapter 1, it was observed that tissues having a high proportion of dividing cells are more susceptible to the cytotoxic effects of anticancer drugs than are tissues with a lower proportion of such cells. The proportion of dividing cells in a tumor or normal tissue is often called the "growth fraction."[6,7] This term has been used differently by different authors, but generally, it is taken to mean that fraction of the total viable cell population that is actually in the active division cycle. The viable tumor cell population consists of those cells in the division cycle (G_1, S, G_2, M) plus those "resting" cells (G_0 cells) that have the potential to divide upon appropriate stimulation. It is very difficult, however, to distinguish between a nondividing cell that has the potential to divide and a nondividing, terminally differentiated cell in a tumor mass or in normal tissue *in vivo*. Since it is the dividing cell that is sensitive to most anticancer drugs, it follows that normal tissues and tumors with high growth fractions are more susceptible to the toxic effects of these

Table 3–1 *Doubling Times of Some Human Tumors*

Tumors	Doubling Time (Days)	Ability of Drugs to Produce a Cure
Burkitt's lymphoma	1.0	+
Choriocarcinoma	1.5	+
Acute lymphocytic leukemia	3–4	+
Hodgkin's disease	3–4	+
Testicular embryonal carcinoma	5–6	+
Colon	80	−
Lung (except small-cell carcinoma)	90	−
Breast	100	+/−

drugs. Since the mass doubling time of a malignant neoplasm is inversely proportional to the growth fraction, it also follows that tumors with shorter mass doubling times are more amenable to treatment with drugs (Table 3–1). The growth fraction of human neoplasms ranges from 20% to 70%, depending on the size of the tumor, the availability of oxygen and nutrients, etc.[6] Normal tissues with a high growth fraction (e.g., bone marrow, gastrointestinal mucosa, and hair follicles) are also the tissues most damaged by cancer chemotherapeutic drugs. For example, the growth fraction of normal bone marrow is about 30%. Thus, during treatment with anticancer drugs, the bone marrow will be damaged at the doses that are needed to kill cancer cells. Due to the types of cells that arise from the marrow (e.g., granulocytes, platelets) bleeding and infection are two of the limiting complications of cancer chemotherapy.

Since the mass doubling time depends on the number of *dividing* cells rather than the total number of cells in a tumor, the mass doubling time and the cell cycle time are not the same unless the growth fraction approaches 100% and cell loss is minimal. A growth fraction this high may be found in certain tumors growing in culture, but it seldom occurs *in vivo*. The growth of a number of experimental tumors *in vivo* may be described by the standard Gompertzian growth curve, as shown in Figure 3–1. The plateau phase of the growth curve appears to result from a decreasing supply of nutrients, which in turn produces a decreasing growth fraction and an increasing rate of cell loss relative to cell proliferation in the tumor. Although similar data on human cancers cannot be easily obtained, the relationship between tumor size, growth fraction, and mass doubling time has been defined for certain experimental tumors by Schabel and his associates in classic studies that are still relevant.[7,8] The data in Table 3–2, for example, indicate that, as a mouse adenocarcinoma increases over an order of magnitude in size, the mass doubling time increases from 0.5 to 7.5 days and the growth fraction falls from 100% to 7%. Interestingly, the difference in the cell cycle time (the time it takes a cell that is programmed to divide to complete the cell cycle) between small and large tumors is not great.

Schabel and his colleagues have also demonstrated in tumor-bearing animals that, as one would predict, small proliferating tumors are the ones most susceptible to chemotherapy. For

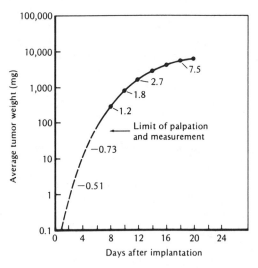

Figure 3–1 Gompertzian curve of tumor growth. The average weight of tumors (calculated from tumor diameters) was determined in 100 BDF₁ mice following the implantation of fragments of adenocarcinoma 755. The line through the observed data (●) and the extrapolation (- - - - -), represent a best-fit Gompertz function as determined by the method of least squares. The numbers next to the curve represent the tumor doubling time (days) at the indicated points. (Adapted from Schabel.[7])

Table 3–2　Relationship Between Tumor Size, Growth Fraction, and Doubling Time in Mouse Adenocarcinoma 755. (Data from Schabel[7])

Tumor Size	Mass Doubling Time	Growth Fraction (%)	Cell Cycle Time (Days)
2 mg	12 hours	100	—
25 mg	0.7 days	61	0.48
250 mg	1.2 days	40	0.57
700 mg	1.8 days	25	0.61
1.3 g	2.7 days	19	0.64
5 g	7.5 days	7	0.69

example, some animal tumors that are very sensitive to antimetabolite drugs in the logarithmic phase of growth become much less sensitive in the plateau phase.[7] Such data indicate the importance of initiating chemotherapy when tumors are still in the proliferating phase. Two other points should be considered here. First, after removal or destruction of large, bulky tumors by surgery or irradiation ("debulking"), the cells remaining may be stimulated to enter the proliferative, drug-sensitive phase and hence become more susceptible to chemotherapy. This phenomenon is sometimes called "recruitment." Second, metastases may initially have a growth fraction and mass doubling time that resemble those of the early stages of the primary tumor (Table 3–3), so they may be more susceptible to anticancer drugs if they are treated early. Thus, chemotherapy is frequently initiated soon after surgery or irradiation, rather than after metastases can be clinically demonstrated.

Total Tumor Burden

Tumor size is another limiting factor to successful chemotherapy in malignant disease. In general, it can be said that large, bulky tumors are not usually curable by chemotherapy. Some of the reasons for this should be obvious from what was said above. Drugs may not be able to penetrate into a solid tumor in amounts sufficient to effect a cell kill. Also, a large percentage of cells in a bulky tumor may be in a nonproliferative stage at the time of treatment and thus survive to reestablish the tumor mass. Of course, it is also true that the larger the tumor the longer it may have been present and there-

fore the higher the probability that it has already metastasized. But there is an additional consideration, related to the sheer number of malignant cells to be eradicated. It is clear that the more cells there are to be killed the more prolonged drug therapy must be, but the drug must eradicate the tumor cells without irreparably damaging the host. The killing of tumor cells by drugs appears to follow first-order kinetics, assuming that the growth fraction and cell cycle time remain relatively constant. This means that a given drug regimen will eliminate a constant *proportion* of neoplastic cells rather than a constant *number* of cells. In other words, it will take just as much drug to lower the tumor cell number from 10^6 to 10^3 cells (a loss of less than 1 mg of tissue) as to lower the number from 10^9 to 10^6 (a loss of 1 g of tissue).

Some of what has just been said is illustrated in Figure 3–2. Here, number of surviving cancer cells is plotted against time-course from the start of treatment. At the time of diagnosis of

Table 3–3　Doubling Times of Primary Tumor and Metastases of the Lewis Lung Carcinoma in the Mouse. (Data from Simpson-Herren et al.[9])

Days After Tumor Implantation	Doubling Time in Days	
	Primary Tumor	Metastases
5	2.1	—
10	3.1	—
15	4.7	0.5
20	7.1	1.4
25	10.7	4.3
30	16.1	13.1

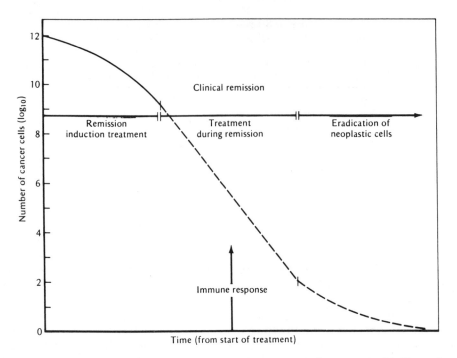

Figure 3–2   Phases of response during the hypothetical complete cure of a tumor. In this illustration, a complete clinical remission is produced when 99.9% of the neoplastic cells are killed. The data deviate from first-order kinetics at the two ends of the response curve because it is likely that the growth fraction and mass doubling time change as the tumor mass decreases from a large, bulky tumor to a smaller tumor. The response curve is also different for the residual cells because they are likely to be less sensitive to the drug or present in sites where drug doesn't penetrate as well. The immune response probably also plays a role in removing cells remaining after chemotherapy. (Adapted from Frei.[10])

a number of disseminated malignant diseases, as many as 10^{12} tumor cells may be present.[10] This may be close to the fatal number for certain tumors.[10] Successful chemotherapy may kill 99.9% of the cells (a "3-log kill") and still leave 10^9 cells in the patient. This number is barely detectible, and clinically, the patient may appear to be in "remission." But it is necessary to continue therapy even in the face of an apparent remission to eliminate the many malignant cells that are still present. One positive factor at this stage is that the cell-kill rate may increase after the initial treatment as a result of the "recruitment" effect (see above). Although a complete clinical remission occurred in the example given in the figure when 99.9% of the tumor cells were killed, to produce a cure, therapy must be continued until the last tumor cell is killed. There is ample experimental evidence that one viable tumor cell can pro-

duce a tumor that will kill a susceptible host animal.[8]

The correct duration of treatment is difficult to estimate and it requires that a number of assumptions be made about the total tumor burden of the patient, the rate of tumor cell kill, the proliferation of tumor cells surviving chemotherapy, and the time for bone marrow and gastrointestinal tract recovery. Ideally, treatment is continued until the last tumor cell is killed. This probably cannot occur without some concomitant action of the patient's own immune defense system against the tumor. If one simply calculates, logistically, how soon a rapidly dividing tumor cell population reestablishes itself if it is allowed to regrow without further treatment, one can easily grasp how enormously difficult it is to kill that last cell (Table 3–4). Even if it were possible to achieve a 5-log kill (i.e., eliminate 99.999% of an initial tumor mass of 10^9 cells), it would take only 16.7 doubling times for the original tumor mass to be reestablished (assuming a growth fraction of 100% and insignificant cell loss). For a tumor like Burkitt's lymphoma, which can double in mass every 24 hours, this would be a very short remission indeed.

Disease-Free Survival Plateau

As noted above, long-term survival or cure implies that all viable surviving cancer cells are eliminated from the body. This usually takes prolonged, follow-up therapy lasting months or sometimes years. To achieve cure, chemotherapy must be carried out empirically, since treatment has to be continued even in the face of an apparent clinical remission. Following effective chemotherapy, the risk for relapse is highest early on and decreases with time. This may be 1 to 4 years, depending on the growth parameters of the tumor; however, for some tumors (e.g., breast cancer) a definitive disease-free plateau is not evident.[11] A few clinical examples will suffice to portray this.

ACUTE LYMPHOCYTIC LEUKEMIA. It became clear in the 1960s that the use of drug combinations such as vincristine and prednisone could induce a high percentage of remission in children with acute lymphocytic leukemia (ALL). However, relapses usually occurred, frequently due to spread to the central nervous system. It became evident that treatment during remission was essential. Then it was shown that 6-MP and methotrexate (MTX) could significantly prolong the duration of complete remission. Experimental animal studies showed that intermittent administration of MTX was better than twice-daily injection,[12] and this idea was soon adopted in the clinic.[13] Thus, induction of remission with vincristine and prednisone, followed by continuous 6-MP and intermittent MTX during remission, led to a significant increase in the number of long-term survivors.[11] However, patients continued to relapse at later times with meningeal infiltration of leukemic cells, presumably because the drugs couldn't penetrate the blood-brain barrier to reach this "pharmacologic sanctuary." This led to the use of irradiation of the central nervous system and intrathecal injection of MTX prophylactically to prevent the occurrence of meningeal leukemia.

The use of L-asparaginase and doxorubicin (Adriamycin) during the first 6 months of remission, together with 6-MP and intermittent MTX, has resulted in a disease-free survival approaching 85% for up to 5 years or more.[11] Nevertheless, it became clear after several years of experience with combination drug regimens that treatment had to be continued for two to three years to assure long-term survival.

DISSEMINATED HODGKIN'S DISEASE. A number of single agents, going back to the 1940s, were found to induce short-term remission in Hodgkin's disease patients. These include nitrogen mustard, vincristine, prednisone, and methotrexate.

In 1963, DeVita and his colleagues introduced MOPP combination chemotherapy.[14]

Table 3–4 *Estimation of Tumor Kill and Recovery with Chemotherapy*

Tumor Kill (%)	Surviving Cells	Viable Mass	Recovery of Tumor (Units in Doubling Times)
Untreated	10^9	1 g	—
50	5×10^8	500 mg	1
90 (1-log)	10^8	100 mg	3.33
99 (2-log)	10^7	10 mg	6.66
99.9 (3-log)	10^6	1 mg	9.99
99.99 (4-log)	10^5	100 μg	13.3
99.999 (5-log)	10^4	10 μg	16.7

MOPP is the acronym for mustargen (nitrogen mustard), Oncovin (vincristine), procarbazine, and prednisone. The rationale for this and other drug combinations was to use agents that were effective as single agents, that had different mechanisms of action, and that had non-overlapping toxicities. This and similar drug combinations, such as Adriamycin, bleomycin, vincristine, and dacarbazine (ABVD), sometimes used as adjuvants to radiotherapy, have been successful in curing about 75% of patients. Again, however, a disease-free survival plateau is achieved. The risk period for failure after a successful treatment is 4 years.[11]

BURKITT'S LYMPHOMA. Burkitt's lymphoma was one of the first malignant neoplasms found to be curable by chemotherapy. A B-cell type lymphoma first discovered as endemic in certain areas of equatorial Africa, Burkitt's lymphoma also occurs in somewhat modified form in temperate climates, including North America. Both forms are curable with combination chemotherapy.[15,16] High-risk patients will usually succumb to this disease within the first 8 months of diagnosis (Fig. 3–3). Thereafter, patients kept in remission achieve a disease-free survival plateau approaching normal life expectancy.

GESTATIONAL CHORIOCARCINOMA. Women who develop gestational choriocarcinoma also are curable with drugs and achieve a disease-free survival plateau indicating that they are cured of their disease after 13 months (Fig. 3–3). This malignant disease was the first example of a cancer cured by chemotherapy. In 1956, Roy Hertz and his colleagues at NIH showed that intensive intermittent methotrexate could induce complete remissions in women with this disease.[17]

Fortunately, in this disease the presence of a definite "tumor marker," human chorionic gonadotropin (hCG), allows accurate follow-up of patients and enables the clinical oncologist to track the drug response and level of tumor burden during and after chemotherapy. Unfortunately, such sensitive and accurate tumor markers are not available for most other cancers (see Chapter 12).

TESTICULAR CANCER. hCG and alpha fetoprotein (AFP) are useful tumor markers in testicular cancer, another highly treatable malignancy. In this case, hCG and AFP can be used to follow response and remission duration, and after about one year of disease-free remission, patients are generally cured. Effective therapy for this disease has been pioneered by Einhorn and his coworkers, and effective combination

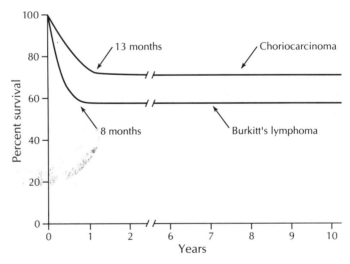

Figure 3–3   Disease-free survival plateaus for choriocarcinoma and Burkitt's lymphoma. Long-term survival after 13 months or 8 months, respectively, usually means the patient is cured.

regimens include cisplatin, vinblastine, and bleomycin (PVB), or cisplatin, VP-16 (etoposide), and bleomycin.[18]

BREAST CANCER. Although breast cancer can be effectively treated, especially if diagnosed early, a clear disease-free survival plateau is not attained. Relapse after effective remission-inducing therapy may occur 5, 10, or even 15 years later, although risk of failure does appear to decrease with time.[11]

Tumor Heterogeneity

Tumors are usually heterogenous populations of cells—some cells are proliferating, some can proliferate but are dormant, others are dying. Within the first two categories, some cells proliferate for one or several generations but will eventually stop (dead-end cells), and others can produce an unlimited line of descendants ("clonogenic" cells). For any tumor therapy to be completely effective, the most invasive, metastatic cells must be killed.

CLONAL DERIVATION OF CANCER. The question is how does so much heterogeneity arise in a population of cancer cells, since there is significant evidence that many human tumors arise from a single cell of origin and thus are clones of the original transformed cell. This evidence derives from studies showing that (1) in many primary cancers, all the cells have the same abnormal chromosome rearrangement—for example, the Philadelphia chromosome in chronic myelocytic leukemia cells; (2) all the cells of a given multiple myeloma produce the same type of immunoglobulin, whereas populations of normal immunoglobulin-producing cells in the body produce many different types; and (3) tumors arising in a woman whose cells are heterozygous for the X chromosome-linked isoenzymes of glucose-6-phosphate dehydrogenase (G-6-PDH) express only one of the two possible isoenzyme types.[19,20] The explanation for the latter finding comes from the observation that only one X chromosome is expressed in the adult female and its expression is randomly determined. Hence, some females who are heterozygous for the G-6-PDH gene will be mosaics in the sense that some cells will express the A-type and some the B-type isoenzyme. Because malignant tumors arising in women with this characteristic usually have only one of the two isozyme types, the implication is that the tumor arose from a single clone of cells. Otherwise, the tumor would be expected to be a mosaic as well. When this criterion is applied, a number of human tumors have been identified as of probable single-clonal origin. It has also been found that, when multiple tumors of the same type arise in the same patient, all the cells of a given tumor contain only one G-6-PDH isoenzyme, but the cells of other tumors may contain the other isoenzyme.[21] This indicates that different primary tumors can arise from different clones of cells.

The hypothesis of single-cell clonal origin of cancer does not explain how the phenotypic characteristics of a cancer can change as it grows and metastasizes in a patient. The explanation for this is probably that neoplastic cells are more genetically unstable than their normal counterparts and go through several "evolutionary" changes as the tumor progresses. Nowell has proposed a model to explain this process.[20] In this model, tumor initiation is postulated as occurring from the interaction of a carcinogenic agent and a susceptible normal cell. The induced change provides some selective growth advantage over adjacent normal cells. Other cells in the same individual may also undergo "initiation" of transformation after exposure to carcinogens, but presumably they never proliferate (i.e., undergo tumor promotion) or they are destroyed before they progress to a clinically detectable tumor. The proliferation of neoplastic cells, after some lag time, leads eventually to genetically variant cells because of the genetic instability of neoplastic cells. This accounts for the aneuploidy of most advanced cancers. Many of these genetic variants are eliminated because of a metabolic disadvantage or an immunologic reaction of the host, but a few tumor cells with an additional selective advantage proliferate and become predominant. As the tumor progresses, there is sequential selection of sublines of cells with increasingly abnormal karyotype, state of differentiation, invasiveness, and metastatic potential. Although many advanced cancers share similar genotypic and phenotypic characteristics (e.g., increased ability to synthesize DNA and to proliferate continuously), tumors of the same histologic type from different patients may have many differences because their microenvironments affect the rate of emergence and type of variant sublines. The fact that most advanced human cancers, even those of the same histologic and tissue type, are aneuploid and have unique biochemistry and immunologic alterations is discouraging from a therapeutic point of view, but it helps explain the vast biochemical heterogeneity of human tumors and the difficulty in developing anticancer drugs that will specifically kill tumors arising from a given cell type.

THERAPEUTIC CONSIDERATIONS IN THE TREATMENT OF METASTASIS. Metastatic cells appear to have a greater genetic instability than nonmetastatic tumor cells. Thus, as one might suspect, even if individual metastases arise from a single clone of cells, for which there is evidence from both human and animal tumors,[22] cellular heterogeneity is likely to arise within a few population doublings. For example, the metastatic properties of tumor cell clones isolated from individual metastatic lung foci of mouse B16 melanoma cells have been examined for their metastatic characteristics.[23] Initially, the cells of a given metastatic focus displayed "intralesional clonal homogeneity," but as the metastatic lesions grew and progressed, they became populated with cells of heterogeneous phenotypes.

Because in most cases of cancer the metastatic lesions kill the patient, it is extremely important to know the best way to treat these lesions. Unfortunately, though metastatic lesions may initially show a homogeneous sensitivity to cancer chemotherapeutic agents, they quickly develop a marked clonal heterogeneity with respect to their chemosensitivity to drugs, such that cells within one metastatic site may vary from cells in other metastatic sites, as well as from the primary tumor, in their drug responsiveness. Such heterogeneity has been seen in animal[22,24] and in human[25] neoplasms.

DRUG-RESISTANT CELLS IN TUMOR CELL POPULATIONS. Even within a primary solid tumor there may be considerable heterogeneity in responsiveness to anticancer drugs.[26] The reasons for this intratumor variability aren't entirely clear, but it is important to remember that tumors are architecturally complex as well as phenotypically complex. Tumor cells in the center of solid tumors are farther away from the blood supply than those at the periphery, and are more likely to be in the resting, or G_0, phase of the cell cycle (see below) than those closer to capillaries. The different locales within a tumor also have different access to extracellular matrix attachment and exposure to growth factors, and different degrees of intratumor infiltration with immune cells. There are, in addition, different cellular phenotypes within a given tumor, including antigen expression, cell membrane composition, metastatic potential, and responsiveness to anticancer drugs.[27]

Some tumors appear to be inherently resistant to most anticancer drugs—for example, squamous cell carcinoma of the lung and colon cancer. Moreover, most, if not all, cancers have lurking in them some cells that are resistant to anticancer drugs or have the ability to become resistant quickly. When the drug-sensitive cells are killed off, these clones of drug-resistant cells may proliferate and become the dominant cell type in a tumor, rendering it insensitive.

This problem of drug resistance is crucial in cancer chemotherapy; in many cases it is the single most important factor in the failure of drug treatment for cancer. Clinical oncologists attempt to circumvent or delay the development of drug resistance by employing drug combinations with agents that have different mechanisms of action. The mechanisms of drug resistance are known for many anticancer drugs, and these are often related to the drugs' mechanisms of action. For example, cells become resistant to methotrexate by increasing their content of the MTX-inhibited enzyme, dihydrofolate reductase. Other mechanisms of drug resistance include decreased drug uptake or increased drug efflux, decreased activity of drug-activating enzymes, increased activity of drug-detoxifying enzymes, decreased binding to the target enzyme, and increased DNA repair. These mechanisms are discussed in detail in Chapter 4.

Cell-cycle Phase

To understand why only certain cells in a tumor are susceptible to drugs and how different drugs act, the phases of the cell cycle must be considered. The cell cycle is divided into a G_1 or intermitotic phase, an S or DNA synthesis phase, a G_2 or premitotic phase, and an M or mitotic phase (Fig. 3–4). In all normal differentiated adult tissues and in most tumors, there is a population of viable cells that is not proliferating. These cells are sometimes said to be in the G_0 phase. An important consideration is that there is, in normal tissue and in tumors, a certain number of viable cells that can proliferate but that are not, for all practical purposes, going to double their DNA content and divide unless stimulated to do so. These nondividing cells are the cells that are most likely to survive chemotherapy and to regenerate the tumor after treatment. Thus, one aim of chemotherapy is to be selectively toxic to the resting tumor cell (as well as to the proliferating tumor

cell), while allowing the resting normal cell to survive.

There is some evidence that anticancer drugs do have some selective toxicity toward malignant cells. For example, Bruce et al.[28] studied the relationship between the dose of various chemotherapeutic agents and their effect on the colony-forming ability of mouse bone marrow cells and AKR lymphoma cells (Fig. 3–5). The ability of intravenously injected bone marrow cells and lymphoma cells, taken from animals 24 hours after drug administration, to form colonies in the spleen of irradiated recipient mice provides a quantitative assay of the number of viable cells that survive chemotherapy and a comparison of the relative toxicities of a given drug for normal bone marrow cells and for malignant cells. Most of the drugs thus assayed are considerably more toxic to lym-

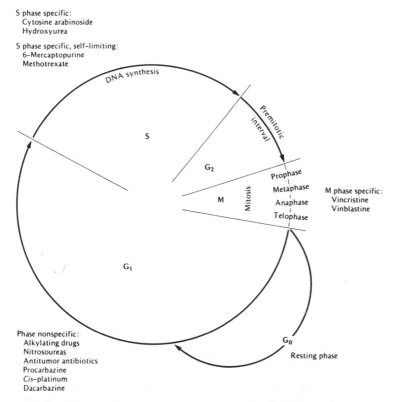

Figure 3–4 The cell cycle and the relationship of antitumor drug action to the cycle. G_1 is the period between mitosis and the beginning of DNA synthesis. Resting cells (cells that are not preparing for cell division) are said to be in a subphase of G_1, G_0. S is the period of DNA synthesis: G_2 the premitotic interval; and M the period of mitosis. Examples of cell-cycle-dependent anticancer drugs are listed next to the phase at which they act. Drugs that are cytotoxic for cells at any point in the cycle are called cycle-phase-nonspecific drugs.

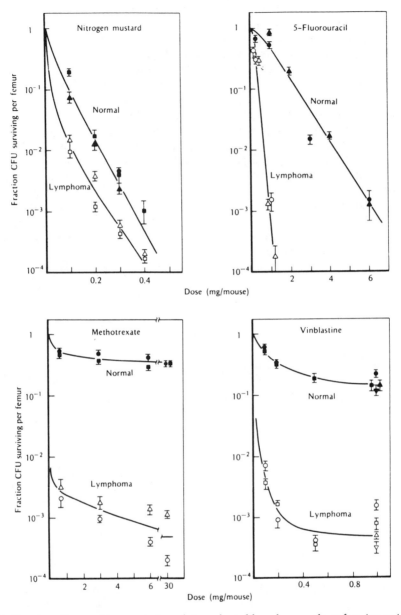

Figure 3–5 Fraction of normal hemopoietic and transplanted lymphoma colony-forming units surviving in femoral marrow 24 hours after drug administration. Anticancer drugs were given to normal mice (solid symbols) or mice that had been injected 1 week earlier with a suspension of lymphoma cells (open symbols). Twenty-four hours after drug administration, femoral marrow suspensions were injected into supralethally irradiated mice. The irradiated animals were killed 10 days later and the number of colony-forming units (CFU) in the spleen were counted. Vinblastine was given as a single dose, and nitrogen mustard, methotrexate, and 5-fluorouracil in divided doses (injected every 4 hours × 6). The numbers on the abscissa represent the total dosage given. (Adapted from Bruce *et al.*[28])

phoma cells than marrow cells. This differential sensitivity is thought to reflect the higher growth fraction and the shorter cell generation time of the lymphoma cells, as compared to the bone marrow cells, so that a higher percentage of bone marrow cells survive a relatively short exposure to the cytotoxic drug. Although nitrogen mustard affects both resting and proliferating cells, its effect is greater on proliferating cells (see Chapter 6) and some differential sensitivity is observed. Such drugs as methotrexate and vinblastine have greater efficacy against the lymphoma cells, but a plateau is reached, probably because the cytotoxicity of these drugs is self-limited and cell-cycle-phase specific. Thus, cells not in the sensitive phase during drug exposure will survive. These results may explain some of the partial selective toxicity seen with the clinical use of anticancer drugs. It should be noted, however, that the data in Figure 3–5 were obtained after a single course of drug treatment. Upon exposure of the bone marrow to cytotoxic drugs, cells in G_0 may be stimulated to proliferate and thus become more sensitive to subsequent drug therapy. Thus, effective scheduling of therapy must allow time for a significant percentage of surviving bone marrow cells to repopulate the marrow before the next course of therapy is initiated. Depending on the toxicity of the drug(s) employed, courses of treatment may have to be scheduled several weeks apart.

Some anticancer drugs are most effective against cells in one phase of the cell cycle. It is generally true, however, even for those drugs that do not have a strict cell-cycle-phase-specific cytotoxicity, that anticancer drugs are more effective against proliferating than against nonproliferating cells. As shown in Figure 3–4, antitumor drugs can be classified as S-phase specific (e.g., cytosine arabinoside, hydroxyurea), S-phase specific, self-limiting (e.g., methotrexate, 6-mercaptopurine), M-phase specific (e.g., vincristine, vinblastine), or cycle-phase nonspecific (e.g., alkylating drugs, antitumor antibiotics). The "S-phase specific, self-limiting" drugs are most effective in S phase but they have another inhibitory action that slows the entry of cells into S phase. The mitotic inhibitors primarily arrest cells in metaphase. The cycle phase nonspecific agents can kill cells in any phase of the cell cycle, but even

they are usually more effective against proliferating cells and may show enhanced activity against cells in a specific phase of the cell cycle.

Drug Scheduling

Regimens for maximum tumor cell kill can be designed when the cell-cycle specificity of anticancer drugs is known. Further optimization may be achieved if a population of tumor cells is "synchronized" to enter the sensitive phase at a given time. An example of how a treatment regimen can be optimized is given in Figure 3–6. Here, mice bearing the L1210 leukemia were treated with the S-phase-specific inhibitor cytosine arabinoside (ara-C), the M-phase inhibitor vinblastine, or a combination of the two.[29] When the two drugs were given simultaneously, a slight decrease in the therapeutic effect was noted, possibly because the cells were prevented from entering the most sensitive phase for each drug when the concentration of that drug was high enough to kill cells. A remarkable synergism is observed, however, if vinblastine is given first followed by ara-C 16 hours later. Vinblastine arrests cells in M phase, producing a "roadblock" behind which the cells that are not killed outright pile up. As the effective concentration of vinblastine decreases (due to its redistribution, metabolism, and excretion), all the blocked but still viable cells are synchronized to enter S phase more or less at the same time. In the L1210 system, maximum synchrony in S phase is achieved about 16 hours after vinblastine injection. Hence, ara-C has its greatest effect at that time. For this type of scheduling to be effective clinically, a concomitant synchronization of bone marrow cells would have to be avoided.

Both experimental and clinical studies have clearly shown that effective drug concentrations must be maintained long enough to "catch" the maximal number of tumor cells in the sensitive phase of the cell cycle for chemotherapy with cell-cycle-phase-specific drugs to be successful. This has been demonstrated in classic studies by Skipper and his associates[30] in the mouse L1210 leukemia system. From the summary of their data in Table 3–5, it can be seen that therapeutic failure may occur, even if large drug doses are employed, unless an appro-

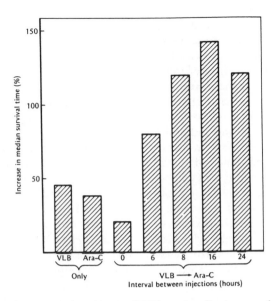

Figure 3–6   Influence of treatment with vinblastine (VLB) on the effectiveness of cytosine arabinoside (ara-C) in leukemic mice. Vinblastine was given 2, 4, 6, 8 and 10 days after inoculation of the mice with L1210 leukemia cells. Cytosine arabinoside was given on the same days at various intervals after vinblastine injection. The median survival time in untreated controls was 9 days after inoculation with tumor cells and the anti-leukemic effect of each treatment protocol is expressed as the percent increase in median survival time over untreated controls. (From Frei[10] after data of Vadlamudi and Goldin.[29])

priate concentration of drug is maintained for the right amount of time. In mice bearing an initial tumor load of 10^5 cells, 15 mg/kg of ara-C administered every 3 hours on days 2 and 6 following inoculation of leukemic cells is required to effect a cure. A 93% cure rate can be obtained if ara-C is given every 3 hours on days 2, 6, and 10. Since the half-life of ara-C in the mouse is short, the drug must be given every 3 hours in order to maintain a concentration that will inhibit DNA synthesis. When ara-C is injected every 3 hours for 24 hours, which is twice the cell-cycle time of L1210 cells, most of the leukemic cells will have entered S phase, the drug-sensitive phase for ara-C. But the tumor will recur following a one-day regimen, since some cells will escape and reestablish the tumor mass. When drug injections are spaced 3 days apart, the tumor is eliminated and sufficient time is allowed for the normal tissues of the mouse to recover from the drug-induced damage. None of the animals inoculated with 10^7 tumor cells are cured even with an intensive drug regimen, which reiterates the difficulties involved in treating individuals with a large tumor load.

Similar therapeutic principles can be demonstrated in studies in which ara-C was used to treat acute myelogenous leukemia in humans.[31] Since ara-C is rapidly deaminated in the liver, the plasma half-life of ara-C in humans is about 10 minutes. The cell-cycle time of acute myelogenous leukemia cells is in the range of 2 to 4 days. One way to provide effective concentrations of ara-C for about twice the cycle time is to give 5-day courses of continuous intravenous infusion every 2 to 3 weeks. The therapeutic results (Table 3–6) were better than those obtained with a daily dosage regimen. Thus, the results from both animal and human studies show that a knowledge of tumor growth kinetics as well as the cell cycle specificity and pharmacokinetics of the drugs employed can be applied clinically to the design of effective chemotherapeutic regimens.

The importance of drug scheduling can be further demonstrated in a treatment regimen designed to remove all tumor cells. This can be visualized in the therapy of an experimental animal leukemia that has a doubling time of 12 hours (Figure 3-7). Here, the number of leukemic cells quadruples every 24 hours to reach

Table 3–5 Effects of Different Therapeutic Schedules in the Treatment of the L1210 Mouse Leukemia with the S-Phase-Specific Drug Cytosine Arabinoside. (Adapted From a Table by Skipper[30])

Size of Inoculum (Cell No.)	Dose (mg/kg)	Schedule of Drug Administration (All Doses Were Begun on Day 2 After Tumor Cell Inoculation)	Cures (%)	Interpretation: Reasons for Success or Failure			
				Success	Failure		
				Clonogenic Leukemia Cells Exposed in S Phase	Gaps in Effective Serum Concentration Too Long	Period of Effective Serum Concentration Too Short	Disease Too Far Advanced
10^5	3000	Single dose	0			X	
	30	Every day (× 15)	0		X		
	500	Every 2 days (× 8)	0		X		
	1500	Every 4 days (× 4)	0		X		
10^5	15	Every 3 hours (× 8) day 2	0			X	
	15	Every 3 hours (× 8) days 2, 6	32	X			
	15	Every 3 hours (× 8) days 2, 6, 10	93	X			
	15	Every 3 hours (× 8) days 2, 6, 10, 14	86	X			
10^7	15	Every 3 hours (× 8) days 2, 6, 10, 14	0				X

Table 3-6 *Effect of Dose Schedule on the Response of Acute Myelogenous Leukemia to Cytarabine (Cytosine Arabinoside).* (From Frei[31])

Schedule	Number of Patients	Patients Achieving Complete Remission(%)	Median Duration of Remission (Months)
Daily dose	98	8–25	7
Five-day infusions every 2 to 3 weeks	85	38	12

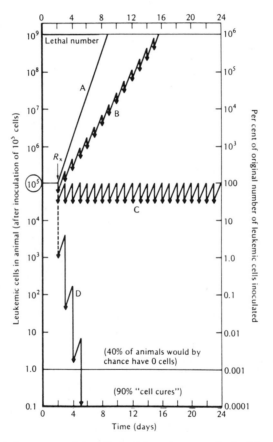

Figure 3-7 Hypothetical illustration of the effect of drug dosage and schedule of administration in an experimental leukemia in animals. Mice are inoculated with 10^5 leukemic cells and various treatment schedules are initiated at day 2 (R_x) after inoculation. (A) In these untreated control animals, the number of leukemic cells quadruples daily until death occurs at about 10^9 cells/mouse. (B) The mice are given a low drug dosage on a long-term basis; the plot represents a daily killing of 50% of the animals' leukemic cells in the presence of a daily quadrupling of the surviving leukemic cells. (C) The result of treatment is sufficient to yield a daily 75% "drug kill" of the leukemic cells. (D) Daily treatment with a high drug dosage in short-term therapy is plotted to represent a 99% daily "drug kill." With no further complications, this treatment schedule would yield cures. (From Skipper[32])

10^9, which is approximately the lethal tumor burden in the mouse. Daily treatment with a drug at a dose that produces a 50% cell kill would only moderately increase the animal's life span. Daily treatment at a dose that produces a 75% kill would allow the host to live out a normal life span if the drug, at the dosage required, was not lethal to the host and if the leukemic cells did not become drug resistant or metastasize to sites where the drug could not penetrate. It should be noted that, in such a situation, the likelihood of one of these events occurring would be extremely high, and would in all probability lead to the failure of therapy. If the mice could tolerate a daily dose of drug that would produce a 99% leukemic cell kill, then 90% of the animals would be cancer-free after four doses. Most human tumors do not have a mass doubling time of 12 hours, but the principles illustrated in this mouse leukemia model should be relevant to cancer in humans. Clinical experience has indicated that prolonged daily administration of drugs is often not as efficacious as intermittent therapy. The reason for this is that time is required for recovery of the host's bone marrow function and immune defense mechanisms before another course of cytotoxic therapy is initiated. Thus, in the treatment of cancer with drugs, success can only be achieved if the time required to restore critical normal functions is significantly shorter than the time required for the tumor to reestablish its original mass.

Application of Cytokinetic Principles in the Treatment of Human Tumors

Most of the examples of tumor growth kinetics and cell-cycle effects presented in this chapter are from animal studies. Although the data obtained in animal systems form the basis for much of the current thinking in human cancer and certainly are relevant to tumor growth and drug action in humans, it must be remembered that cell-cycle kinetics, growth fraction, and drug responsiveness of the most common solid tumors in humans differ from those in animals. With few exceptions, attempts to apply these principles directly to clinical practice so far have not been very successful. Nevertheless, utilization of cell-kinetic parameters to improve a chemotherapeutic response in patients with breast cancer has shown some interesting results. Experimental data have shown the effects of estrogens and antiestrogens on cell proliferation in cultures of human breast cancer cells[33] and the ability of estrogens to stimulate the thymidine labeling index of human breast cancer cells and thereby improve their responsiveness to anticancer drugs.[34,35] Based on these data, therapeutic trials utilizing hormonal synchronization followed by combination chemotherapy have been carried out for advanced breast cancer, with some positive results.[36,37]

The inability to achieve in humans what can be demonstrated in cell culture or animal studies is probably related to (1) the likelihood that most human solid tumors are already at the low growth fraction, plateau phase of the Gompertzian growth curve by the time they are diagnosed; (2) our lack of information on the cytokinetics of human tumors *in vivo;* (3) the importance of factors related to the general metabolic state of the patient; and (4) the apparent innate drug resistance of certain types of human tumors (e.g., adenocarcinoma of the colon).

Circadian Timing of Chemotherapy

Chronobiotic experiments in animals have shown that the time of day that anticancer drugs are administered significantly affects the antitumor response as well as host toxicity of the drugs.[38] This is apparently due to the fact that normal tissues vary in their metabolism and proliferation in a circadian way depending on the daily rhythm of hormone and growth factor release (and probably other factors), whereas tumor tissue varies less so in response to these rhythms. Thus, the susceptibility of normal tissues to the toxic effects of drugs will vary with the time of day, but the susceptibility of tumor cells will not be modulated to the same extent.

This hypothesis has been tested in animal studies and it has now been shown that, for example, the greatest toxicity of Adriamycin is late in the daily activity cycle of rodents while that of cisplatin is near awakening.[38] These results have been extrapolated to clinical trials, with promising results. In a study of 31 patients with advanced ovarian cancer, a circadian schedule infusing Adriamycin in the morning (6:00 to 6:30 A.M.) followed 12 hours later (6:00 P.M. to 6:30 P.M.) by cisplatin caused significantly less toxicity and dosage reductions than when the drugs were given in the reverse order.[38] In another clinical study, the incidence of distal paresthesias and emesis was significantly lower for the platinum analog oxaliplatin when it was given by infusion every 16 hours than when the drug was administered by continuous venous infusion.[39] These clinical investigations support the concept that cell kinetic parameters, as influenced by internal circadian rhythms, are important considerations for designing clinically effective therapeutic regimens.

Host Determinants

General Status of the Patient

Several determinants of the chemotherapeutic response are intrinsic to the host rather than to the tumor cell. One important determinant relates to the general status of patients and their ability to tolerate the cytotoxic effects of the drugs. From the patient's point of view, the important questions are: Will the treatment prolong the period of useful life? Will the quality of that life be acceptable? Will I be able to work, to care for myself, to be in less pain? Unless the answer to at least one of these questions is "yes," drug therapy is not worth very much to the individual cancer patient.

All cancer chemotherapeutic drugs have side effects that must be considered in planning the treatment regimen. During treatment, patients may become nauseated, and with some drugs vomiting is common. With aggressive, highly toxic drug regimens, the patient's mouth may become sore and ulcerated, hair may fall out, infections may occur, or a bleeding tendency may develop. Although many side effects can be minimized with carefully conducted therapeutic regimens, toxic effects like these clearly impose limitations on the use of some drugs, particularly in debilitated patients who tend to have a lower response rate and who tolerate such drugs poorly.

A set of "performance status" criteria established by Karnofsky summarizes the degree to which a patient is compromised. These criteria are useful in evaluating whether or not the disease is progressing both during and after therapy (Table 3–7). If one employs these criteria and conducts examinations for the objective signs of tumor regression (e.g., decrease in

Table 3–7   *Performance Status of Patients With Neoplastic Diseases.* (Adapted from Karnofsky[40])

Definition	Percent	Criteria
Able to carry on normal activity and to work; no special care need	100	Normal; no complaints; no evidence of disease
	90	Able to carry on normal activity; minor signs or symptoms of disease
	80	Normal activity with effort; some signs or symptoms of disease
Unable to work; able to live at home and care for most personal needs; a varying amount of assistance needed	70	Cares for self; unable to carry on normal activity or to do active work
	60	Requires occasional assistance; able to care for most needs
	50	Requires considerable assistance and frequent medical care
Unable to care for self; requires equivalent of institutional or hospital care; disease may be progressing rapidly	40	Disabled; requires special care and assistance
	30	Severely disabled; hospitalization is indicated although death not imminent
	20	Very sick; hospitalization necessary; active supportive treatment necessary
	10	Moribund; fatal processes progressing rapidly

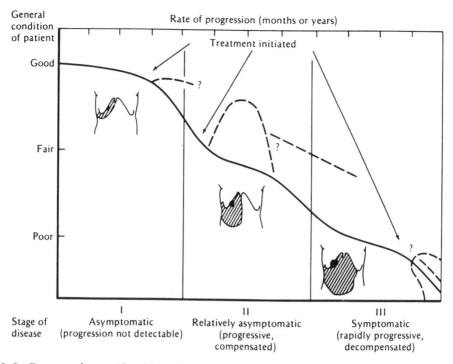

General
condition
of patient

Rate of progression (months or years)

Treatment initiated

Good

Fair

Poor

?

?

?

I	II	III
Stage of	Asymptomatic	Relatively asymptomatic	Symptomatic
disease	(progression not detectable)	(progressive,	(rapidly progressive,
		compensated)	decompensated)

Figure 3–8 Factors to be considered in evaluating the response to an anticancer drug are illustrated by the generalized case of a patient with carcinoma of the colon, with metastases to the liver. *Response evaluation:* This is based on the stage of the disease; survival time; objective and subjective benefits; performance; duration of benefit; and drug toxicity, morbidity, and mortality. The *solid line* traces the natural history of the disease as the patient progresses through the three stages. *Stage I:* The patient is relatively asymptomatic, progression of the disease is not detectable, and control of the disease for an extended period of time would be evidence of benefit from chemotherapy. *Stage II:* The disease is progressive, but the patient is compensated in that he can maintain almost normal activity. A favorable therapeutic response in stage II may represent a temporary suppression of the disease, a significant interruption in its progression, or possibly, even prolonged control. *Stage III:* The disease is symptomatic and rapidly progressive. The liver is the principal site of metastasis in this patient and he progresses to the end stage, with hepatic insufficiency as a likely cause of death. Treatment in stage III may have no effect on the disease, it may prolong life, or it may shorten life because such a seriously debilitated patient may not be able to tolerate therapy with toxic drugs. (From Karnotsky.[41])

tumor size seen on CT scan or X ray; decrease in palpable size of the involved organs, like the spleen; decrease in the number of leukemic blast cells in the bone marrow), the patient's overall clinical response to therapy can be more accurately evaluated. In general, if a patient's performance status is below 40%, it is less that his or her clinical condition can be markedly improved. A generalized example of this type of assessment is given in Figure 3–8. Clearly, the best way to increase survival time is to begin treatment early. By the time the patient's status is poor, chemotherapy may have only a short-range palliative effect. At that point, the clinical decision for or against the initiation of

chemotherapy may be a very difficult one to make, and its possible value to the patient must be weighed against the side effects of the drugs used.

Immunocompetence of the Patient

In addition to the ability of the patient to withstand the cytotoxic effects of the anticancer drugs and the ability of the tissues to recover from these effects, another determinant of the response to chemotherapy is the patient's immune status. Components of the immune system that appear to play a role in the destruction of tumor cells are illustrated in Figure 3–

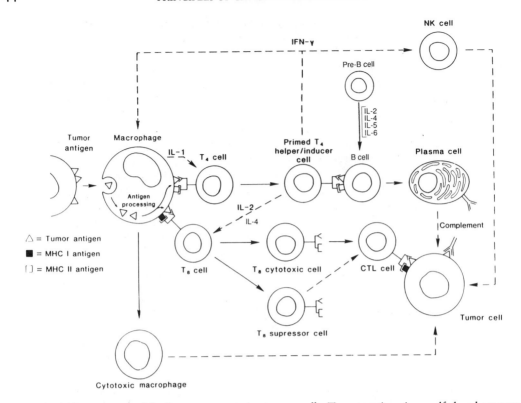

Figure 3–9 Components of the immune response to tumor cells. Tumor antigen is engulfed and processed by macrophages, which, in association with MHC antigen, "present" the foreign antigen to preeffector $T_{helper/inducer}$ and $T_{cytotoxic/suppressor}$ cells. Macrophages also release interleuekin-1 (IL-1), which plays a role in T-cell activation. $T_{helper/inducer}$ cells bear a cell surface antigen, called T4 (CD4), and cytotoxic/suppressor cells bear a T8 (CD8) marker. Activated T4 cells release various lymphokines, including interleukins 2, 4, 5, and 6, which stimulate proliferation and foster activation of T8 cells and which stimulate proliferation and differentiation of B cells into antibody-producing plasma cells. Activated T cells also produce γ-interferon (IFN-γ), which fosters activation of natural killer (NK) cells and macrophages. A subpopulation of T8 cells become suppressor cells, which moderate and dampen the immune reaction. The action of cytolytic lymphocytes (CTL cells) requires recognition of tumor antigen in association with MHC antigen on tumor cells. Activated NK cells appear to be able to kill tumor cells without such MHC restriction. Production of antitumor antibodies is important in two ways: 1) for antibody-dependent, complement-mediated tumor cell killing and 2) for tumor-cell killing by macrophages and lymphocytes of antibody-coated tumor cells, so-called antibody-dependent cellular cytotoxicity (ADCC) reactions. The dotted lines in the figure represent cell–cell interactions, sometimes mediated by secreted factors; solid lines represent proliferation and/or conversion of one cell type into another.

9. The nature of the interaction between the cells of the immune system is complex, but most investigators in tumor immunology would agree that cell-mediated immunity (i.e., the effects initiated by activated macrophages and T lymphocytes) is the most important factor in the immune response to malignant cells. Figure 3-9 presents a scheme of the immune response system to malignant tumor cells. This is a complex system in which both direct cell-ular interactions and humoral factors play a role.[42–47] Our knowledge of this system is continually evolving, and representations like those shown in Figure 3–9 are, at best, oversimplifications. The immune response has several components. These can be described as follows:

1. Macrophage/monocyte system. Circulating phagocytic monocytes and their counterparts in tissue, the macrophages, are the primary responding cell type in the immune system. These cells can bind and internalize antigenic substances present in their environment. The internalized antigens are processed by a mechanism that involves antigen degradation by lysosomal proteases. The processed antigenic peptides are then returned to the cell surface in association with cell surface recognition markers of the major histocompatability (MHC) system. Processed antigen, in conjunction with the MHC marker, is required for activation of T lymphocytes of both the T-helper/inducer type and the T-cytotoxic/suppressor type. In the case of the former, the recognition signal involves MHC class II antigens; in the latter, it involves MHC class I antigens. Activated macrophages also secrete lymphokines such as interleukin-1 (IL-1), which is involved in the activation and proliferation of T lymphocytes.

Macrophages also become active cytotoxic cells by contact with tumor antigen and by the stimulatory effects of γ-interferon (IFN-γ), produced by already activated macrophages and by activated T lymphocytes. Thus, there is an amplification effect moderated by the soluble mediators released by cell types involved in the immune reaction. Cytotoxic macrophages can attack and lyse tumor cells directly.

2. T lymphocytes. The lymphocytic stem cell produced in the bone marrow has two pathways of differentiation. One pathway requires the thymus gland and leads to the generation of cells called thymus-dependent (or T) lymphocytes, which are involved in cell-mediated or delayed immune reactions. Precursor T cells (prothymocytes) migrate to the thymus gland, where they are processed into functionally competent cells and are then released into the circulation, from which they populate the peripheral lymphoid tissue. The second pathway produces "bursal-equivalent" (or B) lymphocytes. The term "bursal equivalent" derives from the fact that this class of cells was first clearly delineated in chickens that have a distinct bursa in which these cells are produced. In higher animals and humans, the equivalent B-lymphocyte-producing tissues appear to be the lymph tissue of the gastrointestinal tract and certain areas of the spleen. Both T and B lymphocytes are present in lymph nodes and spleen, although their relative concentrations vary within these organs. Both types of cells circulate in the blood, but about 70% of circulating lymphocytes are T cells.

A number of subpopulations of human T cells have been defined on a functional basis and on the basis of their cell surface marker antigens.[48] One of these cell populations carries a distinct surface marker called T4 (or CD4). These $T4^+$ cells constitute about 55–65% of peripheral T cells and are the $T_{helper/inducer}$ cells of the immune response system. These cells can respond directly to antigen (although interaction with macrophages is usually involved in the response, as indicated before) or to such lectins as Con A or phytohemagglutinin by undergoing a burst of cell proliferation. These cells provide helper function to other T cells, to B lymphocytes, and to macrophages mediated at least in part by the release of various lymphokines. The $T_{helper/inducer}$ cells do not themselves have a cytolytic effector function, but they play a role in stimulating the generation of cytolytic T cells, which bear a surface marker called T8 (CD8) and can kill tumor cells by mechanisms similar to those for macrophages. It is these $T4^+$ helper/inducer cells that are the target for the AIDS virus, and their loss, as observed in this disease, is devastating to the immune system.

$T_{suppressor}$ cells also have the T8 surface marker. These cells suppress the proliferative response of T cells to alloantigens and the production of immunoglobulin by B lymphocytes, possibly by the release of suppressor factor. Normally, these cells function to modulate the immune response system and prevent overresponse to an antigenic stimulus. However, excessive $T_{suppressor}$ cell activity can produce generalized immunosuppression and decrease the immune response to a number of foreign antigens, including those present on tumor cells. On the other hand, a loss of $T_{suppressor}$ cells has been observed in cases of excessive immune response such as occurs in certain autoimmune diseases, including systemic lupus erythematosus, hemolytic anemia, and inflammatory bowel disease. Thus, the balance of T_{helper} and $T_{suppressor}$ activities regulates the immune response and determines the outcome of antigenic stimulation of the host.

3. B lymphocytes. The B cells also originate in the bone marrow, but mature differently from T cells. They are the precursors of antibody-forming plasma cells. When B cells are stimulated by antigen either directly (a few antigens do not require interaction with T_{helper} cells to elicit antibody formation) or indirectly by T-cell interactions, B cells specifically activated by the antigenic stimulus proliferate and differentiate into immunoglobulin-producing plasma cells.

Activated T_{helper} cells interact with antigen-stimulated B cells in a manner analogous to that of T cell–macrophage interactions. Antigen, processed by B cells and presented on the cell surface together with MHC class II antigens, interacts with receptors on T cells. Contact with $T4^+$ helper cells stimulates B cells to mature, multiply, and differentiate into antibody-secreting plasma cells as well as into a clone of memory B-cells. Lymphokines secreted by $T4^+$ cells aid in this maturation process. A number of lymphokines appear to be involved here, including interleukins IL-2, IL-4, IL-5, and IL-6.

Initially, the activated B cell looks like a primitive blast cell and produces mainly IgM-type immunoglobulin. As it matures to a plasma cell, it produces mainly IgG-type immunoglobulin. Antibody directed against the tumor antigen is released from the expanded clone of plasma cells that are specifically producing it. These antibodies can induce tumor cell killing by means of antibody-mediated, complement-dependent cell lysis. This mechanism of cell killing, however, appears to play a minor role in the immune reaction against cancer. A more active cytotoxic reaction in which antibodies participate is the so-called antibody-dependent, cell-mediated cytotoxicity (ADCC) reaction. Antibody released by plasma cells adheres to antigens on the tumor cell surface, and this attracts cells that have receptors for the Fc portion of IgG. Cells with such Fc receptors on their surface include macrophages, T lymphocytes, and natural killer cells. This mechanism for cell killing is in addition to the direct killing effect of cytolytic T cells. Soluble antitumor antibodies or antigen-antibody complexes, when present in high concentrations, may actually block cell-mediated cytotoxicity by binding recognition sites on cytotoxic cells.

4. *Natural killer cells.* In animals and humans, another population of cells is cytotoxic for tumor cells. These cells appear to belong to the lymphocyte class, but they lack surface markers that clearly place them in a specific category. They are nonphagocytic and nonadherent, they appear to possess Fc receptors after activation, and they have a low density of certain T-cell markers. Thus, these cells are thought to be derived from clones of immature pre-T lymphocytes. Their ability to kill tumor cells does not depend on prior immunization of the host and does not appear to depend on the generation of antitumor antibodies; hence, these cells have been called natural killer (NK) cells.[49] They will kill tumor cells from both syngeneic and heterologous animal species and, in this respect, are rather indiscriminate killer cells. In some animal systems, populations of NK cells have been shown to recognize certain tumor antigens and to have cytotoxic activity against heterologous normal thymus cells, macrophages, and bone marrow cells.[50] It has been postulated that NK cells can recognize several different types of specificities on cells that may have some cross-reactive antigenic determinants. This could explain the broad cytotoxic specificity that NK cells possess. It is of interest that NK cells are stimulated to become active killer cells by IFN-γ, which is released by T cells as well as activated NK cells. The latter mechanism would provide a positive feedback system even in animals lacking a functional thymus gland (e.g., nude mice). The stimulation of NK cells may partly explain the antitumor activity of interferon when injected into animals or cancer patients.

The function of the immune system is clearly important for the patient to have a long-term remission following cancer chemotherapy. A number of studies have shown that patients with any one of a number of neoplasms are less responsive to chemotherapy if tests of their cell-mediated immune function show a decreased responsiveness. For example, patients with acute leukemia who are immunocompetent at the start of chemotherapy and those who convert from immunoincompetence to immunocompetence during therapy are more likely to achieve remissions than those who are immunoincompetent before treatment or convert to that status during therapy.[51,52] The determination of immune status is complicated by (1) the progression of the neoplastic disease process that itself produces immunological deficiency and (2) the immunosuppressive effects of many anticancer drugs. It has been found, however, that intensive intermittent chemotherapy, with a dosage regimen that allows the patient's immune system to recover, may permit the maintenance of immunocompetence between courses of treatment.

Site and Blood Supply of the Neoplasm

If any drug is to be effective, it must be present in sufficient concentration at the site of its action. In cancer chemotherapy, this means that tumor cells, even if they are very sensitive to the administered drug, cannot be destroyed unless they have a good blood supply. Failure of drug therapy may occur when tumors metastasize into the pleural space or the central nervous system. The choroid plexus prevents the attainment of cytotoxic concentrations of many drugs in the cerebrospinal fluid. When tumor cells infiltrate into the central nervous system in leukemia patients, for example, drugs may not reach them in high enough concentration to be effective. For this reason, the "remission maintenance" phase of antileukemic drug therapy now frequently includes the use of intrathecal methotrexate, as noted above.

In addition to the problem of drug delivery to tumors in pharmacologic "sanctuaries," the local determinants of blood flow to a given solid tumor must be considered. A tumor has two types of blood vessels: those recruited from the host's own capillary network by the release of angiogenic factors, and those derived from the preexisting host's vasculature to the tissue in which the tumor arises. Because this "neovascularization" of tumors is not normal, tumor blood vessels may respond differently to neurogenic stimuli and to vasoconstricting or vasodilating drugs, as compared to normal tissue vasculature.[53] In addition, there are variations in hydrostatic pressure in various areas of a tumor. Thus, the heterogeneity in tumor microcirculation within a tumor and from tumor to tumor make it difficult to predict how solid tumors, particularly large tumors with a poorly vascularized necrotic core, will respond to drugs.

Another consideration relating to tumor hemodynamic factors is how immune cells and large molecules—e.g., antitumor antibodies or polypeptides such as tumor necrosis factor—can effectively penetrate a tumor. This becomes important for some of the new strategies for chemotherapy—e.g., drug (or radionuclide) antitumor antibody complexes, biological response modifiers, LAK and TIL cell therapy, gene therapy, and so on (see Chapter 14).

The physiologic factors that contribute to impaired delivery of immune cells and macromolecules to tumor cells include heterogeneous blood supply, elevated interstitial pressure, fluid effusion from the tumor periphery, and large diffusion distances in a big tumor mass.[54]

Several strategies may be thought of to improve pharmacologic delivery of agents to solid tumors, including local heating or vasoactive drugs to improve tumor blood flow, lowering tumor interstitial pressure by shrinking a tumor mass with irradiation, and increasing tumor permeability with lytic enzymes such as hyaluronidase.[54] These approaches remain to be tested in a definitive way in patients.

REFERENCES

1. G. B. Pierce: Differentiation of normal and malignant cells. Fed. Proc. 29:1248 (1970).
2. J. H. Weisberger: "Chemical carcinogenesis," in Cancer Medicine, ed. by J. F. Holland and E. Frei III. Philadelphia: Lea and Febiger, 1973, pp. 45–90.
3. C. G. Zubrod: Chemical control of cancer. Proc. Natl. Acad. Sci. USA 69:1042 (1972).
4. J. Folkman: The vascularization of tumors. Scientific American 234:58 (1976).
5. J. Folkman: What is the evidence that tumors are angiogenesis dependent? J. Natl. Cancer Inst. 82:4 (1990).
6. G. G. Steel: "Cytokinetics of neoplasia," in Cancer Medicine, ed. by J. F. Holland and E. Frei III. Philadelphia: Lea and Febiger, 1973, pp. 125–140.
7. F. M. Schabel, Jr.: The use of tumor growth kinetics in planning "curative" chemotherapy of advanced solid tumors. Cancer Res. 29:2384 (1969).
8. H. E. Skipper, F. M. Schabel, Jr., and W. S. Wilcox: Experimental evaluation of potential anticancer agents. XIII. On the criteria and kinetics associated with "curability" of experimental leukemia. Cancer Chemother. Rept. 35:1 (1964).
9. L. Simpson-Herren, A. H. Sanford, and J. P. Holmquist: Cell population kinetics of transplanted and metastatic Lewis lung carcinoma. Cell Tissue Kinet. 7:349 (1974).
10. E. Frei III: Combination cancer chemotherapy: Presidential address. Cancer Res. 32:2593 (1972).

11. E. Frei III: Curative cancer chemotherapy. *Cancer Res.* 45:6523 (1985).

12. A. Goldin, J. M. Venditti, S. B. Humphreys, and N. Mantel: Modification of treatment schedules in the management of advanced mouse leukemia with amethopterin. *J. Natl. Cancer Inst.* 17:293 (1956).

13. O. S. Selawry, J. Hananian, I. J. Wolman, *et al.*: New treatment schedules with improved survival in childhood leukemia. Intermittent parenteral vs. daily oral administration of methotrexate for maintenance of induced remission. Acute leukemia group B. *J. Am. Med. Assoc.* 194:75 (1965).

14. V. T. DeVita, A. A. Serpick, and P. Carbone: Combination chemotherapy in the treatment of Hodgkin's disease. *Ann. Intern. Med.* 73:881 (1970).

15. D. P. Burkitt: Long-term remissions following one and two dose chemotherapy for African lymphoma. *Cancer* (Phila.) 20:756 (1967).

16. J. L. Ziegler: Burkitt's lymphoma. *New Engl. J. Med.* 305:735 (1981).

17. M. C. Li, R. Hertz, and D. B. Spencer: Effect of methotrexate upon choriocarcinoma and chorioadenoma. *Proc. Soc. Exp. Biol. Med.* 93:361 (1956).

18. P. J. Loehrer, Sr., S. D. Williams, and L. H. Einhorn: Testicular cancer: The quest continues. *J. Natl. Cancer Inst.* 80:1373 (1988).

19. P. J. Fialkow: The origin and development of human tumors studied with cell markers. *New Engl. J. Med.* 291:26 (1974).

20. P. C. Nowell: The clonal evolution of tumor cell populations. *Science* 194:23 (1976).

21. S. B. Baylin, S. H. Hsu, D. S. Gann, R. C. Smallridge, and S. A. Well, Jr.: Inherited medullary thyroid carcinoma: A final monoclonal mutation in one of multiple clones of susceptible cells. *Science* 199:429 (1978).

22. J. E. Talmadge, K. Benedict, J. Madsen, and I. J. Fidler: Development of biological diversity and susceptibility to chemotherapy in murine cancer metastases. *Cancer Res.* 44:3801 (1984).

23. G. Poste, J. Tzeng, J. Doll, R. Greig, D. Rieman, and I. Zeidman: Evolution of tumor cell heterogeneity during progressive growth of individual lung metastases. *Proc. Natl. Acad. Sci. USA* 79:6574 (1982).

24. T. Tsuruo and I. J. Fidler: Differences in drug sensitivity among tumor cells from parental tumors, selected variants, and spontaneous metastases. *Cancer Res.* 41:3058 (1981).

25. N. Tanigawa, Y. Mizuno, T. Hashimura, K. Honda, K. Satomura, Y. Hikasa, O. Niwa, T. Sugahara, O. Yoshida, D. H. Kern, and D. L. Morton: Comparison of drug sensitivity among tumor cells within a tumor, between primary tumor and metastases, and between different metastases in the human tumor colony-forming assay. *Cancer Res.* 44:2309 (1984).

26. G. H. Heppner: Tumor heterogeneity. *Cancer Res.* 44:2259 (1984).

27. F. Valeriote and L. van Putten: Proliferation dependent cytotoxicity of anticancer agents: A review. *Cancer Res.* 35:2619 (1975).

28. W. R. Bruce, B. E. Meeker, and F. A. Valeriote: Comparison of the sensitivity of normal hematopoietic and transplanted lymphoma colony-forming cells to chemotherapeutic agents administered in vitro. *J. Natl. Cancer Inst.* 37:233 (1966).

29. S. Vadlamudi and A. Goldin: Influence of mitotic cycle inhibitors on the antileukemic activity of cytosine arabinoside (NSC-63878) in mice bearing leukemia L1210. *Cancer Chemother. Rept.* 55:547 (1971).

30. H. E. Skipper: Cancer chemotherapy is many things: G. H. A. Clowes Memorial Lecture. *Cancer Res.* 31:1173 (1971).

31. E. Frei III: "Effect of dose and schedule on response," in *Cancer Medicine*, ed. by J. F. Holland and E. Frei III. Philadelphia: Lea and Febiger, 1973, pp. 717–730.

32. H. E. Skipper: The effects of chemotherapy on the kinetics of leukemic cell behavior. *Cancer Res.* 25:1544 (1965).

33. M. Lippman, G. Bolan, and A. A. Huff: The effects of estrogens and antiestrogens on hormone-responsive human breast cancer in long-term tissue culture. *Cancer Res.* 36:4595 (1976).

34. P. F. Conte, G. Fraschini, A. Alama, A. Nicolin, E. Corsaro, G. Canavese, R. Rosso, and B. Drewinko: Chemotherapy following estrogen-induced expansion of the growth fraction of human breast cancer. *Cancer Res.* 45:5926 (1985).

35. V. Hug, D. Johnston, M. Finders, and G. Hortobagyi: Use of growth-stimulatory hormones to improve the in vitro therapeutic index of doxorubicin for human breast tumors. *Cancer Res.* 46:147 (1986).

36. M. D. Lippman, J. Cassidy, M. Wesley, and R. C. Young: A randomized attempt to increase efficacy of cytotoxic chemotherapy in metastatic breast cancer by hormonal synchronization. *J. Clin. Oncol.* 2:28 (1984).

37. J. C. Allegra: Methotrexate and 5-fluorouracil following tamoxifen and premarin in advanced breast cancer. *Semin. Oncol. (Suppl. 2),* 10:23 (1983).

38. W. J. M. Hrushesky: Circadian timing of cancer chemotherapy. *Science* 228:73 (1985).

39. J.-P. Caussanel, F. Levin, S. Brienza, J.-L. Misset, M. Itzhaki, R. Adam, G. Milano, B. Hecquet, G. Mathe: Phase I trial of 5-day continuous venous infusion of oxaliplatin at circadian rhythm-modulated rate compared with constant rate. *J. Natl. Cancer Inst.* 82:1046 (1990).

40. D. A. Karnofsky, W. H. Abelmann, L. F. Craver, and J. H. Burchenal: The use of the nitrogen mustards in the palliative treatment of carcinoma. With particular reference to bronchogenic carcinoma. *Cancer* 1:634 (1948).

41. D. A. Karnofsky: Problems and pitfalls in the evaluation of anticancer drugs. *Cancer* 18:1517 (1965).

42. V. V. Likhite: "On the frontiers of immunology," in *The Handbook of Cancer Immunology*, Vol. 1, ed. by H. Waters. New York: Garland STPM Press, 1978, pp. 1–36.

43. P. Perlmann: "Cellular immunity: Antibody-dependent cytotoxicity (K-cell activity)," in *Clinical Immunology*, ed. by F. H. Bach and R. A. Good. New York: Academic Press, 1976, pp. 107–132.

44. G. Klein: Immune and non-immune control of neoplastic development: Contrasting effects of host and tumor evolution. *Cancer* 45:2486 (1980).

45. F. Melchers and J. Andersson: B cell activation: Three steps and their variations. *Cell* 37:715 (1984).

46. J. Laurence: The immune system in AIDS. *Sci. Am.* 253:84 (1985).

47. R. S. Goodenow, J. M. Vogel, and R. L. Linsk: Histocompatibility antigens on murine tumors. *Science* 230:777 (1985).

48. E. L. Reinherz and S. F. Schlossman: The differentiation and function of human T lymphocytes. *Cell 19:*821 (1980).

49. R. B. Herberman and H. T. Holden: Natural cell-mediated immunity. *Adv. Cancer Res. 27:*305 (1978).

50. M. E. Nunn and R. B. Herberman: Natural cytotoxicity of mouse, rat, and human lymphocytes against heterologous target cells. *J. Natl. Cancer Inst. 62:*765 (1979).

51. E. M. Hersh, J. P. Whitecar, K. B. McCredie, G. P. Bodey, and E. J. Freireich: Chemotherapy, immunocompetence, immunosuppression and prognosis in acute leukemia. *New Engl. J. Med. 285:*1211 (1971).

52. A. R. Cheema and E. M. Hersh: Patient survival after chemotherapy and its relationship to in vitro lymphocyte blastogenesis. *Cancer 28:*851 (1971).

53. R. K. Jain: Determinants of tumor blood flow: A review. *Cancer Res. 48:*2641 (1988).

54. R. K. Jain: Delivery of novel therapeutics agents in tumors: physiological barriers and strategies. *J. Natl. Cancer Inst. 81:*570 (1989).

Resistance to Anticancer Drugs

Intrinsic versus Acquired Drug Resistance

Drug resistance[1-3] is best defined as a state of insensitivity or decreased sensitivity of a population of neoplastic cells to drugs that ordinarily cause cell death. Resistance can be *intrinsic* or *acquired*. A population of cancer cells is said to be intrinsically resistant if it does not respond to initial therapy with a drug or a combination of drugs. In previous chapters we have seen that certain tumors of gestational, embryonal, or lymphocytic cell origin are particularly susceptible to initial treatment with anticancer drugs and chemotherapy may be curative in a relatively high percentage of patients with these tumors (Table 4–1). In contrast to these highly responsive tumors, some tumors are intrinsically resistant to a variety of anticancer drugs and only minimal response or no response is seen with chemotherapy. In most cases the basis for the intrinsic resistance is undefined and probably involves a combination of kinetic factors, such as a low growth fraction as discussed in Chapter 3, and intrinsic biochemical factors, such as a poor ability to transport the drug into the cell or to convert the drug to its active form. Also, as discussed in Chapter 3, cancer cells within the same tumor may be either resistant or responsive to chemotherapy, depending on their location in large solid tumor masses. On the periphery of the tumor, where nutrient and oxygen supply are optimal, rapidly dividing cells may proliferate rapidly and be very responsive to killing by anticancer drugs. In contrast, the cells in the core of the tumor may be largely in the resting, or G_0, phase of growth and thus intrinsically resistant to treatment with anticancer drugs.

In the case of acquired drug resistance, a population of cancer cells that is initially sensitive to the drug undergoes a change in the direction of insensitivity.[2,3] Typically, there is a decrease in tumor mass when drug treatment begins, but eventually tumor growth resumes despite continued treatment with the same anticancer drug. When a cell is partially or completely resistant to an anticancer drug, it is more likely to survive in a drug-containing environment where the drug-sensitive cells are killed. This enrichment of resistant cells in a tumor cell population is called *selection* and the anticancer drug is considered to exert a *selective pressure* that by killing sensitive cells favors the growth of resistant cells.

Although there is good evidence that most tumors develop by expansion from a single clone of cells,[4] it is clear that as a tumor's growth continues, its cells develop differences that can be detected morphologically or by biochemical assays.[5] These cell differences result from mutations that occur at an expected background rate during tumor growth. Some of the biochemical changes that occur in such a spontaneous manner confer drug resistance. The genetic changes that lead to drug resistance occur at a rate of one per every 10^5 to 10^6 cancer cell divisions.[6,7] Thus, by the time a tumor has achieved the size where it is clinically detectable and drug therapy is initiated, it

Table 4–1   *Responsiveness of Tumors to Chemotherapy.* In many of the diseases listed below, treatment routinely includes surgery or both, in addition to chemotherapy.

Group	Responsiveness to Chemotherapy	Neoplastic Disease	Type of Drug Regimen
A	Highly responsive—very sensitive to drugs with good evidence for drug-induced cures (a high percentage of responders achieve normal life expectancy)	Gestational choriocarcinoma Burkitt's lymphoma Hodgkin's disease Wilms' tumor Embryonal rhabdomyosarcoma	Single drug Single drug Combination Combination Combination
B	Responsive—50% or greater response rate (responders definitely have prolonged survival and some patients may achieve normal life expectancy from a combination of drugs and other treatment modalities)	Acute leukemia in children Histiocytic lymphoma Ewing's sarcoma Retinoblastoma Testicular cancer Lymphocytic lymphomas Osteogenic sarcoma	Combination Combination Combination Single drug Combination Combination Single drug
C	Moderately responsive—clinical response is often obtained (responders have increased survival)	Adult acute leukemias Multiple myeloma Breast carcinoma Neuroblastoma Carcinoma of the prostate Endometrial carcinoma Carcinoma of the ovary Lung cancer (small cell, undifferentiated)	Combination Combination Combination Combination Single drug Single drug Single drug Combination
D	Partially responsive—tumor regression observed with chemotherapy in 20% or more of the cases, but complete remission is rare or nonexistent (minimal or no prolongation of survival)	Glioblastoma Adrenocortical carcinoma Pancreatic islet cell carcinoma Colorectal cancer Head and neck cancer	
E	Minimally responsive—objective response observed in fewer than 20% of cases; if there is an effect, it is palliative (no demonstrable prolongation of survival)	Hepatocellular carcinoma Bladder carcinoma Esophageal carcinoma Lung carcinoma (non-small cell) Pancreatic adenocarcinoma Melanoma	Therapeutic protocols are constantly changing as new drugs and drug combinations are evaluated

is a mixed population containing both drug-sensitive cells and drug-resistant cells. The killing of the sensitive cells is accompanied by an initially favorable clinical response, but in subsequent courses of treatment, progressively higher proportions of resistant cells are present in the tumor and the response obtained with the same drug decreases with each course of therapy. It is generally considered that *acquired drug resistance is the most common reason for the failure of drug treatment in cancer patients with initially sensitive tumors.*[8]

When cells acquire the property of drug resistance, they undergo a heritable change. This change in the genetic composition of the tumor cell can occur in two ways:

1. The tumor cell may undergo a *mutation* in the DNA, such as a base deletion, addition, or change (transition or transversion). The mutant protein may be deficient in its ability to interact with the drug directly or to perform some function required for the drug effect. Resistance due to mutation can be readily demonstrated in tumor cells growing *in vitro* and in animal tumor models. Although it stands to reason that mutation accounts for a significant portion of the anticancer drug resistance encountered clinically, it has not been possible to prove a mutational origin of resistance in cancer patients.

2. The tumor cell may undergo *gene amplification*. In this case the gene for a normal protein becomes multiplied. Cells containing more copies of the gene synthesize more of the protein, and they are able to survive in the presence of drug concentrations that would normally be lethal. There is good evidence that gene amplification occurs in the tumors of patients undergoing treatment with anticancer drugs, and gene amplification is likely responsible for a significant percentage of the acquired drug resistance encountered during chemotherapy.

Resistance via Mutation

It is clear from fluctuation tests and other methods that mutations conferring drug resistance occur in tumor cells independent of the presence of an anticancer drug. Thus, in the case of resistance arising via mutation, the only role played by the drug is to provide a selective pressure in favor of the resistant cell by killing the sensitive cells. Many of the anticancer drugs are mutagenic and thus increase the probabilities of many kinds of mutations in a nonspecific manner, but no example is known of a drug that specifically increases the mutation rate at a particular gene locus determining resistance to itself.

It has been shown with cancer cells growing *in vitro* and in animal tumor models that populations of cancer cells become resistant in stepwise fashion. Thus, all of the sensitive cells are not killed during the first course of therapy,

leaving a homogeneously resistant population that does not respond at all to a second course of therapy. Some of the sensitive cells may not be in the growth phases that are optimum for a drug's action during the time that it is present in killing concentrations. Also, because of differences in drug distribution in different regions of a tumor, some of the sensitive cells may not be exposed to killing concentrations of drug. Thus, in addition to a few resistant cells with a high level of resistance, some sensitive cells and cells with low levels of resistance may survive the first course of therapy. As the tumor regrows, the percentage of resistant and partially resistant cells will be higher than it was before each course of therapy, so that there is a progressively diminishing response to the drug.

There is a principle of chemotherapy that issues from this stepwise pattern of resistance development. That is, the higher the concentration of cancer drug that can be achieved within the tumor, the greater the number of sensitive and low-level resistant cells that will be killed. The direct relationship between dose intensity and effectiveness of anticancer drug treatment has been demonstrated in the laboratory.[9] However, to avoid undesirable levels of toxicity, clinicians may wish to use much lower doses than those that can be maximally achieved in the patient. The lower the dosage that is employed, the more cells with intermediate levels of resistance will survive to repopulate the tumor mass and the less effective therapy will be. The relationship between dose intensity and clinical response has been demonstrated in the clinical treatment of a variety of tumors.[10,11]

Combination Chemotherapy

Another principle that emerged from a consideration of the mutational origin of resistance is that of using drug combinations in tumor treatment.[12] The probability of selecting tumor cells that are resistant to therapy is less if two drugs with different mechanisms of action and different biochemical mechanisms of resistance are administered together in combination chemotherapy. When drug combinations were first used to treat cancer, it was thought that all anticancer drug resistance was due to mutation. At that time, it was also not appreciated, as it is now, that some mechanisms of resistance can result in cross-resistance between drugs that are very different in their structures and biochemical mechanisms of action. It was reasoned that if a cell mutates to resistance to one drug at a rate of 10^{-6} and to another drug at a rate of 10^{-6}, then the probability is very small (10^{-12}) that a cell would arise that is resistant to both drugs. Thus, cells resistant to the first drug would be killed by the second drug, and vice versa. Although there are other reasons for combining drugs in chemotherapy, the potential for suppression of resistance was, historically, probably the most important factor that prompted studies of the effects of drug combinations in cancer treatment.[1]

As indicated in Table 4–2, there are multiple ways in which cancer cells develop drug resistance, and a knowledge of cross-resistance patterns among different drugs and drug classes is critical in the design of combination therapeutic protocols. It stands to reason that if a tumor has been treated successfully one time with a single drug or drug combination, the second course of therapy might yield more remissions if it was composed of different drugs that were not cross-resistant with those of the first administration.[13] This procedure, called *alternating non-cross-resistant* chemotherapy, in some cases has been found to yield higher cure rates than repeated treatments with the same drug combination. For example, in one study[14] of 75 patients with advanced (stage IV) Hodgkin's

Table 4–2   Some Mechanisms of Resistance to Anticancer Drugs

Drug	Mechanisms of Resistance
Alkylating agents	Decreased drug uptake Increased DNA repair
Methotrexate	Increased dihydrofolate reductase Altered DHFR with decreased affinity for drug Decreased drug uptake Decreased polyglutamation
Thiopurines (6-MP, 6-thioguanine)	Decreased hypoxanthine-guanine phosphoribosyl transferase Increased alkaline phosphohydrolase Altered PRPP amidotransferase that is less inhibited by analog nucleotide
5-Fluorouracil	Decreased uridine kinase Decreased affinity of thymidylate synthetase for 5-fluorodeoxyuridine monophosphate, the active form of the drug Increased thymidylate synthetase
Cytosine arabinoside	Increased deoxycytidine deaminase Decreased deoxycytidine kinase
Vinca alkaloids	Increased drug efflux
Dactinomycin	Increased drug efflux
Doxorubicin, daunorubicin	Increased drug efflux Decreased daunorubicin reductase
L-asparaginase	Increased asparagine synthetic capacity Development of antibodies to enzyme
Steroid hormones	Decreased receptor Inability to translocate drug-receptor complex to the nucleus

disease, 38 patients were treated with the drug combination MOPP (mechlorethamine, vincristine (Oncovin®), procarbazine, and prednisone) on a once-monthly basis for 12 months, while 37 patients were treated with MOPP every other month and the combination ABVD (doxorubicin (adriamycin), bleomycin, vinblastine, and dacarbazine) on the alternate months. Seventy-one percent of the patients receiving MOPP alone achieved a complete remission of their disease, whereas 92% of those receiving the alternating regimen achieved complete remission. In a more advanced application of this technique, MOPP and the ABV combination are alternated on day 1 and day 8 of each 4-week therapeutic cycle to achieve the maximal kill of both sensitive and resistant cells through the early use of all of the effective drugs.[15]

The treatment of acute lymphocytic leukemia in childhood is a classic example of the value of combination chemotherapy. Initially, treatment was carried out with a single cytotoxic drug, and although remissions were often induced, subsequent courses of therapy with the same drug were progressively less effective, yielding a median survival time of about 6 months. Drug combinations were introduced and there was a marked increase in response rate, but subsequent courses of therapy with the same drug combinations were progressively less effective. As discussed in the last chapter, many factors may account for this eventual therapeutic failure. A few cancer cells, for example, may have invaded the intrathecal space, where they remain protected from most anticancer drugs that do not pass across the choroid plexus into the CSF. Another factor responsible for therapeutic failure is that cells that are highly resistant to both drugs in the combination are selected during repeated courses of therapy.

Elaborate combination drug protocols have been developed to circumvent these problems in treating acute lymphocytic leukemia. A combination of two drugs (often vincristine and prednisone) is administered for a short period to induce remission of the disease. This is followed by long-term treatment with another combination of drugs (e.g., methotrexate and mercaptopurine) with mechanisms of action and resistance that are different from the drugs used to induce remission. This is the so-called maintenance phase of therapy. During this time, the patient also receives a course of intrathecal methotrexate and/or a course of radiotherapy to the head in order to kill cancer cells that have invaded the central nervous system. Because different drugs are employed in maintenance therapy, there is ideally no selective advantage to cells containing mutations that made them resistant to one or both of the drugs used to induce remission. Thus, in the event of a renewal of the disease the induction drugs may be effective at inducing subsequent remissions. This combination chemotherapy approach has been so effective in the treatment of acute lymphocytic leukemia in children that a majority of patients may now expect a complete cure.

Resistance via Gene Amplification

If a drug acts as an inhibitor of an enzyme, then overproduction of the enzyme target may permit the cell to survive in the presence of normally cytotoxic concentrations of drug. Such high levels of enzyme can result from the selection of cells that have undergone spontaneous amplification for the gene encoding the normal wild-type enzyme. Resistance to several clinically useful anticancer drugs has been shown to occur via gene amplification in cultured cells. The example that has been described in greatest detail is the resistance to methotrexate that results from amplification of the gene for dihydrofolate reductase.[16] The pyrimidine analog 5-fluorouracil inhibits thymidylate synthetase, and in cells where that is the primary cytotoxic effect, resistance can arise due to amplification of the thymidylate synthetase gene.[17] Hydroxyurea is an effective antileukemia drug because it inhibits ribonucleotide reductase and resistance can result from overproduction of that enzyme. The anticancer drug PALA (N-(phosphonacetyl)-L-aspartate) is a transition-state analog inhibitor of aspartate transcarbamylase. Resistance to PALA can result from amplification of the gene for CAD (carbamyl-P synthetase, aspartate transcarbamylase, dihydroorotase), which is a multifunctional enzyme that catalyzes the first three reactions of de novo uridine monophosphate biosynthesis.[18]

Methotrexate resistance due to overproduction of dihydrofolate reductase (DHFR) serves as a good example of gene amplification that has a clear relevance to clinical drug resistance. As will be discussed in Chapter 5, methotrexate is a competitive inhibitor of DHFR. Thus, it blocks the conversion of folate to a variety of coenzymes that are required for synthesis of thymidylate, purines, methionine, and glycine, and depletion of these substrates results in inhibition of DNA, RNA, and protein synthesis. Although cultured cells become resistant to methotrexate by at least four biochemical mechanisms (Table 4–2), overproduction of DHFR is the most common mechanism. The resistant cells accumulate high enough levels of DHFR to maintain some free enzyme in the presence of drug.

DHFR Gene Amplification and Methotrexate Resistance

The murine sarcoma 180 (S-180) cell line was the primary experimental system used to demonstrate DHFR gene amplification. In 1961, Hakala and her colleagues[19] demonstrated that S-180 cells selected for resistance to methotrexate had levels of DHFR activity that increased in proportion to the degree of resistance. Fifteen years later, Schimke and his coworkers[20] demonstrated that the increased DHFR activity in the AT-3000 resistant subline of S-180

cells reflected increased levels of enzyme-protein with the same kinetic and physical properties of the wild-type DHFR, and that the increased level of enzyme was due to an increased rate of enzyme synthesis in the resistant cells. The extent of enzyme overproduction can be impressive. It was shown, for example, that in some resistant cells, DHFR can account for 5% or more of the total soluble protein. A [3H] cDNA for DHFR was then used to quantitate the relative levels of DHFR mRNA sequences and gene copies in sensitive and resistant lines.[21] As illustrated in Table 4–3 the specific activity of DHFR in the highly resistant AT-3000 resistant subline was 250-fold that of the sensitive cell line, and this was accounted for by corresponding increases in the relative number of DHFR mRNA sequences and DHFR gene copies.

A second phenomenon of potential clinical importance is illustrated in Table 4–3 by the data for the partially revertant cell line Rev-400. This subline was established by growing the AT-3000 cells in the absence of methotrexate for 400 cell doublings. It is clear that in the absence of the selective pressure of the drug, the number of DHFR gene copies decreases dramatically and this is accompanied by a parallel decrease in the DHFR activity. The Rev-400 cells have reverted toward the drug-sensitive state. The implication for the clinical situation is that resistance that arises via gene am-

Table 4–3   Relative Levels of DHFR Activity, DHFR mRNA and DHFR Gene Copies in Methotrexate Sensitive S-180 Cells, a Drug-Resistant Subline, and a Revertant Subline. The specific activity of DHFR was determined by an immunologic procedure, and the number of DHFR-specific mRNA sequences and gene copies were determined by hybridization with a DHFR-specific [3H]cDNA probe. The S-3 cells are methotrexate-sensitive, the AT-3000 line is highly methotrexate-resistant, and the Rev-400 line is a partial revertant obtained by growing AT-3000 cells in the absence of methotrexate for 400 cell duplications. Each value is expressed relative to that obtained in the drug-sensitive S-3 cells. (From Alt et al.[21])

| S-180 Line | Relative DHFR | | |
	Specific Activity	mRNA Sequences	Gene Copies
S-3	1	1	1
AT-3000	250	220	180
Rev-400	10	7	10

plification during brief exposure of the patient to one treatment regimen may decrease during subsequent treatment with a second non-cross-resistant drug regimen, thus permitting the drugs in the initial treatment regimen to be used again.

The data of Table 4-3 demonstrate clearly that the overproduction of DHFR is due to the selection of cells with an increased number of DHFR genes and that the degree of resistance reflects the gene dosage. In most cases, the resistant cells produce a normal enzyme, but resistance can also reflect the amplification of a gene sequence encoding a mutant enzyme with reduced drug affinity.[22]

Amplification of DHFR genes occurs *in vitro* when the concentration of methotrexate in the medium is increased by stepwise increments. Indeed, it has been shown that amplification events themselves occur in small steps and it may not be possible to achieve a high degree of resistance via gene amplification with a single exposure to a very high concentration of methotrexate.[23] As discussed above with resistance via mutation, the fact that amplification occurs in small steps dictates that anticancer drugs should be administered at the highest possible doses in order to kill the maximum number of low-level resistant cells as possible.

The amplified genes may be located on one chromosome where they appear as regions that are expanded in length and lack the characteristic banding patterns observed in normal chromosomes after staining. These regions are called *homogeneously staining regions,* or HSRs, and they have been shown to contain multiple DHFR genes by *in situ* hybridization with cDNA probes. DHFR genes that are located in HSRs tend to be stably amplified. That is, the number of gene copies does not decline when cells are grown in the absence of drug and the degree of resistance does not decrease. Alternatively, the amplified genes may be located on extrachromosomal elements that often exist in pairs and are called *double minute chromosomes,* or DMs. Amplified DHFR genes located on DMs tend to be unstable in that they are spontaneously eliminated during mitosis when cells are grown under nonselective conditions. Thus, the resistance is unstable and reversion occurs as illustrated for the Rev-400 subline in Table 4-3. As gene amplification is often initially unstable and becomes stable

only when cells are maintained under selective conditions for a long time, prolonged exposure to a single treatment regimen should perhaps be avoided.

It seems quite clear that resistance due to amplification occurs during methotrexate therapy of cancer patients.[24] Figure 4-1 presents a metaphase chromosome plate of a tumor cell containing double minute chromosomes that was cultured from a patient with small-cell cancer of the lung who was treated with methotrexate.[25] When the cells were initially cultured, they had a high level of DHFR activity, elevated amounts of DHFR protein, and an increased number of gene copies relative to a tumor cell line isolated from a patient with small-cell lung cancer who had not been treated with methotrexate.[25] After 6 months of passage in the absence of methotrexate, the tumor cells shown in Figure 4-1 had lost their double minute chromosomes and had reverted from resistance to sensitivity to methotrexate.[25]

One interesting aspect of drug resistance arising as a result of gene amplification is that the rate of resistance development can be affected by drug treatment. As discussed above for resistance arising via mutation and selection, it has been shown that the DHFR gene undergoes spontaneous amplification in the absence of methotrexate[26] and that methotrexate then selects for the resistant cells in the population. For many years, it has been a principle in the field of drug resistance that the presence of drug does not alter the frequency at which the events that determine drug resistance occur. However, it has been shown that transient exposure of cells to the anticancer drug hydroxyurea[27] as well as to a variety of other agents that alter DNA replication or DNA structure, such as tumor promoters[28] or ultraviolet light,[29] enhances the frequency of methotrexate resistance due to DHFR gene amplification. Even submitting cells to hypoxia for a short time prior to methotrexate selection increases the frequency of DHFR gene amplification.[30] As solid tumors may contain regions where there is transient hypoxia, this could contribute to the substantial frequency of spontaneous anticancer drug resistance observed clinically.[31]

These observations lead to a couple conclusions that are relevant to the clinical treatment of cancer. First, as transient inhibition of rep-

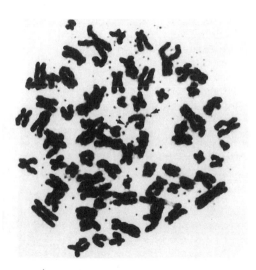

Figure 4–1 Metaphase chromosome plate of a methotrexate-resistant tumor cell isolated from a patient with small cell carcinoma of the lung. The arrows point to double minute chromosomes carrying multiple copies of the DHFR gene. (From Curt et al.[25])

lication favors gene amplification, it is important to ensure that an effective concentration of the anticancer drug is delivered to the tumor for sufficient time to produce cell death. Second, as conditions that damage DNA may facilitate gene amplification, it is possible that DNA-damaging drugs, such as the alkylating agents, have the ability to promote drug resistance when they are used to treat tumors in which a major portion of the cells are actively replicating.[30]

Multidrug Resistance

There are several ways in which cancer cells can develop resistance to multiple anticancer drugs. Most examples involve the development of resistance to several drugs belonging to a particular structural class. However, certain antibiotics and plant alkaloids with very different structures and biochemical mechanisms of action can select for cells that are cross-resistant between drug classes. This *multidrug resistance* (MDR) is obtained through stepwise selection and it reflects the amplification of a gene that encodes a transmembrane protein that pumps the drugs out of the cell. Thus, the resistant cell maintains a lower intracellular drug level than the drug-sensitive parental cells do.

The MDR phenotype was established when it was observed that certain drugs that interact with tubulin, like vinca alkaloids, colchicine, and epipodophyllotoxins, could select for resistance to themselves and to antibiotics, like actinomycin D and anthracyclines, both of which produce their cytotoxic effects via interaction with DNA, but by very different mechanisms.[32,33] Selection with one of the antibiotics, in turn, yields cross-resistance to the vinca alkaloids and colchicine. The only common features are that all of these drugs have a hydrophobic aromatic ring and a tendency to be positively charged at neutral pH.[34] Different drug resistance profiles emerge in different cell lines. Usually MDR cells are most resistant to the drug used for selection,[35] but this does not have to be the case. This is illustrated by the data shown in Table 4–4 for two MDR sublines selected from a drug-sensitive human KB carcinoma cell line.[36] When colchicine was used as the selecting drug, the cells were most resistant to colchicine (1,750-fold) and less resistant to vinblastine (254-fold) and doxorubicin (159-fold). Cells submitted to stepwise selection in vinblastine, however, were more resistant to doxorubicin than to vinblastine or colchicine. To date, there is no satisfactory way to explain either the large variation in cross-resistance profiles or the frequent ability of the selecting drug to select for cells that are more resistant

Table 4–4. *Relative Resistance of Human KB Carcinoma Cells to Three Anticancer Drugs.* Multidrug-resistant sublines were selected from drug-sensitive human KB carcinoma cells (KB-3-1) by stepwise selection with colchicine (KB-C4) or with vinblastine (KB-V1). KB-C4-R and KB-V1-R are revertant lines prepared by growing the multidrug-resistant cells under nonselective conditions. The concentration of each drug required to produce 50% inhibition of growth was determined for each cell line and is expressed relative to the concentration required to inhibit the growth of the drug-sensitive parent KB-3-1 cells. (Data from Cornwell et al.[36])

Cell Line	Relative Resistance		
	Vinblastine	Colchicine	Doxorubicin
KB-3-1	1	1	1
KB-C4	254	1750	159
KB-C4-R	3	6	4
KB-V1	213	170	458
KB-V1-R	1	1	1

to it than to other drugs for which there is cross-resistance.

The P-glycoprotein

Although it was known that multiple drug resistance was due to decreased drug accumulation in the cell, it was not clear for several years whether the decreased accumulation reflected decreased drug uptake or increased drug efflux. The observation that exposure of MDR cells to metabolic inhibitors led to increased intracellular drug levels[37] strongly suggested that the decreased accumulation is due to accelerated drug efflux. It now appears that all of the drugs involved in the MDR phenotype enter cells via unmediated diffusion and exit via an energy-dependent process.[38]

Ling and his colleagues examined the membrane proteins of both drug-sensitive and multidrug-resistant Chinese hamster ovary cells and showed that cell lines with a high level of resistance produce large amounts of a 170,000-dalton glycoprotein that they called P170 or P-glycoprotein.[39,40] It is now clear that P-glycoprotein is overproduced as a result of gene amplification.[41] Multidrug resistance is associated

with the presence of both double-minute chromosomes and homeogeneously staining regions in the same manner as discussed above for methotrexate resistance due to DHFR gene amplification.[35] The degree of P-glycoprotein overproduction correlates well with the degree of drug resistance.[42,43] This was shown both in cell lines at different levels of resistance during stepwise selection and in revertant lines with reduced drug resistance.

P-glycoprotein cDNAs have now been cloned from mouse,[44] human,[45] and other species. A model of the P-glycoprotein based on the deduced amino acid sequence is shown in Figure 4–2.[33] The P-glycoprotein contains about 1,280 amino acids and 12 transmembrane domains are predicted. The left half of the molecule is more than 40% identical with the right half, suggesting that the two halves were generated from a gene duplication. The ATP-binding domains, which are identified by the circles at the inside of the cell membrane in Figure 4–2, share strong homology with the ATP-binding components of a number of bacterial permeases. These permeases are complex systems composed of at least four proteins that transport substrates, such as sugars, amino acids, and peptides, into bacteria. The homology with the permease ATP-binding proteins includes the ATP binding site and extends well beyond it, which suggests that there is a strongly conserved function. A three-dimensional model[46] of the P-glycoprotein is presented in Figure 4–3. The six membrane-spanning loops likely form a pore with the two ATP-binding sites and probably a substrate binding site being located at the inside of the membrane. It is likely that ATP hydrolysis permits a conformational change in the pore such that drug efflux occurs.

Several observations support the proposal that the P-glycoprotein is the transporter responsible for multidrug resistance:

1. P-glycoprotein binds drugs that are transported out of multidrug-resistant cells. This has been demonstrated directly by labeling the P-glycoprotein with a photoaffinity derivative of vinblastine and showing that labeling could be inhibited by some other drugs for which there is cross-resistance.[36]

2. As diagrammed in Figures 4–2 and 4–3, the P-glycoprotein has conserved structural features that are consistent with its being an energy-dependent transporter.

3. The development of multidrug resistance is accompanied by appropriate amplification of the P-glycoprotein gene, and reversion toward drug sensitivity is accompanied by a commensurate reduction in the number of gene copies.

4. The cDNAs for human and mouse *mdr*1 genes coding for P-glycoprotein have been transfected into drug-sensitive cells with conversion of the cells to multidrug resistance.[47,48]

P-glycoprotein and Tumor Response

A major question that can be asked is, What is the normal function of the P-glycoprotein in the nonneoplastic cell? Although P-glycoprotein is expressed at a low level in a variety of cell types, relatively high levels are expressed in kidney, liver, pancreas, small intestine, colon, and adrenal gland. In the cells of the adrenal gland, P-glycoprotein is distributed in all regions of the plasma membrane, but in the other tissues where there is high expression it is localized to the luminal or apical surface of cells. For example, it is found on the brush border of renal proximal tubular cells, on hepatocyte surfaces that line the bile canaliculi and bile ductules, at the pancreatic ductules, and on the luminal surface of villus cells in the intestinal mucosa.[49] Such a localization suggests that P-glycoprotein may have a normal physiologic role in secretion. In the case of the adrenal gland, it is probably used to transport endogenous metabolites. But the presence of P-glycoprotein in organs of elimination, such as the kidney, liver, and bowel, suggests that it may function normally in the elimination of drugs and other xenobiotics from the body. Thus, the multidrug resistance phenotype in the cancer cell could reflect the amplification of genes encoding a protein that is normally involved in drug elimination. It could be that the poor responsiveness (intrinsic resistance) of renal, hepatic, and gastrointestinal adenocarcinomas to chemotherapy (Table 4–1) is due in part to the relatively high normal expression of P-glycoprotein in these tissues.

It is not yet clear how much of the resistance that arises during the therapy of human cancer is due to overexpression of the P-glycoprotein. High levels of P-glycoprotein have been de-

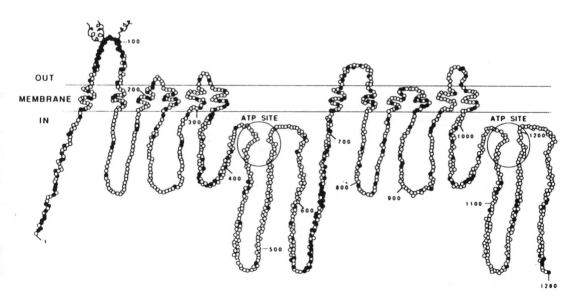

Figure 4–2 Model of P-glycoprotein structure based on amino acid sequence deduced from the cDNA. The amino acids that differ between the mouse and human *mdr* sequences are shown as solid circles. Potential N-linked sugars are indicated as curly lines, and ATP binding sites are circled. (From Gottesman and Pastan[33])

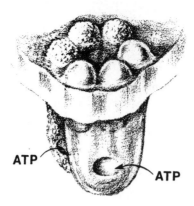

Figure 4–3   Three-dimensional model of P-glycoprotein. The six membrane-spanning loops shown in Figure 4–2 have been arranged to form a central pore in the transporter. Two ATP binding sites lie at the inside surface of the plasma membrane. (Modified from Ames[46])

tected in tumor cells from patients with ovarian cancer, soft tissue sarcoma, and acute myelocytic leukemia.[50–52] But it has been difficult in the clinical setting to design studies that determine how often drug resistance is due to high levels of P-glycoprotein that are observed in surgically resected tumor samples.

As the P-glycoprotein transports anticancer drugs of diverse structure, it was thought likely that other compounds would also be transported, and several noncytotoxic drugs have been tested for their ability to compete for the efflux of drugs involved in multidrug resistance (see Fig. 4–4). The calcium channel blocker verapamil is one such competitor. Figure 4–5 demonstrates the ability of verapamil to increase the intracellular concentration of vinblastine in multidrug-resistant human cells.[53]

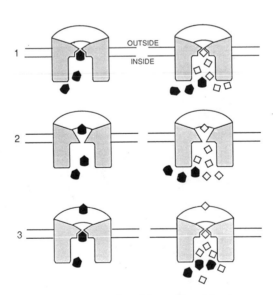

Figure 4–4   Competition for P-glycoprotein-mediated drug efflux. The three stages on the left depict the drug efflux in the absence of a competitor and, on the right, in the presence of a competitor (open squares). Step 1: both the drug and the competitor can occupy the transport site. Step 2: the hydrolysis of ATP then drives a conformational change in the transporter with release of the substrate at the external surface. Step 3: the transporter returns to the substrate-binding conformation. (From Pratt[1])

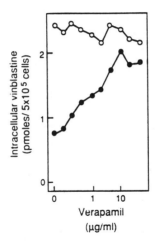

Figure 4–5 Verapamil increases the accumulation of the cytotoxic drug vinblastine in multidrug-resistant cells. Drug-sensitive human KB carcinoma cells (open circles) and a multidrug-resistant subline (closed circles) were incubated for 1 hour with [³H] vinblastine and various concentrations of verapamil. At the end of the incubation, the cells were washed and intracellular radioactivity was assayed. (From Fojo *et al.*[53])

This effect suggests that combined therapy with anticancer drugs and an agent that competes for their efflux might permit treatment of resistant tumors. In some human myeloma cells the level of multidrug resistance has been correlated with P-glycoprotein overexpression,[54] and in an early clinical study, a few patients with drug-resistant, P-glycoprotein-expressing multiple myeloma following multiple courses of therapy with vincristine and doxorubicin demonstrated some clinical response to these drugs when they were administered with verapamil.[55] Because of their own pharmacological effects, verapamil and other efflux competitors, like trifluoperazine and quinidine, are poor candidate compounds for this type of combined drug therapy. It is hoped that pharmacologically inert compounds can be developed that will block the P-glycoprotein-mediated efflux of cytotoxic drugs. If the intrinsic resistance of some cancers (e.g., colon, pancreas, liver) to chemotherapy involves intrinsically high levels of P-glycoprotein expression, then combined therapy with cytotoxic drugs and compounds that block their efflux might yield an increased response to initial therapy.

Other Mechanisms of Multidrug Resistance

If different drugs, through perhaps different mechanisms, influence a common enzymatic process that is required for their killing effect, then alterations in the activity or level of that enzyme may yield a form of multidrug resistance. A number of anticancer drugs of the DNA intercalator (e.g., doxorubicin, m-AMSA) and epipodophyllotoxin (e.g., etoposide, VM-26)[57] classes induce DNA topoisomerase II–mediated cleavage of DNA *in vitro* and in intact cells. The increase in DNA strand breakage is critical for the ultimate killing effects of the drugs. Thus, a reduction in topoisomerase II activity has been shown to correlate with drug resistance in animal tumor cells maintained *in vitro* and *in vivo*.[58,59] It is not yet known whether the topoisomerase II mechanism accounts for any multidrug resistance in tumors of patients who have been treated with these drugs.

Several classes of anticancer drugs (e.g., nitrogen mustards, nitrosoureas) form covalent drug adducts with DNA. These adducts can be excised by the DNA excision and repair systems of mammalian cells,[60] and in bacteria an enhanced ability to excise the alkylated nucleotides from DNA has been shown to account for resistance to the cytotoxicity of alkylating agents (see Chapter 6).[61] Cross-resistance between different classes of alkylating agents has been observed in tumor models,[62,63] but increased DNA repair activity has not been established as the mechanism. Although multidrug resistance via increased excision and repair has not been established in drug-resistant human tumors, it is a possible mechanism.

Cellular Thiols and Multiple Drug Resistance

Important relationships have been noted between cellular reducing capacity as reflected by glutathione (γ-glutamyl-cysteinyl-glycine, GSH) content and sensitivity to the effects of alkylating agents and radiation.[64] GSH helps to protect cells both by reacting with cytotoxic electrophile drug derivatives and by reacting with drug-generated reactive oxygen compounds such as peroxides (Fig. 4–6).[65] Supplementation of cellular GSH has been shown to be radioprotective for human lymphoid cells,[66] and acquired resistance to alkylating agents in tumor models has been associated with increased GSH.[67] As shown in Figure 4–6, glutathione S-transferases are multifunctional enzymes that catalyze the conjugation of electrophilic compounds with GSH, and elevated levels of this enzyme have been associated with resistance to alkylating agents.[68]

It was reasoned that multidrug resistance due to increased GSH might be counteracted by conditions that would lower GSH. This thinking led to the synthesis of butathionine sulfoximine (BSO), a structural analog of γ-glutamylcysteine that irreversibly inhibits γ-glutamylcysteine synthetase (Fig. 4–6), the first enzyme involved in *de novo* GSH biosynthesis.[69] When BSO is administered to mice, there is a marked decrease in glutathione levels in many tissues.[67] GSH depletion with BSO has been reported to increase the *in vitro* cytotoxicity of diverse alkylating agents, such as nitrogen mustard, melphalan, mitomycin, and cis-platin.[65] Similar sensitization to several of these drugs and to radiation has been reported after administration of BSO to rodents *in vivo*.[65] L1210 leukemia cells that were selected for resistance to melphalan were found to have GSH levels that were about twice those of sensitive cells. In mice bearing these melphalan-resistant L1210 leukemia cells, treatment with BSO led to resensitization of the tumor cells to the drug.[70]

An example of BSO-mediated potentiation of cytotoxicity is shown in Figure 4–7.[71] In this

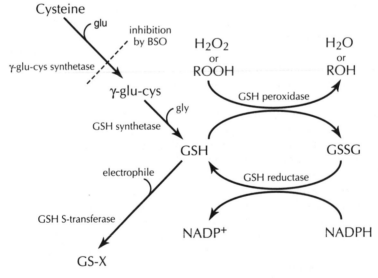

Figure 4–6   Some important reactions involved in the synthesis and function of glutathione in cells. GSH has a detoxifying role as a substrate for glutathione S-transferase, which detoxifies electrophilic compounds, such as reactive forms of alkylating drugs. GSH is also a substrate for glutathione peroxidase, which detoxifies peroxides. Oxidized glutathione (GSSG) is recycled to GSH by glutathione reductase. Cellular GSH levels can be reduced by buthionine sulfoxide (BSO), which inhibits γ-glutamylcysteine synthetase in the *de novo* synthesis pathway. (From Coleman *et al.*[65])

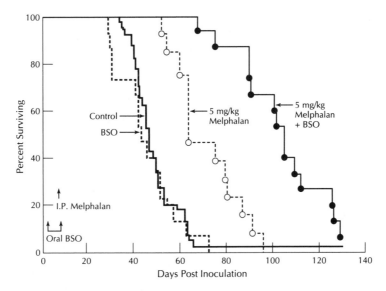

Figure 4-7 Prolonged survival of nude mice inoculated with human ovarian cancer cells by combined treatment with melphalan and BSO. Survival of untreated controls (−), controls given only BSO (- - -), melphalan-treated (5 mg/kg single injection) animals (- - -O- - -), and animals treated with melphalan and BSO. (From Ozols et al.[71])

experiment drug-resistant human ovarian cancer cells were injected into athymic ("nude") mice. The ovarian cancer cell line used in this experiment was established from a patient who was refractory to therapy with the alkylating agents cisplatin and cyclophosphamide. Previous to this experiment, it had been determined that some human ovarian cell lines selected *in vitro* for resistance to melphalan or cisplatin have a two- to three-fold elevation in intracellular GSH compared to the parent drug-sensitive cells, and that depletion of GSH by BSO in these cell lines was accompanied by a marked increase in cytotoxicity.[72] In the experiment of Figure 4-7, nude mice were administered BSO in their drinking water for six days, beginning 3 days after tumor cell inoculation. On day 8 melphalan was administered, and the survival of treated animals and untreated controls was recorded. The survival rate in animals treated with BSO alone was the same as that of untreated controls, and it was demonstrated that BSO lowered the GSH content of the tumor cells by 96% and that of bone marrow cells by 79%, suggesting that some selective antitumor cytotoxicity might be achieved with combination therapy. Treatment with melphalan increased the median survival time by about 20

days, and combination therapy with BSO and melphalan increased median survival by 60 days. These kinds of observations in tumor models suggest that it may be possible to resensitize patients who have developed multidrug resistance via an elevation in GSH levels by using a combination protocol containing a drug that inhibits glutathione synthesis.

Biochemical Mechanisms of Anticancer Drug Resistance

Cancer cells become resistant to anticancer drugs by a wide variety of mechanisms. The major biochemical mechanisms of resistance are summarized in Table 4-5. For most members of the major drug groups, several different mechanisms have been demonstrated. It is fair to say that if resistance could theoretically develop to a drug via any specific mechanism, cancer cells have done so, and it is likely that it has been reported in the literature. In the next section of this book we review each of the anticancer drugs, and where appropriate, specific resistance mechanisms will be summarized.

Table 4–5   Biochemical Mechanisms by Which Tumor Cells Develop Resistance to Anticancer Drugs. Listed on the right column are some drug classes for which the mechanism has been demonstrated.

Mechanism	Drugs
I Decreased intracellular drug level	
a. Increased drug efflux	Anthracyclines, dactinomycin, vinca alkaloids, epipodophyllotoxins
b. Decreased inward transport	Antimetabolites, nitrogen mustards, antibiotics
II Increased drug inactivation	Alkylating agents, antimetabolites, bleomycin
III Decreased conversion of drug to an active form	Antimetabolites
IV Altered amount of target enzyme or receptor	Methotrexate, steroids, hydroxyurea, PALA
V Decreased affinity of target enzyme or receptor for drug	Antimetabolites, hydroxyurea
VI Enhanced repair of drug-induced defect	Alkylating agents, cisplatin
VII Decreased activity of an enzyme required for the killing effect (topoisomerase II)	Doxorubicin, m-AMSA, epipodophyllotoxins

The study of biochemical mechanisms of resistance has contributed immensely to our understanding of how anticancer drugs work at the cellular and molecular level. The study of resistance mechanisms has also led to improvements in therapy. This has occurred by modifying drug structures such that a specific resistance mechanism no longer is effective. There are a few instances in which delineation of a resistance mechanism has led to unique applications of established therapy in order to obtain a selective effect against the resistant cell (e.g., the use of high-dose methotrexate therapy followed by thymidine rescue in certain fluorouracil-resistant tumor cell populations). Finally, as we have seen above with multidrug resistance due to increased drug efflux or to an increased level of GSH, specific approaches can be developed to resensitize certain resistant cell populations.

REFERENCES

1. W. B. Pratt: "Drug resistance," in *Principles of Drug Action*, 3rd ed., ed by W. B. Pratt and P. Taylor. New York: Churchill Livingstone, 1990, pp. 565–637.

2. B. W. Fox and W. Fox (eds.): *Handbook of Experimental Pharmacology*, Vol. 72. *Antitumor Drug Resistance.* New York: Springer-Verlag, 1984.

3. P. V. Woolley and K. D. Tew: *Mechanisms of Drug Resistance in Neoplastic Cells.* New York: Academic Press, 1988.

4. P. J. Fialkow: Clonal origin of human tumors. *Biochim. Biophys. Acta* 458:283 (1976).

5. J. R. Shapiro and W. R. Shapiro: Clonal tumor cell heterogeneity. *Prog. Exptl. Tumor Res.* 27:49 (1984).

6. J. H. Goldie and A. J. Coldman: A mathematic model for relating the drug sensitivity of tumors to their spontaneous mutation rate. *Cancer Treat. Rep.* 63:1727 (1979).

7. R. T. Schimke: Gene amplification in cultured mammalian cells. *Cell* 37:705 (1984).

8. H. E. Skipper and F. M. Schabel: Experimental therapeutics and kinetics: Selection and overgrowth of specifically and permanently drug-resistant tumor cells. *Semin. Hematol.* 5:207 (1978).

9. F. M. Schabel, D. P. Griswold, T. H. Corbett, W. R. Laster, J. G. Mayo, and H. H. Lloyd: "Testing therapeutic hypotheses in mice and man," in *Cancer Drug Development*, Part B: *Methods in Cancer Research*, Vol. 17, ed. by V. DeVita and H. Busch. New York: Academic Press, 1979, pp. 3–51.

10. W. Hryniuk and H. Busch: The importance of dose intensity in chemotherapy of metastatic breast cancer. *J. Clin. Oncol.* 2:1281 (1984).

11. L. Levin and W. M. Hryniuk: Dose intensity analysis of chemotherapy regimens in ovarian carcinoma. *J. Clin. Oncol.* 5:756 (1987).

12. R. E. Wittes and A. Goldin: Unresolved issues in combination chemotherapy. *Cancer Treat. Rep.* 70:105 (1986).

13. J. H. Goldie, A. J. Coldman, and G. A. Gudauskas: Rationale for the use of alternating non-cross-resistant chemotherapy. *Cancer Treat. Rep. 66:*439 (1982).

14. A. Santoro, G. Bonadonna, V. Bonfante, and P. Valagussa: Alternating drug combinations in the treatment of advanced Hodgkin's disease. *New Engl. J. Med. 306:*770 (1982).

15. P. Klimo and J. M. Connors: An update on the Vancouver experience in the management of advanced Hodgkin's disease treated with the MOPP/ABV hybrid program. *Semin. Hematol. 25:*34 (1988).

16. R. T. Schimke: Gene amplification, drug resistance, and cancer. *Cancer Res. 44:*1735 (1984).

17. S. H. Berger, C. H. Jenh, L. F. Johnson, and F. G. Berger: Thymidylate synthetase overproduction and gene amplification in fluorodeoxyuridine-resistant human cells. *Mol. Pharmacol. 28:*461 (1985).

18. G. M. Wahl, R. A. Padgett, and G. R. Stark: Gene amplification causes overproduction of the first three enzymes of UMP synthesis in N-(phosphonoacetyl)-L-aspartate-resistant hamster cells. *J. Biol. Chem. 254:*8679 (1979).

19. M. T. Hakala, S. F. Zakrzewski, and C. A. Nichol: Relation of folic acid reductase to amethopterin resistance in cultured mammalian cells. *J. Biol. Chem. 236:*952 (1961).

20. F. W. Alt, R. E. Kellems, and R. T. Schimke: Synthesis and degradation of folate reductase in sensitive and methotrexate-resistant lines of S-180 cells. *J. Biol. Chem. 251:*3063 (1976).

21. F. W. Alt, R. E. Kellems, J. R. Bertino, and R. T. Schimke: Selective multiplication of dihydrofolate reductase genes in methotrexate-resistant variants of cultured murine cells. *J. Biol. Chem. 253:*1357 (1978).

22. D. A. Haber, S. M. Beverley, M. L. Kiely, and R. T. Schimke: Properties of an altered dihydrofolate reductase encoded by amplified genes in cultured mouse fibroblasts. *J. Biol. Chem. 256:*9501 (1981).

23. H. Rath, T. Tlsty, and R. T. Schimke: Rapid emergence of methotrexate resistance in cultured mouse cells. *Cancer Res. 44:*3303 (1984).

24. R. C. Horns, W. J. Dower, and R. T. Schimke: Gene amplification in a leukemic patient treated with methotrexate. *J. Clin. Oncol. 2:*2 (1984).

25. G. A. Curt, D. M. Carney, K. H. Cowan, J. Jolivet, B. D. Bailey, J. C. Drake, C. S. Koo-Shan, J. D. Mina, and B. A. Chabner: Unstable methotrexate resistance in human small cell carcinoma associated with double minute chromosomes. *New Engl. J. Med. 308:*199 (1983).

26. R. N. Johnston, S. M. Beverley, and R. T. Schimke: Rapid spontaneous dihydrofolate reductase gene amplification shown by fluorescence-activated cell sorting. *Proc. Natl. Acad. Sci. USA 80:*3711 (1983).

27. P. C. Brown, T. D. Tlsty, and R. T. Schimke: Enhancement of methotrexate resistance and dihydrofolate reductase gene amplification by treatment of mouse 3T6 cells with hydroxyurea. *Mol. Cell. Biol. 3:*1097 (1983).

28. A. Varshavsky: Phorbol ester dramatically increases incidence of methotrexate-resistant mouse cells: Possible mechanisms and relevance to tumor promotion. *Cell 251:*561 (1981).

29. T. D. Tlsty, P. C. Brown, and R. T. Schimke: UV irradiation facilitates methotrexate resistance and amplification of the dihydrofolate reductase gene in cultured 3T6 mouse cells. *Mol. Cell. Biol. 4:*1050 (1984).

30. R. T. Schimke, S. Sherwood, R. Johnston, A. Hill, G. Rice, C. Hoy, J. Feder, and P. Farnham: "On the mechanism of induced gene amplification in mammalian cells," in *Mechanisms of Drug Resistance in Neoplastic Cells,* ed. by P. V. Woolley and K. D. Tew. New York: Academic Press, 1988, pp. 29–40.

31. S. E. Salmon, H. W. Hamburger, B. Soehnlen, B. G. M. Durie, D. S. Alberts, and T. E. Moon: Quantitation of differential sensitivity of human-tumor stem cells to anticancer drugs. *New Engl. J. Med. 298:*1321 (1978).

32. G. Bradley, P. F. Juranka, and V. Ling: Mechanism of multidrug resistance. *Biochim. Biophys. Acta. 948:*87 (1988).

33. M. M. Gottesman and I. Pastan: The multidrug transporter, a double-edged sword. *J. Biol. Chem. 263:*12163 (1988).

34. P. Borst: DNA amplification and multidrug resistance. *Nature 309:*580 (1984).

35. J. L. Biedler, M. B. Meyers, and B. A. Spengler: "Cellular concomitants of multidrug resistance," in *Mechanisms of Drug Resistance in Neoplastic Cells,* ed. by P. V. Woolley and K. D. Tew. New York: Academic Press, 1988, pp. 41–68.

36. M. M. Cornwell, A. R. Safa, R. L. Felsted, M. M. Gottesman, and I. Pastan: Membrane vesicles from multidrug-resistant human cancer cells contain a specific 150- to 170-kDa protein detected by photoaffinity labeling. *Proc. Natl. Acad. Sci. USA 83:*3847 (1986).

37. M. Inaba, H. Kobayashi, Y. Sakurai, and R. K. Johnson: Active efflux of daunorubicin and Adriamycin in sensitive and resistant sublines of P388 leukemia. *Cancer Res. 39:*2200 (1979).

38. V. Ling, P. F. Juranka, J. A. Endicott, K. L. Deuchars, and J. H. Gerlach: "Multidrug resistance and P-glycoprotein expression," in *Mechanisms of Drug Resistance in Neoplastic Cells,* ed. by P. V. Woolley and K. D. Tew. New York: Academic Press, 1988, pp. 197–209.

39. R. L. Juliano and V. Ling: A surface glycoprotein modulating drug permeability in Chinese hamster ovary cell mutants. *Biochim. Biophys. Acta. 455:*152 (1976).

40. J. R. Riordan and V. Ling: Purification of P-glycoprotein from plasma membrane vesicles of Chinese hamster ovary cell mutants with reduced colchicine permeability. *J. Biol. Chem. 254:*12701 (1979).

41. I. B. Roninson, H. T. Abelson, D. E. Hausman, N. Howell, and A. Varshavski: Amplification of specific DNA sequences correlates with multidrug resistance in Chinese hamster cells. *Nature 309:*626 (1984).

42. N. D. Kartner, G. Evernden-Porelle, G. Bradley, and V. Ling: Detection of P-glycoprotein in multidrug-resistant cell lines by monoclonal antibodies. *Nature 316:*820 (1985).

43. S. M. Robertson, V. Ling, and C. P. Stanners: Coamplification of double minute chromosomes, multiple drug resistance and cell surface P-glycoprotein in DNA-mediated transformants of mouse cells. *Mol. Cell. Biol. 4:*500 (1984).

44. P. Gros, J. Croop, and D. Housman: Mammalian multidrug resistance gene: Complete DNA sequence indicates strong homology to bacterial transport proteins. *Cell 47:*371 (1986).

45. C. J. Chen, J. E. Chin, K. Ueda, D. P. Clark, I. Pastan, M. M. Gottesman, and I. B. Roninson: Internal duplication and homology with bacterial transport proteins in the

mdr1 (P-glycoprotein) gene from multidrug-resistant human cells. *Cell* 47:381 (1986).

46. G. F. Ames: The basis of multidrug resistance in mammalian cells: Homology with bacterial transport. *Cell* 47:323 (1986).

47. P. Gros, Y. Ben-Neriah, J. Croop, and D. E. Housman: Isolation and expression of a cDNA clone that confers multidrug resistance. *Nature* 323:728 (1986).

48. K. Ueda, C. Cardarelli, M. M. Gottesman, and I. Pastan: Expression of a full-length cDNA for the human "MDR1" gene confers resistance to colchicine, doxorubicin, and vinblastine. *Proc. Natl. Acad. Sci. USA* 84:3004 (1987).

49. F. Thiebault, T. Tsuruo, H. Hamada, M. M. Gottesman, I. Pastan, and M. C. Willingham: Cellular localization of the multidrug-resistance gene product P-glycoprotein in normal human tissues. *Proc. Natl. Acad. Sci. USA* 84:7735 (1987).

50. D. R. Bell, J. H. Gerlach, N. Kartner, R. N. Buick, and V. Ling: Detection of P-glycoprotein in ovarian cancer: A molecular marker associated with multidrug resistance. *J. Clin. Oncol.* 3:311 (1985).

51. J. H. Gerlach, D. R. Bell, C. Karakousis, H. K. Slocum, N. Kartner, Y. M. Rustum, V. Ling, and R. M. Baker: P-glycoprotein in human sarcoma: Evidence for multidrug resistance. *J. Clin. Oncol.* 5:1452 (1987).

52. D. D. F. Ma, R. A. Davey, D. H. Harman, J. P. Isbister, R. D. Scurr, S. M. Mackertich, G. Dowden, and D. R. Bell: Detection of a multidrug resistant phenotype in acute non-lymphoblastic leukemia. *Lancet* 1:135 (1987).

53. A. Fojo, S. Akiyama, M. M. Gottesman, and I. Pastan: Reduced drug accumulation in multiple drug-resistant human KB carcinoma cell lines. *Cancer Res.* 45:3002 (1985).

54. W. S. Dalton, T. M. Grogan, J. A. Rybski, R. J. Scheper, L. Richter, J. Kailey, H. J. Broxterman, H. M. Pinedo, and S. E. Salmon: Immunohistochemical detection and quantitation of P-glycoprotein in multiple drug-resistant human myeloma cells: Association with level of drug resistance and drug accumulation. *Blood* 73:747 (1989).

55. W. S. Dalton, T. M. Grogan, P. S. Meltzer, R. J. Scheper, B. G. M. Durie, C. W. Taylor, T. P. Miller, and S. E. Salmon: Drug-resistance in multiple myeloma and non-Hodgkin's lymphoma: Detection of P-glycoprotein and potential circumvention by addition of verapamil to chemotherapy. *J. Clin. Oncol.* 7:415 (1989).

56. Y. Pommier, J. K. Miford, R. E. Schwartz, L. A. Zwelling, and K. W. Kohn: Effects of the intercalators, 4′-(9-acridinylamino)methanesulfon-*m*-aniside (m-AMSA, amsacrine) and 2-methyl-9-hydroxyellipticinium (2-Me-9-OH-E+) on topoisomerase II–mediated DNA strand cleavage and strand passage. *Biochemistry* 24:6410 (1985).

57. G. L. Chen, L. Yang, T. C. Rowe, B. D. Halligan, K. M. Tewey, and L. F. Liu: Nonintercalative antitumor drugs interfere with the breakage-reunion reaction of mammalian DNA topoisomerase II. *J. Biol. Chem.* 259:13560 (1984).

58. Y. Pommier, D. Kerrigan, R. E. Schwartz, J. A. Swack, and A. McCurdy: Altered DNA topoisomerase II activity in Chinese hamster cells resistant to topoisomerase II inhibitors. *Cancer Res.* 46:3075 (1986).

59. A. M. Deffie, J. K. Batra, and G. J. Goldenberg: Direct correlation between DNA topoisomerase II activity and cytotoxicity in adriamycin-sensitive and -resistant P388 leukemia cell lines. *Cancer Res.* 49:58 (1989).

60. R. A. G. Ewig and K. W. Kohn: DNA damage and repair in mouse leukemia L1210 cells treated with nitrogen mustard, 1,3-bis(2-chloroethyl)-1-nitrosourea, and other nitroureas. *Cancer Res.* 39:1411 (1979).

61. K. W. Kohn, N. H. Steigbigel, and C. L. Spears: Cross-linking and repair of DNA in sensitive and resistant strains of *E. coli* treated with nitrogen mustard. *Proc. Natl. Acad. Sci. USA* 53:1154 (1965).

62. G. J. Goldenberg: The role of drug transport in resistance to nitrogen mustard and other alkylating agents in L5178Y lymphoblasts. *Cancer Res.* 35:1687 (1975).

63. F. M. Schabel, M. W. Trader, W. R. Laster, G. P. Wheeler, and M. H. Witt: Patterns of resistance and therapeutic synergism among alkylating agents. *Antibiot. Chemother.* 23:200 (1978).

64. A. Meister: Selective modification of glutathione metabolism. *Science* 220:472 (1983).

65. C. N. Coleman, E. A. Bump, and R. A. Kramer: Chemical modifiers of cancer treatment. *J. Clin. Oncol.* 6:709 (1988).

66. G. L. Jensen and A. Meister: Radioprotection of human lymphoid cells by exogenously-supplied glutathione is mediated by γ-glutamyl transpeptidase. *Proc. Natl. Acad. Sci. USA* 80:4714 (1983).

67. A. Meister: "Novel drugs that affect glutathione metabolism," in *Mechanisms of Drug Resistance in Neoplastic Cells,* ed. by P. W. Woolley and K. D. Tew. New York: Academic Press, 1988, pp. 99–126.

68. K. D. Tew and M. L. Clapper: "Glutathione S-transferase and anticancer drug resistance," in *Mechanisms of Drug Resistance in Neoplastic Cells,* ed. by P. W. Woolley and K. D. Tew. New York: Academic Press, 1988, pp. 141–159.

69. O. W. Griffith and A. Meister: Potent and specific inhibition of glutathione synthesis by butathionine sulfoximine (S-n-butyl homocysteine sulfoximine). *J. Biol. Chem.* 254:7558 (1979).

70. K. Suzakake, B. J. Petro, and D. T. Vistica: Reduction in glutathione content of L-PAM resistant L1210 cells confers drug sensitivity. *Biochem. Pharmacol.* 31:121 (1982).

71. R. F. Ozols, K. G. Louie, J. Plowman, B. C. Behrens, R. L. Fine, D. Dykes, and T. C. Hamilton: Enhanced melphalan cytotoxicity in human ovarian cancer *in vitro* and in tumor-bearing nude mice by butathione sulfoximine depletion of glutathione. *Biochem. Pharmacol.* 36:147 (1987).

72. J. A. Green, D. T. Vistica, R. C. Young, T. C. Hamilton, A. M. Rogan, and R. F. Ozols: Potentiation of melphalan cytotoxicity in human ovarian cancer cell lines by glutathione depletion. *Cancer Res.* 44:5427 (1984).

The Anticancer Drugs

Antimetabolites

FOLATE ANTAGONISTS
    Methotrexate (MTX, amethopterin)
    Trimetrexate (TMQ)
PYRIMIDINE ANTAGONISTS
    Fluorouracil (FUra, 5-FU)
    Fluorodeoxyuridine (FdUrd, 5-FUdR)
    CB3717
    Azacytidine (Aza-C, 5-AC)

PURINE ANTAGONISTS
    Mercaptopurine (MP, 6-MP)
    Thioguanine (TG, 6-TG)
    Tiazofurin
    Chlorodeoxyadenosine (CdA)
    Pentostatin (2′-deoxycoformycin, dCF)
SUGAR-MODIFIED ANALOGS
    Cytarabine (ara-C)
    Fludarabine (F-ara-A)
RIBONUCLEOTIDE REDUCTASE INHIBITORS
    Hydroxyurea (HU)

Antimetabolites interfere with the production of nucleic acids by one or both of two major mechanisms. Some of these drugs inhibit production of the deoxyribonucleoside triphosphates that are the immediate precursors for DNA synthesis, thus inhibiting the replication process. Although short intervals of DNA synthesis inhibition are not necessarily harmful to cells, extended periods of inhibition are usually cytotoxic. A number of mechanisms have been proposed to explain how persistent DNA synthesis inhibition leads to cell death, as discussed later in this chapter. In addition to preventing the synthesis of normal nucleoside triphosphates, some antimetabolites are sufficiently similar in structure to normal purines or pyrimidines to be able to substitute for them in the anabolic nucleotide pathways. In this case, the nucleotide derivatives of the antimetabolites not only inhibit formation of normal precursors by competition for anabolic enzymes, but are also used as substrates themselves. While the polymerases responsible for making nucleic acids are highly selective, analog triphosphates can nevertheless be incorporated into RNA and DNA, in place of their normal counterparts. The extent of analog incorporation has been correlated with cytotoxicity for some of the antimetabolites, although the exact consequences of analog incorporation are obscure at this time. Whether the major action of a given antimetabolite is through inhibition of nucleotide synthesis or through incorporation into nucleic acids (or both), understanding antimetabolite effects requires some knowledge of the network of processes involved in nucleotide and nucleic acid metabolism. We therefore begin this chapter with a short summary of these metabolic pathways.

Nucleotide and Nucleic Acid Metabolism

The major pathways for synthesis of nucleotides in mammalian cells have been extensively characterized, and both concise[1] and detailed[2]

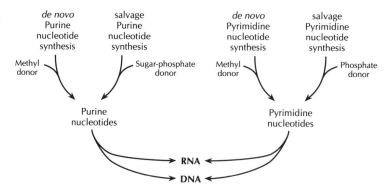

Figure 5–1   Symmetry in nucleotide and nucleic acid synthesis.

reviews are available. Our aim here is to give an overview of the various routes involved, highlighting those points that are related to the actions of antimetabolites. This system is represented in a very simplified form in Figure 5–1. When viewed with a somewhat global perspective, these pathways exhibit a fair degree of symmetry. For example, synthesis of both RNA and DNA requires two purine and two pyrimidine nucleoside triphosphates, each of which can be derived from either a *"de novo"* pathway (newly made) or a "salvage" pathway (recycling of partially degraded nucleotides). Studies on a large number of normal and neoplastic cells indicate that in most normal tissues the *de novo* purine pathway is relatively inactive, while tumors tend to rely on this pathway quite heavily, thus providing strong rationale for choosing *de novo* purine biosynthesis as a therapeutic target.[3]

De novo *Pathways*

De novo purine nucleotide synthesis, summarized in Figure 5–2, begins with the attachment of an amine group to an activated ribose derivative, phosphoribosyl pyrophosphate (PRPP), by the enzyme PRPP amidotransferase. This first step is quite sensitive to feedback inhibition by purine nucleotides and their analogs, and is a target of the thiopurines, 6-mercaptopurine (6-MP) and 6-thioguanine (6-TG). Atoms that make up the purine ring come from a variety of metabolic sources, such as amino acids and CO_2, which serve many other functions within the cell. One of these sources, the pool of reduced folates, is particularly critical.

Reduced folates exist in several intracellular forms whose major anabolic function is to act as a methyl group donor in both purine and thymidine synthesis. In the purine pathway, reduced folates pick up and deliver methyl groups without a change in their own oxidation status, and therefore are needed only in catalytic amounts for this purpose. They are also used in the production of thymidine nucleotides, in a stoichiometric manner. Methotrexate and trimetrexate inhibit folate interconversion and consequently antagonize both purine and thymidine production.

Upon closure of the purine ring structure, the first complete purine nucleotide, inosine monophosphate (IMP), is formed. This molecule represents a branch point in purine biosynthesis, giving rise to separate routes to guanine and adenine ribonucleotides. Both of these pathways are inhibited by 6-MP; the first enzyme in the guanine pathway, IMP dehydrogenase, is more selectively inhibited by 6-TG and tiazofurin.

The step at which *ribo*nucleoside diphosphates are converted to *deoxyribo*nucleoside diphosphates, through the action of ribonucleotide reductase, is controlled by a complex combination of feedback loops, and is affected to some extent by almost all of the antimetabolites. Although changes in this activity are probably incidental for most drugs, there are some for which effects on ribonucleotide reduction are thought to be important, such as chlorodeoxyadenosine, fludarabine, and pentostatin. Finally, triphosphate derivatives of 6-MP, 6-TG, chlorodeoxyadenosine, and fludarabine can antagonize nucleic acid synthesis both by inhibition of the polymerases involved and by incorporation into nucleic acids in place of endogenous purines.

In contrast to the piecewise assembly of the purine ring, *de novo* formation of the pyrimidine ring structure is largely accomplished in one step via the condensation of two major precursor molecules by the enzyme aspartate carbamoyltransferase. An inhibitor of this enzyme has been synthesized and tested as an anticancer drug. This agent, N-phosphonoacetyl-L-aspartate (PALA), has shown some activity against tumors *in vivo,* although it may be more useful as a modulator of the action of other antimetabolites.[4] The steps in the pyrimidine nucleotide synthesis scheme that are most frequently relevant to therapeutics are in the upper right-hand portion of Figure 5–3, involving deoxyuridine and thymidine nucleotides. The importance of these steps is due to the unique presence of thymidine in DNA and the close link between DNA synthesis and cellular proliferation. The key enzyme in this part of

the pathway for producing thymidine nucleotides is thymidylate synthase. The conversion of dUMP to TMP by thymidylate synthase is inhibited both directly and indirectly by several antimetabolites, and will be addressed in much greater detail later in this chapter. In addition to having an enzyme that provides thymidine nucleotides, cells also possess systems for excluding dUTP from DNA. One such activity is dUTPase, which specifically degrades dUTP to dUMP. This not only limits the opportunity for dUTP to be used as a substrate for DNA polymerases, but also serves to enhance availability of dUMP, the substrate for thymidylate synthase.

Salvage Pathways

Construction of purine and pyrimidine rings from small precursors is a complex process requiring considerable energy, and the continuous need for these molecules in RNA and DNA synthesis is a potentially serious drain on cel-

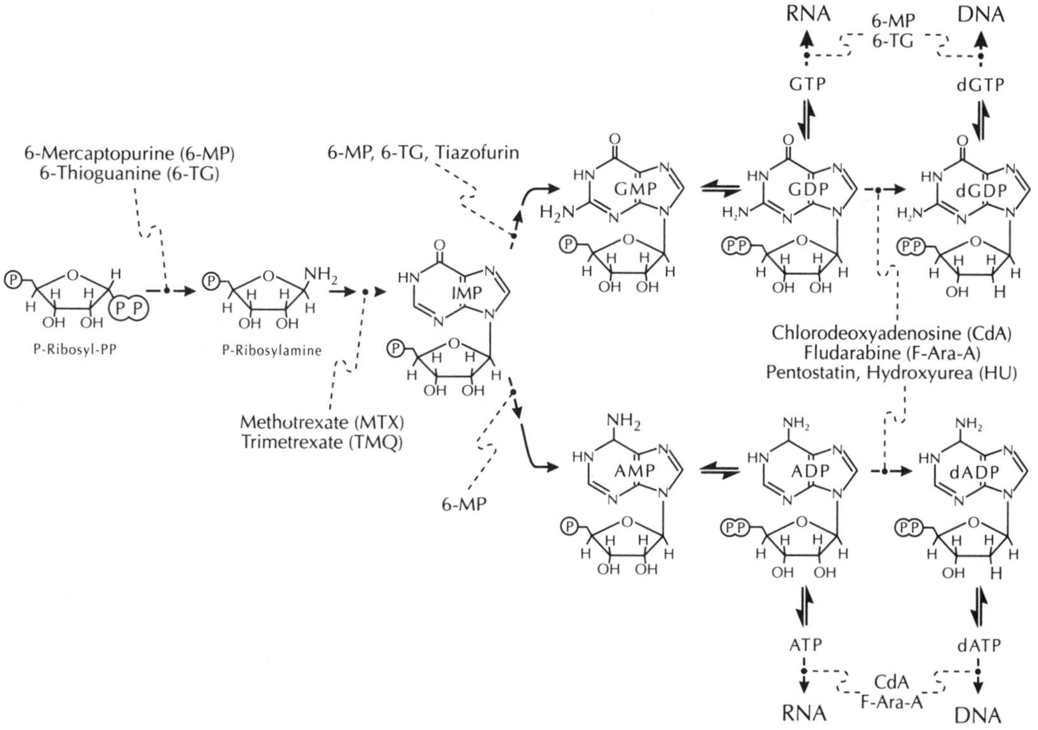

Figure 5–2 Inhibition of *de novo* purine synthesis by antimetabolites. Sites of drug inhibition are indicated by dashed lines.

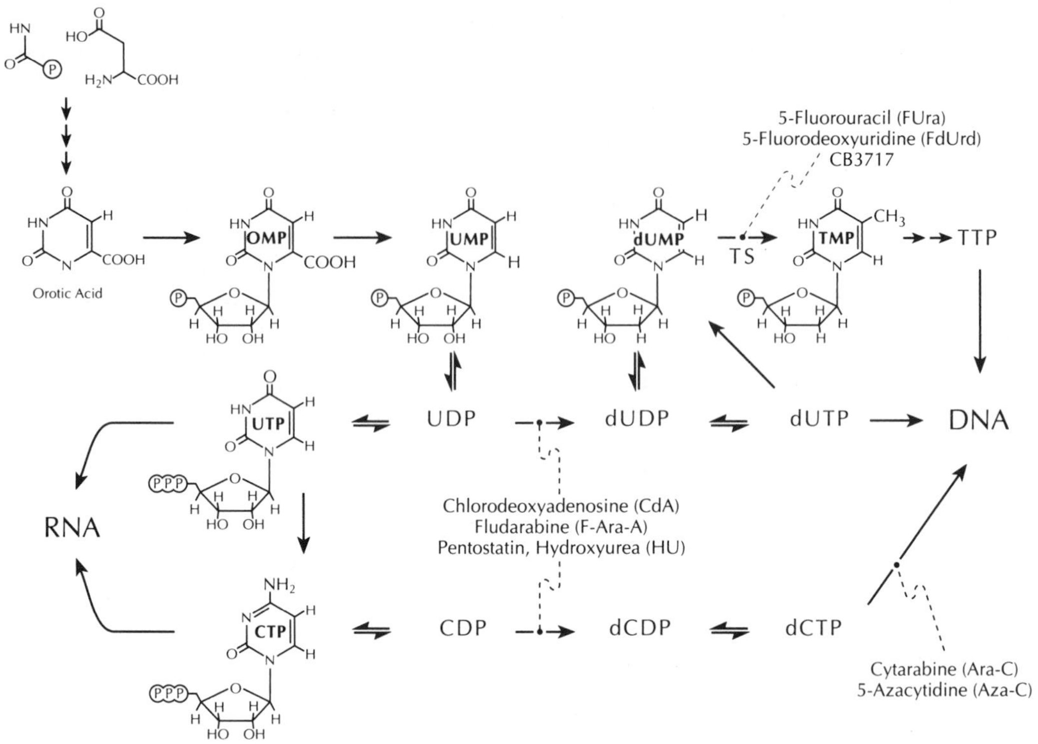

Orotic Acid → OMP → UMP → dUMP → TMP → → TTP

5-Fluorouracil (FUra)
5-Fluorodeoxyuridine (FdUrd)
CB3717

TS

UTP ⇌ UDP → dUDP ⇌ dUTP → DNA

RNA

CTP ⇌ CDP → dCDP ⇌ dCTP

Chlorodeoxyadenosine (CdA)
Fludarabine (F-Ara-A)
Pentostatin, Hydroxyurea (HU)

Cytarabine (Ara-C)
5-Azacytidine (Aza-C)

Figure 5–3 Inhibition of *de novo* pyrimidine synthesis by antimetabolites. Sites of drug inhibition are indicated by dashed lines. Incorporation of dUTP into DNA is miniscule under normal conditions but can become significant upon inhibition of thymidylate synthase (TS), which creates an abnormally high ratio of dUTP to TTP.

lular resources, especially in the more rapidly proliferating normal tissues. Fortunately, efficient systems have evolved for recycling bases and nucleosides present in physiological fluids by converting them back to nucleotides in a single step. Because many antimetabolites are also bases or nucleosides they, too, are frequently substrates for the "salvage" enzymes. In fact, the biological activity of several antimetabolites is completely dependent on their activation by salvage enzymes, and attenuation or deletion of one of these enzymes is a common mechanism of resistance to certain antimetabolites.

The activities of the salvage enzymes are summarized in Table 5–1. The phosphoribosyltransferases catalyze the fusion of purine or pyrimidine bases with 1-phosphoribosyl-5-pyrophosphate (PRPP) to form 5'-ribonucleotides, which can then be further anabolized by the reactions described in the *de novo* synthesis

schemes, above. Although the supply of PRPP is probably not a limiting factor for drug activation in most cases, it has been shown in some circumstances that treatments that elevate PRPP levels can enhance anabolism of drugs that are substrates for phosphoribosyl transferases. The other important salvage enzymes are the nucleoside kinases, which transfer a phosphate group from a donor (such as ATP) to the 5' position of ribo- or deoxyribonucleosides, to form the corresponding ribo- or deoxyribonucleotide.

In addition to their role in activating antimetabolites, salvage pathways are also necessary to consider in chemotherapy, because their endogenous function, recovery of normal nucleotides, can oppose antimetabolite action. For example: The major metabolic consequences of methotrexate treatment are to inhibit purine and thymidine nucleotide synthesis; this blockade can be circumvented if hypoxanthine and thymidine are salvaged by HPRTase and thymidine kinase, respectively. Whereas the circulating levels of endogenous bases and nucleosides are not extremely high under normal conditions, they can be elevated significantly in cancer patients undergoing treatment (as the nucleic acids from dead tumor and host cells are degraded) and thus become an important factor in drug treatment.

Catabolic Pathways

Even though recovery of bases and nucleosides by salvage enzymes is beneficial and reasonably efficient, cells must still have a means of disposing of any excess amounts of these molecules. Figure 5–4 gives an overview of the major processes by which purines and pyrimidines are degraded in humans, and also points out the role of this system in eliminating some of the most commonly used antimetabolites, as well.

One of the most important catabolic reactions is conversion of nucleosides to bases by various nucleoside phosphorylases. Although this reaction is reversible *in vitro,* in intact tissues it is usually slanted heavily in the catabolic direction. Enzymes have been found that can

Table 5–1   Salvage Pathway Synthesis of Purine and Pyrimidine Nucleotides.
Phosphoribosyl transferases (top) and nucleoside kinases (bottom) convert bases and nucleosides into nucleotides for re-use in nucleic acid synthesis. Most antimetabolites (bold type) are activated by these pathways. Deficiencies of these enzymes are often associated with resistance to the drugs that use them for anabolism.

Purine or Pyrimdine Base	Phosphoribosyl Transferase	Ribonucleotide
Adenine	APRTase	AMP
Hypoxanthine	HPRTase	IMP
Guanine	HPRTase	GMP
6-Mercaptopurine (6-MP)	**HPRTase**	**Thio-IMP**
6-Thioguanine (6-MP)	**HPRTase**	**Thio-GMP**
Orotic Acid	OPRTase	OMP
Uracil	OPRTase	UMP
5-Fluorouracil (FUra)	**OPRTase**	**FUMP**

Purine or Pyrimdine Nucleoside	Nucleoside Kinase	5′-Nucleotide
Adenosine	Ado kinase	AMP
Deoxyadenosine	Ado kinase	dAMP
Chlorodeoxyadenosine (CdA)	**Ado kinase**	**CldAMP**
Uridine	Urd kinase	UMP
Cytidine	Urd kinase	CMP
5-Azacytidine (aza-C)	**Urd kinase**	**Aza-CMP**
Deoxyadenosine	dCyd kinase	dAMP
Deoxycytidine	dCyd kinase	dCMP
Deoxyguanosine	dCyd kinase	dGMP
Cytarabine (ara-C)	**dCyd kinase**	**Ara-CMP**
Fludarabine (F-ara-A)	**dCyd kinase**	**F-Ara-AMP**
Thymidine	dThd kinase	dTMP
Deoxyuridine	dThd kinase	dUMP
Fluorodeoxyuridine (FdUrd)	**dThd kinase**	**FdUMP**

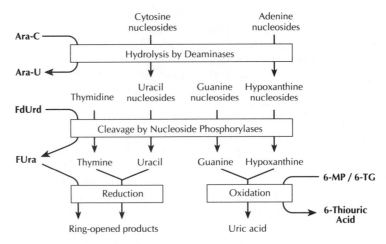

Figure 5–4 Catabolic pathways for purines and pyrimidines. Conversion of nucleosides to bases is potentially reversible, although this equilibrium is usually slanted toward the catabolic reaction *in vivo*. Reduction and oxidation of the bases are effectively irreversible, as is deamination. The role of these enzymes in elimination of the most commonly used antimetabolites is shown in bold type. Competition for degradation between drugs and endogenous bases or nucleosides can prolong the duration of action of the drugs.

cleave thymine-, uracil-, guanine-, and hypoxanthine-containing nucleosides, but cytosine- and adenine-containing nucleosides are not subject to phosphorylase cleavage to any significant extent in mammalian cells. In order for cytosine or adenine nucleosides to be degraded, they must first be deaminated to uracil or hypoxanthine nucleosides, respectively. This deamination can occur at either the nucleoside or nucleotide level, through the action of separate, specific enzymes.

The purine and pyrimidine bases formed by phosphorylase action can still be salvaged by phosphoribosyl transferases, as discussed in the preceding section, and the degradative process is not really irreversible until these bases are processed further. The pyrimidines are usually reduced in two successive steps by dihydrouracil dehydrogenase, resulting in scission of the ring structure and formation of carboxylic acids. On the purine side, guanine and hypoxanthine are each converted to xanthine, by guanine deaminase and xanthine oxidase, respectively. Xanthine is then subject to further metabolism by xanthine oxidase, to form uric acid, which is the major end product of this pathway in humans.

Uric acid has a relatively low solubility in aqueous solution, and, because of this, precipitation from bodily fluids can be problematic.

Individuals who overproduce uric acid as the result of an inherited metabolic defect (gout) accumulate uric acid crystals in their synovial fluid, which causes a painful inflammatory response. A more serious situation can occur in patients undergoing successful cancer treatments, due to the sudden death and lysis of large numbers of tumor cells (tumor lysis syndrome). As RNA and DNA are released and degraded from these cells, the circulating level of uric acid can rise sharply and crystals of uric acid may start to form in the renal tubules.

Allopurinol   Hypoxanthine

This potentially life-threatening event can be prevented by administration of allopurinol, an analog of hypoxanthine, which inhibits xanthine oxidase.

Folate Antagonists

The importance of folates in tumor cell growth was brought into focus by Farber and coworkers,[5] who demonstrated in 1948 that treatment of leukemic children with the folate antagonist 4-amino-folic acid (aminopterin) induced remission of the disease, while administration of naturally occurring folate derivatives (which increased the availability of folates in the patients) had the adverse effect of accelerating the disease process. Shortly thereafter another analog, methotrexate (4-amino-10-methyl-folic acid, MTX), was found to be similarly effective as aminopterin, but less toxic. Although folate metabolism has been studied intensively since that time, and many other antifolates have been made and tested, methotrexate continues to be a first-line agent in the treatment of breast cancer, osteogenic sarcoma, and leukemias.

The Role of Folates in Cellular Metabolism

Folates exist within mammalian cells in many different forms. The core structure for all of these forms, folic acid, is not useful to mammalian cells in its fully oxidized native state. To perform its function as a coenzyme it must be reduced in two successive steps by dihydrofolate reductase (DHFR) to form 7,8-dihydrofolate and then 5,6,7,8-tetrahydrofolate (Figure 5–5). The latter, fully reduced form is the one that picks up and delivers single carbon units in various metabolic processes.

Folic acid (Pteroyl-L-Glutamic acid)

The single carbon units to be transferred by tetrahydrofolate can be attached to the folate structure at the N-5 or N-10 position (or both, forming an extra ring). Also, just as the main part of the molecule can assume different oxidation states, so too can the added carbon unit. In most of these steps the carbon transfer occurs without changing the oxidation status of the folate ring. If this were universally true, then cells would require only a catalytic amount of tetrahydrofolates, which could probably be met from dietary sources. However, the carbon transfer catalyzed by thymidylate synthase, conversion of dUMP to TMP, is accompanied by oxidation of the folate ring, yielding one dihydrofolate molecule per molecule of TMP produced. Therefore, cells must use DHFR to convert dihydrofolate back to tetrahydrofolate. The primary biochemical effect of methotrexate in mammalian cells is to inhibit DHFR activity. Once this inhibition occurs, and the preexisting pool of tetrahydrofolates is used up by TMP synthesis, de novo purine and thymidine nucleotide production cease.

Biochemical Determinants of Methotrexate Action

The factors that influence the effectiveness of methotrexate treatment in a given cell type can be divided into two broad categories. In one group are those factors that concentrate the drug intracellularly, such as transmembrane transport and metabolic conversion to higher-molecular-weight species (polyglutamates) that are preferentially retained within the cell. Factors in the second group include changes in the amount of DHFR present and structural alterations in the DHFR molecule that diminish methotrexate binding and determine how well intracellular methotrexate is able to inhibit de novo nucleotide synthesis.

At the plasma concentrations achieved following conventional dosing regimens (in the range of 1–10 μM), methotrexate primarily enters and leaves the cell via the same specific, saturable transport system used by natural reduced folates.[6] Alternative influx/efflux mechanisms may also be involved to some extent.[7] Cells selected for methotrexate resistance in vitro often have altered transport systems[8] and transport alterations often have also been found to be a common cause of resistance in model animal tumors in vivo.[9]

Once folates or their analogs reach the interior of a cell, their glutamate moieties are modified by the addition of glutamyl polymers. The sequential addition of glutamate molecules is catalyzed by folylpolyglutamyl synthetase, resulting in products containing up to a dozen glutamyl residues.[10] Due to the large size and highly charged nature of these polyglutamate derivatives, they are unable to exit the cell by

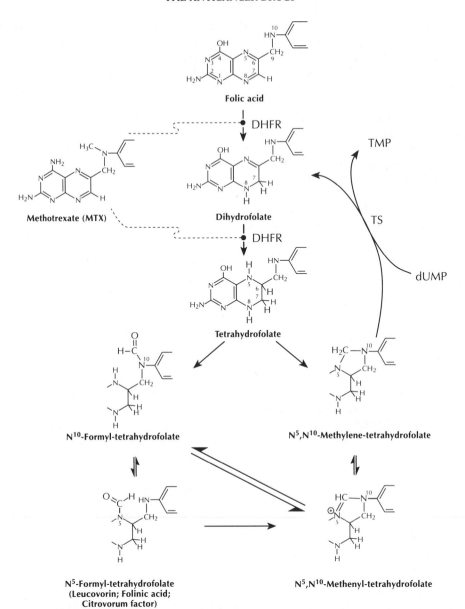

Figure 5–5　Folate interconversions and inhibition by methotrexate. Folic acid is converted in two steps by dihydrofolate reductase (DHFR) to the fully reduced form, tetrahydrofolate. This conversion is blocked by methotrexate. Consumption of methyl-bearing reduced folates, by the action of thymidylate synthase (TS), results in an inadequate source of methyl donors for purine and thymidylate synthesis.

passive diffusion and are also poor substrates for the folate efflux system. As a result, significant intracellular accumulation of folates and their analogs can occur, the magnitude of which is dictated by both the rate of extension of the polyglutamyl chain and by the rate of degradation of these polymers by γ-glutamyl hydrolase.[11] Although polyglutamylated folates are not efficiently used by the folate transport system, these conjugates are as good (or better) than their unconjugated counterparts at interacting with DHFR and thymidylate synthase.[12] It is therefore not surprising that the cytotoxic effects of methotrexate sometimes reflect its ability to be converted to polyglutamylated forms.

As discussed in detail in Chapter 4, cells can also be resistant to methotrexate because of an increase in the intracellular level of the target enzyme, DHFR. This increase is due to amplification of the number of copies of the DHFR structural gene. In the clinical setting, several cases have been documented in which there seems to be a correlation between lack of response to methotrexate treatment and the presence of amplified DHFR genes in tumor cells.[13] As better techniques for the controlled insertion of genes into mammalian cells and for introduction of altered cells into the body (e.g., via bone-marrow transplants) are developed, it may be possible to insert amplified DHFR genes into sensitive host tissues and protect them from the effects of intensive chemotherapy.[14]

In addition to the quantitative changes in the status of DHFR genes brought about by the continued presence of methotrexate, qualitative changes in the DHFR gene (i.e., structural mutations) can occur. The mutant reductases have altered kinetic properties[15] and specific base changes responsible for mutant enzymes have been identified.[16,17] Although such mutations have been observed in various experimental systems, there is no clear indication at this time that simple point mutations are a major cause of clinical resistance to methotrexate.

Pharmacology of MTX

CONVENTIONAL DOSE VS. "HIGH DOSE" ADMINISTRATION WITH LEUCOVORIN RESCUE. The demonstration that host tissues can be rescued from the harmful effects of intense methotrexate treatments by providing them with the reduced folate leucovorin (N^5-formyl-tetrahydrofolate, Figure 5-5), which circumvents methotrexate-induced inhibition of DHFR,[18] raised the possibility that these normal tissues could be protected from the lethal effects of methotrexate. The protection afforded by leucovorin appears to be selective in that it does not diminish the antitumor effect of methotrexate in model systems. Two arguments have been used to explain selective rescue by leucovorin. In one argument, tumor cells became resistant to methotrexate by virtue of diminished folate transport capacity, which limits their uptake of the drug at low concentrations. In the presence of high methotrexate concentrations, the drug gains access to both host and tumor cells by passive diffusion through the cell membrane, providing much greater tumor-cell kill but also putting host tissues at serious risk. When leucovorin is subsequently administered at relatively low concentrations, only the host cells (which are transport-competent) are able to utilize it, leaving the tumor cells to die.

A more recent explanation is based on differential reactivation of DHFR in host and tumor cells.[19] Although methotrexate and its polyglutamates bind tightly to DHFR, they can be displaced from the enzyme by tetrahydrofolates. In normal tissues there is relatively little accumulation of methotrexate polyglutamates and, as a result, administration of a modest concentration of leucovorin can produce enough intracellular reduced folates to regenerate a significant amount of DHFR activity. Tumor cells, on the other hand, generally accumulate sufficiently high levels of methotrexate polyglutamates so as to minimize displacement (and, therefore, rescue) by tetrahydrofolates derived from leucovorin.

Despite the theoretical advantages of using high-dose methotrexate followed by leucovorin rescue, it is still unclear if the benefits of this therapeutic approach outweigh its drawbacks.[20] Although it may be superior to conventional methotrexate administration in maintenance therapy for acute leukemia and for treatment of osteogenic sarcoma, it has shown no advantage in a variety of other human tumor types. Furthermore, it is a more expensive and technically demanding mode of treatment than conventional therapy. Additional clinical trials will be needed to resolve this issue.

ABSORPTION, DISTRIBUTION, AND ELIMINATION. Methotrexate can be administered by the oral, intravenous, intraarterial, or intrathecal route (Table 5-2). Although absorption of orally administered drug is efficient at low doses (≤ 12 mg/m^2) it is variable and incomplete at higher doses.[21,22] This is most likely due to its dependence on a saturable folate carrier.[23] At higher doses methotrexate is probably taken up by passive diffusion. Methotrexate distribution in tissues seems to reflect both the abil-

Table 5–2   Pharmacology of Methotrexate

Administration Regimen	Principal Indications	Toxicities	Other Characteristics
Chronic oral	Gestational choriocarcinoma	Bone-marrow depression, hepatic fibrosis	
Intermittent oral or intravenous	Acute lymphocytic leukemia, breast cancer	Bone-marrow depression, mucositis	
Intrathecal	Acute lymphocytic leukemia	Neurotoxicity (acute and delayed)	Prevents CNS relapse
High-dose intravenous	Osteogenic sarcoma	Mucositis, renal failure, neurotoxicity (acute and delayed), elevated hepatic enzymes	Requires leucovorin rescue

ity of the cell to transport the drug and the cellular level of dihydrofolate reductase. Very little methotrexate passes into the cerebrospinal fluid at concentrations achieved with conventional dose regimens. Since meningeal recurrence of leukemia is a serious threat, intrathecally delivered methotrexate and cranial irradiation have been used as prophylactic measures to prevent it. One apparent benefit of high-dose methotrexate regimens is that they permit high concentrations of the drug to reach the CNS, potentially obviating the need for these other measures.

Fifty percent of the drug is bound to serum protein, and its apparent volume of distribution is in the range of 67–91% of body weight.[24] Autoradiographic studies in mice reveal high concentrations of the drug in the kidney, intestinal epithelium, and the liver.[25] Drug accumulation in these organs is correlated with their high content of dihydrofolate reductase.[26] Methotrexate can also be sequestered in fluids such as ascites and pleural effusions.[27] If large volumes of of these fluids are present, a substantial amount of drug can accumulate there, and its prolonged release back into the general circulation can cause low (but toxic) drug levels to be maintained long after administration has been stopped.

In humans, methotrexate is excreted, predominantly as the unchanged drug, via the kidney by a combination of glomerular filtration and active tubular transport.[28] There appears to be appreciable enterohepatic circulation of the unchanged drug, since most of the drug secreted into the intestine in the bile is reabsorbed, with an average of only 2% of a dose appearing in the feces over a 4-day period.[29] When radiolabeled drug is given to patients at conventional doses, drug metabolism accounts for about 10% of the total radioactivity recovered in the urine. In mice, the intestinal bacteria may convert some of the drug to 4-amino-4-deoxy-N^{10}-methylpteroic acid, a less active compound.[30] There is significant oxidation of methotrexate to 7-hydroxy-methotrexate by hepatic aldehyde oxidase in some animals (e.g., rabbits and guinea pigs),[31] but this metabolite has not been observed in the urine of humans receiving conventional doses of the drug. Significant amounts of 7-hydroxy-methotrexate, however, are excreted after high-dose methotrexate therapy in humans.[32] Thus, 7-hydroxy-methotrexate production is dose dependent, and presumably the enzyme system catalyzing the reaction has a low affinity for the drug. It has been suggested that this 7-hydroxy compound, which is less soluble in water than methotrexate, may contribute to the nephrotoxicity observed in patients on high-dose therapy.[32]

It is difficult to summarize concisely the complex pharmacokinetics of methotrexate. The plasma disappearance curve has been characterized as triphasic with half-lives of 0.75, 3.5, and 27 hours.[29] In addition, long-term retention of methotrexate in tissues like the kidney and the liver accounts for the exceedingly slow terminal loss of the drug from the body. The pharmacokinetics reflect cellular transport, dihydrofolate reductase levels, enterohepatic circulation, third-space accumulation, as well as significant metabolism when high doses of the drug are given. It is important to understand this complex pharmacology, since toxicity depends upon the duration of exposure to inhibitory levels of methotrexate. The appropriate dose of leucovorin and the duration of its administration in rescue protocols also depend upon the pharmacokinetics of the drug. Given the complexity of the kinetics and the toxicity of methotrexate, measurement of its plasma concentration during treatment can be quite valuable. Enzymatic assays and immunoassays are available to the clinician for this purpose.

Clinical Use and Toxicity

Methotrexate is used to treat a wide variety of neoplastic diseases.[33] It is the drug of choice for the treatment of gestational choriocarcinoma, with cures being obtained in a substantial number of patients.[34] Methotrexate is very useful in the management of acute lymphocytic leukemia of childhood, where it is given at low doses for maintenance of remission (by combined systemic and intrathecal routes), or at high doses (by the systemic route only).[35] Both conventional and high-dose methotrexate regimens are used with significant success to treat patients with osteogenic sarcoma and with more modest success against head and neck cancer.[20] Methotrexate is also used effectively in combination with other drugs for the adjuvant therapy of breast cancer.[36] Although cyclophosphamide is the drug of choice in Burkitt's lymphoma, methotrexate has been used effectively in this disease. Remissions of significant duration are achieved in mycosis fungoides patients. Methotrexate is considered to produce objective responses in some patients with lung cancer, epidermal carcinomas of the cervix, and a few other solid tumors.[33]

Methotrexate is occasionally used to treat some non-neoplastic diseases. In low doses, it has a well-established role in the treatment of severe psoriasis and psoriatic arthritis.[37] After systematic administration, some methotrexate is distributed to the skin,[38] where it inhibits DNA synthesis in the rapidly proliferating psoriatic epidermal cells.[39] The mechanism of its effect in psoriatic arthritis, however, is not clear. Because it is immunosuppressive,[40] methotrexate had been used in the past to treat several diseases thought to have an immunological etiology, including Wegener's granulomatosis, systemic lupus erythematosis, and chronic rheumatoid arthritis.[41]

Toxic effects occur with conventional methotrexate therapy and with high-dose administration, but the latter is of particular interest with respect to pharmacological monitoring of therapy. In high-dose protocols, the patient is exposed to potentially lethal concentrations of the drug and the physician must rescue normal tissues with leucovorin. Patients who experience toxic reactions after high-dose therapy clearly have higher average blood levels of the drug than those who do not experience toxic reactions. This relationship is shown in Figure 5–6, where the vertically striped area of the graph represents the range of serum methotrexate levels observed in patients who did not have a toxic reaction and the diagonally striped area the serum levels in patients who did have a toxic reaction during leucovorin rescue.[42] Such high-risk patients can usually be identified by observing their serum methotrexate levels at 24 and 48 hours after treatment, to detect an unusually long half-life of the drug during this time.[36] Monitoring drug levels is therefore a vital part of this therapeutic regimen. Any condition that impairs renal excretion of the drug increases the risk of toxicity. The patient's renal status should be carefully monitored, and both adequate hydration and alkalinization of the urine are necessary to ensure efficient drug clearance.

The two major sites of methotrexate toxicity are the bone marrow and the endothelium of the oropharynx and gastrointestinal tract. The severity of the clinical effects depends to a great extent on the duration of exposure to inhibitory levels of the drug and not on the peak plasma level. All of the stem-cell types of the marrow can be affected, to produce leukopenia, thrombocytopenia, and, with long-term administration, anemia. After a single dose, granulocyte and platelet count depression is usually maximal at about day 10. As with almost all the anticancer drugs, methotrexate therapy must be modified according to the patient's hematological status, and leukocyte and platelet counts must be rigorously monitored. The endothelium of the oropharynx and gas-

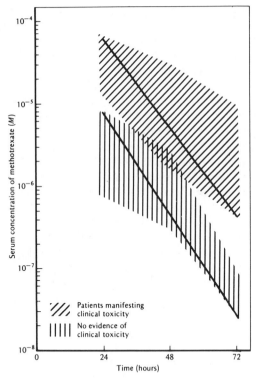

Figure 5–6 Methotrexate serum levels in patients who developed clinical toxicity and in those who did not after high-dose therapy. Serum levels of methotrexate were determined by microbiological assay 24, 48, and 72 hours after the start of a 4-hour, high-dose (8 g/m²) methotrexate infusion. Patients received leucovorin (9–15 mg) 2 hours after completion of the methotrexate infusion and every 6 hours for an additional 12 doses. Clinical toxicity was defined a oral mucositis, fever, hematological depression, and/or generalized rash. (From Nirenberg *et al.*[42])

trointestinal tract is particularly sensitive to methotrexate. Oral damage may range from mild erythema of the buccal mucosa to extensive ulceration of the oropharynx, and the effect on the intestinal tract ranges from mild diarrhea to severe ulceration and bleeding. Oral mucositis is prognostic of a more severe reaction if the drug is continued. Therapy must be interrupted if diarrhea and ulcerative stomatitis occur.

Because most of the methotrexate administered is excreted by the kidney unchanged, impaired renal function can delay excretion and

increase the risk of toxic reactions. This is especially important in high-dose therapy when both creatinine clearance and blood methotrexate levels should be monitored. Methotrexate itself causes kidney damage, which is a frequent complication of high-dose therapy.[43] The mechanism of the renal toxicity, which is manifested by elevated serum creatinine and decreased creatinine clearance, has been studied in animal models. Crystalline deposits of methotrexate and methotrexate-derived material have been demonstrated in the renal tubules of rhesus monkeys, and most of the non-protein-bound drug remaining in the monkey kidney after 24 hours (77%) represents the 7-hydroxymethotrexate metabolite.[32] The presence of crystalline deposits is not surprising, since methotrexate has a low aqueous solubility and the solubility of the 7-hydroxy metabolite in water is even lower. At our current level of understanding, most of the nephrotoxicity would appear to be due to the deposition of crystals in the renal tubules. Both the drug and its metabolite are more soluble at higher pH and the risk of nephrotoxicity can be minimized in patients on high-dose therapy by alkalinizing the urine and ensuring good urine flow.[44]

High dose methotrexate can cause transient elevations in hepatic enzymes, indicative of hepatotoxicity. A second type of hepatotoxicity occurs in low-dosage therapy, as in the treatment of psoriasis, with about a 3% incidence of severe hepatic pathology, including cirrhosis.[45,46] The mechanism of the effect is not known. It is also not known why the problem is more commonly seen with continuous, low-dose therapy than with intermittent administration.[21,46] Chronic use of methotrexate in maintenance therapy of acute lymphocytic leukemia has also been associated with liver pathology, including portal fibrosis.[47]

Methotrexate can cause a reversible pulmonary syndrome, which has been observed primarily in children undergoing maintenance therapy. The syndrome is rapidly progressive, with cough, dyspnea, fever, and cyanosis. Radiographic findings include diffuse bilateral pulmonary infiltrates, which are predominantly interstitial; the syndrome must be differentiated from an infectious process, particularly the interstitial pneumonia caused by

Pneumocystis carinii.[48] Although eosinophilia has been observed in some cases, and it has been suggested that the syndrome represents a hypersensitivity reaction, the mechanism is not known. Furthermore, this syndrome will often not reappear upon retreatment, as would be expected in the case of hypersensitivity.[44]

Nausea and anorexia frequently occur as acute side effects of methotrexate therapy. Various skin rashes have also been reported, the most common being a maculopapular rash occurring in the upper trunk and neck, with an incidence that is possibly as high as 10% to 20%.[41] Protection from solar exposure may prevent these reactions. Alopecia and osteoporosis can occur in methotrexate therapy. Methotrexate is an abortifacient and has been shown to be teratogenic in rats, and thus it should not be given to pregnant psoriatic patients. The physician should advise female cancer patients of childbearing age of these potential effects.

Intrathecal and high-dose administration of methotrexate is accompanied by a range of neurotoxicities.[49] Acute manifestations (within hours to a few days after treatment) can include headache, nausea, disorientation, and other symptoms associated with elevated intracranial pressure. Within a few days to a few weeks, subacute toxicity may be seen as evidenced by motor deficits. Long-term delayed toxicity can arise in the form of encephalopathy. Whereas the acute and subacute complications are often rapidly reversible upon discontinuation of the drug, the delayed encephalopathic phenomenon reverses over a much longer period of time, if at all.

The average age of patients who experience neurotoxicity is significantly higher than that of patients who do not. This may, in part, reflect the fact that the intrathecal drug dosage is sometimes determined on the basis of body surface area, a calculation that could yield higher doses in relation to cerebrospinal fluid volume in older children and adults. Meningeal leukemia can alter cerebrospinal fluid dynamics, and this may also predispose patients to neurotoxicity. There is evidence that patients who experience neurotoxicity have a more prolonged exposure to higher cerebrospinal fluid levels of the drug than have nontoxic patients.[50]

Trimetrexate: A "Nonclassical" Folate Antagonist

Trimetrexate is one of a series of lipophilic DHFR inhibitors that were synthesized with the aim of circumventing methotrexate resistance due to transport deficiency.[51] It was thought that the lipid nature of these compounds would allow them to be taken up by passive diffusion. This appears to be the case to some extent, although trimetrexate is also taken up through a relatively low-affinity carrier separate from the folate transport system.[52] The structure of trimetrexate is quite different from the folate analogs that preceded it, in that its main ring structure is a 2,4-diaminoquinazoline (rather than a pteridine) and that it completely lacks a glutamate residue. For this reason, it is called a "nonclassical" antifolate.

Trimetrexate (TMQ)

Early studies indicated that, as hoped, some cells that were resistant to methotrexate were still quite sensitive to trimetrexate.[52] In addition, trimetrexate appeared to have a broader spectrum of activity in model systems than did methotrexate.[53] Phase II clinical studies of trimetrexate are still under way, and although it has shown some activity against breast, non-small-cell lung, and head and neck tumors, it is not yet clear if this drug will be sufficiently superior to methotrexate to supplant it in the treatment of these or other neoplasms.[53,54]

Pyrimidine Antagonists

Whereas folate antagonists affect thymidine nucleotide production *indirectly,* other commonly used anticancer drugs are *direct* inhibitors of thymidylate synthase, the key enzyme in this process (see Fig. 5-3). The most impor-

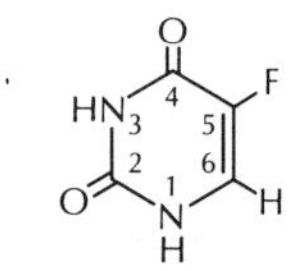

5-Fluorouracil
(FUra)

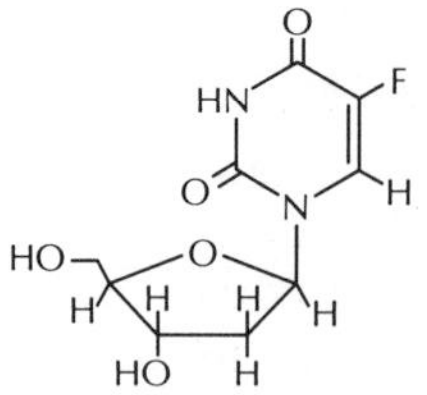

5-Fluorodeoxyuridine
(FdUrd)

tant members of this group are 5-fluorouracil (FUra) and its nucleoside derivative, 5-fluoro-2′-deoxyuridine (FdUrd).

Sites and Determinants of Fluoropyrimidine Action

In contrast to methotrexate, whose effects are in one way or another attributable to inhibition of a single enzyme (DHFR), the fluoropyrimidines are more typical of the antimetabolite class in that they can induce multiple biochemical lesions, any one of which has the potential to be cytotoxic.

INHIBITION OF THYMIDINE NUCLEOTIDE SYNTHESIS. Of the biochemical effects known to result from fluoropyrimidine treatment, direct inhibition of thymidylate synthase is the best characterized one (Fig. 5–7A). This inhibition occurs when the enzyme attempts to use fluorodeoxyuridine monophosphate (FdUMP) as a substrate.[55] Ordinarily, thymidylate synthase catalyzes the methylation of dUMP in a multistep process, summarized in Fig. 5–8A. When FdUMP is utilized instead, the process becomes frozen at an intermediate step, trapping the enzyme, the pseudosubstrate, and the folate cofactor in a covalent ternary complex (Fig. 5–8B). Although this complex can dissociate very slowly,[56] it is sufficiently stable so as to effectively prevent the trapped enzyme molecule from making any significant contribution toward TMP production. Because steady-state pools of thymidine nucleotides are small, DNA synthesis is inhibited until the drug is withdrawn and new thymidylate synthase can be made.

Although FUra and FdUrd can both be con-

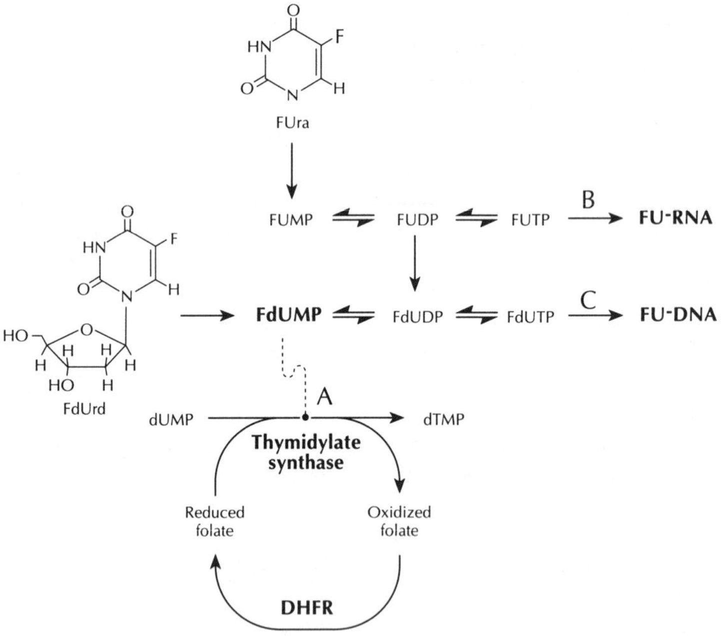

Figure 5–7   Sites of fluoropyrimidine action. Both 5-fluorouracil (FUra) and 5-fluorodeoxyuridine (FdUrd) can be metabolized to 5-fluorodeoxyuridine monophosphate (FdUMP), which inhibits thymidylate synthase and, consequently, DNA synthesis (A). FUra can also be metabolized to the ribonucleoside triphosphate, FUTP, and incorporated into various types of RNA, inhibiting their metabolism and function (B). Both drugs can be converted to the deoxyribonucleoside triphosphate, FdUTP, which is incorporated into DNA (C).

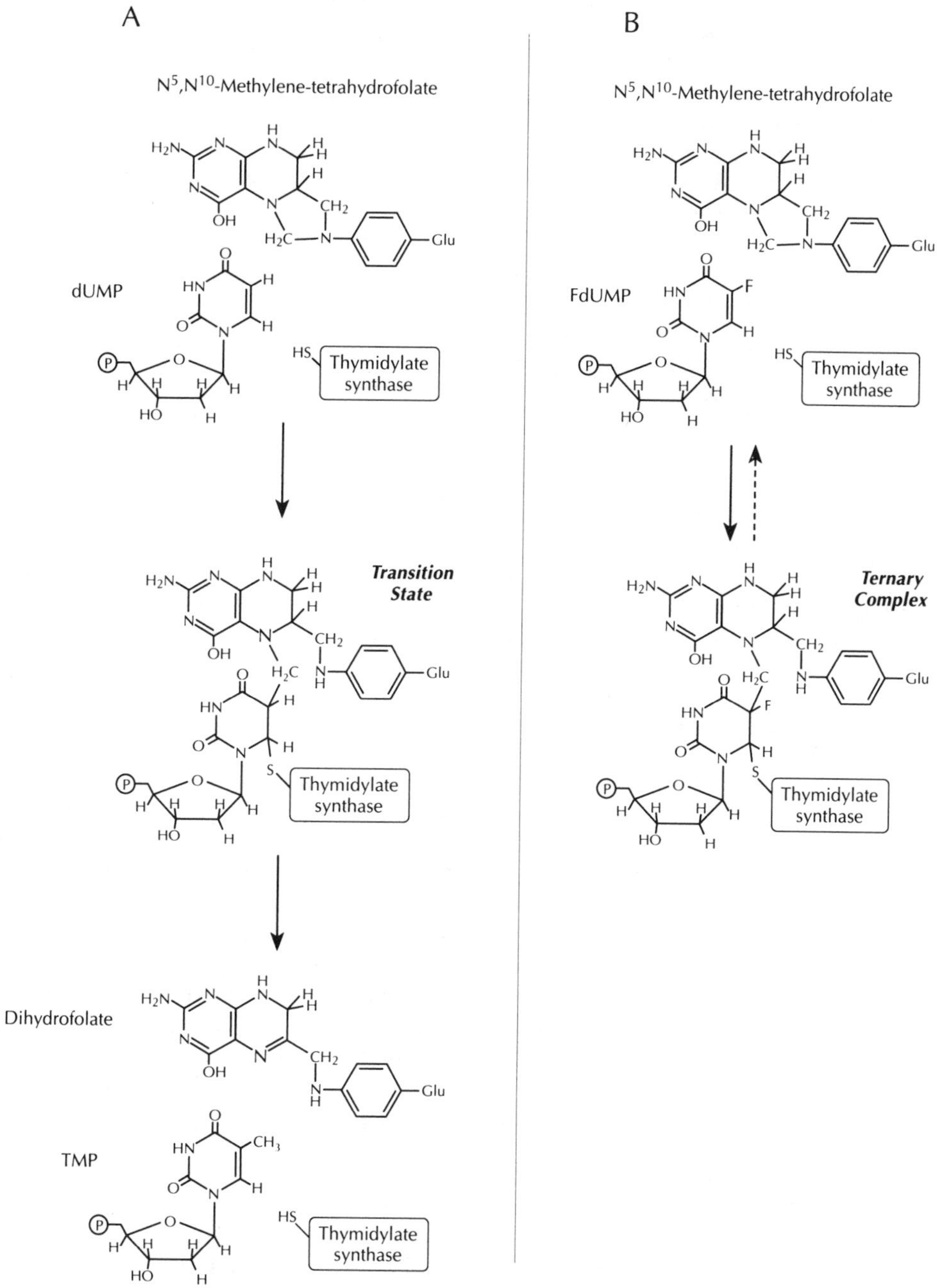

Figure 5-8 Inhibition of thymdylate synthase (TS) by FdUMP. (A) Normal conversion of dUMP to TMP by TS involves formation of a transition state complex containing the enzyme, the substrate and the reduced folate methyl donor. This structure decomposes into product (TMP), oxidized cofactor (dihyrofolate), and free enzyme. (B) when FdUMP is used in place of dUMP the reaction fails because the fluorine atom, unlike the hydrogen atom in dUMP, cannot be easily abstracted. Instead, a stable ternary complex is formed that decomposes very slowly, thereby trapping and inactivating the enzyme.

verted to FdUMP in intact mammalian cells, FdUrd is typically a much more potent inhibitor of thymidylate synthase activity, often being effective in the low-nanomolar-concentration range. This is because only one step is required to metabolize FdUrd to FdUMP (i.e., phosphorylation by thymidine kinase), whereas conversion of FUra to FdUMP is a multistep process (see Fig. 5–7). As a result, thymidylate synthase inhibition by FUra usually requires micromolar concentrations of that drug. When such concentrations are applied, other active metabolites are also produced in significant quantities, most notably fluorouridine triphosphate (FUTP), which can become incorporated into RNA in place of UTP (Fig. 5–7B).

INCORPORATION INTO NUCLEIC ACIDS. Because ribosomal RNA is the most abundant type of RNA, effects of FUra incorporation were first noted in this species. Wilkinson and Pitot observed that FUra treatment can inhibit the endonuclease-catalyzed conversion of 45S ribosomal RNA precursors to their normal 28S and 18S mature products.[57] Although this inhibition is significant under some circumstances, several studies have demonstrated that RNA-directed cytotoxicity can occur under conditions during which rRNA function and cellular content are essentially normal,[58] thus implicating other RNA species as targets for FUra. Several properties of mRNA can be affected by FUra incorporation, including transcription,[59] intracellular distribution,[60] and translation.[61] Although the molecular basis for disruption of RNA function by FUra incorporation is not completely understood, studies on self-splicing *Tetrahymena* RNA suggest that the base-pairing properties of the incorporated analog are sufficiently different from those of uracil so as to distort or destroy intramolecular interactions that are necessary for maintaining biologically active conformations.[62]

In contrast to the relatively high level of FUra incorporation into RNA, its incorporation into DNA is much smaller. In fact, for many years it was assumed that FUra was not incorporated into DNA to any significant degree. However, in the early 1980s sensitive methodology emerged that permitted the detection of FUra in DNA, albeit at low levels (typically on the order of 0.01–0.001% replace-ment of thymine).[63,64] Evaluating the biological significance of FUra incorporation into DNA has been difficult, since the frequency of this event tends to parallel the magnitude of FUra's other effects. Furthermore, since it is possible that cytotoxicity might be related to the rate and efficiency of excision of FUra from DNA, it is not clear that the steady-state level of FUra incorporation is necessarily the most informative parameter to reflect the biological impact of this phenomenon.[58,65]

RESISTANCE. Several factors can influence the degree to which a particular fluoropyrimidine treatment inhibits TMP synthesis. As is the case with all antimetabolites, alterations in the enzymatic pathways by which the administered drug is converted to active metabolites can influence its actions. Thus, deficiencies in thymidine kinase and orotic acid phosphoribosyl transferase have been shown to be responsible for resistance to FdUrd and FUra, respectively, in cell culture systems.[66] While anabolic defects can affect all of the potentially cytotoxic mechanisms of these drugs, other factors are more specifically related to thymidylate synthase inhibition. For example, the quantity[67,68] and quality[69] of the target enzyme are critical determinants of the extent of inhibition of thymidylate synthesis. It has also been recognized that availability of the reduced folate cofactor has a profound impact on the effectiveness of thymidylate synthase inhibition by fluoropyrimidines.[70] This knowledge has been applied to the design of clinical treatment protocols and the increased efficacy of fluoropyrimidine treatment by concurrent administration of a reduced folate (leucovorin) represents a significant advance in the use of these drugs.[71]

RELATIVE IMPORTANCE OF RNA- AND DNA-DIRECTED MECHANISMS OF FURA. Numerous studies have been performed with the aim of determining whether RNA- or DNA-directed effects are more important in mediating the antitumor (and host-toxic) effects of FUra. Currently available information suggests that thymidylate synthase inhibition (and subsequent DNA synthesis inhibition) is the lesion to which tumor-cell kill can most often be attributed. This statement is based both on biochemical data from studies on human tumors[72,73] and on the improved therapeutic response obtained when leucovorin is combined with FUra, as discussed above. However, if thymidylate synthase inhibition were the only important mechanism in FUra-induced cytotoxicity, then exogenously supplied thymidine would always protect cells from FUra. Not only does thymidine fail to act as a universal antidote to FUra, it can enhance that drug's cytotoxic effects in some cases.[74,75] It is therefore probable that FUra's primary cytotoxic mechanism is not the same in all cell lines, and that this heterogeneity is the basis for the wide variability of response to FUra treatment observed *in vivo*.

Pharmacology of the Fluoropyrimidines

ABSORPTION, DISTRIBUTION, AND ELIMINATION. Fluorouracil is usually administered parenterally, since absorption from the gastrointestinal tract is incomplete and unpredictable.[76] For many years FUra has been given by bolus IV injection or by short infusions. Typical bolus regimens result in peak plasma concentrations in the range of 0.1–1 mM, occurring within minutes of administration, followed by a biphasic elimination profile with a terminal half-life of 10–20 minutes.[77] Because of the rapid disappearance of FUra from the circulation, plasma levels that result from daily bolus injections fluctuate over several orders of magnitude. Since DNA synthesis inhibition is an effect aimed primarily at cells in the S phase of the cell cycle, this fluctuation presents a significant therapeutic problem: tumor cells not in S phase at the time of treatment are unlikely to be exposed to an effective concentration of the drug at the stage of their cell cycle when they would be most sensitive to it. Protocols using continuous infusions of FUra were developed to overcome this potential problem.

Various continuous infusion schedules have been used for FUra, ranging from one day to several weeks.[78] The steady-state plasma concentrations achieved on these schedules vary somewhat, due to the nonlinear pharmacokinetics of FUra,[79] but are generally in a range of 1–10 micromolar.[78] Design of infusion protocols was initially limited by the need to execute them in an inpatient setting, although improvements in the design of vascular access de-

vices and portable pumping systems have now made it practical to conduct IV infusions for any period of time. Such advances also permit extended intraarterial infusions of FdUrd, especially for the regional treatment of primary or metastatic tumors in the liver. Other routes of administration for FUra include intraperitoneal injection for the treatment of disseminated abdominal tumors[80] and topical application. FUra distributes into most extracellular fluids, including cerebrospinal fluid, ascites fluid and pleural effusions,[81] with an apparent volume of distribution corresponding to about that of extracellular water (about 25% of total body water).[82]

Elimination of FUra is primarily accomplished through metabolism, with only a small fraction of the drug being excreted unchanged. Both anabolic and catabolic processes contribute to disappearance of the drug from plasma, although catabolism by the enzyme dihydrouracil dehydrogenase is the key step in the ultimate disposition of FUra.[83] This enzyme converts FUra to the 5,6-dihydro derivative, after which the ring is split to form α-fluoro-β-ureidopropionic acid. These intermediates are then catabolized to α-fluoro-β-alanine, ammonia, urea, and carbon dioxide, as in the degradation of uracil. Both the toxicity and antitumor effects of FUra are potentiated if catabolism is blocked by dihydrouracil dehydrogenase inhibition. The liver is the major site of FUra inactivation, although it has been deduced that nonhepatic sites of metabolism are also important.[79]

Clinical Use and Toxicity

FUra is used to treat several of the most commonly occurring types of solid tumors, including colorectal, breast, head and neck, gastric, and pancreatic cancers.[66] FUra, given topically, is also used for the treatment of solar keratoses and multiple superficial basal cell carcinomas, but it is not recommended for invasive skin cancer. Topical FUra permits the selective resolution of the malignant or premalignant lesion, with minimal effects of adjacent normal skin.

Many strategies have been devised to enhance FUra's clinical activity, based on mechanistic information. Some of these approaches

Table 5–3   Fluoropyrimidine Toxicities. Dose-limiting lesions are shown in bold type

Mode of Administration	Fluorouracil	Fluorodeoxyuridine
Bolus intravenous	**Bone-marrow depression** mucositis, nausea, vomiting, alopecia, acute cerebellar dysfunction	—
Continuous infusion (intravenous)	**Mucositis, diarrhea,** dermopathy ("hand-foot" syndrome), bone marrow depression (mild)	—
Continuous infusion (hepatic arterial)	**Mucositis,** nausea, vomiting, diarrhea, cholestatic jaundice, elevated liver enzymes	**Biliary sclerosis,** elevated liver enzymes

involve a combination of FUra with other cytotoxic agents (e.g., methotrexate), while others combine FUra with agents that are themselves not toxic, but that modulate FUra's cytotoxic effects.[77] The most successful of these strategies has been the enhancement of FUra activity against colorectal tumors by combination with leucovorin, which enhances formation of the ternary complex shown in Figure 5–8.[84] Response rates with this regimen have been reported to be as high as 45%, compared to about 15–20% with FUra alone.[85]

Nausea, vomiting, anorexia, stomatitis, and diarrhea can occur during systemic therapy with FUra, the frequency of side effects varying with the treatment schedule employed (Table 5–3). FUra is more toxic to proliferating than to nonproliferating cells, and clinical toxicity is more pronounced in tissues with a high growth fraction. Stomatitis and diarrhea are the most common dose-limiting toxicities when FUra is given by continuous infusion. Effects on the alimentary canal can proceed to severe ulceration of the oropharynx and bowel. When the drug is administered by repetitive bolus injection the most serious toxicity is bone-marrow depression, manifested by leukopenia and somewhat less often by thrombocytopenia and anemia. The lowest granulocyte count usually occurs in 7 to 14 days. Alopecia, thinning of the skin, nail changes, dermatitis, and photosensitivity (manifested by erythema or increased skin pigmentation) can also occur. Erythematous desquamation of the palms and soles ("hand-foot" syndrome) often occurs following extended infusions of fluorouracil.

Fluorouracil also produces an acute cerebellar syndrome in less than 1% of patients (the incidence may be higher with intensive daily treatment regimens).[86] The clinical picture includes ataxia of the trunk or extremities, nystagmus, slurred speech, and dizziness. The syndrome is reversible, with symptom abatement occurring 1 to 6 weeks after therapy is discontinued. Extreme caution must be used in FUra therapy of patients who are severely debilitated or who have markedly impaired hepatic or renal function. Teratogenicity is a risk, since fetal malformations have been observed in mice and rats.

Other Antagonists of Pyrimidine Metabolism

CB3717 (N[10]-PROPARGYL-5,8-DIDEAZAFOLIC ACID) Both the antifolates and the fluoropyrimidines have the ultimate effect of depriving cells of thymidine nucleotides, through divergent mechanisms. The interactivity of folate and thymidylate metabolism is emphasized by the properties of a new class of compounds that can inhibit both thymidylate synthase and DHFR. The best characterized of these agents is N[10]-propargyl-5,8-dideazafolic acid, which, in the absence of a commonly accepted trivial name, will be referred to here by the manufacturer's identifier, CB3717.

CB3717 is one of a series of quinazoline an-

CB3717 (N[10]-Propargyl-5,8-dideazafolic Acid)

alogs that were synthesized with different substituents at the N^{10} position.[87] In view of the antifolate activity of the related compound, trimetrexate, it was not surprising that the members of this series inhibited DHFR. As was the case with trimetrexate, it was anticipated that the more lipophilic nature of these compounds might allow them to bypass folate transport and, therefore, to be effective against cells resistant to methotrexate by virtue of reduced uptake. In addition, it was found that these compounds directly inhibit thymidylate synthase and, in the case of CB3717, do so with great selectivity (i.e., with relatively little effect on DHFR).[87] This observation raised the possibility that CB3717 might also be effective against tumor cells whose methotrexate resistance was due to DHFR overproduction, since DHFR would not be its major target. The realization of these predictions in a series of human tumor cell lines[88] has led to considerable interest in the clinical evaluation of CB3717 and related drugs.

Phase I and II trials indicate that CB3717 may be useful for treating ovarian and breast cancers and mesothelioma.[89] Renal toxicity was dose-limiting under the conditions used for these studies, and hepatotoxicity and malaise were frequently observed as well. Work is continuing to try to improve the clinical application of this compound (e.g., by using urinary alkalinization to reduce nephrotoxicity), as well as on the development of other related drugs.

AZACYTIDINE. Unlike the other pyrimidine antagonists covered in this section, the activity of 5-azacytidine (aza-C) is unrelated to thymidine nucleotide metabolism. Rather, aza-C appears to exert its effects as a consequence of being incorporated into RNA and DNA in place of cytosine. The acute cytotoxicity of this drug has been attributed to its disruption of various RNA functions.[90] Aza-C is known to be chemically unstable in neutral or alkaline solutions, resulting in a spontaneous ring-opening reaction, and it has been suggested that the decomposition of incorporated analog may be responsible for its effect on RNA.[91]

Much greater attention has been given to the effects of aza-C incorporation on DNA methylation. It has been well established that the transcriptional activity of many genes is closely

5-Azacytidine (Aza-C)

correlated with the methylation status of nearby cytosine residues.[92] This methylation pattern is preserved though generations of cell division by the action of a methyltransferase whose activity is noncompetitively inhibited if it attempts to methylate an aza-C residue. Extensive incorporation of aza-C into DNA results in decreased DNA methylation and, concomitantly, major alterations in gene expression and differentiation status.[93] Although the changes in gene expression that result from aza-C treatment appear to be nonrandom, it has not yet been determined why this drug has a selective effect on some genes but not others. Elucidation of the basis of this phenomenon would likely lead to novel and therapeutically valuable applications.

Aza-C has limited clinical activity and is under continued evaluation for use against acute nonlymphocytic leukemia.[94] Due to its instability in solution, it must be freshly prepared for parenteral administration.

Purine Antagonists

The two major drugs in this category are the thiopurines 6-mercaptopurine (6-MP) and 6-thioguanine (6-TG), which are analogs of hypoxanthine and guanine, respectively.

6-Mercaptopurine (6-MP) Hypoxanthine

6-Thioguanine (6-TG) Guanine

The thiopurines are similar to FUra in the sense that they cause nucleotide synthesis inhibition as well as being incorporated into nucleic acids. With FUra, however, these two actions are somewhat independent, since the major effect on nucleotide metabolism concerns DNA synthesis while the major site of analog incorporation is into RNA. 6-MP and 6-TG inhibit the synthesis of both ribo- and deoxyribonucleotides, and can be incorporated to a significant extent into both RNA and DNA. As a result, these mechanisms can interact with each other in complex ways.

Sites and Determinants of Thiopurine Action

INHIBITION OF PURINE SYNTHESIS. Metabolic activation of the thiopurines usually proceeds through the salvage enzyme HPRTase, which produces thioinosine monophosphate (thio-IMP) from 6-MP and thioguanosine monophosphate (thio-GMP) from 6-TG (Fig. 5–9). Each of these species can inhibit *de novo* purine synthesis at several points, most notably at the first committed step in the purine pathway (PRPP amidotransferase) and at the branch point where IMP is channeled toward guanine nucleotide synthesis (IMP dehydrogenase). Thio-IMP and thio-GMP are subject to further anabolism along the routes ordinarily used by guanine nucleotides and are ultimately converted to thioguanosine triphosphate (thio-GTP) and thiodeoxyguanosine triphosphate (thio-dGTP), which can then be incorporated into nucleic acids.

On the surface, it is not clear why inhibition

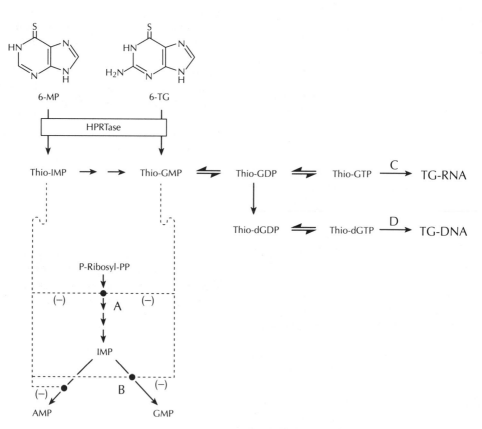

Figure 5–9   Sites of thiopurine action. 6-Mercaptopurine (6-MP) and 6-thioguanine (6-TG) are both anabolized to ribonucleoside monophosphates (thio-IMP and thio-GMP, respectively) by hypoxanthine phosphoribosyl transferase (HPRTase). These metabolites inhibit the first step in the *de novo* purine synthesis pathway (PRPP amidotransferase, A) and the key step in guanine nucleotide biosynthesis, IMP dehydrogenase (B). The TG derivatives are also converted to triphosphates that can be incorporated into RNA (C) and DNA (D).

of the *de novo* purine synthesis pathway should be selectively toxic to neoplastic cells, since normal cells also require purines for their existence. However, it has been observed that there is a close correlation between proliferative status and some of the enzyme activities in this pathway, especially IMP dehydrogenase.[95] It has been proposed that the neoplastic state is characterized by a shift in the overall metabolic program of the cell, part of which results in the expression of different isoenzymes than are expressed in the untransformed state.[96] It has been reported that at least two isoenzymes for IMP dehydrogenase exist in humans,[97] and it is possible that the activity or expression of these forms may be differentially affected by antimetabolites. It is also known that several proteins (including the *ras* oncogene) mediate intracellular signaling in a GTP-dependent manner, and it is possible that GTP depletion might alter signal transduction. In any case, although the mechanistic reasons are undefined, purine synthesis inhibitors exhibit significant antitumor activity *in vivo*.

INCORPORATION INTO NUCLEIC ACIDS. Because 6-MP is an analog of hypoxanthine, its metabolites cannot be incorporated directly; they must first merge with the anabolic pathway for 6-TG-containing nucleotides, by conversion of thio-IMP to thio-GMP (Fig. 5–9). Both agents are therefore incorporated in the same form, as 6-TG derivatives. Although incorporation into RNA can be significant, and can inhibit rRNA maturation,[98] most studies have focused on the biological effects of DNA incorporation.

Unlike the situation with FdUTP, there is no specific, active mechanism for excluding thio-dGTP from DNA. Furthermore, thio-dGTP is nearly as good a substrate for DNA synthesis as dGTP in cell-free systems.[99,100] As a result, 6-TG and 6-MP can be incorporated into cellular DNA to a much greater extent than FUra or FdUrd. As much as 1–2% of the guanine moieties in cellular DNA can be replaced by 6-TG.[101,102] The consequences of 6-TG incorporation into DNA are not realized immediately. Exposure conditions that cause extensive substitution by 6-TG during the S phase of a given cell cycle often have little effect on progression through that cycle.[103,104] During the next cycle,

however, cells become arrested in late-S and G2 phases.[104,105] This arrest is associated with a severe and specific form of DNA damage in which one chromatid on each chromosome is preferentially disrupted, a pattern consistent with the failure of the 6-TG-containing strand to function properly as a replication template.[105] Although the mechanism of this disruption is not precisely understood, it has been shown that the presence of incorporated 6-TG can antagonize sequence-specific binding of proteins to DNA,[106] and it has been proposed that 6-TG incorporation may inhibit the function of chromosomal replication origins.[107]

INTERACTIONS BETWEEN THIOPURINE MECHANISMS. 6-MP and 6-TG are sometimes referred to as "self-limiting" drugs, because their biochemical effects can antagonize one another. That is, incorporation of the drug into DNA can be decreased when total DNA synthesis is inhibited by purine starvation. The degree to which such interactions actually take place is highly variable, and can depend on the concentration of the drug and the particular cell line or tissue being studied. Owing to the dose-dependence of these interactions, it has been observed in some systems that 6-MP[108] and 6-TG[109] are actually less cytotoxic at high concentrations than they are at lower concentrations, presumably due to prevention of analog incorporation into DNA by purine-synthesis inhibition.

In addition, although we have referred to 6-MP and 6-TG as if their actions were identical, there are circumstances in which their primary cytotoxic mechanisms are clearly different.[110] It has been shown that resistance to one of them does not necessarily confer resistance to the other, and that combinations of 6-MP and 6-TG can be synergistically effective against tumors *in vivo*.[111] Each of these observations implies that the two agents were not acting in exactly the same manner in that system. The most likely reason for these differences is that, although more than one of the thiopurine metabolites can inhibit *de novo* purine synthesis, the most potent one (thio-IMP) is unique to 6-MP.

Owing to the factors discussed above, it is difficult to predict which thiopurine mechanism (i.e., inhibition of purine synthesis or incorporation into DNA) is primarily responsible for killing leukemic cells in humans, under the exposure conditions achieved using standard treatment protocols. The major mechanism may even vary from patient to patient, depending on the spectrum of metabolites generated in each case. It may be possible to obtain some mechanistic information by observing the type of cell-cycle arrest resulting from thiopurine treatments, since each of the two mechanisms appears to cause its own characteristic pattern of cytokinetic disturbance.[112]

RESISTANCE. For either purine synthesis inhibition or DNA incorporation to take place, efficient generation and maintenance of nucleotide forms of 6-MP or 6-TG is necessary. Resistance to 6-MP and 6-TG *in vitro* is often due to deletion of the first enzyme in the anabolic pathway, HPRTase. Because this lesion is so common in cell-culture systems, the frequency of occurrence of 6-TG-resistant cells has often been used as an index of the mutagenic effect of various chemical and physical insults.

A very different pattern is seen in humans receiving thiopurine therapy, where HPRTase deficiency does not consistently correlate with resistance.[113] An alternative mechanism of resistance was identified in cell culture, characterized by a sharp elevation in membrane-bound alkaline phosphatase activity.[114] It was hypothesized that this catabolic activity could protect tumor cells by antagonizing the accumulation of thiopurine nucleotides. Although increased alkaline phosphatase activity was elevated at the time of relapse in some patients undergoing therapy with 6-MP, neither this factor nor HPRTase activity was a strong correlate of drug sensitivity in this study.[115]

The failure to identify a single, major mechanism of thiopurine resistance may stem from our lack of knowledge about which cytotoxic mechanisms of these drugs are actually active in humans, as discussed above. It is possible that cells may become resistant not only by decreasing the *occurrence* of purine starvation or analog incorporation, but also by altering their *response* to these insults. Prediction (and prevention) of resistance may therefore require more information about the identity of the active cytotoxic mechanism in each individual patient, as well as a better understand-

ing of how these initial lesions ultimately kill cells.

Pharmacology of the Thiopurines

ABSORPTION, DISTRIBUTION, AND ELIMINATION. Although 6-MP is incompletely and variably absorbed in the gastrointestinal tract,[116] the drug is routinely given orally. The total urinary excretion of the drug and its metabolites after an oral dose is only 50% of that recovered after intravenous administration.[116] 6-Mercaptopurine is widely distributed in the body tissues, but the level achieved in the cerebrospinal fluid is only a small fraction of that of the plasma (2% at 30 minutes after injection).[116] The volume of distribution exceeds the total body water and the drug is about 20% bound to plasma protein. After a single intravenous injection, the half-life in children (21 minutes) is shorter than the half-life in adults (47 minutes).[116] The drug is extensively metabolized, and the forms recovered in the urine include the unchanged compound ($<5\%$), 6-thiouric acid, and methylated and desulfurated compounds.[116]

6-Thioguanine is also given orally, and peak plasma levels occur at about 8 hours.[117] In humans, the plasma half-life after a single intravenous injection varies considerably, with a median of 80 minutes.[117] Initial plasma levels correlate with dosage, but plasma half-life does not. Some unchanged thioguanine appears in the urine during the first 2 hours after an intravenous dose, but thereafter only metabolites are excreted. After oral administration, there is no significant excretion of the unchanged drug, and a variable portion of the ingested drug (24% to 46%) can be recovered in the urine as metabolites (6-methylthioguanine, 6-thiouric acid, and desulfurated metabolites).[117] Thioguanine is not extensively deaminated, and only a small amount is converted to a 6-thiouric acid; thus, in contrast to 6-MP and azathioprine, it can be used in combination with allopurinol without the dosage being reduced.

Clinical Use and Toxicity

Mercaptopurine and thioguanine are used primarily to treat acute leukemias, and response rates are higher in children than in adults

Table 5–4 *Pharmacology of the Thiopurines.* Dose-limiting lesions are shown in bold type

Drug	Principal Indications	Toxicities	Other Characteristics
6-Mercaptopurine	Acute lymphocytic leukemia	**Bone-marrow depression,** nausea, vomiting, stomatitis, hepatotoxicity, hyperuricemia	Used at reduced dosage when combined with allopurinol, to avoid tumor lysis syndrome
6-Thioguanine	Acute nonlymphocytic leukemia	**Bone-marrow depression,** nausea, vomiting	No dose adjustment necessary when used with allopurinol

(Table 5–4). Cross-resistance between the two drugs occurs. These drugs occasionally cause nausea, vomiting, and anorexia. In contrast to methotrexate, however, oral lesions are rarely seen. Bone-marrow depression is the principal toxic effect of both drugs. The maximum effect on the blood count may be delayed, and it is important to discontinue these drugs temporarily if there is an abnormally large fall in the leukocyte count or abnormal depression of the bone marrow. Some patients receiving 6-MP (and perhaps 6-TG) develop jaundice or other evidence of liver damage.[118] This complication has been observed in nonleukemic patients who have received 6-MP,[119] and it is clearly drug related. Unexpected, severe liver toxicity, manifested by a clinical picture of cholestasis, has been reported when 6-MP was used in combination therapy with adriamycin.[120] Renal toxicity has not been reported with conventional therapy, but hematuria and crystalluria have occurred after high-dose parenteral 6-MP.[121] The crystals in the urine contained 6-MP and a very small amount of 6-thiouric acid.

Allopurinol is sometimes added to 6-MP regimens, to prevent the hyperuricemia and uricosuria that follow the marked cell kill consequent to the therapy of leukemias and lymphomas. Since allopurinol partially blocks 6-MP catabolism by inhibiting xanthine oxidase, the antitumor effect and the toxicity of 6-MP are greater in this combination than when 6-MP is given alone.[122] Thus, when these two drugs are used together, the dosage of 6-MP is reduced to no more than one-third the usual amount.[123]

Other Purine Antagonists

TIAZOFURIN. Tiazofurin is an investigational agent that was originally synthesized as part of a program to obtain improved analogs of the antiviral drug ribavirin.[124]

In human cells tiazofurin can be anabolized by at least two enzymes, adenosine kinase and

Tiazofurin
(2-β-D-ribofuranosylthiazole-
4-carboxamide)

Ribavirin

5′-nucleotidase, to form the 5′-monophosphate.[125] This monophosphate is then converted to the critical metabolite, thiazole-4-carboxamide adenine dinucleotide, which is a potent inhibitor of IMP dehydrogenase[126] (Fig. 5–10). Tiazofurin-induced cytotoxicity appears to be closely related to the extent of intracellular accumulation of the dinucleotide, and its preferential anabolism in leukemic cells (compared to normal leukocytes) may be one basis for therapeutic selectivity.[127] Another important factor in determining the effectiveness of tiazofurin treatment is the degree to which cells can circumvent guanine nucleotide depletion, by salvage-pathway conversion of guanine to GMP (see Table 5–1). It has been shown that allopurinol treatment reduces guanine salvage in human leukemic cells, presumably by preventing degradation of hypoxanthine, which competes with guanine for phosphoribosylation.[128] Resistance to tiazofurin has been found to be multifactorial and can include elevated levels of IMP dehydrogenase, decreased transport and anabolism of the drug, and increased guanine salvage.[129]

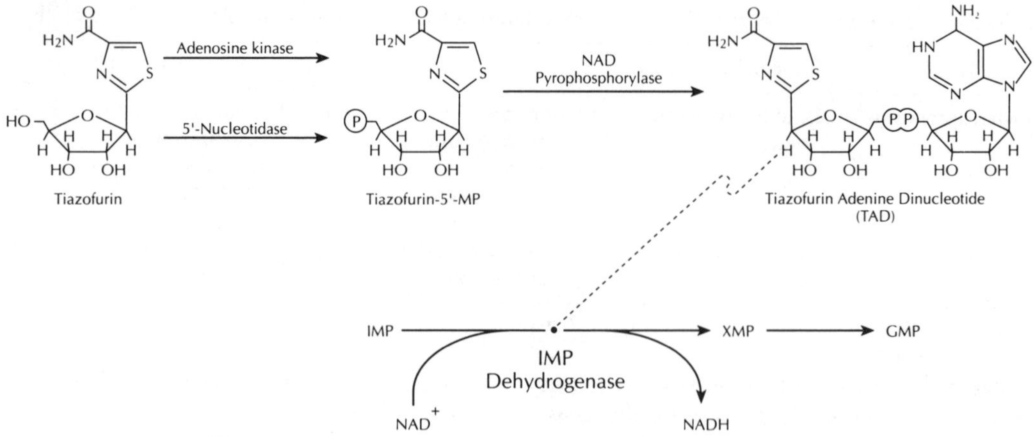

Figure 5–10 Tiazofurin anabolism and site of action. Tiazofurin is converted in two steps to the NAD analog, tiazofurin adenine dinucleotide, which exerts its major metabolic effect by blocking IMP dehydrogenase

Phase I and II clinical trials indicate that, although tiazofurin appears to be ineffective against various solid tumors, it has significant activity against some leukemias, especially chronic granulocytic leukemia.[130-132] Tiazofurin has been administered by both short (30-minute) and long (5-day) IV infusions and has a terminal elimination half-life of about 7–8 hours.[133,134] Renal excretion accounts for the majority of tiazofurin elimination, with 50–85% of the unchanged drug being recovered from urine.[134] In rhesus monkeys tiazofurin was found to have good access to the central nervous system, with the area under the time-concentration curve for CSF ranging from 14% to 51% of that for plasma.[135] More limited data in humans also reveal the presence of substantial levels of the drug in CSF.[134] Dose-limiting toxicities were primarily nonhematological, with neurotoxicity and pleuropericarditis being most severe.[132-134] A "viral-like" syndrome was also reported, which included malaise, myalgias, muscle weakness, headaches, fever, nausea, and vomiting.[133]

CHLORODEOXYADENOSINE. Clinical use of adenine nucleoside analogs has been hampered by their extensive degradation by adenosine deaminase. It was found that halogen substituents at the 2 position of the adenine ring resulted in resistance to deamination, and of the analogs in this series that were tested for antitumor effects, 2-chlorodeoxyadenosine (CdA) showed the greatest activity.[130]

Two sites of action have been identified for CdA, both of which depend on its anabolism to 2-chlorodeoxyadenosine-5'-triphosphate (Cl-dATP). The first mechanism is allosteric inhi-

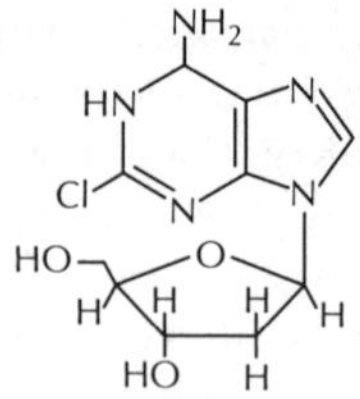

2-Chlorodeoxyadenosine (CdA)

bition of ribonucleotide reductase by Cl-dATP, which, like dATP, decreases conversion of all four ribonucleoside diphosphates to their 2'-deoxy counterparts. dCTP is the triphosphate whose pool size was most affected in a human T-lymphoblastic cell line treated with CdA.[136] Co-incubation with deoxycytidine reversed dCTP depletion in these cells, but only partially prevented CdA-induced DNA synthesis inhibition, indicating that one or more other mechanisms were also active. A second site of action appears to be Cl-dATP-mediated inhibition of DNA-strand elongation. Using synthetic primer-template substrates, it was shown that Cl-dATP caused pausing and termination of DNA-strand synthesis catalyzed by human DNA polymerases α, β, and γ, in a sequence- and enzyme-dependent manner.[137,138]

Chlorodeoxyadenosine causes extensive DNA damage, the pattern of which varies among cell lines. The mechanism by which this damage occurs is undefined, although the finding that CdA causes DNA damage and lethality in both proliferating and quiescent cells[139] indicates that interference with replicative DNA synthesis is not the sole site of action of this drug. As discussed in more detail in the last part of this chapter, it has been proposed that nucleotide pool imbalances caused by CdA (and other antimetabolites) may trigger a programmed cellular suicide response.[140,141]

Clinical studies with CdA have been limited but quite promising, primarily in the treatment of indolent B-cell lymphocytic leukemias such as hairy cell leukemia and chronic lymphocytic leukemia.[142,143] In one of these studies, a single course (7-day continuous IV infusion) of CdA resulted in complete responses in 11 out of 12 patients with hairy cell leukemia,[142] and these responses appear to be longer lasting than those obtained with other agents. Responses were also obtained in pediatric patients with relapsed or refractory acute lymphocytic leukemia.[144] The dose-limiting toxicity arising from infusions of CdA is relatively mild bone-marrow suppression.[145] Further evaluation of CdA in Phase II and III clinical trials is continuing.

PENTOSTATIN. The finding that lack of adenosine deaminase activity is the basis for some immunodeficiency syndromes[146,147] has led to development of adenosine deaminase inhibitors as agents for treatment of lymphocytic neoplasms. Pentostatin is a natural product (isolated from *Streptomyces antibioticus*) whose structure resembles the transition state intermediate in the adenosine deaminase-catalyzed conversion of adenosine to inosine,[148] inhibiting this reaction with a K_i on the order of 10^{-11} M.[149,150]

Pentostatin (2'-deoxycoformycin, dCF)

Intracellular accumulation of dATP resulting from pentostatin treatment appears to be important in causing cytotoxicity in some cases, possibly due to the allosteric effects of dATP on ribonucleotide reductase, leading to decreased synthesis of the other deoxynucleotides.[151] Not all cases of pentostatin-induced cell death are consistent with this model, however, and other mechanisms have been proposed to explain pentostatin's actions, including depletion of NAD, inhibition of S-adenosylhomocysteine hydrolase, and depletion of ATP.[152]

Disappearance of pentostatin from plasma is biphasic with a terminal half-life that ranges from 5 to 15 hours following bolus IV administration.[153,154] Renal excretion is the major mode of elimination.[153] Pentostatin has been used most successfully against hairy cell leukemia, with overall response rates >80% in several studies.[155] Moreover, these responses have been much more durable than those obtained with other treatments.[156] Significant activity has also been seen in patients with B-cell chronic lymphocytic leukemias.[155] Pentostatin has modest activity against mature T-cell leukemias.[157] Toxicities from pentostatin treatment are varied and somewhat unpredictable. Lymphopenia is often encountered, leading to potentially serious infections. Acute renal failure and neurological toxicities (including seizures and coma) are less common but can be life-threatening.[152]

Sugar-modified Analogs

When the therapeutic value of compounds containing modified purine or pyrimidine ring structures became apparent in the late 1950s,

Cytarabine (Cytosine arabinoside, Ara-C)

screening programs were initiated to identify other types of analogs that might give new leads for the development of antitumor drugs. One series of agents tested as part of this program was derived from a nucleoside analog, isolated from a Carribbean sponge, in which the sugar moiety (rather than the base portion) was altered.[158] The cytosine-containing analog (cytarabine; ara-C) proved to be the most efficacious member of this series and is in wide use today for the treatment of leukemias.

Sites and Determinants of Cytarabine Action

Unlike most other commonly used antimetabolites, ara-C appears to direct its action exclusively toward DNA function and synthesis, having little or no effect on RNA. The triphosphate form of the parent drug, ara-CTP, is a competitive inhibitor of DNA polymerases. Inhibition of DNA synthesis by ara-C (as well as by other agents) can result in the abnormal re-replication ("endoreduplication") of certain segments of the genome within a single S phase.[159] In addition, ara-CTP is a substrate for DNA polymerases and can be incorporated in place of dCTP. The relative biological impact of DNA synthesis inhibition versus incorporation of ara-C into DNA was investigated by combining ara-C with a direct-acting DNA polymerase inhibitor, aphidicolin.[160] It was found that aphidicolin cotreatment significantly antagonized both ara-C incorporation into DNA and cell kill, strongly suggesting that the cytotoxic importance of DNA-synthesis inhibition induced by exposure to ara-C alone is secondary to that of analog incorporation, in the cell line used in that study.

INCORPORATION INTO DNA. Although ara-CTP can be used as a substrate by DNA polymerases, the sugar modification in ara-C has a substantial impact on the efficiency of this process, much more so than in the case of the base-modified drugs. This effect is most noticeable when a DNA synthesis system attempts to incorporate ara-C moieties into consecutive sites.[161] At relatively low concentrations of ara-C the endogenous substrate, dCTP, is able to effectively compete with ara-CTP for incorporation. DNA synthesis probably stalls to some degree after each ara-CTP is added to the nascent chain, but elongation is generally able to continue. Under these conditions most of the incorporated ara-C has been found to located internally, within an intact DNA chain.[162] At higher ara-C levels the probability of two or more ara-CTP molecules being incorporated in a row is elevated and, correspondingly, so is the fraction of incorporated ara-C residues located at the 3' end of DNA chains, indicative of drug-induced termination of strand elongation.[162] Such termination is likely to be irrecoverable and probably represents a lethal lesion.

Even in those cases where cells are able to successfully complete a round of synthesis in the presence of ara-CTP, they face a severe challenge during the next S phase, when they must replicate an ara-C-containing template. A single ara-C unit within the template is sufficient to inhibit the elongation capacity of several DNA polymerases.[163] Interestingly, strand synthesis in this case is not inhibited until after addition of the G residue opposite the incorporated ara-C. In contrast, more drastic template lesions usually prevent insertion of the complimentary nucleotide. As is the case with the other incorporated analogs, the cellular reaction to inclusion of ara-C is poorly understood, and variations in this reaction might be partially responsible for heterogeneity of clinical response to ara-C.

METABOLISM AND RESISTANCE. Whereas bases such as FUra, 6-MP, and 6-TG typically enter cells by diffusion, intracellular access for ara-C is dependent upon the transport system used by several different nucleosides.[164,165] Once inside the cell, ara-C follows the pathways normally utilized by deoxycytidine for both activation and degradation (Fig. 5–11). Much of the drug is immediately converted to the inactive metabolite, ara-U, by deoxycytidine deaminase. For the ara-C molecules that escape inactivation at this stage, the first anabolic enzyme is deoxycytidine kinase. This enzyme, which can also phosphorylate dideoxycytidine, deoxyadenosine, and deoxyguanosine (and some of their analogs), probably represents the overall rate-limiting step in ara-C activation.[91] The resultant monophosphate, ara-CMP, is either inactivated by dCMP deaminase or further activated by dCMP kinase to ara-CDP. The relatively nonspecific enzyme, nucleoside diphosphate kinase, completes the activation process by producing ara-CTP.

Ara-C resistance in experimental situations has been associated with decreased transport or deoxycytidine kinase activity, and with increased deaminase activity.[166] In contrast, it is much harder to attribute resistance in vivo to any one of these factors by itself. Rather, it has

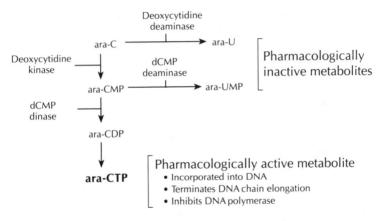

Figure 5–11   Metabolism and biochemical effects of cytarabine (ara-C).

been found that observation of the net result of these processes—i.e., the rise and fall of intracellular ara-CTP levels, is more informative. In patients with *refractory* acute leukemia who received high doses of ara-C upon relapse, there was a significant correlation between the area under the ara-CTP concentration versus time curve and clinical response rate.[167] On the basis of findings such as these, protocols using ara-C are being designed for such patients with the aim of individualizing dose schedules to achieve preselected ara-CTP concentrations in the target cell population.[168]

In patients with *newly diagnosed* acute leukemias, the relationship between response rate and ara-CTP levels is not as well established at this time. It is unclear if this is due to fundamental biological differences between the leukemic cells in such patients compared to those experiencing relapse, or to statistical factors arising from the relatively small number of newly diagnosed patients who fail treatment.[166] Alternatively, there seems to be a significant correlation between specific cytogenetic changes and response to ara-C in this population.[169] While the mechanistic implications of these changes are beyond our understanding at the present time, they may still provide an important practical means of predicting response (and therefore guiding therapeutic strategy) in individual patients.

Pharmacology and Toxicity of Cytarabine

ABSORPTION, DISTRIBUTION, AND ELIMINATION. Cytarabine is very poorly absorbed (less than 20%) after oral administration in humans, and it is routinely given parenterally. Conventional dosing regimens call for 100–200 mg/m^2/day to be given by continuous IV infusion for 5 to 10 days, resulting in plasma drug concentrations in the range of 0.5–1.0 μM.[170] Because the K_m for activation of ara-C by deoxycytidine kinase is on the order of 20 μM and because of the possibility of clinical resistance due to decreased influx of the drug, high-dose regimens were developed in which 3 gm/m^2 of ara-C is given in short (1–3 hours) infusions every 12 hours, for up to 6 days.[91,171] Such schedules result in plasma concentrations in excess of 100 μM during the infusion, a level at which transport does not limit uptake.[171] Low-dose regimens for ara-C (5–30 mg/m^2/day) have also been used in patients with preleukemic syndromes and in patients at high risk for toxicity from conventional therapy.[172,173] Intrathecal administration is also used for meningeal leukemia and lymphoma.[174]

The apparent volume of distribution of ara-C is approximately that of total body water.[175] Ara-C is also able to reach the central nervous system reasonably well, with drug levels in CSF reaching 6–40% of those found in plasma, when measured during the infusion.[176-178] Ara-C is more persistent in CSF than in plasma (probably due to the lack of deaminase activity in the central nervous system), and CSF levels were found to exceed plasma levels by several-fold shortly after infusions were stopped.[176,177] Metabolic deamination accounts for 70–90% of ara-C elimination, with most of the drug being excreted as ara-U.[176,179] Spleen and liver are the major sites of deamination, although significant deaminase activity was also detected in several other human tissues.[180] Elimination kinetics were similar following either conventional or high-dose regimens. In each case an initial half-life of 10–15 minutes was observed, followed by a second phase with a half-life of 1.5–2.5 hours.[176,179]

CLINICAL USE AND TOXICITY. Cytarabine has a potent myelosuppressive action and it is used primarily in combination with daunorubicin to treat acute nonlymphocytic leukemia. It is occasionally used to treat acute lymphocytic leukemia, and high-dose protocols are under investigation for treatment of advanced non-Hodgkin's lymphoma and chronic myelocytic leukemia.[171] Ara-C has not been found useful against solid tumors.

The principal toxicities of ara-C are leukopenia (primarily granulocytopenia) and thrombocytopenia. Anemia and megaloblastosis occur in roughly 15% of patients and are reversible on cessation of therapy. Oral inflammation and ulceration has been observed in about 10% of patients. Acute effects include nausea, vomiting, and diarrhea, and thrombophlebitis at the site of injection. High-dose regimens can induce significant neurologic toxicities, including seizures, cerebral and cerebellar dysfunction, and peripheral neuropathy.[174] These effects appear to be related to both age and dose.

Other Sugar-Modified Analogs

FLUDARABINE. Of the series of synthetic analogs having modifications in both the base and sugar moieties, fludarabine (2-fluoro-ara-A) is

Fludarabine (2-fluoro-ara-A)

the one that currently shows the most promise as a therapeutic agent.

Like ara-C, fludarabine is anabolized by the sequential action of deoxycytidine kinase and other kinases to the triphosphate form, which interferes with DNA synthesis both by competitive inhibition of replicative DNA polymerases and by incorporation into nascent DNA.[181] Unlike ara-C, more than 90% of the fludarabine molecules that become incorporated into DNA in intact cells are found at 3′ termini, indicating that fludarabine is much more likely to cause chain termination than ara-C.[182] Experiments using synthetic primer-template substrates with purified polymerases also showed that fludarabine triphosphate is an effective chain terminator.[137,182] In addition, it was found that incorporated fludarabine monophosphate moieties apparently inhibit the proofreading exonuclease activity of DNA polymerase ϵ.[182] Another property of fludarabine that is in sharp contrast to ara-C is its ability to be incorporated into RNA, resulting in inhibited transcription.[183] It is not clear at this time whether RNA incorporation plays a significant role in fludarabine-induced cytotoxicity.

Because fludarabine is poorly soluble in aqueous solutions it is administered as the 5′ monophosphate (fludarabine phosphate), which is rapidly dephosphorylated back to fludarabine in vivo.[184,185] A variety of schedules have been used in Phase I and II studies with fludarabine, ranging from single IV bolus injections to 5-day continuous infusions. An oral dosage form is under development, based on encouraging preliminary results in dogs.[186]

Elimination pharmacokinetics of fludarabine have been described in the context of both two- and three-compartment models.[185,187] In both cases the terminal half-life is on the order of 9–10 hours, preceded by a faster phase with a half-life of 1–2 hours. Volumes of distribution were significantly higher than total body water, suggesting some degree of tissue binding of the drug. Although excreted drug accounted for only 24% of administered dose in one study,[185] renal function appears to be an important factor in patient tolerance to fludarabine.[187,188] This may be related to elimination of a toxic metabolite, 2-fluoroadenine. Mammalian enzymes do not convert fludarabine to 2-fluoroadenine, but it has been shown that bacterial purine nucleoside phosphorylase can accomplish this conversion efficiently and it has been proposed that enteric flora might produce a significant amount of 2-fluoroadenine.[130] The overall metabolic profile of fludarabine has not been well characterized in humans.

Fludarabine has been shown to be very effective against chronic lymphocytic leukemia, yielding a response rate of >80% in previously untreated patients.[189] In addition, responses to fludarabine appear to be of longer duration than those obtained following conventional treatments. Responses in patients with non-Hodgkin's lymphoma have also been encouraging, particularly in those cases classified as having low-grade histologies.[190] Moderate to severe myelosuppression has been observed at most of the dose levels tested so far.[188,191,192] Severe neurologic toxicity also occurs, especially at higher doses.[192,193] This toxicity has a delayed onset (3–6 weeks) and is characterized by the eventual appearance of blindness, coma, and paralysis.[193]

Ribonucleotide Reductase Inhibitors

Hydroxyurea

Ribonucleotide reductase occupies a unique position in nucleotide metabolism in that it is the only highly regulated enzyme whose activity is involved in the *de novo* synthesis of all of the precursors used in DNA synthesis, by converting *ribo*nucleoside diphosphates to *deoxyribonucleotide* diphosphates. It is therefore not surprising that this enzyme is closely linked to proliferative status in tumor cells[96] and that it is a target for anticancer drugs. Mammalian ribonucleotide reductase is composed of two protein dimer subunits, designated M1 and M2.[194] M1 contains binding sites for both nucleoside diphosphates (substrates) and nucleoside triphosphates (allosteric effectors). The pattern of allosteric regulation of ribonucleotide reductase activity (summarized in Fig. 5–12) is quite complex and involves at least four different triphosphates, of which dATP is the most influential. As noted earlier in this chapter, accumulation of dATP as a result of either disease states or pharmacological treatments (e.g., with pentostatin) can profoundly inhibit deoxyribonucleotide production and DNA synthesis in some cell types. In addition, some of the antimetabolites (chlorodeoxyadenosine, fludara-

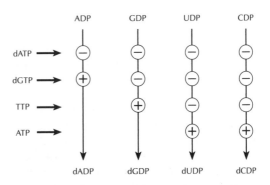

Figure 5–12   Allosteric control of ribonucleotide reductase activity. Ribonucleotide reductase catalyzes the conversion of ribonucleoside diphosphates to the corresponding deoxyribonucleoside diphosphates. The triphosphates in the left-hand column exert positive or negative allosteric control over these reactions, as indicated.[194]

bine) are deoxyadenosine analogs that, when anabolized to the triphosphate form, can mimic dATP and inhibit ribonucleotide reduction.

The M2 subunit of ribonucleotide reductase contains two moieties that are critical for the enzyme's catalytic activity: a tyrosyl free radical, which is thought to initiate the reaction by abstracting a hydrogen atom from the substrate, and a nonheme iron center, which is needed to generate and stabilize the tyrosyl radical.[195] A number of compounds have been identified that inhibit ribonucleotide reductase by destabilizing the iron center and thereby inactivating the M2 subunit, including a variety of N-hydroxylated species, guanazole, thiosemicarbazones, and an endogenously produced molecule, nitric oxide.[196–198] Of these, only hydroxyurea has been used routinely in the clinic.

$$\begin{array}{c} O \quad H \\ \| \quad | \\ H_2N-C-N-OH \end{array}$$

Hydroxyurea (HU)

Hydroxyurea is well absorbed from the gastrointestinal tract, and it is routinely given orally. Peak plasma concentrations are achieved in 80 minutes to about 2 hours, and the plasma half-life in man is about 3 hours.[199] At doses of 40 to 80 mg/kg, the drug has been shown to enter the cerebrospinal fluid.[199] The primary route of elimination appears to be renal, but only an average of 30% (range in ten patients of 10–94%) of an oral or an intravenous dose has been accounted for in the urine.[200] Hydroxyurea should be used with caution in patients with compromised renal function.

Hydroxyurea is used primarily to treat busulfan-resistant chronic granulocytic leukemia.[201-203] It can also be given to prevent the effects of leukostasis in leukemia patients.[204] Based on reports that it sensitized cultured cells to killing by X rays,[205] hydroxyurea has been used in combination with radiotherapy for the treatment of head and neck cancer[206,207] and cervical cancer.[208-210] Other indications include psoriasis[211] and polycythemia vera.[212]

Mild nausea and vomiting are experienced by most patients receiving this drug.[201,213] The major dose-limiting toxicity is bone-marrow depression, with leukopenia and, less commonly, thrombocytopenia and anemia.[213] Megaloblastosis in the marrow is common.[213] In most cases, the marrow depression is rapidly reversible on cessation of therapy. Stomatitis and gastrointestinal ulceration may occur when particularly large amounts of drug are given. Nephrotoxicity and neurotoxicity have been reported on rare occasions, but the latter complication (manifested by headache, dizziness, disorientation, and convulsions) has not been proven to be drug related. Dermatological reactions in patients on long-term maintenance therapy include increased pigmentation, scaling and atrophy of the skin, partial alopecia, nail changes, and erythema of the face and hands.[214] The histological changes in the epidermis are similar to those seen in lichen planus.[214] Hydroxyurea is known to be teratogenic in animals, including primates, and this effect must be considered when women of childbearing age are treated.[215] When hydroxyurea therapy is combined with radiotherapy, mucosal reactions in the radiation field may be more severe.[206]

Why Do Antimetabolites Kill Cells?

For every drug discussed in this chapter, one or more biochemical lesions were identified that appear to be related to its cytotoxic mechanism. In many cases, these initial lesions resulted in DNA-synthesis inhibition that could be reversed either by removing the drug or by providing the bases or nucleosides necessary to circumvent the drug-induced metabolic block. Although it is clear that sustained DNA synthesis inhibition precludes cellular proliferation, it is not clear what events occur during temporary DNA synthesis inhibition that permanently halt proliferation, even after the blockade is relieved. Whereas most investigations on the selectivity of anticancer drugs have focused on their initial effects, it seems likely that differences in cells' *response* to these initial lesions, which ultimately lead to cell death, may also determine the selectivity of their cytotoxic effects.

Thymineless Death

One of the first important studies in this area concerned the effects of thymidine nucleotide deprivation on growth and viability of E. coli thymine auxotrophs.[216,217] Incubation of these bacteria in thymine-free medium not only inhibited cell growth, it also induced cell death, as evidenced by a decrease in the fraction of cells able to form colonies when plated onto thymine-replete dishes. It was unexpectedly found that induction of this "thymineless death" was dependent upon continued RNA and protein synthesis during thymine deprivation, implying that conversion of DNA synthesis inhibition into a lethal insult is an active process requiring the participation of one or more induced or activated enzymes.

Subsequent investigations in a variety of prokaryotic and eukaryotic systems revealed that a persistent correlate of cell death due to thymine deprivation is DNA damage manifested as mutagenesis, recombinogenesis, single-strand breaks, double-strand breaks, and other lesions.[218] One mechanism proposed to account for such damage is based on observations that under normal circumstances deoxyuridine triphosphate (dUTP) will occasionally be misincorporated into DNA in place of thymidine triphosphate (TTP), and that most cells possess an excision repair system that digests and then resynthesizes the stretch of DNA containing the mistake. When the ratio of dUTP to TTP is extraordinarily high (e.g., following thymidylate synthase inhibition), the repair system may wind up inserting more uracil than it removes during each attempt at resynthesizing the excised region, leading to a futile cycle of misincorporation → misrepair → misincorporation, etc.[219] This could lead to saturation of the repair process, accumulation of unrepaired single-strand regions, and, eventually, to double-strand breaks.

Although good evidence was presented to support the uracil misrepair mechanism in some systems,[220-222] other reports are inconsistent with this hypothesis. For example, in studies using both wild-type and TS-negative mutants of a murine mammary carcinoma cell line it was found that thymidylate deprivation induced a substantial number of nonrandomly distributed double-strand DNA breaks without causing a concomitant increase of uracil content in DNA.[223] Furthermore, similar patterns of damage resulted from treatment with 2-chlorodeoxyadenosine, which causes DNA-synthesis inhibition without depleting TTP.[141] These findings led the authors to propose that a general cellular response to nucleotide pool imbalances is induction of an endonuclease activity, which is responsible for double-strand-break formation.[224] Although this mechanism still requires more substantiation, it seems clear that the sequelae of thymidylate synthase inhibition that led to DNA damage and cell death may well vary from one cell line to another.

Programmed Cell Death

In some cells drug treatment and other stimuli can trigger a series of events that appear to constitute a cellular suicide process, culminating in degradation of DNA down to oligonucleosomal fragments. This programmed mode of cell death has been named "apoptosis" and is distinguished from unprogrammed cell death (necrosis) by several biochemical and morphological characteristics.[225] Although apoptosis is sometimes a response to noxious treatments, it also occurs as part of the normal process of vertebrate development.[226]

The biochemical basis of apoptosis is largely unknown. The enzyme responsible for the DNA damage leading to oligonucleosomal fragments is a calcium-magnesium-dependent endonuclease that is activated when intracellular calcium levels rise.[227,228] Attempts at defining a genetic basis for control of this program have led to the identification of genes associated with apoptosis,[229] although inhibition of RNA and protein synthesis do not always prevent apoptosis, demonstrating that induction of new gene products is not obligatory for this process.[230] Apoptosis occurs in many different cell types, but it appears to be especially prominent in cells sensitive to endocrine manipulation, such as lymphoblasts and thymocytes. In cells that are prone to this response there seems to be little pharmacological specificity for induction of apoptosis, as evidenced by the mechanistic diversity of the drugs (including antimetabolites) that produce oligonucleosomal fragments.[231] In such cells apoptosis therefore appears to be a very general response to stress.

Another phenomenon that has been referred to as programmed cell death is related to activation of poly(ADP-ribose) polymerase,[232] which catalyzes the formation of ADP-ribose polymers on histones and certain other nuclear proteins (including itself), using NAD as a substrate.[233] Such conjugations result in significant changes in chromatin structure and modulations of the activity of several enzymes, including DNA ligase and DNA topoisomerases.[234] Poly(ADP-ribose) polymerase activity requires a free DNA end, as would be found at single- or double-strand break sites,[235,236] and this enzyme has been strongly implicated in the repair of various kinds of DNA damage.[237] Regeneration of NAD after the addition of each ADP-ribose moiety is energetically costly and, since poly(ADP-ribose) polymers turn over rapidly, it has been proposed that the induction of a large number of DNA strand breaks could sufficiently enhance poly(ADP-ribose) activity to create a lethal energy deficit.[232] Subsequent cell death might then be considered a "suicide" response in which the organism is better served by the destruction of heavily damaged cells than it would be by attempting to salvage such cells at the risk of mutagenesis.

Most investigations on the role of poly(ADP-ribosylation) in drug-induced cytotoxicity have focused on alkylators and other directly acting DNA-damaging agents. Although antimetabolites are less well studied in this regard, there is evidence to support the involvement of this process in cytotoxicity induced in noncycling human lymphocytes by pentostatin and chlorodeoxyadenosine.[139] It is not known if effects on poly(ADP-ribosylation) are significant in antimetabolite-induced cell death in cycling cells. However, it is conceivable that some of the known consequences of antimetabolite treatment (such as prolonged inhibition of replication fork movement, chain termination, and induction of excision repair systems) might provide a source of free DNA ends for activation of poly(ADP-ribose) polymerase.

Although it is not clear if there is a connection between apoptosis and poly(ADP-ribose) polymerase activity, it has been found that calcium-magnesium-dependent endonuclease can be inactivated by poly(ADP-ribosylation),[238] and it is possible that the two systems are related in some way. For example, if the endonuclease is constitutively suppressed by poly(ADP-ribosylation), then induction of enough DNA damage to saturate poly(ADP-ribose) formation might result in disinhibition of the endonuclease, leading to even more DNA degradation.[237]

Summary

The existence of ordered responses to the initial lesions caused by antimetabolites implies that drug-induced cell death is a regulated process. Various mechanisms involving the generation of DNA damage have been proposed to explain how cell death occurs following antimetabolite treatment, although it remains largely unknown how the primary drug lesions are detected and acted upon by the cell. It is possible that multiple cell-death mechanisms exist and that different ones may be induced by different drugs or even by the same drug in different cell lines. Variations in this process among normal and neoplastic cell types may provide a basis for explaining some cases of differential drug sensitivity and may ultimately represent a site for therapeutic intervention.[239]

REFERENCES

1. R. L. P. Adams, J. T. Knowler, and D. P. Leader: "The metabolism of nucleotides," in *The Biochemistry of the Nucleic Acids*. New York: Chapman and Hall, 1986, pp. 120–135.

2. J. F. Henderson and A. R. P. Paterson: *Nucleotide Metabolism*. New York: Academic Press, 1973.

3. R. C. Jackson and R. J. Harkrader: "The contributions of de novo and salvage pathways of nucleotide biosynthesis in normal and malignant cells," in *Nucleosides and Cancer Treatment,* ed. by M. H. N. Tattersall and R. M. Fox. Sydney: Academic Press, 1981, pp. 18–31.

4. B. Leyland-Jones, G. C. Hoo, J. L. Grem, G. Sarosy, M. P. Dearing, W. P. Henry, and M. C. Christian: "Investigational new agents," in *Cancer Chemotherapy: Principles and Practice,* ed. by B. A. Chabner and J. M. Collins. Philadelphia: J.B. Lippincott, 1990, pp. 514–519.

5. S. Farber, L. K. Diamond, R. D. Mercer, R. F. Sylvester and J. A. Wolff: Temporary remissions in acute leukemia in children produced by folic acid antagonist 4-amino-pteroyl-glutamic acid (aminopterin). *New Engl. J. Med.* 238:787 (1948).

6. I. D. Goldman, N. S. Lichtenstein, and V. T. Oliverio: Carrier-mediated transport of the folic acid analogue, methotrexate, in the L1210 leukemia cell. *J. Biol. Chem.* 243:5007 (1968).

7. M. Dembo and F. M. Sirotnak: "Membrane transport of folate compounds in mammalian cells," in *Folate Antagonists as Therapeutic Agents,* ed. by F. M. Sirotnak, J. J. Burchall, W. D. Ensminger, and J. A. Montgomery. New York: Academic Press, 1984, pp. 184–196.

8. D. Kessel, T. C. Hall, D. Roberts, and I. Wodinsky: Uptake as a determinant of methotrexate response in mouse leukemias. *Science* 150:752 (1965).

9. F. M. Sirotnak, D. M. Moccio, L. E. Kelleher, and L. J. Goutas: Relative frequency and kinetic properties of transport-defective phenotypes among methotrexate-resistant L1210 clonal cell lines derived in vivo. *Cancer Res.* 41:4447 (1981).

10. L. H. Matherly, R. L. Seither, and I. D. Goldman: Metabolism of the diaminoantifolates: Biosynthesis and pharmacology of the 7-hydroxyl and polyglutamyl metabolites of methotrexate and related antifolates. *Pharmacol. Ther.* 35:27 (1987).

11. J. Galivan, T. Johnson, M. Rhee, J. J. McGuire, D. Priest, and V. Kesevan: The role of folylpolyglutamate synthetase and gamma-glutamyl hydrolase in altering cellular folyl- and antifolylpolyglutamates. *Adv. Enzyme. Regul.* 26:147 (1987).

12. C. J. Allegra: "Antifolates," in *Cancer Chemotherapy: Principles and Practice,* ed. by B. A. Chabner and J. M. Collins. Philadelphia: J.B. Lippincott, 1990, pp. 110–153.

13. R. F. Ozols and K. Cowan: New aspects of clinical drug resistance: The role of gene amplification and the reversal of resistance in drug refractory cancer. *Important Adv. Oncol.* 129–157 (1986).

14. J. R. Bertino: "Turning the tables"—making normal marrow resistant to chemotherapy [editorial; comment]. *J. Natl. Cancer Inst.* 82:1234 (1990).

15. A. L. Albrecht and J. L. Biedler: "Acquired resistance of tumor cells to folate antagonists," in *Folate Antagonists as Therapeutic Agents,* ed. by F. M. Sirotnak, J. J. Burchall, W. D. Ensminger, and J. A. Montgomery. New York: Academic Press, 1984, pp. 332–333.

16. A. P. Dicker, M. Volkenandt, B. I. Schweitzer, D. Banerjee, and J. R. Bertino: Identification and characteriza-

tion of a mutation in the dihydrofolate reductase gene from the methotrexate-resistant Chinese hamster ovary cell line Pro-3 MtxRIII. *J. Biol. Chem.* 265:8317 (1990).

17. S. Srimatkandada, B. I. Schweitzer, B. A. Moroson, S. Dube, and J. R. Bertino: Amplification of a polymorphic dihydrofolate reductase gene expressing an enzyme with decreased binding to methotrexate in a human colon carcinoma cell line, HCT-8R4, resistant to this drug. *J. Biol. Chem.* 264:3524 (1989).

18. A. Goldin, J. M. Venditti, I. Kline, and N. Mantel: Eradication of leukemic cells (L1210) by methotrexate and methotrexate plus *Citrovorum* factor. *Nature* 212:1548 (1966).

19. L. H. Matherly, C. K. Barlowe, and I. D. Goldman: Antifolate polyglutamylation and competitive drug displacement at dihydrofolate reductase as important elements in leucovorin rescue in L1210 cells. *Cancer Res.* 46:588 (1986).

20. S. P. Ackland and R. L. Schilsky: High-dose methotrexate: A critical reappraisal. *J. Clin. Oncol.* 5:2017 (1987).

21. S. H. Wan, D. H. Huffman, D. L. Azarnoff, R. Stephens, and B. Hoogstraten: Effect of route of administration and effusions on methotrexate pharmacokinetics. *Cancer Res.* 34:3487 (1974).

22. F. M. Balis, J. L. Savitch, and W. A. Bleyer: Pharmacokinetics of oral methotrexate in children. *Cancer Res.* 43:2342 (1983).

23. W. B. Strum: A pH-dependent, carrier-mediated transport system for the folate analog, amethopterin, in rat jejunum. *J. Pharmacol. Exp. Ther.* 203:640 (1977).

24. E. S. Henderson, R. H. Adamson, and V. T. Oliverio: The metabolic fate of tritiated methotrexate. II. Absorption and excretion in man. *Cancer Res.* 25:1018 (1965).

25. Z. Darzynkiewicz, A. W. Rogers, E. A. Barnard, D. H. Wang, and W. C. Werkheiser: Autoradiography with tritiated methotrexate and the cellular distribution of folate reductase. *Science* 151:1528 (1966).

26. J. R. Bertino: The mechanism of action of the folate antagonists in man. *Cancer Res.* 23:1286 (1963).

27. B. A. Chabner, R. G. Stoller, K. Hande, S. Jacobs, and R. C. Young: Methotrexate disposition in humans: Case studies in ovarian cancer and following high-dose infusion. *Drug Metab. Rev.* 8:107 (1978).

28. D. G. Liegler, E. S. Henderson, M. A. Hahn, and V. T. Oliverio: The effect of organic acids on renal clearance of methotrexate in man. *Clin. Pharmacol. Ther.* 10:849 (1969).

29. D. H. Huffman, S. H. Wan, D. L. Azarnoff, and B. Hogstraten: Pharmacokinetics of methotrexate. *Clin. Pharmacol. Ther.* 14:572 (1973).

30. D. M. Valerino, D. G. Johns, D. S. Zaharko, and V. T. Oliverio: Studies of the metabolism of methotrexate by intestinal flora. I. Identification and study of biological properties of the metabolite 4-amino-4-deoxy-N 10-methylpteroic acid. *Biochem. Pharmacol.* 21:821 (1972).

31. D. G. Johns, A. T. Ianotti, A. C. Sartorelli, B. A. Booth, and J. R. Bertino: The identity of rabbit liver methotrexate oxidase. *Biochim. Biophys. Acta* 105:380 (1965).

32. S. A. Jacobs, R. G. Stoller, B. A. Chabner, and D. G. Johns: 7-Hydroxymethotrexate as a urinary metabolite in human subjects and rhesus monkeys receiving high dose methotrexate. *J. Clin. Invest.* 57:534 (1976).

33. M. H. N. Tattersall: "Clinical utility of methotrexate in neoplastic disease," in *Folate Antagonists as Therapeutic Agents,* ed. by F. M. Sirotnak, J. J. Burchall, W. D. Ensminger, and J. A. Montgomery. New York: Academic Press, 1984, pp. 166–191.

34. R. Hertz, G. T. Ross, and M. B. Lipsett: Chemotherapy in women with trophoblastic disease: Choriocarcinoma, chorioadenoma destruens, and complicated hydatidiform mole. *Ann. N.Y. Acad. Sci.* 114:881 (1964).

35. O. G. Jonsson and B. A. Kamen: Methotrexate and childhood leukemia. *Cancer Invest.* 9:53 (1991).

36. R. G. Stoller, K. R. Hande, S. A. Jacobs, S. A. Rosenberg, and B. A. Chabner: Use of plasma pharmacokinetics to predict and prevent methotrexate toxicity. *New Engl. J. Med.* 297:630 (1977).

37. G. D. Weinstein: Methotrexate. *Ann. Intern. Med.* 86:199 (1977).

38. L. L. Anderson, G. J. Collins, Y. Ojima, and R. D. Sullivan: A study of the distribution of methotrexate in human tissues and tumors. *Cancer Res.* 30:1344 (1970).

39. G. D. Weinstein, G. Goldfaden, and P. Frost: Methotrexate. Mechanism of action on DNA synthesis in psoriasis. *Arch. Dermatol.* 104:236 (1971).

40. S. R. Kaplan and P. Calabresi: Drug therapy: Immunosuppressive agents (second of two parts). *New Engl. J. Med.* 289:1234 (1973).

41. J. R. Bertino: "Folate antagonists" in *Antineoplastic and Immunosuppressive Agents.* Part II, ed. by A. C. Sartorelli and D. G. Johns. Berlin: Springer-Verlag, 1975, pp. 468–483.

42. A. Nirenberg, C. Mosende, B. M. Mehta, A. L. Gisolfi, and G. Rosen: High-dose methotrexate with citrovorum factor rescue: predictive value of serum methotrexate concentrations and corrective measures to avert toxicity. *Cancer Treat. Rep.* 61:779 (1977).

43. P. T. Condit, R. E. Chanes, and W. Joel: Renal toxicity of methotrexate. *Cancer* 23:126 (1969).

44. W. D. Ensminger: "Clinical pharmacology of folate analogs," in *Folate Antagonists as Therapeutic Agents,* ed. by F. M. Sirotnak, J. J. Burchall, W. D. Ensminger, and J. A. Montgomery. New York: Academic Press, 1984, pp. 133–165.

45. H. H. Roenigk, Jr., W. F. Bergfeld, R. St. Jacques, F. J. Owens, and W. A. Hawk: Hepatotoxicity of methotrexate in the treatment of psoriasis. *Arch. Dermatol.* 103:250 (1971).

46. M. G. Dahl, M. M. Gregory, and P. J. Scheuer: Liver damage due to methotrexate in patients with psoriasis. *Br. Med. J.* 1:625 (1971).

47. M. Nesbit, W. Krivit, R. Heyn, and H. Sharp: Acute and chronic effects of methotrexate on hepatic, pulmonary, and skeletal systems. *Cancer* 37:1048 (1976).

48. C. S. Everts, J. L. Westcott, and D. G. Bragg: Methotrexate therapy and pulmonary disease. *Radiology* 107:539 (1973).

49. W. A. Bleyer: Neurologic sequelae of methotrexate and ionizing radiation: A new classification. *Cancer Treat. Rep. 65 (Suppl. 1):*89 (1981).

50. P. A. Pizzo, D. G. Poplack, and W. A. Bleyer: Neurotoxicities of current leukemia therapy. *Am. J. Pediatr. Hematol. Oncol.* 1:127 (1979).

51. *E. F. Elslager, J. L. Johnson, and L. M. Werbel:* Folate antagonists. 20. Synthesis and antitumor and antima-

larial properties of trimetrexate and related 6-[(phenylam-ino)methyl]-2,4-quinazolinediamines. *J. Med. Chem.* 26:1753 (1983).

52. B. A. Kamen, B. Eibl, A. Cashmore, and J. Bertino: Uptake and efficacy of trimetrexate (TMQ, 2,4-diamino-5-methyl-6-[(3,4,5-trimethoxyanilino)methyl] quinazoline), a non-classical antifolate in methotrexate-resistant leukemia cells in vitro. *Biochem. Pharmacol.* 33:1697 (1984).

53. J. T. Lin and J. R. Bertino: Trimetrexate: A second generation folate antagonist in clinical trial. *J. Clin. Oncol.* 5:2032 (1987).

54. J. R. Bertino: Trimetrexate: overall clinical results. *Semin. Oncol.* 15:50 (1988).

55. K. M. Ivanetich and D. V. Santi: Thymidylate synthase and fluorouracil. *Adv. Exp. Med. Biol.* 244:113 (1988).

56. W. L. Washtien and D. V. Santi: Assay of intracellular free and macromolecular-bound metabolites of 5-fluorodeoxyuridine and 5-fluorouracil. *Cancer Res.* 39:3397 (1979).

57. D. S. Wilkinson and H. C. Pitot: Inhibition of ribosomal ribonucleic acid maturation in Novikoff hepatoma cells by 5-fluorouracil and 5-fluorouridine. *J. Biol. Chem.* 248:63 (1973).

58. W. B. Parker and Y. C. Cheng: Metabolism and mechanism of action of 5-fluorouracil. *Pharmacol. Ther.* 48:381 (1990).

59. T. Iwata, T. Watanabe, and D. W. Kufe: Effects of 5-fluorouracil on globin mRNA synthesis in murine erythroleukemia cells. *Biochemistry* 25:2703 (1986).

60. R. D. Armstrong, M. Lewis, S. G. Stern, and E. C. Cadman: Acute effect of 5-fluorouracil on cytoplasmic and nuclear dihydrofolate reductase messenger RNA metabolism. *J. Biol. Chem.* 261:7366 (1986).

61. B. J. Dolnick and J. J. Pink: Effects of 5-fluorouracil on dihydrofolate reductase and dihydrofolate reductase mRNA from methotrexate-resistant KB cells. *J. Biol. Chem.* 260:3006 (1985).

62. P. V. Danenberg, L. C. Shea, and K. Danenberg: Effect of 5-fluorouracil substitution on the self-splicing activity of *Tetrahymena* ribosomal RNA. *Cancer Res.* 50:1757 (1990).

63. D. W. Kufe, P. Scott, R. Fram, and P. Major: Biologic effect of 5-fluoro-2'-deoxyuridine incorporation in L1210 deoxyribonucleic acid. *Biochem. Pharmacol.* 32:1337 (1983).

64. J. D. Schuetz, H. J. Wallace, and R. B. Diasio: 5-Fluorouracil incorporation into DNA of CF-1 mouse bone marrow cells as a possible mechanism of toxicity. *Cancer Res.* 44:1358 (1984).

65. H. A. Ingraham, B. Y. Tseng, and M. Goulian: Nucleotide levels and incorporation of 5-fluorouracil and uracil into DNA of cells treated with 5-fluorodeoxyuridine. *Mol. Pharmacol.* 21:211 (1982).

66. J. L. Grem: "Fluorinated pyrimidines," in *Cancer Chemotherapy: Principles and Practice,* ed. by B. A. Chabner and J. M. Collins. Philadelphia: J.B. Lippincott, 1990, pp. 189–190.

67. W. L. Washtien: Thymidylate synthetase levels as a factor in 5-fluorodeoxyuridine and methotrexate cytotoxicity in gastrointestinal tumor cells. *Mol. Pharmacol.* 21:723 (1982).

68. S. H. Berger and F. G. Berger: Thymidylate synthase as a determinant of 5-fluoro-2'-deoxyuridine response in human colonic tumor cell lines. *Mol. Pharmacol.* 34:474 (1988).

69. S. H. Berger, K. W. Barbour, and F. G. Berger: A naturally occurring variation in thymidylate synthase structure is associated with a reduced response to 5-fluoro-2'-deoxyuridine in a human colon tumor cell line. *Mol. Pharmacol.* 34:480 (1988).

70. B. Ullman, M. Lee, D. W. Martin, Jr., and D. V. Santi: Cytotoxicity of 5-fluoro-2'-deoxyuridine: Requirement for reduced folate cofactors and antagonism by methotrexate. *Proc. Natl. Acad. Sci. USA* 75:980 (1978).

71. J. L. Grem, D. F. Hoth, J. M. Hamilton, S. A. King, and B. Leyland-Jones: Overview of current status and future direction of clinical trials with 5-fluorouracil in combination with folinic acid. *Cancer Treat. Rep.* 71:1249 (1987).

72. C. P. Spears, B. G. Gustavsson, M. Berne, R. Frösing, L. Bernstein, and A. A. Hayes: Mechanisms of innate resistance to thymidylate synthase inhibition after 5-fluorouracil. *Cancer Res.* 48:5894 (1988).

73. P. J. Houghton, J. A. Houghton, B. J. Hazelton, and S. Radparvar: Biochemical mechanisms in colon xenografts: Thymidylate synthase as a target for therapy. *Invest. New Drugs* 7:59 (1989).

74. J. Maybaum, B. Ullman, H. G. Mandel, J. L. Day, and W. Sadee: Regulation of RNA- and DNA-directed actions of 5-fluoropyrimidines in mouse T-lymphoma (S-49) cells. *Cancer Res.* 40:4209 (1980).

75. W. L. Washtien: Comparison of 5-fluorouracil metabolism in two gastrointestinal tumor cell lines. *Cancer Res.* 44:909 (1984).

76. H. W. Bruckner and W. A. Creasey: The administration of 5-fluorouracil by mouth. *Cancer* 33:14 (1974).

77. H. M. Pinedo and G. F. Peters: Fluorouracil: Biochemistry and pharmacology. *J. Clin. Oncol.* 6:1653 (1988).

78. B. Ardalan, S. Waldman, and L. Sklaver: "The pyrimidine antagonists: 5-fluorouracil and floxuridine," in *Cancer Chemotherapy by Infusion,* ed. by J. J. Lokich. Chicago: Precept Press, 1990, pp. 85–121.

79. J. M. Collins, R. L. Dedrick, F. G. King, J. L. Speyer, and C. E. Myers: Nonlinear pharmacokinetic models for 5-fluorouracil in man: intravenous and intraperitoneal routes. *Clin. Pharmacol. Ther.* 28:235 (1980).

80. J. L. Speyer, J. M. Collins, R. L. Dedrick, M. F. Brennan, A. R. Buckpitt, H. Londer, V. T. DeVita, Jr., and C. E. Myers: Phase I and pharmacological studies of 5-fluorouracil administered intraperitoneally. *Cancer Res.* 40:567 (1980).

81. B. Clarkson, A. O'Connor, L. Winston and D. Hutchison: The physiologic disposition of 5-fluorouracil and 5-fluoro-2'-deoxyuridine in man. *Clin. Pharmacol. Ther.* 5:581 (1964).

82. W. E. MacMillan, W. H. Wolberg, and P. G. Welling: Pharmacokinetics of fluorouracil in humans. *Cancer Res.* 38:3479 (1978).

83. R. B. Diasio and B. E. Harris: Clinical pharmacology of 5-fluorouracil. *Clin. Pharmacokinet.* 16:215 (1989).

84. R. G. Moran and K. Keyomarsi: Biochemical rationale for the synergism of 5-fluorouracil and folinic acid. *NCI Monogr.* 159 (1987).

85. S. G. Arbuck: Overview of clinical trials using 5-fluorouracil and leucovorin for the treatment of colorectal cancer. *Cancer* 63:1036 (1989).

86. H. D. Weiss, M. D. Walker, and P. H. Wiernik: Neurotoxicity of commonly used antineoplastic agents (first of two parts). *New Engl. J. Med.* 291:75 (1974).

87. T. R. Jones, A. H. Calvert, A. L. Jackman, S. J. Brown, M. Jones, and K. R. Harrap: A potent antitumour quinazoline inhibitor of thymidylate synthetase: Synthesis, biological properties and therapeutic results in mice. *Eur. J. Cancer* 17:11 (1981).

88. H. Diddens, D. Niethammer, and R. C. Jackson: Patterns of cross-resistance to the antifolate drugs trimetrexate, metoprine, homofolate, and CB3717 in human lymphoma and osteosarcoma cells resistant to methotrexate. *Cancer Res.* 43:5286 (1983).

89. A. H. Calvert, D. R. Newell, A. L. Jackman, L. A. Gumbrell, E. Sikora, B. Grzelakowska-Sztabert, J. A. Bishop, I. R. Judson, S. J. Harland, and K. R. Harrap: Recent preclinical and clinical studies with the thymidylate synthase inhibitor N10-propargyl-5,8-dideazafolic acid (CB 3717). *NCI Monogr.* 213 (1987).

90. A. B. Glover and B. Leyland-Jones: Biochemistry of azacitidine: A review. *Cancer Treat. Rep.* 71:959 (1987).

91. B. A. Chabner: "Cytidine analogues," in *Cancer Chemotherapy: Principles and Practice*, ed. by B. A. Chabner and J. M. Collins. Philadelphia: J.B. Lippincott, 1990, pp. 169–170.

92. P. A. Jones: DNA methylation and cancer. *Cancer Res.* 46:461 (1986).

93. P. A. Jones: Altering gene expression with 5-azacytidine. *Cell* 40:485 (1985).

94. A. B. Glover, B. R. Leyland-Jones, H. G. Chun, B. Davies, and D. F. Hoth: Azacytidine: 10 years later. *Cancer Treat. Rep.* 71:737 (1987).

95. R. C. Jackson, G. Weber, and H. P. Morris: IMP dehydrogenase, an enzyme linked with proliferation and malignancy. *Nature* 256:331 (1975).

96. G. Weber: Biochemical strategy of cancer cells and the design of chemotherapy: G.H.A. Clowes Memorial Lecture. *Cancer Res.* 43:3466 (1983).

97. Y. Natsumeda, S. Ohno, H. Kawasaki, Y. Konno, G. Weber, and K. Suzuki: Two distinct cDNAs for human IMP dehydrogenase. *J. Biol. Chem.* 265:5292 (1990).

98. J. W. Weiss and H. C. Pitot: Inhibition of ribosomal RNA maturation in Novikoff hepatoma cells by toyocamycin, tubercidin, and 6-thioguanosine. *Cancer Res.* 34:581 (1974).

99. S. Yoshida, M. Yamada, S. Masaki, and M. Saneyoshi: Utilization of 2'-deoxy-6-thioguanosine 5'-triphosphate in DNA synthesis in vitro by DNA polymerase alpha from calf thymus. *Cancer Res.* 39:3955 (1979).

100. Y. H. Ling, J. A. Nelson, Y. C. Cheng, R. S. Anderson, and K. L. Beattie: 2'-Deoxy-6-thioguanosine 5'-triphosphate as a substrate for purified human DNA polymerases and calf thymus terminal deoxynucleotidyltransferase in vitro. *Mol. Pharmacol.* 40:508 (1991).

101. S. Drake, R. L. Burns, and J. A. Nelson: Metabolism and mechanisms of action of 9-(tetrahydro-2-furyl)-6-mercaptopurine in Chinese hamster ovary cells. *Chem. Biol. Interact.* 41:105 (1982).

102. N. T. Christie, S. Drake, R. E. Meyn, and J. A. Nelson: 6-Thioguanine-induced DNA damage as a determinant of cytotoxicity in cultured Chinese hamster ovary cells. *Cancer Res.* 44:3665 (1984).

103. S. C. Barranco and R. M. Humphrey: The effects of beta-2'-deoxythioguanosine on survival and progression in mammalian cells. *Cancer Res.* 31:583 (1971).

104. L. L. Wotring and J. L. Roti Roti: Thioguanine-induced S and G2 blocks and their significance to the mechanism of cytotoxicity. *Cancer Res.* 40:1458 (1980).

105. J. Maybaum and H. G. Mandel: Unilateral chromatid damage: A new basis for 6-thioguanine cytotoxicity. *Cancer Res.* 43:3852 (1983).

106. L. M. Iwaniec, J. J. Kroll, W. M. Roethel, and J. Maybaum: Selective inhibition of sequence-specific protein/DNA interactions by incorporation of 6-thioguanine: Cleavage by restriction endonucleases. *Mol. Pharmacol.* 39:299 (1991).

107. J. Maybaum, A. N. Bainnson, W. M. Roethel, S. Ajmera, L. M. Iwaniec, D. R. TerBush and J. J. Kroll: Effects of incorporation of 6-thioguanine into SV40 DNA. *Mol. Pharmacol.* 32:606 (1987).

108. S. Matsumura, T. Hoshino, M. Weizsaecker, and D. F. Deen: Paradoxical behavior of 6-mercaptopurine as a cytotoxic agent: Decreasing cell kill with increasing drug dose. *Cancer Treat. Rep.* 67:475 (1983).

109. J. Maybaum, C. W. Morgans, and L. A. Hink: Comparison of in vivo and in vitro effects of continuous exposure of L1210 cells to 6-thioguanine. *Cancer Res.* 47:3083 (1987).

110. J. Maybaum, L. A. Hink, W. M. Roethel, and H. G. Mandel: Dissimilar actions of 6-mercaptopurine and 6-thioguanine in Chinese hamster ovary cells. *Biochem. Pharmacol.* 34:3677 (1985).

111. J. F. Henderson and I. G. Junga: Potentiation of carcinostasis by combinations of thioguanine and 6-mercaptopurine. *Biochem. Pharmacol.* 5:167 (1960).

112. J. Maybaum, P. Ting, and C. E. Rogers: Prediction of thioguanine-induced cytotoxicity by dual-parameter flow cytometric analysis. *Cancer Chemother. Pharmacol.* 24:291 (1989).

113. J. D. Davidson: Formal discussion on resistance to purine antagonists in experimental leukemia systems. *Cancer Res.* 25:1606 (1965).

114. M. K. Wolpert, S. P. Damle, J. E. Brown, E. Sznycer, K. C. Agrawal, and A. C. Sartorelli: The role of phosphohydrolases in the mechanism of resistance of neoplastic cells to 6-thiopurines. *Cancer Res.* 31:1620 (1971).

115. S. Zimm, G. Reaman, R. F. Murphy, and D. G. Poplack: Biochemical parameters of mercaptopurine activity in patients with acute lymphoblastic leukemia. *Cancer Res.* 46:1495 (1986).

116. T. L. Loo, J. K. Luce, M. P. Sullivan, and E. Frei: Clinical pharmacologic observations on 6-mercaptopurine and 6-methylthiopurine ribonucleoside. *Clin. Pharmacol. Ther.* 9:180 (1968).

117. G. A. LePage and J. P. Whitecar, Jr.: Pharmacology of 6-thioguanine in man. *Cancer Res.* 31:1627 (1971).

118. J. H. Burchenal and R. R. Ellison: The purine and pyrimidine antagonists. *Clin. Pharmacol. Ther.* 2:523 (1961).

119. J. Shorey, S. Schenker, W. N. Suki, and B. Combes:

Hepatotoxicity of mercaptopurine. *Arch. Intern. Med.* 122:54 (1968).

120. V. Rodriguez, G. P. Bodey, K. B. McCredie, E. J. Freireich, R. A. Minow, J. H. Casey, and M. Luna: Combination 6-mercaptopurine-adriamycin in refractory adult acute leukemia. *Clin. Pharmacol. Ther.* 18:462 (1975).

121. M. J. Duttera, R. L. Carolla, J. F. Gallelli, D. S. Gullion, D. E. Keim, and E. S. Henderson: Hematuria and crystalluria after high-dose 6-mercaptopurine administration. *New Engl. J. Med.* 287:292 (1972).

122. G. B. Elion, S. Callahan, H. Nathan, S. Bieber, R. W. Rundles and G. H. Hitchings: Potentiation by inhibition of drug degradation: 6-Substituted purines and xanthine oxidase. *Biochem. Pharmacol.* 12:85 (1963).

123. A. S. Levine, H. L. Sharp, J. Mitchell, W. Krivit, and M. E. Nesbit: Combination therapy with 6-mercaptopurine (NSC-755) and allopurinol (NSC-1390) during induction and maintenance of remission of acute leukemia in children. *Cancer Chemother. Rep.* 53:53 (1969).

124. P. C. Srivastava, M. V. Pickering, L. B. Allen, D. G. Streeter, M. T. Campbell, J. T. Witkowski, R. W. Sidwell, and R. K. Robins: Synthesis and antiviral activity of certain thiazole C-nucleosides. *J. Med. Chem.* 20:256 (1977).

125. A. Fridland, M. C. Connelly, and T. J. Robbins: Tiazofurin metabolism in human lymphoblastoid cells: Evidence for phosphorylation by adenosine kinase and 5'-nucleotidase. *Cancer Res.* 46:532 (1986).

126. D. A. Cooney, H. N. Jayaram, G. Gebeyehu, C. R. Betts, J. A. Kelley, V. E. Marquez, and D. G. Johns: The conversion of 2-beta-D-ribofuranosylthiazole-4-carboxamide to an analogue of NAD with potent IMP dehydrogenase-inhibitory properties. *Biochem. Pharmacol.* 31:2133 (1982).

127. H. N. Jayaram, K. Pillwein, C. R. Nichols, R. Hoffman, and G. Weber: Selective sensitivity to tiazofurin of human leukemic cells. *Biochem. Pharmacol.* 35:2029 (1986).

128. G. Weber: Critical issues in chemotherapy with tiazofurin. *Adv. Enzyme. Regul.* 29:75 (1989).

129. H. N. Jayaram, K. Pillwein, M. S. Lui, M. A. Faderan, and G. Weber: Mechanism of resistance to tiazofurin in hepatoma 3924A. *Biochem. Pharmacol.* 35:587 (1986).

130. W. Plunkett and P. P. Saunders: Metabolism and action of purine nucleoside analogs. *Pharmacol. Ther.* 49:239 (1991).

131. G. J. Tricot, H. N. Jayaram, E. Lapis, Y. Natsumeda, C. R. Nichols, P. Kneebone, N. Heerema, G. Weber, and R. Hoffman: Biochemically directed therapy of leukemia with tiazofurin, a selective blocker of inosine 5'-phosphate dehydrogenase activity. *Cancer Res.* 49:3696 (1989).

132. G. Tricot, H. N. Jayaram, G. Weber, and R. Hoffman: Tiazofurin: Biological effects and clinical uses. *Int. J. Cell Cloning* 8:161 (1990).

133. T. J. Melink, D. D. Von Hoff, J. G. Kuhn, M. R. Hersh, L. A. Sternson, T. F. Patton, R. Siegler, D. H. Boldt, and G. M. Clark: Phase I evaluation and pharmacokinetics of tiazofurin (2-beta-D-ribofuranosylthiazole-4-carboxamide, NSC 286193). *Cancer Res.* 45:2859 (1985).

134. D. L. Trump, K. D. Tutsch, J. M. Koeller, and D. C. Tormey: Phase I clinical study with pharmacokinetic analysis of 2-beta-D-ribofuranosylthiazole-4-carboxamide (NSC 286193) administered as a five-day infusion. *Cancer Res.* 45:2853 (1985).

135. J. J. Grygiel, F. M. Balis, J. M. Collins, C. M. Lester, and D. G. Poplack: Pharmacokinetics of tiazofurin in the plasma and cerebrospinal fluid of rhesus monkeys. *Cancer Res.* 45:2037 (1985).

136. J. Griffig, R. Koob, and R. L. Blakley: Mechanisms of inhibition of DNA synthesis by 2-chlorodeoxyadenosine in human lymphoblastic cells. *Cancer Res.* 49:6923 (1989).

137. W. B. Parker, A. R. Bapat, J.-X. Shen, A. J. Townsend, and Y.-C. Cheng: Interaction of 2-halogenated dATP analogs (F, Cl, and Br) with human DNA polymerases, DNA primase, and ribonucleotide reductase. *Mol. Pharmacol.* 34:485 (1988).

138. P. Hentosh, R. Koob, and R. L. Blakley: Incorporation of 2-halogeno-2'-deoxyadenosine 5-triphosphates into DNA during replication by human polymerases alpha and beta. *J. Biol. Chem.* 265:4033 (1990).

139. S. Seto, C. J. Carrera, M. Kubota, D. B. Wasson, and D. A. Carson: Mechanism of deoxyadenosine and 2-chlorodeoxyadenosine toxicity to nondividing human lymphocytes. *J. Clin. Invest.* 75:377 (1985).

140. D. A. Carson, C. J. Carrera, D. B. Wasson, and H. Yamanaka: Programmed cell death and adenine deoxynucleotide metabolism in human lymphocytes. *Adv. Enzyme. Regul.* 27:395 (1988).

141. Y. Hirota, A. Yoshioka, S. Tanaka, K. Watanabe, T. Otani, J. Minowada, A. Matsuda, T. Ueda, and Y. Wataya: Imbalance of deoxyribonucleoside triphosphates, DNA double-strand breaks, and cell death caused by 2-chlorodeoxyadenosine in mouse FM3A cells. *Cancer Res.* 49:915 (1989).

142. L. D. Piro, C. J. Carrera, D. A. Carson, and E. Beutler: Lasting remissions in hairy-cell leukemia induced by a single infusion of 2-chlorodeoxyadenosine. *New Engl. J. Med.* 322:1117 (1990).

143. L. D. Piro, C. J. Carrera, E. Beutler, and D. A. Carson: 2-Chlorodeoxyadenosine: An effective new agent for the treatment of chronic lymphocytic leukemia. *Blood* 72:1069 (1988).

144. V. M. Santana, J. Mirro, Jr., F. C. Harwood, J. Cherrie, M. Schell, D. Kalwinsky, and R. L. Blakley: A phase I clinical trial of 2-chlorodeoxyadenosine in pediatric patients with acute leukemia. *J. Clin. Oncol.* 9:416 (1991).

145. D. A. Carson, D. B. Wasson, and E. Beutler: Antileukemic and immunosuppressive activity of 2-chloro-2'-deoxyadenosine. *Proc. Natl. Acad. Sci. USA* 81:2232 (1984).

146. E. R. Giblett, J. E. Anderson, F. Cohen, B. Pollara, and H. J. Meuwissen: Adenosine-deaminase deficiency in two patients with severely impaired cellular immunity. *Lancet* 2:1067 (1972).

147. B. S. Mitchell and W. N. Kelley: Purinogenic immunodeficiency diseases: Clinical features and molecular mechanisms. *Ann. Intern. Med.* 92:826 (1980).

148. R. Wolfenden, D. F. Wentworth, and G. N. Mitchell: Influence of substituent ribose on transition state affinity in reactions catalyzed by adenosine deaminase. *Biochemistry* 16:5071 (1977).

149. J. Constine, R. I. Glazer, and D. G. Johns: Adenosine deaminase inhibitors: Differential effects on multiple forms of adenosine deaminase. *Biochem. Biophys. Res. Comm.* 85:198 (1978).

150. R. P. Agarwal, T. Spector, and R. E. Parks, Jr.: Tight-binding inhibitors—IV. Inhibition of adenosine de-

aminases by various inhibitors. *Biochem. Pharmacol.* 26:359 (1977).

151. A. Cohen, R. Hirschhorn, S. D. Horowitz, A. Rubinstein, S. H. Polmar, R. Hong, and D. W. Martin, Jr.: Deoxyadenosine triphosphate as a potentially toxic metabolite in adenosine deaminase deficiency. *Proc. Natl. Acad. Sci. USA 75*:472 (1978).

152. P. J. O'Dwyer, B. Wagner, B. Leyland-Jones, R. E. Wittes, B. D. Cheson, and D. F. Hoth: 2'-Deoxycoformycin (pentostatin) for lymphoid malignancies. Rational development of an active new drug. *Ann. Intern. Med. 108*:733 (1988).

153. P. P. Major, R. P. Agarwal, and D. W. Kufe: Clinical pharmacology of deoxycoformycin. *Blood 58*:91 (1981).

154. J. F. Smyth, R. M. Paine, A. L. Jackman, K. R. Harrap, M. M. Chassin, R. H. Adamson, and D. G. Johns: The clinical pharmacology of the adenosine deaminase inhibitor 2'-deoxycoformycin. *Cancer Chemother. Pharmacol. 5*:93 (1980).

155. C. Dearden and D. Catovsky: Deoxycoformycin in the treatment of mature B-cell malignancies. *Br. J. Cancer 62*:4 (1990).

156. P. A. Cassileth, B. Cheuvart, A. S. Spiers, D. P. Harrington, F. J. Cummings, R. S. Neiman, J. M. Bennett, and M. J. O'Connell: Pentostatin induces durable remissions in hairy cell leukemia. *J. Clin. Oncol. 9*:243 (1991).

157. C. Dearden, E. Matutes, and D. Catovsky: Deoxycoformycin in the treatment of mature T-cell leukaemias. *Br. J. Cancer 64*:903 (1991).

158. S. S. Cohen: Introduction to the biochemistry of D-arabinosyl nucleosides. *Prog. Nucleic Acid Res. Mol. Biol. 5*:1 (1966).

159. D. M. Woodcock, R. M. Fox, and I. A. Cooper: Evidence for a new mechanism of cytotoxicity of 1-beta-D arabinofuranosylcytosine. *Cancer Res. 39*:1418 (1979).

160. D. W. Kufe, D. Munroe, D. Herrick, E. Egan, and D. Spriggs: Effects of 1-beta-D-arabinofuranosylcytosine incorporation on eukaryotic DNA template function. *Mol. Pharmacol. 26*:128 (1984).

161. A. J. Townsend and Y.-C. Cheng: Sequence specific effects of ara-5-aza-CTP and ara-CTP on DNA synthesis by purified human DNA polymerase in vitro: Visualization of chain elongation on a defined template. *Mol. Pharmacol. 32*:330 (1987).

162. P. P. Major, E. M. Egan, D. J. Herrick, and D. W. Kufe: Effect of ara-C incorporation on deoxyribonucleic acid synthesis in cells. *Biochem. Pharmacol. 31*:2937 (1982).

163. T. Mikita and G. P. Beardsley: Functional consequences of the arabinosylcytosine structural lesion in DNA. *Biochemistry 27*:4698 (1988).

164. P. G. Plagemann, R. Marz, and R. M. Wohlhueter: Transport and metabolism of deoxycytidine and 1-beta-D-arabinofuranosylcytosine into cultured Novikoff rat hepatoma cells, relationship to phosphorylation, and regulation of triphosphate synthesis. *Cancer Res. 38*:978 (1978).

165. J. S. Wiley, J. Taupin, G. P. Jamieson, M. Snook, W. H. Sawyer, and L. R. Finch: Cytosine arabinoside transport and metabolism in acute leukemias and T cell lymphoblastic lymphoma. *J. Clin. Invest. 75*:632 (1985).

166. E. H. Estey, M. J. Keating, K. B. McCredie, E. J. Freireich, and W. Plunkett: Cellular ara-CTP pharmaco-

kinetics, response, and karyotype in newly diagnosed acute myelogenous leukemia. *Leukemia 4*:95 (1990).

167. E. Estey, W. Plunkett, D. Dixon, M. Keating, K. McCredie, and E. J. Freireich: Variables predicting response to high dose cytosine arabinoside therapy in patients with refractory acute leukemia. *Leukemia 1*:580 (1987).

168. V. Heinemann, E. Estey, M. J. Keating, and W. Plunkett: Patient-specific dose rate for continuous infusion high-dose cytarabine in relapsed acute myelogenous leukemia. *J. Clin. Oncol. 7*:622 (1989).

169. M. J. Keating, T. L. Smith, H. Kantarjian, A. Cork, R. Walters, J.M. Trujillo, K. B. McCredie, E. A. Gehan, and E. J. Freireich: Cytogenetic pattern in acute myelogenous leukemia: A major reproducible determinant of outcome. *Leukemia 2*:403 (1988).

170. W. Hiddemann: Cytosine arabinoside in the treatment of acute myeloid leukemia: The role and place of high-dose regimens. *Ann. Hematol. 62*:119 (1991).

171. B. J. Bolwell, P. A. Cassileth, and R. P. Gale: High dose cytarabine: A review. *Leukemia 2*:253 (1988).

172. B. J. Bolwell, P. A. Cassileth, and R. P. Gale: Low dose cytosine arabinoside in myelodysplasia and acute myelogenous leukemia: A review. *Leukemia 1*:575 (1987).

173. J. S. Wisch, J. D. Griffin, and D. W. Kufe: Response of preleukemic syndromes to continuous infusion of low-dose cytarabine. *New Engl. J. Med. 309*:1599 (1983).

174. W. J. Baker, G. L. Royer, Jr., and R. B. Weiss: Cytarabine and neurologic toxicity. *J. Clin. Oncol. 9*:679 (1991).

175. R. van Prooijen, E. van der Kleijn, and C. Haanen: Pharmacokinetics of cytosine arabinoside in acute myeloid leukemia. *Clin. Pharmacol. Ther. 21*:744 (1977).

176. D. H. Ho and E. Frei: Clinical pharmacology of 1-beta-d-arabinofuranosyl cytosine. *Clin. Pharmacol. Ther. 12*:944 (1971).

177. M. L. Slevin, E. M. Piall, G. W. Aherne, V. J. Harvey, A. Johnston, and T. A. Lister: Effect of dose and schedule on pharmacokinetics of high-dose cytosine arabinoside in plasma and cerebrospinal fluid. *J. Clin. Oncol. 1*:546 (1983).

178. H. Breithaupt, H. Pralle, T. Eckhardt, M. von Hattingberg, J. Schick, and H. Loffler: Clinical results and pharmacokinetics of high-dose cytosine arabinoside (HD ARA-C). *Cancer 50*:1248 (1982).

179. S. H. Wan, D. H. Huffman, D. L. Azarnoff, B. Hoogstraten, and W. E. Larsen: Pharmacokinetics of 1-beta-D-arabinofuranosylcytosine in humans. *Cancer Res. 34*:392 (1974).

180. D. H. Ho: Distribution of kinase and deaminase of 1-beta-D-arabinofuranosylcytosine in tissues of man and mouse. *Cancer Res. 33*:2816 (1973).

181. W. Plunkett, P. Huang, and V. Gandhi: Metabolism and action of fludarabine phosphate. *Semin. Oncol. 17*:3 (1990).

182. P. Huang, S. Chubb, and W. Plunkett: Termination of DNA synthesis by 9-beta-D-arabinofuranosyl-2-fluoroadenine. A mechanism for cytotoxicity. *J. Biol. Chem. 265*:16617 (1990).

183. P. Huang and W. Plunkett: Action of 9-beta-D-arabinofuranosyl-2-fluoroadenine on RNA metabolism. *Mol. Pharmacol. 39*:449 (1991).

184. P. E. Noker, G. F. Duncan, S. M. El Dareer, and D. L. Hill: Disposition of 9-beta-D-arabinofuranosyl-2-fluo-

roadenine 5′-phosphate in mice and dogs. *Cancer Treat. Rep.* 67:445 (1983).

185. M. R. Hersh, J. G. Kuhn, J. L. Phillips, G. Clark, T. M. Ludden, and D. D. Von Hoff: Pharmacokinetic study of fludarabine phosphate (NSC 312887). *Cancer Chemother. Pharmacol.* 17:277 (1986).

186. B. D. Cheson: Issues for the future development of fludarabine phosphate. *Semin. Oncol.* 17:71 (1990).

187. L. Malspeis, M. R. Grever, A. E. Staubus and D. Young: Pharmacokinetics of 2-F-ara-A (9-beta-D-arabinofuranosyl-2-fluoroadenine) in cancer patients during the phase I clinical investigation of fludarabine phosphate. *Semin. Oncol.* 17:18 (1990).

188. M. Grever, J. Leiby, E. Kraut, E. Metz, J. Neidhart, S. Balcerzak, and L. Malspeis: A comprehensive phase I and II clinical investigation of fludarabine phosphate. *Semin. Oncol.* 17:39 (1990).

189. M. J. Keating: Fludarabine phosphate in the treatment of chronic lymphocytic leukemia. *Semin. Oncol.* 17:49 (1990).

190. H. Hochster and P. Cassileth: Fludarabine phosphate therapy of non-Hodgkin's lymphoma. *Semin. Oncol.* 17:63 (1990).

191. J. J. Hutton, D. D. Von Hoff, J. Kuhn, J. Phillips, M. Hersh, and G. Clark: Phase I clinical investigation of 9-beta-D-arabinofuranosyl-2-fluoroadenine 5′-monophosphate (NSC 312887), a new purine antimetabolite. *Cancer Res.* 44:4183 (1984).

192. D. R. Spriggs, E. Stopa, R. J. Mayer, W. Schoene, and D. W. Kufe: Fludarabine phosphate (NSC 312878) infusions for the treatment of acute leukemia: Phase I and neuropathological study. *Cancer Res.* 46:5953 (1986).

193. R. P. Warrell, Jr., and E. Berman: Phase I and II study of fludarabine phosphate in leukemia: therapeutic efficacy with delayed central nervous system toxicity. *J. Clin. Oncol.* 4:74 (1986).

194. J. A. Wright, A. K. Chan, B. K. Choy, R. A. Hurta, G. A. McClarty, and A. Y. Tagger: Regulation and drug resistance mechanisms of mammalian ribonucleotide reductase, and the significance to DNA synthesis. *Biochem. Cell Biol.* 68:1364 (1990).

195. J. Stubbe: Ribonucleotide reductases. *Adv. Enzymol. Relat. Areas Mol. Biol.* 63:349 (1990).

196. J. G. Cory and G. L. Carter: Drug action on ribonucleotide reductase. *Adv. Enzyme. Regul.* 24:385 (1985).

197. G. A. McClarty, A. K. Chan, B. K. Choy, and J. A. Wright: Increased ferritin gene expression is associated with increased ribonucleotide reductase gene expression and the establishment of hydroxyurea resistance in mammalian cells. *J. Biol. Chem.* 265:7539 (1990).

198. N. S. Kwon, D. J. Stuehr, and C. F. Nathan: Inhibition of tumor cell ribonucleotide reductase by macrophage-derived nitric oxide. *J. Exp. Med.* 174:761 (1991).

199. G. L. Beckloff, H. J. Lerner, D. Frost, F. M. Russo-Alesi, and S. Gitomer: Hydroxyurea (NSC-32065) in biologic fluids: Dose-concentration relationship. *Cancer Chemother. Rep.* 48:57 (1965).

200. B. H. Bolton, L. A. Woods, D. T. Kaung, and R. L. Lawton: A simple method of colorimetric analysis for hydroxyurea (NSC-32065). *Cancer Chemother. Rep.* 46:1 (1965).

201. J. H. Schwartz and G. P. Cannellos: Hydroxyurea in the management of the hematologic complications of chronic granulocytic leukemia. *Blood* 46:11 (1975).

202. R. W. Bolin, W. A. Robinson, J. Sutherland, and R. F. Hamman: Busulfan versus hydroxyurea in long-term therapy of chronic myelogenous leukemia. *Cancer* 50:1683 (1982).

203. B. J. Kennedy: Hydroxyurea therapy in chronic myelogenous leukemia. *Cancer* 29:1052 (1972).

204. F. M. Grund, J. O. Armitage, and P. Burns: Hydroxyurea in the prevention of the effects of leukostasis in acute leukemia. *Arch. Intern. Med.* 137:1246 (1977).

205. W. K. Sinclair: The combined effect of hydroxyurea and x-rays on Chinese hamster cells in vitro. *Cancer Res.* 28:198 (1968).

206. D. H. Hussey and J. P. Abrams: Combined therapy in advanced head and neck cancer: Hydroxyurea and radiotherapy. *Prog. Clin. Cancer* 6:79 (1975).

207. S. Stefani, R. W. Eells, and J. Abbate: Hydroxyurea and radiotherapy in head and neck cancer. Results of a prospective controlled study in 126 patients. *Radiology* 101:391 (1971).

208. M. S. Piver, J. J. Barlow, V. Vongtama, and L. Blumenson: Hydroxyurea as a radiation sensitizer in women with carcinoma of the uterine cervix. *Am. J. Obstet. Gynecol.* 129:379 (1977).

209. M. M. Hreshchyshyn, B. S. Aron, R. C. Boronow, E. W. Franklin, H. M. Shingleton, and J. A. Blessing: Hydroxyurea or placebo combined with radiation to treat stages IIIB and IV cervical cancer confined to the pelvis. *Int. J. Radiat. Oncol. Biol. Phys.* 5:317 (1979).

210. M. S. Piver, V. Vongtama, and L. J. Emrich: Hydroxyurea plus pelvic radiation versus placebo plus pelvic radiation in surgically staged stage IIIB cervical cancer. *J. Surg. Oncol.* 35:129 (1987).

211. U. W. Leavell, Jr., and J. W. Yarbro: Hydroxyurea. A new treatment for psoriasis. *Arch. Dermatol.* 102:144 (1970).

212. R. Sharon, I. Tatarsky, and Y. Ben-Arieh: Treatment of polycythemia vera with hydroxyurea. *Cancer* 57:718 (1986).

213. K. M. Griffith: Hydroxyurea (NSC-32065): Results of a Phase I Study. *Cancer Chemother. Rep.* 40:33 (1964).

214. B. J. Kennedy, L. R. Smith, and R. W. Goltz: Skin changes secondary to hydroxyurea therapy. *Arch. Dermatol.* 111:183 (1975).

215. J. G. Wilson, W. J. Scott, E. J. Ritter, and R. Fradkin: Comparative distribution and embryotoxicity of hydroxyurea in pregnant rats and rhesus monkeys. *Teratology* 11:169 (1975).

216. S. S. Cohen: On the nature of thymineless death. *Ann. N.Y. Acad. Sci.* 186:292 (1971).

217. S. S. Cohen and H. D. Barner: Studies on unbalanced growth in *Esherichia coli. Proc. Natl. Acad. Sci. USA* 40:885 (1954).

218. B. J. Barclay, B. A. Kunz, J. G. Little, and R. H. Haynes: Genetic and biochemical consequences of thymidylate stress. *Can. J. Biochem.* 60:172 (1982).

219. M. Goulian, B. M. Bleile, L. M. Dickey, R. H. Grafstrom, H. A. Ingraham, S. A. Neynaber, M. S. Peterson, and B. Y. Tseng: Mechanism of thymineless death. *Adv. Exp. Med. Biol.* 195:89 (1986).

220. H. A. Ingraham, L. Dickey, and M. Goulian: DNA

fragmentation and cytotoxicity from increased cellular deoxyuridylate. *Biochemistry 25*:3225 (1986).

221. M. Goulian, B. Bleile, and B. Y. Tseng: The effect of methotrexate on levels of dUTP in animal cells. *J. Biol. Chem. 255*:10630 (1980).

222. R. G. Richards, L. C. Sowers, J. Laszlo, and W. D. Sedwick: The occurrence and consequences of deoxyuridine in DNA. *Adv. Enzyme. Regul. 22*:157 (1984).

223. D. Ayusawa, K. Shimizu, H. Koyama, K. Takeishi, and T. Seno: Accumulation of DNA strand breaks during thymineless death in thymidylate synthase-negative mutants of mouse FM3A cells. *J. Biol. Chem. 258*:12448 (1983).

224. A. Yoshioka, S. Tanaka, O. Hiraoka, Y. Koyama, Y. Hirota, and Y. Wataya: Deoxyribonucleoside-triphosphate imbalance death: deoxyadenosine-induced dNTP imbalance and DNA double strand breaks in mouse FM3A cells and the mechanism of cell death. *Biochem. Biophys. Res. Comm. 146*:258 (1987).

225. A. H. Wyllie, J. F. Kerr, and A. R. Currie: Cell death: The significance of apoptosis. *Int. Rev. Cytol. 68*:251 (1980).

226. T. G. Cotter, S. V. Lennon, J. G. Glynn, and S. J. Martin: Cell death via apoptosis and its relationship to growth, development and differentiation of both tumour and normal cells. *Anticancer Res. 10*:1153 (1990).

227. D. J. McConkey, P. Nicotera, P. Hartzell, G. Bellomo, A. H. Wyllie, and S. Orrenius: Glucocorticoids activate a suicide process in thymocytes through an elevation of cytosolic Ca^{2+} concentration. *Arch. Biochem. Biophys. 269*:365 (1989).

228. J. J. Cohen and R. C. Duke: Glucocorticoid activation of a calcium-dependent endonuclease in thymocyte nuclei leads to cell death. *J. Immunol. 132*:38 (1984).

229. R. Buttyan, C. A. Olsson, J. Pintar, C. Chang, M. Bandyk, P. Y. Ng, and I. S. Sawczuk: Induction of the TRPM-2 gene in cells undergoing programmed death. *Mol. Cell. Biol. 9*:3473 (1989).

230. S. H. Kaufmann: Induction of endonucleolytic DNA cleavage in human acute myelogenous leukemia cells by etoposide, camptothecin, and other cytotoxic anticancer drugs: A cautionary note. *Cancer Res. 49*:5870 (1989).

231. M. A. Barry, C. A. Behnke, and A. Eastman: Activation of programmed cell death (apoptosis) by cisplatin, other anticancer drugs, toxins and hyperthermia. *Biochem. Pharmacol. 40*:2353 (1990).

232. D. A. Carson, S. Seto, D. B. Wasson, and C. J. Carrera: DNA strand breaks, NAD metabolism, and programmed cell death. *Exp. Cell Res. 164*:273 (1986).

233. T. Boulikas: Relation between carcinogenesis, chromatin structure and poly(ADP-ribosylation) [review]. *Anticancer Res. 11*:489 (1991).

234. N. A. Berger: Symposium: Cellular response to DNA damage: The role of poly(ADP-ribose). *Radiat. Res. 101*:4 (1985).

235. R. C. Benjamin and D. M. Gill: Poly(ADP-ribose) synthesis in vitro programmed by damaged DNA. A comparison of DNA molecules containing different types of strand breaks. *J. Biol. Chem. 255*:10502 (1980).

236. R. C. Benjamin and D. M. Gill: ADP-ribosylation in mammalian cell ghosts. Dependence of poly(ADP-ribose) synthesis on strand breakage in DNA. *J. Biol. Chem. 255*:10493 (1980).

237. J. E. Cleaver, C. Borek, K. Milam, and W. F. Morgan: The role of poly(ADP-ribose) synthesis in toxicity and repair of DNA damage. *Pharmacol. Ther. 31*:269 (1987).

238. Y. Tanaka, K. Yoshihara, A. Itaya, T. Kamiya, and S. S. Koide: Mechanism of the inhibition of Ca^{2+}, Mg^{2+}-dependent endonuclease of bull seminal plasma induced by ADP-ribosylation. *J. Biol. Chem. 259*:6579 (1984).

239. C. Dive and J. A. Hickman: Drug-target interactions: Only the first step in the commitment to a programmed cell death? *Br. J. Cancer 64*:192 (1991).

CHAPTER 6

Covalent DNA-Binding Drugs

NITROGEN MUSTARDS
Mechlorethamine (HN$_2$, nitrogen mustard)
Chlorambucil
Melphalan (L-phenylalanine mustard, L-PAM)
Cyclophosphamide
Ifosfamide
AZIRIDINES
Thiotepa (thio-TEPA)
Altretamine (hexamethylmelamine)
Mitomycin (mitomycin C)
ALKANE SULFONATES
Busulfan

NITROSOUREAS
Carmustine (BCNU)
Lomustine (CCNU)
Semustine (methyl-CCNU)
Streptozotocin
PLATINUM COMPOUNDS
Cisplatin (cis-DDP)
Carboplatin
METHYLATING AGENTS
Dacarbazine
Procarbazine

Nitrogen Mustards

Since nitrogen mustard was first used in the treatment of a patient with lymphosarcoma in 1942 (see Chapter 2), many alkylating agents have been synthesized and tested for antitumor activity. All these compounds are capable of reacting in a manner such that an alkyl group or a substituted alkyl group becomes covalently linked to cellular constituents. The reaction is called alkylation; hence the name for this group of drugs. The nitrogen mustards are one of five major classes of anticancer drugs that act as DNA cross-linkers. These drugs include the nitrogen mustards, the aziridines, the alkane sulfonates, the nitrosoureas, and several platinum compounds. The latter group cross-links DNA by a mechanism different from alkylation. The structures of the major nitrogen mustards in clinical use are shown in Figure 6–1. The mechanism of action of nitrogen and

sulfur mustards was studied before that of the other alkylating agents, and these compounds are used here to describe the alkylation reaction and the biological consequences of alkylation. The other alkylating agents react with DNA in a similar manner with similar consequences. All of these agents are mutagenic and carcinogenic as well as cytotoxic.

Mechanism of Action

THE CHEMICAL REACTION. The alkylating agents are highly reactive compounds that form covalent bonds with a number of nucleophilic groups.[1] The proposed mechanism of action for mechlorethamine is shown in Figure 6–2. At neutral or alkaline pH, one of the chlorethyl side chains undergoes a cyclization, releasing chloride ion and forming an immonium-ion intermediate. This strained three-membered ring is highly reactive and can at-

108

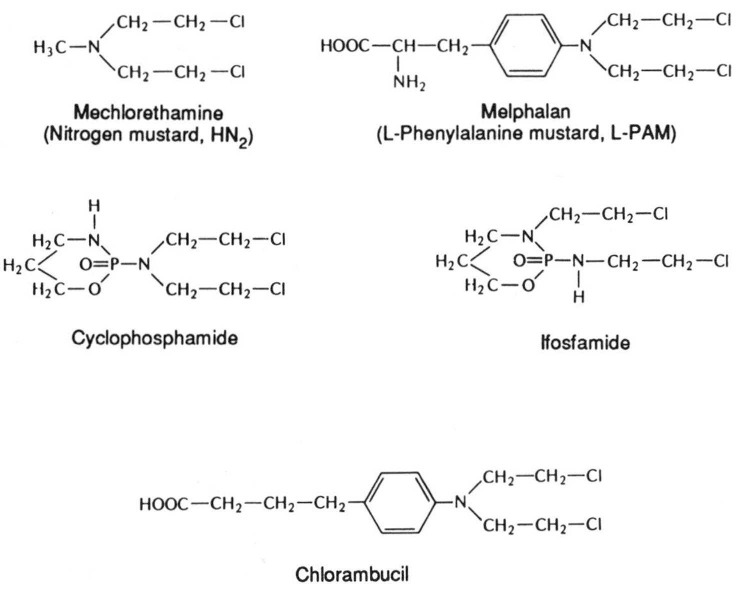

Figure 6–1 Structures of the nitrogen mustards in clinical use.

tack nucleophilic groups. It is possible that, in some cases, the reaction may proceed through a unimolecular ring opening of the immonium ion, with formation of a carbonium-ion intermediate as noted within the brackets in Figure 6–2. Such nucleophilic groups as amino, carboxyl, sulfhydryl, or imidazole moieties in proteins and nucleic acids can be alkylated. One favored reaction of major importance in the cytotoxic effect of the mustards is the formation of a covalent bond between the drug and the 7-nitrogen group of guanine. After forming a covalent bond with one molecule, the bifunctional alkylating agents (those containing two reactive chlorethyl side chains) can then undergo a similar cyclization of the second side chain and form a covalent bond with another nucleophilic group. This second reaction could involve the 7-nitrogen of another guanine or some other nucleophilic moiety.

This sequence of reactions can have a number of results. For example, reaction with another guanine (or possibly less favored reactions with adenine or cytosine) may result in cross-linking between DNA strands or linking between bases within the same strand of DNA. The second side chain may react with water, a weak nucleophile, to produce monoalkylated DNA guanine units. Thus, DNA alkylation may have several different biological effects.

The nitrogen mustards are both mutagens and carcinogens. Experiments with monofunctional alkylating agents have demonstrated that a guanine with the agent covalently bonded to its 7-nitrogen can form anomalous base pairs with thymine. One major mutagenic effect of the mustards seems to involve subsequent transitions from guanine-cytosine to adenine-thymine base pairs.[2] Depurination of the DNA, with splitting of the imidazole ring, can also occur to produce strand scission owing to the weakening of the sugar-phosphate backbone of DNA. Strand scission also occurs as a result of endonuclease attack when the cell attempts to repair the segment of DNA containing the drug adduct.

The nucleophilic groups of proteins, RNA, and many other molecules can also serve as substrates for chemical attack by alkylating agents. Since many cellular constituents can be alkylated, it might be assumed that the cytotoxity of the alkylating agents is the result of the deleterious effects of many diverse insults. Indeed, these agents at high concentration affect a number of biochemical events in the cell.[3] In intact mammalian cells, however, there is evidence that the cytotoxicity of the nitrogen mustards at therapeutic levels is mainly due to an inhibition of DNA replication. It has been demonstrated, for example, that nitrogen mus-

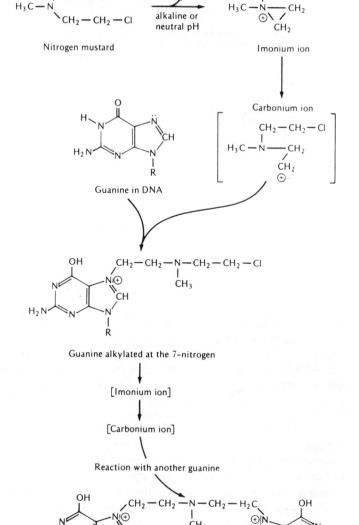

Figure 6-2 The mechanism by which nitrogen mustard becomes covalently bonded to the 7-nitrogens of two guanines. In solution, the drug forms a reactive cyclic intermediate that reacts with the 7-nitrogen of a guanine residue in DNA to form a covalent linkage. The second arm can then cyclize and react with nucleophilic groups such as a second guanine moiety in an opposite DNA strand or in the same strand. Reactions between DNA and RNA and between DNA and protein also occur.

tard in low doses inhibits DNA synthesis in cultured mammalian cells more rapidly and to a greater extent than it inhibits RNA or protein synthesis.[4] In studies with other difunctional alkylating agents, it has been shown that DNA synthesis is preferentially inhibited in tumor cells *in vivo* (e.g., sarcoma 180)[5] and in intact bacteria.[6]

THE CROSS-LINKING OF DNA. Although alkylating agents at high doses will inhibit a number of reactions necessary for the synthesis of DNA by mammalian cells and bacteria, it is the interaction between the drug and DNA itself that is the most meaningful with respect to the major cytotoxic effect. Alkylation of the DNA decreases its ability to act as a template for

DNA synthesis.[7,8] The possibility that alkylating agents may form cross-links between the two DNA strands in the double helix was suggested by the observation that DNA treated with nitrogen mustard is converted to a reversibly denaturable form.[9] The type of experiment[10] that suggests this (Fig. 6–3) and the interpretation of the data is as follows: DNA purified from *Bacillus subtilis* is treated with various concentrations of nitrogen mustard, adjusted to alkaline pH for a short time, neutralized, and dialyzed against a buffer. When normal, double-stranded, helical DNA is made alkaline, the DNA denatures to yield two separated strands. When the solution is neutralized, portions of the DNA strands containing appropriate hydrogen-bonding sequences come into opposition on a random basis, and partial renaturation takes place (Fig. 6–3B). The partially renatured DNA solution contains a large amount of single-stranded DNA. Single-stranded DNA absorbs more light at 260 mμ than the native, double-stranded DNA. This can be seen in the melting curve of the treated DNA (Fig. 6–3A) as an elevated base line of absorbance at temperatures lower than that at which thermal transition from double-stranded to single-stranded DNA occurs. This base line is much lower in samples exposed to nitrogen mustard prior to denaturation in alkali and subsequent neutralization. The drug effect is outlined in Figure 6–3C. Nitrogen mustard has formed a cross-link between the two strands of DNA. In the alkali, hydrogen bonding is disrupted, and strand separation takes place. Strands that are cross-linked by the drug, however, are oriented so that renaturation is more complete than with the control DNA, where appropriate sequences for hydrogen-bonding must come into apposition on a purely random basis. In other words, the two drug-linked strands are able to "zip up" in their normal base-pairing relationships.

Other experiments designed to demonstrate that bifunctional alkylating agents form cross-links between the two strands of the DNA helix have confirmed this hypothesis. Interstrand cross-linking is certainly not the only biologically important reaction between the drug and DNA. Some of the diguanyl derivatives formed when alkylating drugs react with DNA represent intrastrand cross-linkages.[11,12] But several times more monoalkylation products than dialkylation products are formed.[11] It is important to understand this cross-linking in order to understand the bifunctional nature of nitrogen mustard cytotoxicity. As shown with sulfur mustards in Figure 6–4, compounds with two reactive chloroethyl side arms are considerably more cytotoxic (sometimes 100-fold more) than monofunctional compounds.[13] A number of studies have shown a direct correlation between the degree of interstrand cross-linking in tumor cells and cytotoxic response after exposure to alkylating agents both *in vitro*[14,15] and *in vivo*.[16]

EXCISION REPAIR OF ALKYLATED DNA. Both bacterial and mammalian cells can repair DNA damage due to alkylation.[17] The repair process involves a number of different enzymes. The endonucleases recognize the drug-modified DNA and cut the DNA at the site of the damage. The damaged segment of DNA is then degraded by exonucleases, and a repair polymerase synthesizes a new segment, using the opposing DNA strand as a template. The original double-stranded DNA is reconstituted when the newly synthesized segment is covalently linked to the preexisting strand by a ligase enzyme. The entire process is called *excision repair*, and two pathways have been identified in mammalian cells.[18] In the so-called *short-patch* mechanism only three or four nucleotides are excised, and in *long-patch* repair up to 120 nucleotides are excised. Most drug-induced DNA damage is repaired by the short-patch mechanism.

The repair process is nicely demonstrated in experiments with a strain of *Escherichia coli* resistant to both alkylating agents and ultraviolet radiation (ultraviolet radiation produces covalent interstrand cross-linking between thymidine residues). In the resistant bacteria the alkylation reactions proceed as in drug-sensitive strains, but the excision repair system cuts out the diguanyl residues and restores functional DNA to the cell (Fig. 6-5).[19] In mammalian cells exposed to alkylating agents, the excision repair activity may be a significant factor contributing to the cytotoxic threshold for both alkylating agents and radiation. It has been

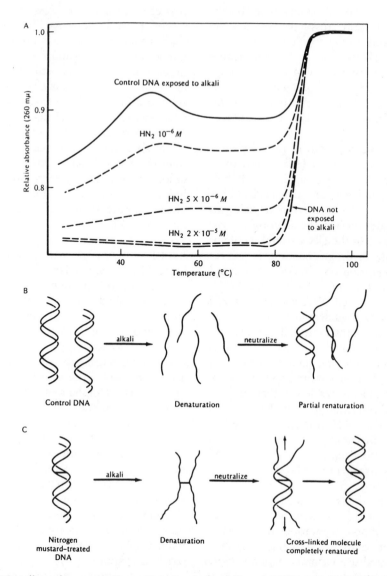

Figure 6–3 The effect of interstrand cross-linkage on the ability of DNA to renature. (A) Purified *Bacillus subtilis* DNA or samples of the same DNA treated with various concentrations of nitrogen mustard were made alkaline for 1.5 minutes, neutralized, and dialyzed against buffer. Melting curves were then carried out on each DNA sample. The graph shows the absorbance of each sample at 260 mμ, expressed as a fraction of the absorbance of fully denatured DNA, versus temperature. Solid line, control DNA treated with alkali and neutralized; dotted lines, DNA treated with various concentrations of nitrogen mustard and then alkali and neutralized; dashed line, untreated DNA (i.e., no drug or alkali treatment). (From Kohn *et al.*[10]) (B) A schematic presentation of the response of normal double-stranded DNA to alkali treatment and neutralization. In alkali, the native DNA denatures; upon neutralization, partial renaturation takes place as possible hydrogen-bonding sequences on the single strands become opposed to one another in a random fashion. (C) A schematic presentation of the response to denaturation and renaturation of DNA that has been cross-linked by nitrogen mustard. Under alkaline conditions, hydrogen bonding of the double-stranded DNA is broken, but the strands are held together by the drug. On neutralization, complete renaturation takes place ("zipping up" process indicated by the vertical arrows) because the complementary DNA strands are able to reassume the "correct" hydrogen-bonding sequence.

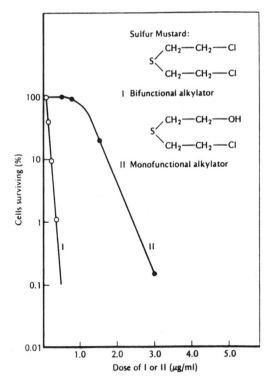

Figure 6–4 Comparison of the effects of a monofunctional and a bifunctional alkylating agent on the survival of HeLa cells. Cultures were exposed to either sulfur mustard (I, a bifunctional agent with two chlorethyl groups) or to half-mustard (II, a monofunctional agent with one chlorethyl group) and the number of surviving cells were determined. (Adapted from Roberts *et al.*[13])

shown in a rodent leukemia cell line, for example, that cross-links formed at subtoxic doses of mechlorethamine were fully repaired by 24 hours, but at cytotoxic doses, the cross-links were not fully repaired within the same period after drug treatment.[20]

Both bacteria and mammalian cells that have an unusual sensitivity to ultraviolet radiation also have an increased sensitivity to alkylating agents.[21,22] These very sensitive cells have deficient repair mechanisms and cannot excise the alkylated regions of their DNA. Patients with xeroderma pigmentosum have defective excision repair, and fibroblasts from these patients are highly sensitive to the cytotoxic and mutagenic affects of alkylating agents when compared to fibroblasts obtained from normal controls.[22] The fact that the sensitivity of a cell to

an alkylating drug varies inversely with its ability to repair drug-induced DNA damage is a powerful argument in support of the proposal that DNA damage is the critical event responsible for cytotoxicity.

RESISTANCE. Although tumor cells selected for resistance to an alkylating agent sometimes have increased excision repair activity,[20] this mechanism may not be a major factor in the development of clinical resistance to these drugs.[17] Two mechanisms of resistance that may very well be clinically important are increased drug inactivation due to reaction with cellular thiols and decreased drug uptake.

In Chapter 4, we have discussed a form of multiple drug resistance based on elevated cellular content of glutathione (GSH), a compound that reacts with the cytotoxic electro-

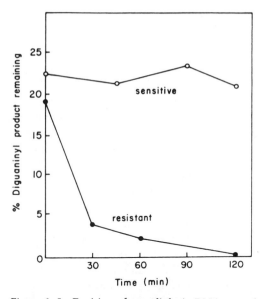

Figure 6–5 Excision of cross-links in DNA treated with an alkylating agent. Cultures of a sensitive and a resistant strain of *E. coli* were treated briefly with [35S]mustard gas, a potent bifunctional alkylating agent. The cultures were diluted and aerated to remove the toxic gas, then sampled at various times. DNA was extracted and hydrolyzed to remove purine residues. Diguanyl and guanine residues were separated, and their radioactivity was determined. The graph shows the bifunctionally alkylated guanine as a percentage of total alkylated guanine, representing the degree of cross-linking of the DNA *in vivo*. (From Venitt[19])

philic derivatives of alkylating agents (see Fig. 6–2) and detoxifies them.[23] The enzyme that catalyzes the conjugation of electrophilic compounds with GSH is glutathione S-transferase (see Fig. 4–6 for reactions), and increased levels of this enzyme have been associated with resistance to alkylating drugs in model tumor systems.[24] These observations led to the development of butathionine sulfoximine (BSO), an inhibitor of γ-glutamlycysteine synthetase, a key enzyme in the pathway of de novo GSH biosynthesis.[25] Depletion of GSH with BSO can increase the in vitro cytotoxicity of several DNA cross-linking drugs, such as nitrogen mustard, melphalan, mitomycin, and cisplatin.[26] Chapter 4 described a study in which combination treatment with BSO and melphalan lowered cellular GSH and potentiated cytotoxicity in drug-resistant human ovarian cells growing in nude mice (see Fig. 4–7).[27,28] Although studies such as these raise the hope that such an approach may render human tumors that are resistant to alkylating agents again responsive to therapy, it should be cautioned that it is not known whether elevated levels of GSH are an important factor in clinical resistance or not.

In several studies it has been shown that tumor cell lines resistant to nitrogen mustards take up the drug at a slower rate than that of the drug-sensitive parent cells.[29] The decrease in drug uptake, however, is not usually enough to account for all the resistance on this basis alone. In a study employing Ehrlich ascites cells, for example, uptake of drug into the resistant line was one-half that of the sensitive line, but resistance to the drug was 10- to 100-fold.[30]. Nitrogen mustard is actively transported into cells,[30,31] and at least two separate transport systems have been identified in human lymphocytes. One, a high-affinity, low-capacity system, is utilized at low drug concentrations and is shared with choline; the other is a lower-affinity, high-capacity system that is operative at high drug concentrations and is unrelated to choline transport.

Resistance mechanisms such as increased excision repair and increased cellular glutathione would be expected to yield cross-resistance among a variety of DNA cross-linking drugs. Resistance due to decreased drug uptake would yield cross-resistance only if the same uptake mechanism was shared by different drug classes. Mechlorethamine-resistant cells with decreased drug uptake may show a low degree of cross-resistance to other alkylating agents, but resistance is only partial and most of the other drugs seem to be taken up by different mechanisms.[32] Although cross-resistance can be elicited in animal tumor models, tumor cells selected for resistance to one alkylating agent can show cross-resistance to another agent and simultaneously respond like the drug-sensitive parent line to many other alkylating drugs.[33]

The level of cross-resistance among alkylating agents is generally low in human tumor cells,[34,35] and clinically, different alkylating agents can be used in retreatment protocols. Because additive or synergistic effects can be obtained with combinations of alkylating agents against experimental tumors in vivo[33] and because there is a relative lack of cross-resistance among the agents,[34,35] high-dose alkylating agent combination regimens (e.g., cyclophosphamide, cisplatin, carmustine, and melphalan) have been administered to patients with advanced cancers.[36] Such combinations are administered with the goal of total tumor cell eradication and the expectation of simultaneous eradication of the normal marrow. At the termination of the high-dose chemotherapy protocol, bone marrow cells obtained from the patient prior to therapy are transplanted back (autologous bone marrow transplantation) to reestablish normal marrow function (see Chapter 13).

PROLIFERATION DEPENDENCY OF THE ALKYLATING AGENTS. As mentioned in Chapter 3, the alkylating agents are generally considered to be cell-cycle-phase nonspecific. Although these drugs interact with the DNA of resting cells as well as the DNA of proliferating cells during any phase of the replication cycle, it is also clear that they are most cytotoxic to rapidly proliferating cells.[37] Some data suggest that when proliferating cells are exposed to low doses of sulfur mustard during S phase or late in G_1 (see Fig. 3–4) the cytotoxic effects are more severe than when cells are exposed at other times in the cell cycle.[13] Thus, although DNA alkylation can occur anytime, its biological consequences are more severe when it occurs during DNA synthesis. This implies that a moderate amount of alkylation is less damaging when the cell is not synthesizing DNA, probably because cells exposed to the drug earlier in G_1 would have sufficient time to repair some of the DNA damage before the next DNA synthesis phase and thus would be less affected. Nonproliferating cells (those in the so-called G_0 state) would have an extended period for DNA repair before irreversible damage occurred and thus escape even more of the drug effect. If the "resting" cells are recruited into division before significant repair takes place, they are irreversibly damaged. Thus, the alkylating agents are said to be proliferation dependent but cell-cycle-phase nonspecific (subject to the modifications noted above). The amount of damage will depend to a significant extent on the growth fraction of the tumor.

Pharmacology of the Nitrogen Mustards

REACTIVITY DIFFERENCES AMONG THE NITROGEN MUSTARDS. A number of modified mustards have been synthesized in an attempt to obtain an anticancer drug that will preferentially localize in a particular tissue. Melphalan (L-phenylalanine mustard) is an example of such a compound. Since phenylalanine is a precursor of melanin, it was postulated that a phenylalanine mustard might preferentially accumulate in melanomas and thereby produce a selective effect. Drugs containing pyrimidines (e.g., uracil mustard), phenylbutyric acid (chlorambucil), amino acids, and steroids have been developed under similar rationales to achieve greater selectivity of action. Although the goal of a "site-directed" mustard effect has not been achieved, a few of these compounds have chemical and pharmacological properties that make them very useful in the treatment of cancer.

Some of the problems associated with the clinical use of mechlorethamine (nitrogen mustard) are due to its high chemical reactivity. At physiological pH, this compound can rapidly cyclize to react with water or blood and tissue constituents. But the placement of an aromatic ring next to the nitrogen (see Fig. 6–1), as in melphalan and chlorambucil, alters the rate of alkylation. Because of the electron-withdrawing effect of the ring moiety, the rate of cyclization (immonium ion formation) in these

modified nitrogen mustards is slow, rendering them much less reactive than mechlorethamine. This decreased reactivity allows time for absorption and wide distribution before extensive alkylation occurs. Thus, these drugs can be given orally, whereas mechlorethamine can only be given intravenously. Although the chemical reaction is slower, these drugs alkylate DNA and other cellular constituents in a manner similar to that of mechlorethamine, and their biological effect is the same.

Cyclophosphamide, another modified mustard, was developed in the hope that it might be preferentially activated in neoplastic cells. Relatively high phosphatase and phosphoramidase activities have been found in some tumors, and it was postulated that the cleavage of the phosphamide ring would produce an active compound within the tumor cells. Although selectivity was not achieved, the drug is clinically useful. Cyclophosphamide itself is not active, but it undergoes a microsomal cytochrome P-450-dependent metabolic activation in the liver. Ifosfamide is a structural analog of cyclophosphamide (Fig. 6–1) that is activated in the same manner as the parent compound is.

ADMINISTRATION. The principal routes of administration of the nitrogen mustards are listed in Table 6–1. The route of administration is determined by the aqueous solubility, the vesicant properties of these drugs, and the rate at which chemical transformation to the active intermediate takes place. As an example, the hydrochloride salt of mechlorethamine is readily soluble in water, it is rapidly activated, and it is a potent vesicant. It is thus provided as a powder that must be dissolved in sterile distilled water and immediately injected into the patient. Because mechlorethamine is a potent vesicant, care should be taken to avoid contact with the skin of both the patient and the person administering the drug. Great care should also be taken to avoid extravasation of the drug into the tissue at the injection site. The safest way to administer the drug is to inject the fresh solution directly into the tubing of a rapidly flowing intravenous infusion, and gloves should be worn during preparation of the drug solution and injection. It stands to reason that this drug, which reacts rapidly with tissue com-

Table 6–1   *Pharmacology of the Nitrogen Mustards*

Drug	Principal Route of Administration	Plasma Half-Life	Pharmacological Characteristics
Mechlorethamine	Intravenous	Very short (minute)	Very rapid action; potent vesicant effect
Chlorambucil	Oral	1.5 hours	Slow rate of conversion to carbonium ion
Melphalan	Oral	1.5 hours	
Cyclophosphamide	Oral or intravenous	7 hours	Must be metabolized in the liver before they are active
Ifosphamide	Intravenous	7 hours	

ponents and is not cell-cycle-phase dependent, has an immediate chemical effect. The other mustard-type alkylating drugs are more lipophilic and slower reacting than nitrogen mustard. They can be given orally, since absorption and distribution in the body can occur before they react with nucleophilic groups.

Experiments in animals have shown that over 90% of the mechlorethamine administered disappears from the plasma within 4 minutes.[38] Because of the rapid reaction rate of mechlorethamine, tissues closer (in the direction of blood flow) to an intraarterial injection site will be exposed to a somewhat higher concentration of the drug than those farther away. In some unusual cases, the rapid reactivity of mechlorethamine has been exploited in therapy by delivering the drug directly into arteries supplying the area in which the tumor is localized. When a tumor is localized in an extremity, higher local drug concentrations can be achieved by limb perfusion, and the concentration of drug in the bone marrow is relatively low, yielding increased selective toxicity.

METABOLISM AND EXCRETION. Because of the reactivity of nitrogen mustard, various byproducts of the drug are formed in the body and very little unchanged drug appears in the urine.

Chlorambucil is rapidly and completely (80%) absorbed from the gastrointestinal tract, with peak plasma concentration being achieved in about 1 hour.[39] A significant portion of the drug is oxidized at the butyric acid side chain to yield phenylacetic acid mustard, which is also an active DNA cross-linking agent and contributes significantly to the activity of the

drug.[40] The terminal phase plasma half-life (Table 6–1) of the parent drug is 1.5 hours and the half-life of the phenylacetic acid metabolite is about 2.5 hours.[39] Very little of the drug is recovered in the urine.[39]

In contrast to chlorambucil, the bioavailability of melphalan after oral administration is extremely variable and the drug undergoes rapid chemical degradation with little active metabolism.[41] Ten to 15 percent of the drug is excreted intact in the urine.[41] When melphalan is administered with prednisone in intermittent therapy of multiple myeloma, the area under the plasma concentration-time curve increases by nearly 45% by the fourth course of drug administration.[42] The pharmacological basis for this increase is not known, but the increased potential cytotoxicity may contribute significantly to the clinical efficacy of this treatment regimen. Melphalan enters tumor cells by utilizing two amino acid transport systems: the sodium-independent, L amino acid system transports leucine and glutamine, and the sodium-dependent, ASC system transports alanine, serine, and cysteine.[29] High concentrations of leucine and glutamine can protect against melphalan cytotoxicity,[43] and in most cells the L system appears to be the dominant uptake mechanism.[29] Melphalan uptake by breast cancer cells is also inhibited by the antiestrogen tamoxifen.[44]

Cyclophosphamide and ifosfamide are unique among the clinically useful mustards in that they must be metabolically activated in the liver before they can alkylate cellular constituents. Cyclophosphamide itself is not cytotoxic to cells in culture, but serum from animals that have been treated with the drug is cytotoxic and cultured cells are killed when they are incubated with both the drug and a liver homogenate, which can convert it to an active form.[45] Cyclophosphamide is converted by the hepatic mixed-function oxidase system to 4-hydroxycyclophosphamide.[46] As shown in Figure 6–6, this product is in equilibrium with its acyclic tautomeric form, aldophosphamide. 4-Ketocyclophosphamide and carboxyphosphamide are produced by further enzymatic oxidation. Although these are the major metabolites of the drug, neither compound is significantly cytotoxic either *in vivo* or *in vitro*.[47] In addition to these inactive metabolites, however, some phosphoramide mustard and acrolein are formed from aldophosphamide by a β-elimination reaction; the phosphoramide mustard is a potent alkylating agent and is cytotoxic.[46] Phosphoramide mustard can itself decompose to nornitrogen mustard.

One might expect that if the initial step in the metabolic activation of cyclophosphamide occurs predominantly in the liver, this organ might be exposed to a higher concentration of the toxic end products phosphoramide mustard and acrolein. Although hepatotoxicity has been reported, it is rare and it is not clear whether significant amounts of cytotoxic end products are produced in the liver. It would seem probable that some of the hydroxyphosphamide (and its tautomer aldophosphamide) formed in the liver returns to the bloodstream to be carried throughout the body. Significant chemical cleavage of aldophosphamide to phosphoramide mustard and acrolein could then occur in the blood, in tissues, and in tumor cells. Thus, one can perhaps think of the liver as effecting the slow release of the active metabolite precursor. It has been proposed that the liver may tend to escape exposure to high concentrations of the toxic products because of its high activity of aldehyde dehydrogenase,[48]

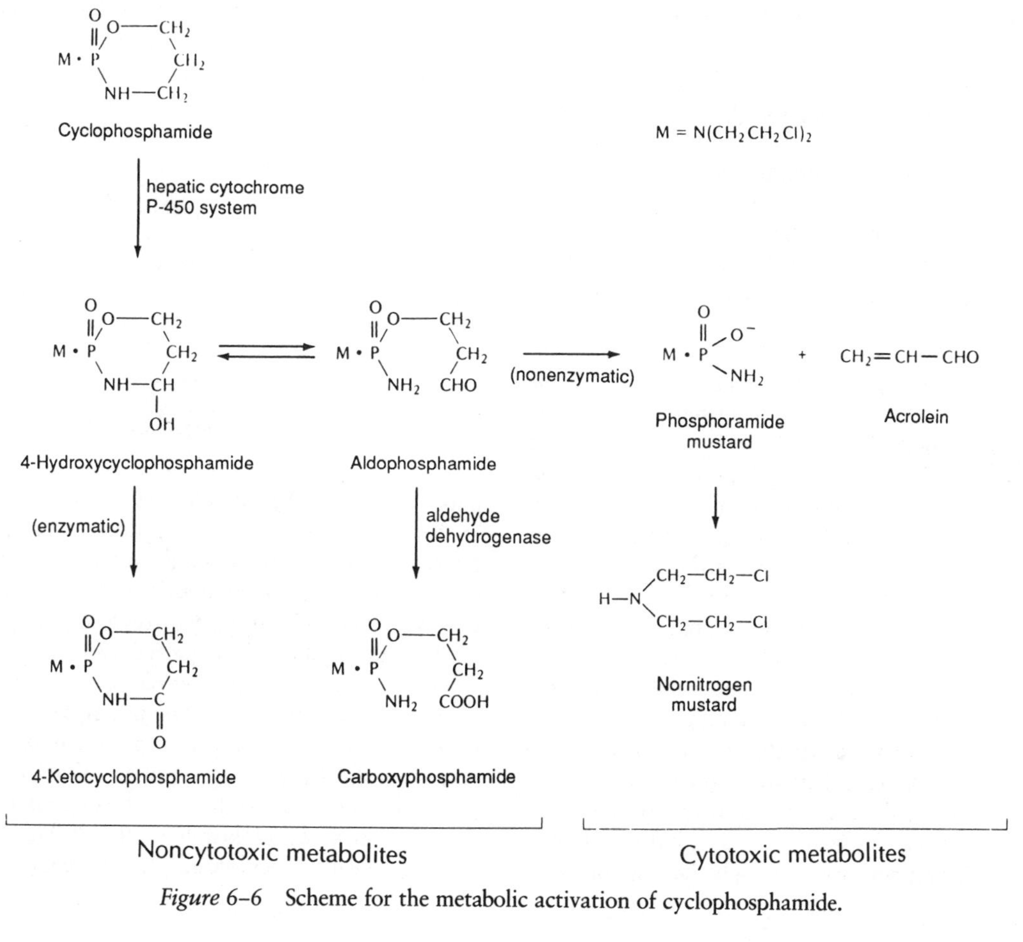

Figure 6–6 Scheme for the metabolic activation of cyclophosphamide.

an enzyme that converts aldophosphamide to the noncytotoxic compound carboxyphosphamide.[49] Some of the selective action of the cyclophosphamide in various tissues may perhaps be attributed to the balance between the enzymatic production (due to oxidation) of nontoxic metabolite (carboxyphosphamide) and the chemical production (due to nonenzymatic breakdown) of the cytotoxic end products.[49]

Acrolein and phosphoramide mustard are produced in equimolar amounts. One might expect that acrolein would contribute to the final cytotoxicity of cyclophosphamide, especially if aldophosphamide is broken down in the tumor cell. Acrolein is not as toxic as phosphoramide mustard in bioassay, however, and there is evidence that phosphoramide mustard is the major cytotoxic end product of cyclophosphamide.[46]

Since the initial step in the activation of cyclophosphamide involves the hepatic cytochrome P-450 metabolizing system, one might predict that drugs that affect the activity of this system could modify the toxic and therapeutic effects of cyclophosphamide. In humans, cyclophosphamide can apparently increase its own rate of metabolism. In patients who have received no medication, the plasma half-life of cyclophosphamide is about 7 hours on the first day of therapy, decreasing by about 30% to 40% on the third to fifth day.[50] The fact that cyclophosphamide induces its own drug metabolizing enzymes[51,52] may account for the high variability in half-lives reported for the drug. Phenobarbital and other drugs that induce the hepatic drug metabolizing system can alter the plasma half-life of cyclophosphamide, but the therapeutic effect of cyclophosphamide is apparently not significantly affected.[51,53] Allopurinol, a drug that prevents hyperuricemia during cancer chemotherapy, inhibits microsomal drug metabolism in humans.[54] Pretreatment with allopurinol increases the half-life of cyclophosphamide in patients, but total plasma alkylating activity does not really change.[50] Thus, it appears that although the half-life of cyclophosphamide is affected by drugs that act upon the hepatic drug metabolizing system, the area under the concentration versus time curve for plasma alkylating activity (that is, the total alkylating activity to which the patient is exposed) does not change significantly over a fourfold range of cyclophosphamide half-lives.[50,51] Since the patient is exposed to approximately the same total alkylating activity, the toxic and therapeutic effects do not change appreciably.

Cyclophosphamide is well absorbed from the gastrointestinal tract, with the oral and intravenous routes being equivalent with respect to the area under the plasma concentration versus time curve.[55] Estimates of the terminal phase plasma half-life have varied from 3 to 12 hours in various studies, with the mean being around 7 hours.[56] Clinically, more important than the half-life of the parent drug is the half-life of plasma alkylating activity, which is about 8.8 hours.[57] About 60% of the drug is excreted in the urine over 24 to 48 hours, mostly as metabolites.[56] (A detailed review of the complex metabolism and pharmacokinetics of cyclophosphamide is found in ref. 58.)

Ifosfamide is metabolized by the hepatic cytochrome P-450 system and it undergoes the same metabolic conversions as cyclophosphamide to yield acrolein and the principal active metabolite isophosphoramide mustard.[59] As with cyclophosphamide, estimates of the

Phosphoramide mustard

Isophosphoramide mustard

plasma half-life of ifosfamide vary widely, but at doses below 3.8 g/m^2, it appears to have a pharmacokinetic profile similar to that of cyclophosphamide.[60] At higher doses, the half-life may be longer. With both of these drugs, patients with significantly impaired liver function should be regarded as having reduced biotransformation and activation. The principal difference between the two drugs is that the hydroxylation of the 4-carbon of the ring of ifosfamide proceeds more slowly than the analogous hydroxylation of cyclophosphamide (see Fig. 6–6). As a result, dechloroethylation reactions, which play a small role in cyclophosphamide metabolism, become quantitatively important pathways for ifosfamide metabolism. Since dechlorethylation inactivates the drug, a smaller proportion of ifosfamide is ultimately converted to cytotoxic compounds and larger doses are used clinically.

Use and Toxicity of the Nitrogen Mustards

MECHLORETHAMINE. Mechlorethamine is now used mainly in the treatment of Hodgkin's lymphoma as part of the MOPP regimen[61] (this regimen combines mechlorethamine, vincristine (Oncovin®), procarbazine, and prednisone). The rationale behind this and other drug combinations is discussed in Chapter 10. With considerably less predictable efficacy, mechlorethamine has been used in other types of lymphomas. It is sometimes used topically in dilute solution to treat mycosis fungoides, and allergic sensitization to the chlorethyl side chain may occur when the drug is administered this way.[62]

Mechlorethamine therapy is frequently accompanied by nausea and vomiting. Vomiting is apparently mediated through the central nervous system, and antiemetic therapy may help alleviate it. Other acute side effects (Table 6–2) are local reactions, which can occur if there is extravasation during administration, and phlebitis, which is also a consequence of the highly irritating properties of the drug. If extravasation occurs, the area should be infiltrated with isotonic sodium thiosulfite, which reacts with the electrophilic drug derivatives. As with all the alkylating agents, the bone marrow is depressed. It is more difficult to control the degree of marrow depression produced by this drug than that produced by the slower acting, orally administered mustards. After an injection of mechlorethamine, marrow depression reaches a maximum in 1 to 2 weeks, and another course of therapy is not usually begun until marrow function has returned (commonly 4 to 6 weeks). Infection and bleeding can occur as a consequence of severe leukopenia and thrombocytopenia. Alopecia occurs, but not as frequently as with cyclosphosphamide therapy. Women should be warned that menstrual irregularities may occur, and the drug should be considered a teratogen and should not be given to pregnant patients. Like all of the other drugs presented in this chapter, the alkylating agents are carcinogens,[63] and therapy with all of the alkylating agents has been associated with the production of second malignancy, most commonly acute leukemia.[64,65]

CHLORAMBUCIL. Chlorambucil is given by daily oral administration, usually for at least 3 to 6 weeks. Compared to mechlorethamine, the extent of its toxicity is easier to control. As a

Table 6–2   *Some Major Untoward Effects of the Nitrogen Mustards.* The usual dose-limiting toxicity is in bold type.

Drug	Principal Toxicities	
	Acute	Delayed
Mechlorethamine	Severe nausea and vomiting; phlebitis and local reaction	**Bone marrow depression,** amenorrhea
Chlorambucil	Nausea and vomiting	**Bone marrow depression**
Melphalan	Mild nausea	**Bone marrow depression**
Cyclophosphamide	Nausea and vomiting	**Bone marrow depression,** hemorrhagic cystitis, alopecia, amenorrhea, sterility, water retention
Ifosphamide with mesna	Nausea and vomiting	**Bone marrow depression,** hemorrhagic cystitis, alopecia, neurotoxicity, water retention

consequence, bone-marrow function is usually less depressed. Chlorambucil is used primarily to treat chronic lymphocytic leukemia,[66] and occasionally to treat patients with lymphomas[67] or carcinoma of the breast or ovary. Chlorambucil is the drug of choice for treating patients with primary (Waldenstrom's) macroglobulinemia. As with other alkylating agents, chlorambucil can cause aspermia,[68] amenorrhea, and acute myelogenous leukemia.[69] Hepatotoxicity and pulmonary fibrosis occur rarely.

MELPHALAN. Melphalan is principally used to treat multiple myeloma;[70] it is also used to treat ovarian[71] and breast tumors.[72] In the treatment of ovarian cancer, intraperitoneal administration allows a much higher local concentration of drug with a tripling of the maximum tolerated dose.[71] The major toxicity of melphalan is bone marrow depression, and as with all these drugs, leukocyte and platelet counts must be very carefully monitored during therapy. Other effects include sterility, amenorrhea,[72] and acute nonlymphocytic leukemia.[73]

CYCLOPHOSPHAMIDE. Cyclophosphamide is the most commonly used alkylating agent, having a broad application in cancer chemotherapy and in the treatment of such non-neoplastic conditions as severe rheumatoid arthritis.[74] It can be given either orally or intravenously, and its side effects are easier to control than those of mechlorethamine. Cyclophosphamide is used in combination drug regimens to treat a wide variety of cancers, including lymphoid tumors (e.g., Hodgkin's disease, non-Hodgkin's lymphoma, diffuse large-cell lymphoma, Burkitt's lymphoma), myeloma, several developmental tumors (e.g., embryonal rhabdomyosarcoma, Ewing's sarcoma, osteogenic sarcoma, Wilms' tumor, neuroblastoma, retinoblastoma), and carcinomas of the breast, lung, ovary, and endometrium.

One side effect of cyclophosphamide, immunosuppression, led to its use to prevent transplant rejection.[75,76] Although more effective drugs have largely replaced cyclophosphamide in the prevention of allograft rejection, it is still used in combination with corticosteroids to treat a few non-neoplastic diseases thought to have an immunological etiology, including

Wegener's granulomatosis, idiopathic thrombocytopenic purpura, childhood nephrosis, and severe rheumatoid arthritis.[77] Cyclophosphamide can markedly depress the primary humoral response when it is given with a sensitizing dose of antigen, and it partially inhibits the secondary response as well.[78] Cellular immune reactions are also inhibited. In patients given cyclophosphamide as immunosuppressive therapy, the number of both the B and T lymphocytes in the peripheral blood is diminished, with the B lymphocytes being depressed earlier.[79]

The toxicity and clinical use of cyclophosphamide have been reviewed by Gershwin et al.[78] Cyclophosphamide frequently causes nausea and vomiting, particularly when it is given intravenously. It is not a vesicant. The dose-limiting toxicity is bone marrow suppression, but the effect on the leukocyte count is much more profound than the effect on the platelet count.[80] After a course of therapy, the nadir in the leukocyte and platelet counts is achieved in about 12 days, with substantial recovery occurring by 3 to 4 weeks.[80] The relative platelet-sparing effect of cyclophosphamide is attractive for its use in combination drug regimens. As with any drug that profoundly depresses the immune response, infection is a risk. Alopecia occurs frequently with cyclophosphamide.[80] Hair growth reoccurs, but there may be a change in pigmentation.[81] Amenorrhea is common and occurs at a lower dose in patients over 40 years of age than in younger patients.[82] Reduced sperm count or aspermia occurs commonly in males.[83] Electrocardiogram changes and serum enzyme alterations compatible with myocardial toxicity occur in some patients receiving high-dose therapy.[80] Interstitial pneumonitis and pulmonary fibrosis are rare complications of cyclophosphamide therapy.[84] As with other alkylating agents, this drug is carcinogenic,[73] mutagenic, and teratoganic.

A major side effect of cyclophosphamide is hemorrhagic cystitis, which occurs in about 10% of patients who are adequately hydrated and treated with normal doses. With high-dose therapy, the incidence is considerably higher. The cystitis ranges from microhematuria to frank hemorrhage and may progress with long-term therapy to urinary-bladder fibrosis and telangiectasia.[85] As mentioned above, a significant portion of a dose of cyclophosphamide is excreted into the urine as the active alkylating species phosphoramide mustard and acrolein. In contrast to the antitumor cytotoxicity, which is mainly due to phosphoramide mustard,[46] the cystitis appears to be caused by acrolein.[86] The problem of cystitis can be reduced by ensuring good fluid intake and frequent voiding, and it can be prevented by administration of compounds like N-acetyl-cysteine or mesna, both of which react with acrolein and detoxify it. As with all patients who are treated with ifosfamide, patients receiving high-dose cyclophosphamide should receive mesna as well (see next section for description of mesna action). Long-term cyclophosphamide therapy can be followed by the development of bladder cancer,[87] and it has been shown in animal models that the development of bladder tumors can be prevented by concomitant administration of mesna.[88]

Water intoxication may also occur at high drug dosage, and this has been correlated temporally with the excretion of active metabolite.[89] The water retention appears to be due to inappropriate antidiuretic hormone secretion and possibly to a direct effect on the renal distal tubule. This syndrome, which is reversible upon withdrawal of the drug, is especially important, since these patients are vigorously hydrated to prevent hemorrhagic cystitis and uric acid lithiasis. Hyponatremia and seizures have occurred as a consequence of water retention. Treatment with furosamide can prevent the water retention.[90]

IFOSFAMIDE. Given their structural and mechanistic similarities, it is not surprising that ifosfamide (given virtually always with mesna) has a broad antitumor activity similar to that of cyclophosphamide.[91] The indications for the use of the two drugs clinically are essentially the same, although ifosfamide (in combination drug therapy) has elicited responses in tumors pretreated with cyclophosphamide,[91] suggesting that, in contrast to *in vitro* studies, clinical cross-resistance may not be complete.

Because of the difference in the metabolism of the two drugs discussed above, the pattern of toxicity for ifosfamide is different from that of cyclophosphamide. The slower rate of hydroxylation of ifosfamide leads to increased

inactivation via dechloroethylation,[92] and consequently, higher drug doses are employed. When the toxicities of ifosfamide and cyclophosphamide were compared as single agents at a dose ratio of 5 to 1, the incidence of bone marrow depression and alopecia were found to be the same.[93] However, cystitis occurred in 18% of patients after ifosfamide, as opposed to 6% after cyclophosphamide. Thus, ifosfamide is less myelosuppressive, and in the absence of concomitant administration of mesna, the dose-limiting toxicity is cystitis. When mesna is administered as well, the dose-limiting toxicity is usually bone marrow depression.

Concomitant administration of mesna markedly reduces the severity and incidence of cystitis both in patients receiving initial treatment and in patients who have experienced cystitis with previous oxazaphosphorine therapy.[94,95] Mesna is sodium 2-mercaptoethane sulfonate and it inactivates alkylating metabolites in the urine, much as reduced glutathione inactivates alkylating species inside tumor cells (Fig. 6–7). The compound is administered intravenously and it dimerizes in the serum to an inactive disulfide that does not inactivate the circulating drug metabolites. Thus, mesna does not affect the antitumor activity or clinical effect of ifosfamide or cyclophosphamide. Mesna disulfide has a short half-life because it is rapidly eliminated by the kidneys, mostly via glomerular filtration. After filtration, it is reduced by gluta-

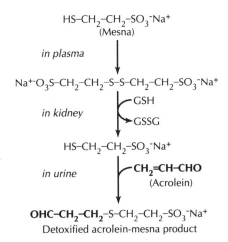

Figure 6–7 Detoxification of acrolein in the urine by mesna. GSH, reduced glutathione; GSSG, oxidized glutathione.

thione in the kidney to the free thiol compound, which reacts with and detoxifies the alkylating derivatives of cyclophosphamide and ifosphamide in the urine.[96] Mesna is given intravenously at the same time as ifosfamide, and again 4 and 8 hours later. As with cyclophosphamide, good hydration of the patient is important.

Like patients receiving cyclophosphamide, patients receiving ifosfamide can retain water due to inappropriate ADH secretion; consequently, there is the potential for hyponatremia and rarely seizures. Rarely, ifosfamide causes renal damage with Fanconi syndrome, even when mesna is administered concomitantly.[97] Neurotoxicity has been reported in as many as 30% of patients receiving high-dose ifosfamide therapy. The spectrum of toxicity ranges from subclinical EEG changes and mild motor dysfunction to severe motor disturbances, including seizures, cerebellar signs, and cranial nerve dysfunction. Neurotoxicity has been correlated with impairment of both hepatic function and renal function.[98] Neurotoxicity has not been seen with cyclophosphamide, and it is thought to be related to the dechloroethylation that occurs with ifosfamide, leading to the presence in the plasma of chloroacetaldehyde, a potential neurotoxin.[99]

Aziridines (Ethylenimines)

Several compounds that contain three-membered aziridine rings (see Fig. 6–8) have been synthesized and found to be active antitumor drugs. Triethylenemelamine (TEM) and thiotepa (triethylenethiophosphoramide) were the first to be used clinically. Thiotepa still has a limited clinical use in the United States, and trenimon, a third compound in this group, is occasionally used in Europe. The three-membered aziridine ring is structurally analogous to the immonium-ion intermediate formed from the nitrogen mustards (Fig. 6–2). Altretamine (hexamethylmelamine) is a nonclassical alkylating agent. It does not have an aziridine ring structure, but it is a structural analog of triethylenemelamine, and for that reason, it is considered here. Mitomycin is an antibiotic that contains an aziridine ring and acts through a unique mechanism as a bifunctional alkylator.

Thiotepa

The mechanism of action of thiotepa is similar to that of the nitrogen mustards, although it is more reactive at acid pH, whereas the mustards are more reactive at alkaline pH. In contrast to

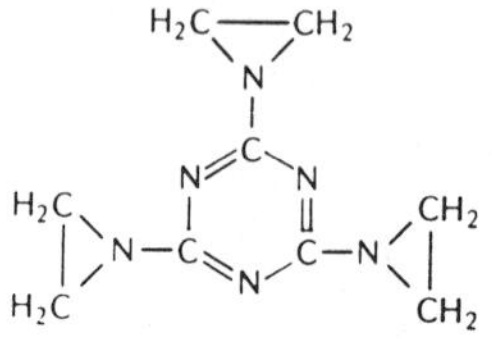

Triethylenemelamine
(TEM)

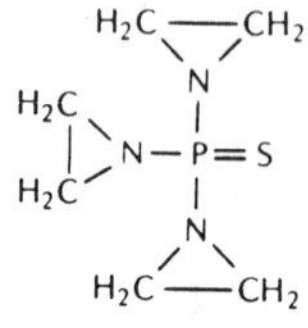

Thio-tepa
(Triethlyenethiophosphoramide, Thio-TEPA)

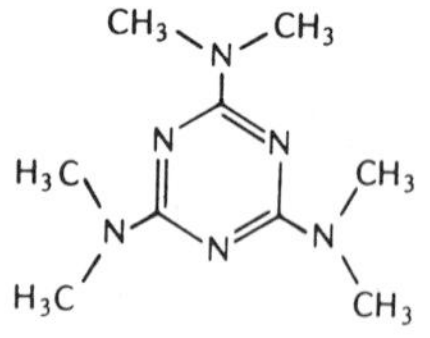

Altretamine
(Hexamethylmelamine)

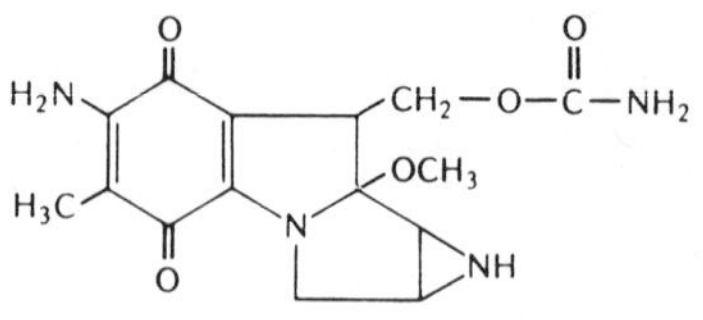

Mitomycin
(Mitomycin C)

Figure 6–8 Structures of drugs in the aziridine (ethylenimine) class of alkylating agents.

the immonium ion formed by the mustards, the aziridine moieties are not charged and the reactivity results from the strain on the three-member ring structures. The general pharmacology of thiotepa has not been worked out in detail.[100] The drug is unstable in acid and poorly absorbed from the gastrointestinal tract. After intravenous injection of radiolabeled drug, the plasma level falls by 90% in 1 to 4 hours and 60% to 85% of the radioactivity is recovered in the urine within 24 hours, with less than 1% representing the parent compound.[101] Thiotepa is now only rarely administered systemically. The drug is used topically, by direct instillation, to treat papillary carcinoma of the bladder, and this is its major clinical application. By intracavitary administration, it is also used to treat ascites caused by tumor metastases in the peritoneum.

When it is given systematically, bone marrow depression is the major toxic effect. Anorexia, nausea, and vomiting occur often, and local pain may be experienced at the injection site. When the drug is given by direct installation into the bladder, there is sufficient absorption of the drug through the bladder mucosa to cause transient myelosuppression in 18% of patients.[102] The risk of myelosuppression may be increased if there is bilateral vesicoureteral reflux.[103]

Altretamine (Hexamethylmelamine)

MECHANISM OF ACTION. Hexamethylmelamine (HMM) itself does not have cytotoxic activity, but it is converted by liver microsomes and an NADPH-generating system to cytotoxic products.[104] The drug undergoes a series of cytochrome P-450-mediated oxidative N-demethylation reactions,[105] to produce active metabolites that bind covalently to DNA and proteins.[106] The major cytotoxic product appears to be hydroxymethylpentamethylmelamine (HMPMM).[107,108] It has been proposed that covalent binding is due to the formation of a reactive iminium species (Fig. 6–9) that reacts with nucleophiles.[105] Although formaldehyde is formed during the demethylation reactions, it does not contribute to HMM cytotoxicity.[109,110] Despite the fact that HMM metabolism yields reactive alkylating species, it has not yet been demonstrated that cytotoxicity is due

to alkylation. The reaction scheme shown in Figure 6–9 suggests that only monoalkylation products would be formed, but it is possible that a small amount of bifunctional alkylation also occurs. This is suggested by the fact that the synthetic dihydroxymethyl compound (N,N'-dihydroxymethltetramethylmelamine) is cytotoxic[110] and has the potential for forming bifunctional cross-links.

PHARMACOLOGY. Because of its poor aqueous solubility, HMM is given orally (Table 6–3), although a parenteral formulation is available for investigational use.[111] The systemic bioavailability of the parent drug after oral administration is low and erratic.[112] The drug apparently traverses the intestine by simple diffusion,[29] but there is then extensive metabolism (both by cytochrome P-450 enzymes in the gut wall and as a result of first-pass metabolism in the liver[113]) that contributes to low blood levels of the unaltered compound.

After oral administration to humans, peak plasma levels are achieved in 1 to 4 hours.[114] A small amount of unaltered drug may be found in the plasma 2 hours after administration, but thereafter HMM is present only in metabolized form.[115] Soon after the administration of HMM-methyl-^{14}C to patients, radioactivity appears in both the respired air ($^{14}CO_2$) and the urine.[116] No respiratory $^{14}CO_2$ is found after administration of HMM labeled with ^{14}C in the triazene ring, and approximately 90% of the radioactivity is excreted in the urine within 72 hours.[114] These studies show that HMM is rapidly demethylated and excreted in the urine as several demethylated metabolites. The triazene ring does not undergo cleavage, and although some of the drug can be recovered in the bile, it is reabsorbed and there is no fecal elimination.[114] The plasma half-life of radioactivity from the ring-labeled compound is about 13 hours.[114] The ring-labeled compound becomes covalently bound to tissue macromolecules, with the highest levels of covalent binding being found in the liver and small intestine,[117] the major sites of metabolism. It has been shown in rodents that pretreatment with phenobarbital, an inducer of hepatic microsomal drug metabolism, reduces both the plasma AUC and cytotoxicity of hexamethylmelamine.[118] In contrast, cimetidine, an inhibitor of

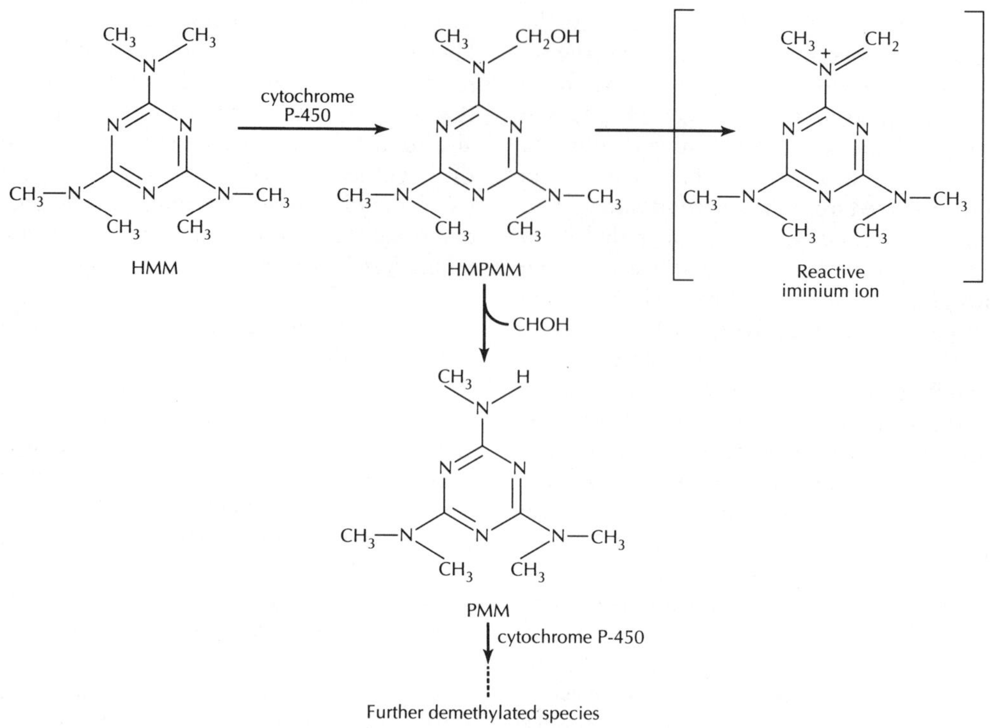

Figure 6–9 Metabolic activation of hexamethylmelamine (HMM) to a potential cytotoxic iminium ion. HMM is oxidized by cytochrome P-450 to hydroxymethylpentamethylmelamine (HMPMM), which can either be converted to pentamethylmelamine (PMM) with the elimination of formaldehyde or can form a proposed iminium ion intermediate that would react with nucleophiles. PMM is converted by successive N-demethylation steps to a variety of demethylated products.

the cytochrome P-450 system, increases both HMM half-life and toxicity.[119]

CLINICAL USE AND TOXICITY. In single agent trials, HMM is active against a number of cancers, including ovarian adenocarcinoma, metastatic small-cell carcinoma of the lung, metastatic breast cancer, and refractory lymphoma.[112,120] Clinically, HMM has elicited responses in patients with advanced ovarian cancer that is resistant to other alkylating agents.[121]

Nausea and vomiting occur commonly and are often the dose-limiting toxicity (Table 6–4).[120] As nausea and vomiting occur after intravenous administration,[111] they appear to be due to an effect on the central nervous system. Anorexia and weight loss may occur. Bone marrow depression is moderate after prolonged administration, with leukopenia being more common than thrombocytopenia. Bone marrow depression is rarely dose-limiting. Neuro-

toxicity (consisting of mood alterations and, less commonly, hallucinations) and peripheral neuropathy occur in a substantial percentage of patients during prolonged therapy and disappear when the drug is withdrawn.[120]

Mitomycin

The mitomycins and their close structural analogs, the porfiromycins, are derived from *Streptomyces* species. Of the several mitomycins, only mitomycin C is used clinically in the United States, and the generic name mitomycin is used for this compound. Mitomycin contains several potentially biologically active groups, such as the aziridine ring, the C-10 carbamate group, and the quinone moiety (Fig. 6–8). Like the other alkylating agents discussed in this chapter, mitomycin cross-links DNA.

MECHANISM OF ACTION. Mitomycin selectively inhibits DNA synthesis in both bacteria

Table 6–3 *Pharmacology of the Aziridines and Alkane Sulfonates*

Drug	Principal Route of Administration	Plasma Half-Life	Pharmacological Characteristics
Aziridines			
Thiotepa	Intravesical	Rapid (<1 hour)	Absorption from bladder can be enough to cause myelosuppression
Altretamine (Hydroxymethylmelamine)	Oral	Rapid metabolism	Rapid demethylation by cytochrome P-450 to its active form
Mitomycin	Intravenous	Rapid (<1 hour)	Bioreductive alkylation. The quinone moiety of the drug is enzymatically reduced to yield an active bioalkylating species
Alkane sulfonates			
Busulfan	Oral	2.5 hours	Selective bone marrow cytotoxicity affecting granulocytes much more than lymphocytes

and tumor cells.[122] This inhibition is the result of DNA alkylation and cross-linking. The production of interstrand cross-links was first shown by DNA-melting experiments similar to the experiment shown in Figure 6–3.[123] Subsequently, DNA cross-linking was demonstrated directly by isolation of the cross-linked product from the DNA of rats injected with the drug.[124] Mitomycin has no effect on purified DNA *in vitro* unless a cell extract is added. It has been shown that mitomycin is activated by chemical or enzymatic reduction of the quinone group[125] (see Fig. 6–10). The C-1 aziridine and the C-10 carbamate groups can be regarded as masked

Table 6–4 *Some Major Untoward Effects of the Aziridines and Alkane Sulfonates.* The usual dose-limiting toxicity is in bold type.

Drug	Principal Toxicities	
	Acute	Delayed
Aziridines		
Thiotepa	Anorexia, nausea, vomiting	**Bone marrow depression**
Altretamine	**Nausea and vomiting**	Neurotoxicity, bone marrow depression (leukopenia more severe than thrombocytopenia)
Mitomycin	Nausea and vomiting, tissue necrosis after extravasation	**Bone marrow depression,** alopecia, stomatitis, diarrhea, interstitial pneumonitis, cardiotoxicity (with doxorubicin), nephrotoxicity, hemolytic-uremic syndrome, hepatotoxicity
Alkane sulfonates		
Busulfan	Nausea and vomiting	**Bone marrow depression, pulmonary infiltration and fibrosis,** diarrhea, impotence, sterility, amenorrhea

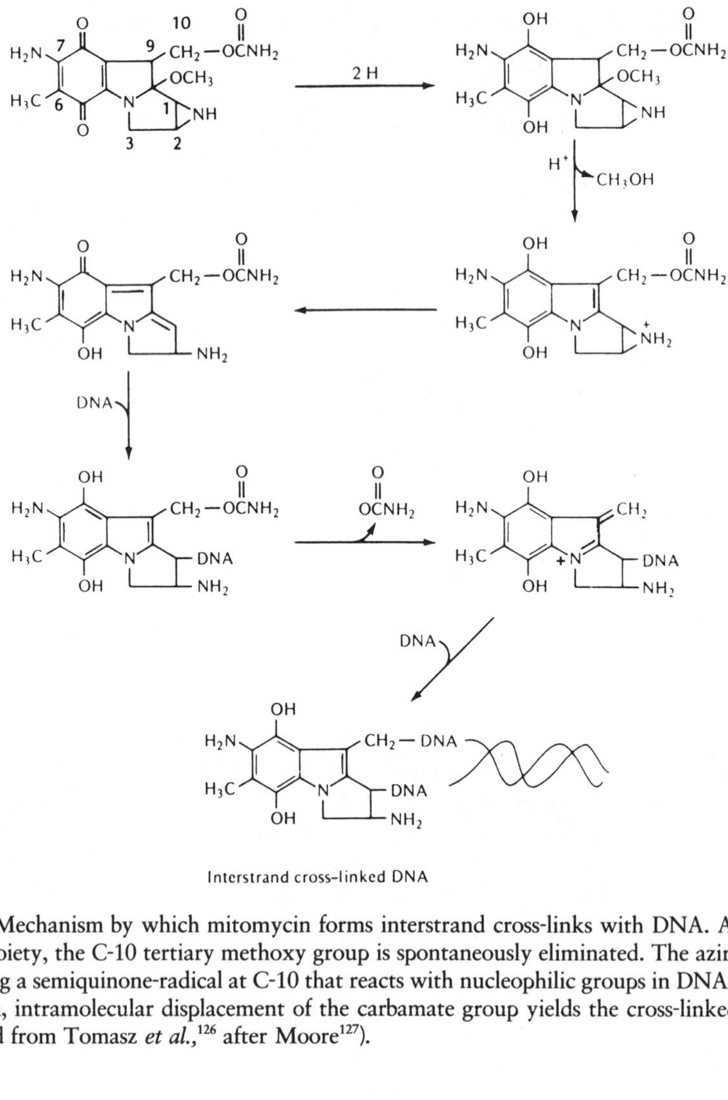

Figure 6–10 Mechanism by which mitomycin forms interstrand cross-links with DNA. After reduction of the quinone moiety, the C-10 tertiary methoxy group is spontaneously eliminated. The aziridine ring is then broken, creating a semiquinone-radical at C-10 that reacts with nucleophilic groups in DNA (most commonly guanine). Then, intramolecular displacement of the carbamate group yields the cross-linked DNA–drug adduct. (Modified from Tomasz et al.,[126] after Moore[127]).

alkylating functions that are activated upon reduction of the quinone and consequent spontaneous elimination of methanol.[126,127] Figure 6–10 presents a two-electron reduction to the dihydroquinone, but there is also evidence that one-electron reduction to the semiquinone is sufficient to activate both the C-1 and C-10 electrophilic centers.[128] In the reaction scheme shown in Figure 6–10, the aziridine ring and the C-10 carbamate are the leaving groups that are displaced by nucleophilic groups in opposite DNA strands to create a bifunctional alkylation. Extensive monofunctional alkylation also occurs. This whole process is called *bioreductive alkylation.*[129]

Reductive activation of mitomycin to the se-miquinone can be carried out by a variety of enzymes, including NADPH-cytochrome *c* reductase,[130] xanthine oxidase,[131] and quinone reductase.[130] Both microsomal and nuclear subcellular fractions carry out the reduction.[129] Under aerobic conditions, the quinone radical formed from one-electron reduction can transfer its electron to oxygen, generating superoxide anion and subsequently other active oxygen species.[132] This would be expected to regenerate the oxidized quinone and decrease the extent of DNA cross-linking. Thus, it was reasoned that mitomycin C might be more active in hypoxic cells than in cells growing under aerobic conditions, and with a mammary tumor cell line, this has been found to be the case.[133] Interestingly, it has been shown that treatment of the mammary tumor cells with dicoumarol, an inhibitor of quinone reductase, increases the toxicity of mitomycin to hypoxic cells, while protecting well-oxygenated cells from mitomycin cytotoxicity.[134] Although the basis for this modulation of cytotoxicity under aerobic and hypoxic conditions is not clear, the possibility arises that agents which undergo bioreductive activation, like mitomycin C, may be used to gain enhanced toxicity against cells in hypoxic regions of solid tumor masses.[129]

The reaction of reduced mitomycin with DNA is highly selective to guanine N^2 positions.[135] After reduction, the reduced mitomycin appears to sit in the minor groove where it reacts with the N^2 positions of two guanine moieties in separate DNA strands, with the resulting bifunctional drug adduct producing minimal distortion of DNA structure.[124] There is a requirement for a CG•CG duplex sequence for the cross-linking reaction with the reduced drug.[136] Mitomycin produces more monoalkylation than bialkylation products, but it is the latter that are considered most important for the cytotoxicity. As a result of alkylation, mitomycin is mutagenic and carcinogenic. The drug also produces chromosome breakage.

Resistance can result from both decreased reductive activation and increased excision repair.[137,138] Examination of several Chinese hamster ovary cell lines with different degrees of resistance showed a correlation with both bioreduction and excision repair activities, with the most resistant cells being bioreduction deficient and repair proficient.[138] Tumor cells selected for resistance to mitomycin have showed decreased drug uptake, cross-resistance with both anthracyclines and vinca alkaloids, and reversal of resistance with verapamil, suggesting a multidrug resistance (MDR) phenotype due to increased P-glycoprotein[139] (see Chapter 4). Other alkylating agents do not select for the MDR phenotype.

PHARMACOLOGY. Since gastrointestinal absorption of mitomycin is not reliable,[140] the drug is given intravenously. The drug rapidly disappears from the plasma, with a terminal phase half-life of about 50 minutes.[141] Urinary recovery is limited to a maximum of 15% of a dose, and decreased renal function does not significantly affect elimination of the drug.[142] Although cumulative toxicity tends to occur after repeated administration of mitomycin, the pharmacokinetic profile does not change with repeated administration.[143] Some studies suggest that the total body clearance is higher and the AUC is lower in patients receiving mitomycin in combination therapy, rather than as a single drug.[144] The basis for such a difference is unknown. As discussed above in the section concerned with bioreductive activation of the drug, mitomycin is metabolized through reduction of the quinone moiety in the liver and elsewhere in the body.[142]

CLINICAL USE AND TOXICITY. Mitomycin is a highly toxic antibiotic that appears to have some activity against carcinomas of the stomach, colon, pancreas, breast, lung, and head and neck.[145] Remissions following therapy are generally limited and of short duration. Like thiotepa, mitomycin is sometimes given by direct intravesicular installation to treat papillary carcinoma of the bladder. Very little drug is adsorbed from the bladder.[146]

After intravenous administration, mitomycin can produce fever, nausea, and vomiting, and inadvertent extravasation into soft tissue produces a chronic painful ulceration similar to that seen with adriamycin.[147] The most significant and frequent toxicity is a delayed, cumulative myelosuppression with both leukopenia and thrombocytopenia.[145] Stomatitis and diarrhea can occur, and occasionally alopecia and rash may occur. At cumulative doses higher than 30 mg/m^2, mitomycin causes interstitial pneumonitis,[148] cardiotoxicity,[149] and nephrotoxicity,[150] each at an overall incidence of less than 10%. The nephrotoxicity may be related to immune complex formation, and it is often associated with microangiopathic hemolytic anemia in a syndrome called the hemolytic-uremic syndrome.[149] The basis for the interstitial pneumonitis and cardiotoxicity are unknown, but a number of investigators have speculated that they may be due to the generation of active oxygen species as a result of autoxidation of the reduced quinone under aerobic conditions.[149] Some patients receiving intensive mitomycin therapy have developed a syndrome of hepatic veno-occlusive disease characterized by progressive abnormalities in liver function, abdominal pain, and ascites.[151] Because the pneumonitis, the cardiotoxicity, the hemolytic-uremic syndrome, and the hepatic veno-occlusive disease are all potentially fatal complications, one can appreciate why mitomycin is considered one of the most toxic anticancer drugs in clinical use.

Alkane Sulfonates

Busulfan

MECHANISM OF ACTION. Busulfan is a bifunctional alkylating agent that reacts with nucleophiles by an S_N2 mechanism.[100] Thus, the rate-limiting step depends upon the concentrations of both the drug and the nucleophile, in contrast to most of the nitrogen mustards where the rate-limiting step is the unimolecular formation of ethylene immonium ion (Fig. 6–2). The alkyl-oxy bonds of busulfan split and react with the N-7 position of guanine residues in

$$H_3C-\overset{\overset{O}{\|}}{\underset{\underset{O}{\|}}{S}}-O-CH_2-CH_2-CH_2-CH_2-O-\overset{\overset{O}{\|}}{\underset{\underset{O}{\|}}{S}}-CH_3$$

Busulfan

DNA to form a diguanyl derivative.[152] It has been shown by the alkaline elution technique that DNA interstrand cross-links are formed.[153] The significance of the DNA alkylation for the cytotoxic effect is supported by experiments that demonstrated cross-sensitivity and cross-resistance to ultraviolet radiation, nitrogen mustard, and some alkane sulfonates.[154,155] This presumably reflects the cells' ability to repair the DNA damage inflicted by any one of these three mechanisms. Busulfan enters cells by diffusion,[29] and resistance appears to reflect more rapid removal of the DNA cross-links.[156]

PHARMACOLOGY AND TOXICITY. Busulfan has a cytotoxic effect on early hemotopoeitic stem cells[157] that is much greater on cells of myeloid lineage than it is on lymphoid cells. This selective effect led to its well-established use in the treatment of chronic granulocytic leukemia.[158] It has also been used in high-dose combination with cyclophosphamide to condition patients for allogeneic marrow transplantation.[159]

Busulfan is well absorbed from the gastrointestinal tract and is routinely given orally. Peak plasma levels of the unaltered drug are achieved in 1 to 2 hours and the plasma levels decline with a half-life of 2.5 hours.[160] Less than 50% of the total dose of radioactive drug is excreted in the urine,[161] virtually all in the form of metabolites, including methanesulfonic acid and several metabolites derived from the alkylating butylene moiety.[162]

The most common toxic effects are those resulting from bone marrow depression, and either bone-marrow depression or pulmonary toxicity may be dose-limiting. Clinically evident pulmonary disease characteristically appears after long-term therapy. Pulmonary symptoms (dyspnea, dry cough), infiltrates on chest roentgenograms, and abnormalities in pulmonary function tests develop in a few patients who receive the drug.[163,164] In some of the affected individuals, the syndrome progresses to a fatal pulmonary fibrosis despite withdrawal of the drug. Patients should be carefully monitored with serial chest roentgenograms and pulmonary function tests, because the pulmonary status can stabilize if the drug is stopped before the onset of clinical symptoms.[163,164] This condition is sometimes called "busulfan lung," and the basis for it is unknown. It is interesting that studies of the tissue distribution of radiolabeled busulfan in the rat showed the highest levels in kidney, liver, and lung,[165] raising the possibility that direct alkylation of lung tissue may trigger the process. Busulfan can also cause diarrhea, impotence, sterility, and amenorrhea. Rarely an Adisonian-like syndrome with increased skin pigmentation has been reported. Busulfan causes chromosomal aberrations in vivo in man,[100] and some patients develop nonlymphocytic leukemia as a side effect.[166]

The Nitrosoureas

A large number of nitrosourea compounds have been synthesized and tested for antitumor activity. Four compounds that are available for clinical use in the United States are shown in Figure 6–11. Carmustine, which contains two

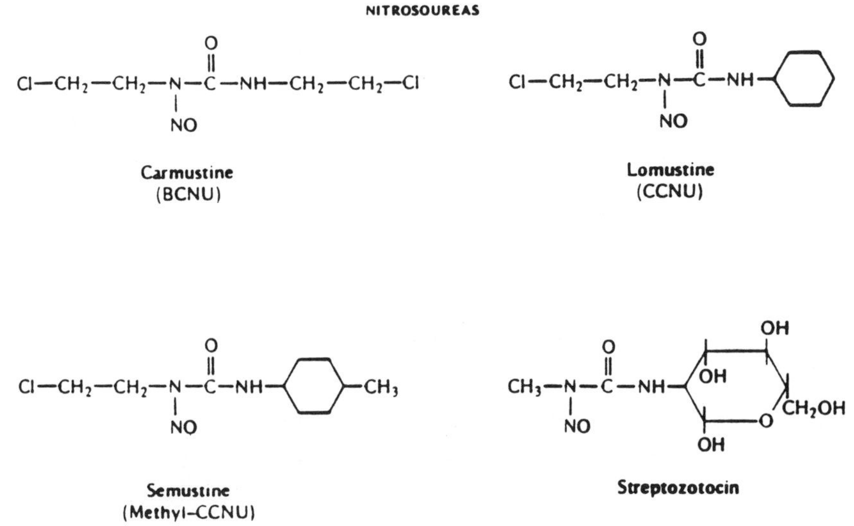

NITROSOUREAS

Figure 6–11 Structures of the nitrosoureas in clinical use.

chloroethyl side chains, is also called BCNU (for bischloroethylnitrosourea). Lomustine (cyclohexylchloroethylnitrosourea, CCNU) and the investigational drug semustine (methyl-CCNU) each contain only one chloroethyl side chain. Streptozotocin is an antibiotic isolated from *Streptomyces achromogenes,* consisting of a nitrosourea moiety with a methyl group on one end and a glucosamine on the other. Chlorozotocin is a synthetic analog of streptozotocin in which the methyl group has been replaced by a chloroethyl moiety. These drugs are all bifunctional alkylating agents.

MECHANISM OF ACTION. The mechanism of action of the chloroethyl nitrosourea compounds (carmustine, lomustine, and semustine) is not as well understood as that of the nitrogen mustards. It is clear that these drugs are both alkylating and carbamoylating agents— that is, they react with a variety of groups to attach an alkyl $(R-CH_2-)$ or a carbamoyl
$$(R-N-C-)$$
moiety. Some of these reactions are shown in Figure 6–12.

The nitrosoureas are unstable, and they decompose to alkylating and carbamoylating intermediates in aqueous media. The mechanism of decomposition presented here is that proposed by Reed *et al.*[167] At physiological pH, the principal products of nitrosourea decomposition are an isocyanate and 2-chloroethyl diazene hydroxide.[167,168] At lower pH, a different decomposition pathway predominates. Here, a chloride ion is lost, with the production of an isocyanate and ethylenediazohydroxide.[169] The pathway shown in the figure is important, because the spontaneous decomposition of the 2-chloroethyl diazene hydroxide yields the 2-chloroethyl carbonium ion, which is the major alkylating moiety. Further reaction of the chloroethyl carbonium ion in aqueous solution of physiological pH generates chloroethanol, vinyl chloride, acetaldehyde, and dichloroethane.[170] Reaction of the chloroethyl carbonium ion with cellular constituents results in alkylation of nucleic acids and proteins.

Importantly, it has been shown that all of the nitrosoureas, even those bearing a single alkylating function (e.g., lomustine and semustine, which have only one chloroethyl moiety), can produce interstrand cross-links in DNA.[171] Initially, there is chloroethylation of a guanine moiety in one strand of DNA. This reaction occurs rapidly (within minutes), and it is followed by a slow rearrangement and reaction with the opposite strand to form a cross-link.[172] In contrast to the nitrogen mustards, it is the O^6 position on guanine that is the preferred site of attack by nitrosoureas, and guaninines in the midst of a run of guanines in DNA are more

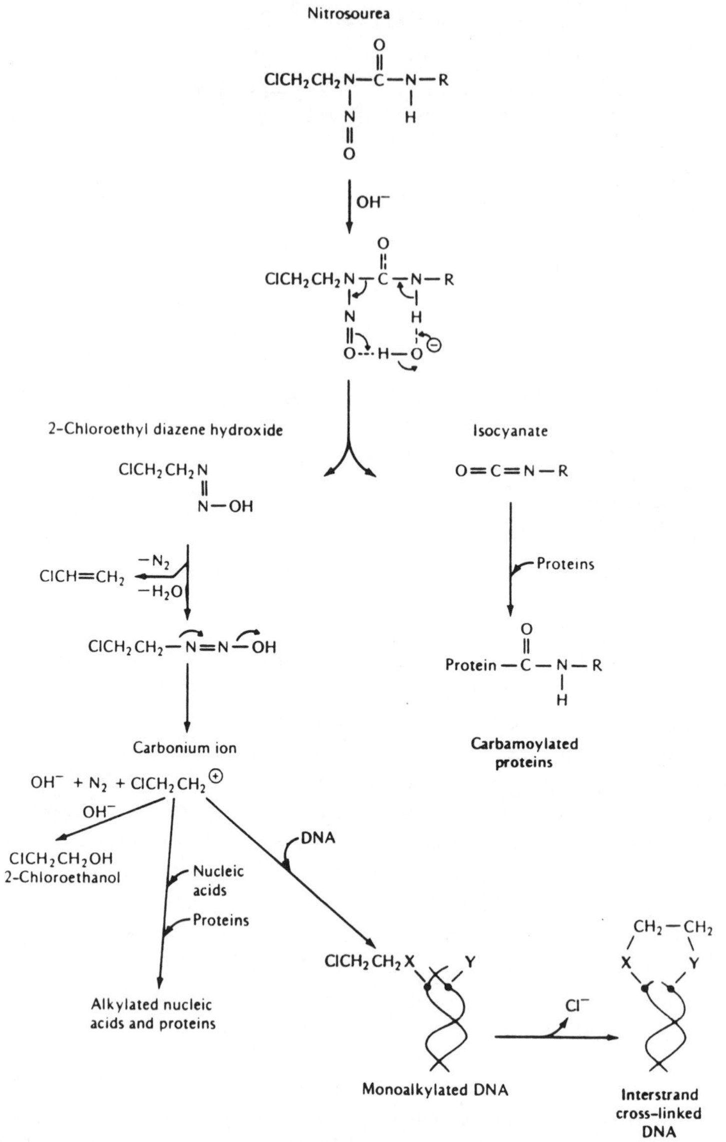

Nitrosourea

Figure 6–12   Mechanisms of alkylation and carbamoylation by nitrosoureas. The reaction scheme at the top of the figure is from Reed et al.,[167] who have proposed that base abstraction of the N-3 hydrogen at physiological pH produces an unstable intermediate, which rapidly decomposes to yield the corresponding alkyl isocyanate and 2-chloroethyl diazene hydroxide. Spontaneous decomposition of the latter compound yields the reactive 2-chloroethyl carbonium ion. The proposed cross-alkylation mechanism is shown at the bottom of the figure. Here, the carbonium ion attacks the O^6-position of a guanine (X) in one DNA strand, and this is followed by the slow elimination of the chloride ion and a second alkylation of base Y in the other strand. In addition to alkylation, the nitrosoureas also extensively carbamoylate cellular constituents via the isocyanate.

susceptible to alkylation, both at the N-7 and O^6 positions.[173] After the initial rapid alkylating event, either repair of the lesion by alkyltransferase[174] or reaction with a nucleophile, such as the glutathione thiolate anion,[175] can prevent subsequent DNA cross-linking in vitro. This suggests that both alkyltransferase and glutathione might serve to attenuate the extent of nitrosourea-induced DNA cross-linkage in tumor cells.

The importance of alkylation of the O^6 position of guanine for nitrosourea cytotoxicity was established by correlating cytotoxicity with the activity of the DNA repair enzyme O^6-alkylguanine-DNA alkyltransferase.[176] For example, in one study examining five human glial cell lines with different sensitivities to nitrosoureas, a quantitative correlation was found between cytotoxicity, extent of interstrand cross-linkage, and repair of O^6-methylguanine.[177] This emphasizes the importance of alkyltransferase activity in determining response to nitrosoureas, with sensitive cells being found to have no or low activity and resistant cells having high activity.[178] Indeed, transfection of alkyltransferase into nitrosourea sensitive cells confers resistance.[179] It is possible that O^6-alkylguanine-DNA alkyltransferase could be a clinically useful predictor of nitrosourea response and that the development of inhibitors of the enzyme could prove useful in potentiating the antitumor effect.

In addition to cross-linking of DNA, extensive carbamoylation occurs through the isocyanate released from the nitrosoureas. In a study of the reaction of CCNU with L1210 leukemia cells, it was found that proteins were extensively carbamoylated, whereas negligible carbamoylation of nucleic acids occurred.[180] Carbamoylation predominantly involves the reaction of the isocyanate moiety with the ϵ-amino group of lysine.[181] However, it is clear that the carbamoylating activity of the nitrosoureas does not play a major role in determining either their cytotoxicity[182] or their myelotoxicity.[183]

Streptozotocin differs from the other nitrosoureas in clinical use in that it has very low bone marrow toxicity and it has a pronounced diabetogenic action. Streptozotocin is composed of a methylnitrosourea moiety attached to the C-2 of glucose. When administered intravenously to rats, it was found to cause the clinical symptoms of diabetes and a marked decrease in, or complete absence of, secretory granules in the β-cells of the pancreatic islets of Langerhans.[184] This led to its unique use in the treatment of pancreatic islet-cell carcinoma.[185]

Chlorozotocin was developed in an attempt to increase the antitumor activity of streptozotocin by substituting its methyl group with the chloroethyl side chain that is present in other nitrosoureas, while maintaining the low

marrow toxicity of the parent drug. Chlorozotocin has high alkylating activity and low carbamoylating activity,[183] and it is not diabetogenic.[186] This suggests that the diabetogenic effect of streptozotocin is related to specific uptake of the drug into the pancreas and subsequent carbamoylation. In contrast, myelosuppression of nitrosoureas correlates with alkylating activity,[187] and the relative lack of myelosuppression on the part of streptozotocin and chlorozotocin must be related to decreased entry of these hydrophilic, sugar-substituted molecules into bone marrow cells as opposed to the other nitrosoureas, which are lipophilic.

PHARMACOLOGY OF THE NITROSOUREAS. Carmustine, lomustine, and semustine are all rapidly absorbed from the gastrointestinal tract and the latter two drugs are routinely administered orally (Table 6–5). Because of rapid metabolism, carmustine is administered intravenously. These drugs are very lipophilic; thus, they distribute widely in the tissues[188,189] and they have a large apparent volume of distribution.[190] Because of rapid chemical decomposition, metabolism and distribution from the central compartment, the plasma half-lives of the parent drugs are short (minutes).[190,191] Consistent with their lipophilicity, a portion of these drugs in the serum distributes into the hydrophobic core region of lipoproteins where it is protected from aqueous chemical decomposition.[192]

The lipophilic nature of these drugs permits them to readily pass across the blood-brain barrier into the cerebrospinal fluid where the level of radioactivity from the chloroethyl moiety of lomustine, for example, is about 30% of the plasma concentration. The lipophilicity of the drugs also facilitates their passage into brain tumor tissue where drug concentrations can exceed those of plasma.[194,195] The passage of these drugs into the CSF and brain tumors is unusual for anticancer drugs and has led to the important clinical application of the nitrosoureas in the treatment of brain tumors and meningeal leukemia.

Carmustine (BCNU) is metabolized by an NADPH-dependent microsomal enzyme system in liver and lung to 1,3-bis(2-chloroethyl)urea, a compound with very little antitumor activity.[196] The rates of microsomal metabolism are fast enough to allow a signifi-

Table 6–5   Pharmacology of the Nitrosoureas

Drug	Principal Route of Administration	Plasma Half-Life	Pharmacological Characteristics
Carmustine (BCNU)	Intravenous	10–20 minutes (for parent drug)	Very lipophilic, good penetration into brain tissue, rapid metabolism to an inactive product
Lomustine (CCNU) Semustine (methyl-CCNU)	Oral	1–3 hours (for active metabolites)	Very lipophilic, good penetration into brain tissue, rapidly hydroxylated to products that retain cytotoxic activity
Streptozotocin	Intravenous	15 minutes (for parent drug)	The drug is taken into and retained in the β-cells of the islets of Langerhans

cant portion of the carmustine to be metabolized before chemical decomposition of the drug occurs. Pretreatment of rats with phenobarbital increases the rate of metabolism and decreases the antitumor activity of carmustine.[197] Lomustine and semustine are substrates for a different microsomal enzyme system that hydroxylates the ring moiety.[196] Several hydroxylated metabolites are produced,[198] and they retain alkylating and antitumor activity.[199] Indeed, most of the biological effect of lomustine and semustine in the body seems to be due to generation of chlorethyl carbonium ion from the ring hydroxylated metabolites. The ring hydroxylation occurs during the "first pass" of the drugs through the gut wall and liver.[200] The chemical decomposition products and metabolites of the nitrosoureas are excreted by the kidneys.

Streptozotocin is administered intravenously, it has a serum half-life of only 15 minutes, and the metabolites are excreted by the kidney.[201] An important aspect of the drug's distribution is its retention in the β-cells of the islets of Langerhans.[202] After injection of streptozotocin with a carbon-14 methyl group label into rats, high levels of radioactivity are retained in islet cell tissue, but when the label is at the 1 position of the sugar or on the carbonyl, the level of islet cell radioactivity is low. This difference may reflect an ability of the compound to methylate nucleophilic groups. The glucosamine portion of the drug is important in providing some specificity of uptake into the β-cell.

USE AND TOXICITY. Carmustine, lomustine, and semustine are used to treat tumors in the central nervous system, both primary brain tumors (experience with these drugs in the treatment of gliomas has been quite extensive[203,204]) and tumors of metastatic origin. They have significant activity in Hodgkin's disease and melanoma, and they are useful in secondary therapy of non-Hodgkin's lymphomas, myeloma, and lung and colorectal cancers.[203,205] Streptozotocin is employed clinically in the treatment of metastatic islet cell carcinoma of the pancreas.[185,206]

The nitrosoureas frequently produce nausea and vomiting, which usually occurs well after drug absorption (e.g., 4 to 6 hours after administration of lomustine) as a direct CNS-mediated effect.[207] The nausea and vomiting persist less than 24 hours; this time can be reduced, however, with antiemetics and by fasting prior to drug administration. Intravenous administration of carmustine causes local pain, and phlebitis can occur. The drug should be infused slowly to avoid pain at the injection site. High-dose administration of carmustine may cause hypotension, tachycardia, flushing and confusion, as well as nausea and vomiting.[190] The major toxic effects of nitrosoureas are leukopenia and thrombocytopenia (Table 6–6). Bone marrow toxicity is delayed, dose-related, dose-limiting, and cumulative. Thrombocytopenia occurs 3 to 5 weeks after a dose with a low point of 1 to 2 weeks' duration. Leukopenia occurs 4 to 6 weeks after a dose with a low point of similar duration. The reason for the

Table 6–6 *Some Major Untoward Effects of the Nitrosoureas.* The usual dose-limiting toxicity is in bold type

| | Principal Toxicities | |
Drug	Acute	Delayed
Carmustine (BCNU)	Nausea and vomiting, phlebitis. Hypotension, tachycardia and flushing with high-dose administration	**Delayed and cumulative thrombocytopenia and leukopenia,** pulmonary fibrosis, renal damage, reversible hepatotoxicity, CNS toxicity, leukemia
Lomustine (CCNU) Semustine (methyl-CCNU)	Nausea and vomiting	**Delayed and cumulative thrombocytopenia and leukopenia,** pulmonary fibrosis, renal damage, reversible hepatotoxicity, CNS toxicity, leukemia
Streptozotocin	Nausea and vomiting	**Renal damage (reversible)**, hepatotoxicity, hyperglycemia, hypoglycemia, anemia

delay in myelosuppression is not clear. In nitrosourea therapy, the drug is given as a single dose and a second course is not given for 6 weeks. The cumulative hematological toxicity is manifested on subsequent courses of therapy by more profound drops in cell count at a given dose level, the same degree of thrombocytopenia and leukopenia at lower dose levels, or a longer period of myelosuppression.[207] The nitrosoureas are occasionally nephrotoxic[208] and hepatotoxic, they can cause pulmonary fibrosis,[209] and carmustine has been associated with central nervous system toxicity (dizziness and ataxia).[210] The drugs are both mutagenic and carcinogenic.

Nausea and vomiting occur in virtually all patients receiving streptozotocin.[185] A dangerous acute toxicity of streptozotocin is insulin shock. In one study, renal toxicity was observed in 65% of the patients, hepatotoxicity in 67% and hematological toxicity (usually anemia) in 20%.[185] The renal toxicity is usually reversible and is dose-limiting. Bone marrow depression is not a frequent problem when streptozotocin is administered alone but it is a problem when the drug is administered with other myelotoxic drugs.[206]

Platinum Compounds

Cis-diamminedichloroplatinum(II) (DDP) is known by the generic name cisplatin (see Fig. 6–13),[211] and it is one of a number of platinum

coordination complexes with antitumor activity. The potential of cisplatin as an antitumor agent was recognized through an observation made by Rosenberg *et al.*[212] that certain group VII′b transition metal compounds inhibit bacterial division. Their study had been designed to explore the possible effects of an electric field on the growth of *E. coli*, but they noted that the bacteria ceased dividing and grew in the form of long filaments. It became clear that cell division was being inhibited by an electrolysis product of the platinum electrode. In a subse-

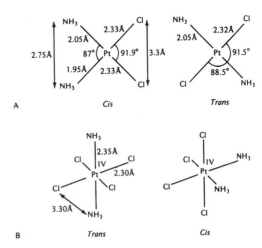

Figure 6–13 Structure of the *cis*-isomer and *trans*-isomer of (A) diamminedichloroplatinum(II) and (B) diamminetetrachloroplatinum(IV). Cisplatin is the *cis*-isomer of diamminedichloroplatinum(II). (From Tomson[211])

quent study, it was shown that a platinum compound was more effective than several other group VIIIb transition metal compounds in inhibiting cell division in cultures of gram-negative bacili.[213] *Cis*-diamminetetrachloroplatinum(IV) was then synthesized and shown to cause filamentous growth, whereas the *trans*-isomer had no effect.[214] Several platinum(IV) complexes have been synthesized as potential drugs, but it appears that in the reducing environment of the cell interior, these compounds are reduced to platinum(II) complexes and it is this latter oxidation state that is the biologically active form.[215] In 1970, Rosenberg and his colleagues tested the antitumor activity of several platinum compounds and demonstrated that cisplatin was extremely effective against sarcoma 180 and L1210 leukemia in mice.[216] The efficacy of cisplatin has now been established in a variety of animal tumor models and in human cancer. Although a number of platinum coordination complexes have been shown to be active in experimental systems. Cisplatin and carboplatin are the only two that are ap-

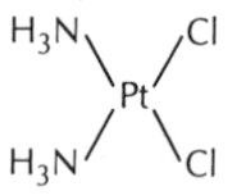

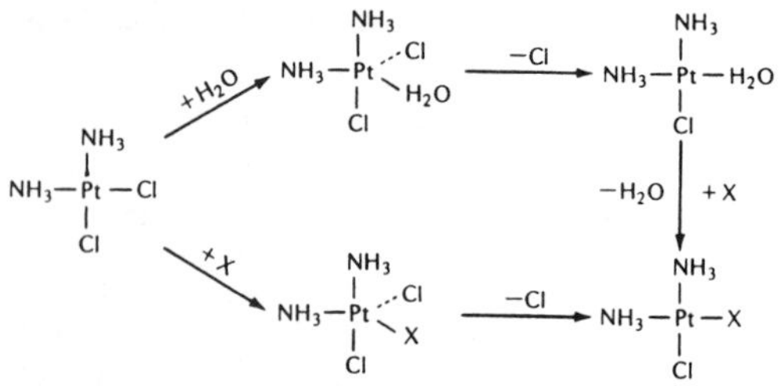

Figure 6–14 Two mechanisms by which cisplatin reacts with a nucleophile (X). The upper path involves the production of an aquo intermediate, the lower a direct replacement mechanism.

Cisplatin 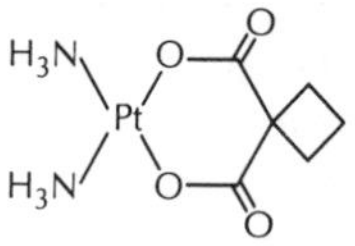   Carboplatin

proved for clinical use in the United States. The chemistry and biological effects of cisplatin[217,218] and carboplatin[219] have been reviewed in detail.

Mechanism of Action

THE CHEMICAL REACTION. Several chemical requirements for the antitumor activity of platinum(II) complexes have been established. Since all the *trans*-compounds tested have been ineffective, the *cis*-configuration appears to be required. Both *cis*- and *trans*-isomers exchange chloride ions for such nucleophilic groups as RS^-, $R-S-CH_3$, $\geqslant N$, and $R-NH_2$ to form links that can be very stable. The substitution of planar platinum(II) compounds, such as cisplatin, may follow one of two pathways in aqueous solution.[211] As shown in Figure 6–14, a chloride ion may be replaced by water to produce a hydrated intermediate, the solvent

molecule being subsequently eliminated by an incoming nucleophile. In most cases, reactions in the cell are thought to proceed in this manner via the formation of aquo species. In some cases, there may be direct replacement of the leaving group without the participation of the solvent. Several reacting species of the complex exist in water solution as defined by the equilibria:

$$Pt(NH_3)_2Cl_2 + H_2O \rightarrow$$
$$[Pt(NH_3)_2Cl(H_2O)]^+ + Cl^-$$
$$[Pt(NH_3)_2Cl(H_2O)]^+ + H_2O \rightarrow$$
$$[Pt(NH_3)_2(H_2O)_2]^{++} + Cl^-$$

Addition of chloride ion to the medium displaces this equilibrium to the left, and thus the reactivity of DDP will depend upon the chloride-ion concentration of the environment. In a high-chloride medium, such as isotonic saline, the species $Pt(NH_3)_2Cl_2$ will predominate, replacement of chloride will tend to be suppressed, and displacement will be effected only by the strongest nucleophiles, such as sulfur. Platinum(II) complexes with antitumor activity contain chloride, bromide, oxalate, or malonate as leaving groups.[220] Complexes with more labile ligands, such as nitrate ion, hydrolyze too rapidly to permit them to be useful *in vivo*, and other ligands, such as cyanide ion, bind too tightly to platinum to be active.[220] Only neutral platinum(II) complexes are known to possess antitumor activity, and to be active the complex should contain relatively inert carrier ligands, such as amine groups. Structure-activity studies have shown that minor variations in the structure of the amine ligands can have a profound effect on the antitumor activity and the toxicity of platinum complexes.[221]

Cis- and *trans-*diamminedichloroplatinum(II) exchange their chloride ions for nucleophilic groups by a similar mechanism, and no known differences in chemical reactivity underlie the marked difference in their biological efficacy. It is clear from Figure 6–13A, however, that the two compounds are very different stereochemically; thus, any molecular explanation of the cytotoxicity of cisplatin must eventually account for the inactivity of the *trans-*isomer.

THE INTERACTION WITH DNA. There is considerable evidence that DNA is the principal target for the cytotoxic action of cisplatin.[222] To possess antitumor activity, a platinum compound must have two relatively labile *cis-*oriented leaving groups. The lack of activity of monodentate platinum has led to the conclusion that cytotoxicity results from the formation of a bidentate lesion.[222] The principal sites of reaction at physiological pH are the N7 atoms of guanine and adenine. Regardless of whether it is purified DNA,[223] intact cells,[224] or tumor-bearing patients[225] that are exposed to cisplatin, the principal coordinate is an intrastrand cross-link formed by binding of the drug to two neighboring guanines (pGpG). For example, in a study in which the DNA adducts were analyzed in white cells of cancer patients treated with cisplatin, 65% of the adducts represented intrastrand cross-links on pGpG, 22% intrastrand cross-links on pApG (but not pGpA) sequences, and 13% a mixture of other adducts.[225] Less than one percent represented monofunctionally bound drug. The formation of cross-links is a relatively slow process, and after exposure of DNA to cisplatin and removal of the drug, the level of cross-linkage increases over a period of several hours.[226] This kind of observation and other data have led to the proposal that the drug reacts rapidly to form a monoadduct and then slowly forms the second adduct to create the cross-link.[227] Cisplatin and carboplatin appear to differ principally in their rates of reaction with DNA. Cisplatin has a faster rate of aquation and forms cross-links faster than carboplatin, but once bound to DNA in equal amounts, both drugs yield equivalent cytotoxicity.[228]

A major question that is not completely resolved is whether it is the DNA-interstrand cross-links or the intrastrand cross-links that are primarily responsible for the cytotoxicity of the platinum compounds. DNA-interstrand cross-links represent less than 1% of the total platination,[226] and there is evidence that intrastrand cross-linkage is sufficient for cytotoxicity.[222] In forming the intrastrand pGpG cross-links, cisplatin causes a major bending of the DNA duplex toward the major groove.[229] This structural distortion may be sufficient to inhibit DNA synthesis. For example, in experiments where DNA polymerase I was used to synthesize duplex DNA on a cisplatin-treated single-stranded template, second strand synthesis was blocked by the presence of platinum on the template strand.[230] This and other evidence[231] have led to the impression that intrastrand cross-linkage accounts for inhibition of DNA replication. In studies on cancer patients, it has been found that the formation of intrastrand DNA adducts correlates with the clinical response to cisplatin therapy.[232]

In addition to DNA–DNA cross-links, DNA–protein cross-linking occurs. The cytotoxicity of *cis-* versus *trans-*platinum(II), however, does not correlate with the extent of DNA–protein cross-linking.[233] In summary, there is considerable evidence that cisplatin exerts its cytotoxic effect through binding to DNA. The critical interactions with DNA are likely to be intrastrand cross-links (predominantly between the 7-nitrogens of neighboring guanines), and the difference between the cytotoxicity produced by the *cis-* and *trans-*isomers has not been adequately explained at either the molecular or the cellular level.

RESISTANCE. No clear-cut dominant mechanism of resistance to cisplatin has been identified. Often, resistant cells have an increased capacity to repair intrastrand adducts,[17] but in many studies the increase in repair capacity has not been sufficient to explain the extent of resistance.[234] It has also been reported that a cell line that is hypersensitive to killing by both UV light and mitomycin C is very sensitive to cisplatin and has a decreased ability to repair DNA cross-links.[235] Taken together, these results demonstrate the importance of DNA cross-linking in the cytotoxicity of the drug, and they suggest that DNA repair activity is one of the major determinants of tumor response to cisplatin therapy.[236] Sometimes, cells with increased repair activity are cross-resistant with other classes of DNA cross-linking drugs, and in other cases no cross-resistance exists.

Cisplatin reacts readily with compounds containing SH groups. Thus, resistance in some cell lines has been found to correlate with increased glutathione content,[237] and in some cases, glutathione depletion with butathionine sulfoximine (see Chapter 4) has resulted in reversal of resistance.[238] It has been suggested that quenching of the platinum compounds by reaction with nucleophilic SH groups in glutathione may be a major determinant of tumor response to initial therapy. This argument has been elaborated in detail for a variety of anticancer drugs, including the nitrogen mustards and nitrosoureas.[239] It was highlighted for platinum compounds by experiments suggesting that thiourea stops the delayed formation of DNA cross-links from cisplatin:DNA monoadducts.[240]

Another thiol-containing modifier of drug response is the metal-binding protein metallothionein. Metallothionein is a 6–7 kDa protein in which about 30% of the amino acids are cysteine. It has been found that tumors grown from cells with a high level of metallothionein have a decreased therapeutic response to cisplatin in comparison to tumors grown from the parent cells with a low level of metallothionein.[241] It was also found that human ovarian carcinoma cells selected for overexpression of metallothionein by stepwise selection in medium containing cadmium or zinc were resistant to cisplatin.[242] The levels of glutathione in these cells were also elevated, but the role of metallothionein was proven when it was demonstrated that transfection of mouse cells with the metallothionein cDNA conferred resistance to cisplatin as well as to melphalan and chlorambucil.[243]

Clearly, a number of factors, including DNA repair capacity, glutathione levels, and metallothionein induction, can affect the sensitivity of human cells to the platinum compounds. No dominant resistance mechanism has been identified in human tumors, and it may be that all of these factors contribute simultaneously to resistance in the same tumor cell.

Pharmacology of Cisplatin and Carboplatin

Cisplatin is administered intravenously and by local introduction into the bladder and into the peritoneal space. For intravenous infusion, the drug is supplied as a lyophilized powder containing sodium chloride, mannitol, and hydrochloric acid for pH adjustment.[244] It is reconstituted with 10 ml of sterile water for injection. The solution is stable at room temperature for at least 8 hours, but if this preparation is diluted into a solution with a low concentration of chloride (e.g., 5% dextrose for infusion), the drug is converted to the aquo forms.[245] Further conversion to the biologically inactive neutral hydroxyl ligands also occurs very slowly in such solutions,[246] but this has not been demonstrated to occur to a significant extent under clinical conditions of administration. After administration, the high chloride concentration of the plasma and extracellular fluid favors the persistence of unaltered cisplatin, which, as a neutral species, can cross cell membranes. The relatively low chloride concentration of the intracellular milieu favors the formation of the reactive mono- and diaquated species. Cisplatin is sometimes reconstituted in hypertonic saline solution and administered to patients who are receiving normal saline hydration. With the resulting saline diuresis, there is less nephrotoxicity because the chloride ion reduces reaction with renal tissue. Under these conditions of high saline diuresis, the pharmacokinetics of the drug are unchanged.[247] Cisplatin forms a precipitate with aluminium, and needles and intravenous sets containing aluminium should not be employed during preparation of the drug solution or during infusion.

After intravenous infusion, the level of ultrafilterable drug (i.e., non-protein-bound drug) in the plasma declines with an initial half-life of 20–40 minutes, followed by a period of very slow decline.[248,249] After high-dose administration, the initial half-life is about 50% longer.[250] Cisplatin binds extensively (90%) to plasma protein[251] in a manner that is often considered to represent irreversible reaction with plasma

Table 6-7   Pharmacology of the Platinum Compounds

Drug	Principal Route of Administration	Plasma Half-Life	Pharmacological Characteristics
Cisplatin	Intravenous; intraperitoneal	20–40 minutes	Rapid aquation and reaction with plasma protein and renal tissue (nephrotoxic). Thirty percent excreted in urine in first 24 hours
Carboplatin	Intravenous	2–3 hours	Slow aquation and slow reaction. Little drug reacts with kidney tissue (not nephrotoxic) and more is excreted in the urine (60–70%) in the first 24 hours

protein thiols. It has been shown, however, that much of the protein-bound platinum in the plasma can still react with a strong nucleophile, such as diethyldithiocarbamate.[252] Thus, the protein binding is slowly reversible, yielding an active electrophile. The principal route of elimination is renal, predominantly via glomerular filtration, but with some tubular secretion.[253] About 30% of the radiolabeled drug is recovered in the urine within the first 24 hours.[251]

Carboplatin generates a reactive species via aquation much more slowly than does cisplatin,[228] and because of this, its pharmacokinetic and toxicologic characteristics are different (Table 6–7). The rate of the initial decline in the plasma level of ultrafilterable platinum is much slower (half-life 2–3 hours) with carboplatin than with cisplatin, and twice as much carboplatin (60–70%) is recovered in the urine in the first 24 hours.[254,255] Thus, less of the drug reacts with plasma protein and more is excreted in the urine as the unreacted parent compound. Because the drug passing through the kidney is not aquated, it does not react extensively with renal tissue, as cisplatin does. As a result, the dose-limiting toxicity of carboplatin is myelosuppression rather than nephrotoxicity. In patients with compromised renal function, the dosage of carboplatin must be reduced to limit the extent of thrombocytopenia.[256]

Use and Toxicity of the Platinum Compounds

Cisplatin is one of the most frequently used anticancer drugs. It is an effective component of combination drug protocols used to treat a variety of human malignancies, most notably tumors of the testis, ovary, head and neck, lung, and bladder.[257-259] The major delayed toxic effects of cisplatin are nephrotoxicity, peripheral neuropathy, and ototoxicity, with nephrotoxicity often being dose-limiting (Table 6–8). Carboplatin was introduced with the view of reducing the toxic potential of the parent drug. Carboplatin has the same spectrum of antitu-

Table 6-8   Some Major Untoward Effects of the Platinum Drugs. The usual dose-limiting toxicity is in bold type

Drug	Principal Toxicities	
	Acute	Delayed
Cisplatin	Severe nausea and vomiting; anaphylatic reactions	**Nephrotoxicity;** hypomagnesemia, ototoxicity, peripheral neuropathy, bone marrow depression
Carboplatin	Moderate nausea and vomiting	**Bone marrow depression,** low potential for ototoxicity and peripheral neuropathy

mor activity as cisplatin, but it is less nephro-toxic, neurotoxic, and ototoxic, and perhaps causes less emesis. Its dose-limiting toxicity is myelosuppression, a side effect that is not a major problem with cisplatin administration. Because carboplatin is not a more active anti-cancer agent than cisplatin, because it has a high (probably total) cross-resistance with cis-platin, and because it induces more myelosup-pression, its role in therapy is limited to that of an alternative to cisplatin in (1) patients with preexisting renal dysfunction; (2) patients with a clear predisposition for neurotoxicity or oto-toxicity; and (3) people who cannot receive the vigorous hydration that accompanies cisplatin administration.[260]

Nausea and vomiting occur in virtually all patients receiving cisplatin, within 1 hour after drug administration, and last from 4 to 6 hours (and occasionally up to a week in especially sensitive patients).[244] The major untoward ef-fect of cisplatin is nephrotoxicity.[261] Clearly dose related, this nephrotoxicity is manifested by a decrease in creatinine clearance and elec-trolyte imbalances, in particular hypomagne-semia. The nephrotoxicity is initiated by an impairment of proximal tubular function. The proximal tubular cells appear to concentrate the drug, with the majority being bound to macromolecules, including both protein and DNA.[262] Long-term renal impairment is accom-panied by damage to the distal tubules and col-lecting ducts as well. A study in rats has shown that two cis-platinum compounds with antitu-mor activity are also nephrotoxic, whereas the corresponding trans-isomers were neither ac-tive nor nephrotoxic.[264] Thus, it is reasonable to predict that the molecular mechanism of tu-bular damage is similar to that of the antitu-mor effect. Therapy with other nephrotoxic drugs, such as aminoglycoside antibiotics, can augment the nephrotoxicity of cisplatin.

Both animal studies and human trials showed that nephrotoxicity can be reduced by a variety of approaches. Renal failure can be prevented in rats by pretreatment with furose-mide,[265] and studies in dogs show that prehy-dration and mannitol-induced diuresis can prevent nephrotoxicity.[266] It has been demon-strated in clinical trial that prehydration and concomitant osmotic mannitol diuresis de-creases nephrotoxicity of cisplatin in pa-tients.[267] Thus, patients are routinely hydrated by the infusion of 1 to 2 liters of fluid prior to drug administration and adequate hydration must be maintained for the next 24 hours. The drug is infused in 5% dextrose in ½ or ⅓ N sa-line, often with mannitol added. When cis-platin is administered in high-dose therapy, in-fusion of the drug in 3% saline together with extensive saline hydration essentially prevents the nephrotoxicity.[268] Hypertonic saline does not provide protection against the nonrenal toxicities of cisplatin.

Thiol-containing compounds such as thio-sulfate,[269] diethyldithiocarbamate,[270] and or-ganic thiophosphates[271] have been administered along with cisplatin to prevent the nephrotox-icity and thus allow increased cisplatin dosage. These compounds do not readily penetrate into cells, but they are excreted by the kidney where they react with and inactivate the cisplatinum. This approach may prove to be especially use-ful with intraperitoneal cisplatin therapy. Ovarian carcinoma can remain confined to the peritoneal cavity for a significant portion of its growth, and direct installation of drugs into the intraperitoneal space allows much higher local drug concentration at the tumor site.[272] Absorption of drug into the circulation and the consequent systemic toxicity limits the intra-peritoneal dosage. The dosage of cisplatin that can be administered into the peritoneal space is increased markedly, however, when the patient is also treated intravenously with an agent, such as sodium thiosulfate, that protects against cisplatin-induced nephrotoxicity.[273]

Cisplatin produces a dose-dependent ototox-icity that may be manifested by tinnitus or hearing loss or both.[274] The hearing loss is most pronounced at high frequencies (over 4000 Hz),[274] although an occasional patient may ex-perience a decrement in the speech range.[275] The high frequency hearing loss is apparently irreversible in some patients;[275] the mechanism is unknown. The cisplatin-induced pathology has been studied in both monkeys and guinea pigs in whom pronounced morphological changes and loss of the outer hair cells were ob-served in the lower turns of the organ of Corti.[276-278] Fosfomycin, an antibiotic that in-hibits aminoglycoside-induced ototoxicity, also reduces cisplatin ototoxicity in guinea pigs.[274] Patients receiving cisplatin should have audiometric testing, particularly if they are being treated with other potentially ototoxic drugs (e.g., aminoglycoside antibiotics or furosemide).

Although cisplatin produces myelosuppression, the degree of leukocytopenia and thrombocytopenia is usually moderate.[244] There have been several reports of patients experiencing anaphylactic types of reactions to cisplatin.[244] The reaction in one patient was clearly shown to represent an atopic hypersensitivity, as confirmed by the development of wheal and flare on skin testing.[280] Skin tests with cisplatin analogs showed that neither the chloride nor the amine groups in cisplatin were essential for reactivity, but in this atopic hypersensitivity, there was no cross-reaction with three other platinum complexes of known antitumor activity.[280] In addition to acting as a hapten and binding to proteins to induce allergic reactions, cisplatin itself is immunosuppressive.

Cisplatin causes a neurotoxicity that most commonly presents as a peripheral neuropathy with sensations of numbness or paresthesias in the hands, feet, arms, and legs.[281] In most cases, cessation of cisplatin is followed by recovery. The incidence of neuropathy is unclear, but it's probably in the range of 10%.[281] Rarely, patients have experienced optic neuritis, blurring of vision, and papilledema.[281]

Carboplatin causes mild to moderate nausea and vomiting. At usual dosage, it is not nephrotoxic, ototoxic, or neurotoxic, allowing it to be administered to patients who cannot receive cisplatin because of renal disease, neurotoxicity, or ototoxicity.[219] Carboplatin produces a dose-related and dose-limiting myelosuppression, with thrombocytopenia being more pronounced than leukopenia.[256]

Methylating Agents

Dacarbazine

Dacarbazine was originally synthesized as an analog of 5-aminoimidazole-4-carboxamide (AIC), an intermediate in purine biosynthesis.[282] Although the goal was to inhibit purine biosynthesis, dacarbazine is cytotoxic because it is metabolized to an active species that methylates DNA.

MECHANISM OF ACTION. Dacarbazine itself has essentially no *in vitro* toxicity, but if the drug is incubated with a hepatic microsomal fraction and NADPH, the drug is converted to a cytotoxic form.[283] Dacarbazine undergoes cytochrome P-450-mediated oxidative N-demethylation in the liver, as shown in Figure 6–15. The first product in the pathway is the relatively stable hydroxymethyl compound, which can be transported from the liver to other tissues via the systemic circulation.[284] Loss of formaldehyde generates 5-(3-methyltriazeno)-imidazole-4-carboxamide, and this is followed by spontaneous rearrangement to 5-aminoimi-

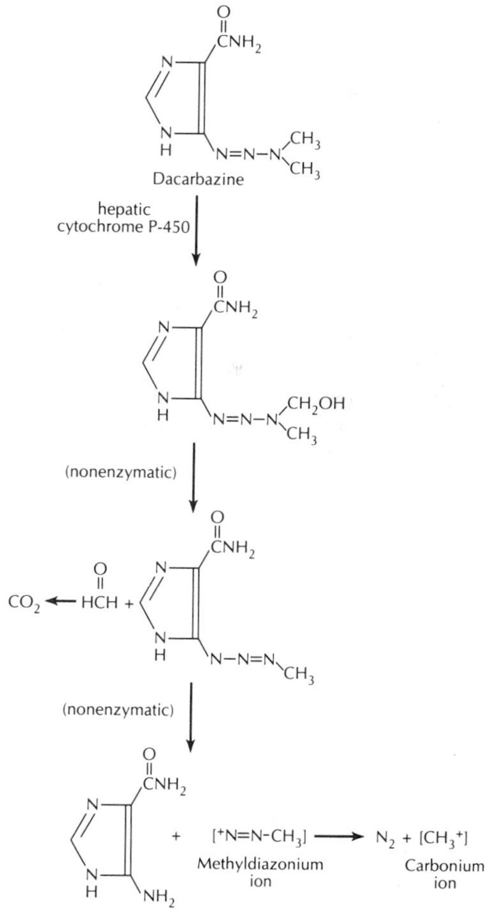

Figure 6–15 Scheme for the metabolism of decarbazine.

dazole-4-carboximide (AIC) with elimination of the methyldiazonium cation, which is the active methylating agent. Methylation of DNA and RNA occurs, with 7-methylguanine being the predominant product.[284] Very small amounts of the promutagenic base O^6-methylguanine are also produced. It is reasonably presumed that the cytotoxicity of dacarbazine, like its mutagenic and carcinogenic effects, results from DNA methylation. However, other effects on DNA synthesis could occur. Treatment of cells with dacarbazine, for example, causes DNA fragmentation in cells that are synthesizing new DNA,[285] and when the repair of dacarbazine-induced DNA lesions is inhibited, the cytotoxicity of the drug is increased.[286] The mechanisms by which tumor cells develop resistance to dacarbazine are unknown.

PHARMACOLOGY. Absorption of dacarbazine from the gastrointestinal tract is slow and incomplete;[287] thus, the drug is administered intravenously (Table 6–9). Dacarbazine can decompose in the presence of light, but solutions of the drug are stable enough under normal lighting conditions such that elaborate precautions to prevent light exposure during preparation of the drug solution and injection are not necessary.[288]

After intravenous injection, the plasma levels of the drug fall in a biphasic manner, with the slow phase having a half-life of 40 minutes by HPLC measurement of the unaltered drug[289] versus a half-life of 5 hours by measuring disappearance of radioactivity from ^{14}C-labeled drug.[290] As described above, dacarbazine undergoes oxidative N-demethylation, predominantly in the liver.[284,290] Forty to 50 percent of a dose is excreted in 6 hours as the unchanged drug and 10% to 20% as AIC (Fig. 6–15).[287,289,290] Small amounts of the hydroxymethyl metabolite, as well as the major 7-methylguanine reaction product, have also been identified in urine.[284,291] There is little plasma binding of dacarbazine (20%),[287] and the volume of distribution is 0.6 l/kg.[289] The highest levels of DNA methylation are in liver, followed by kidney and lung.[284]

USE AND TOXICITY. Dacarbazine is used in single drug and combination drug treatment of metastatic malignant melanoma, where the overall objective response rate to dacarbazine alone is 10–19%.[292] Dacarbazine is used in combination drug therapy of Hodgkin's disease (as part of the ABVD regimen) and soft tissue sarcomas.[293] Virtually all patients receiving dacarbazine experience nausea and vomiting that diminish with subsequent doses. Anorexia and diarrhea are also fairly common initially, and some patients experience pain along the injected vein.

The most common delayed toxicity is bone marrow depression, which is dose-limiting (Table 6–10).[293] Both leukopenia and thrombocytopenia occur, and the depression is usually mild to moderate in extent. Some patients experience a flulike syndrome of fever, myalgia, and malaise, which usually occurs about 7 days after treatment and may last 1 to 2 weeks. Rarely, patients experience hepatotoxicity, which can be fatal.[294] This probably reflects an allergic hepatic thrombophlebitis (Budd-Chiari syndrome) with secondary liver cell necrosis.[295]

Table 6–9 *Pharmacology of Dacarbazine and Procarbazine*

Drug	Principal Route of Administration	Plasma Half-Life	Pharmacological Characteristics
Dacarbazine	Intravenous	40 minutes	A prodrug that is activated by oxidative N-demethylation in the liver
Procarbazine	Oral	7 minutes	A prodrug that is converted by cytochrome P-450 or monoamine oxidase to azoprocarbazine, which is further metabolized by cytochrome P-450 to alkylating species. A weak monoamine oxidase inhibitor

Table 6–10   Some Major Untoward Effects of Dacarbazine and Procarbazine. The usual dose-limiting toxicity is in bold type

Drug	Principal Toxicities	
	Acute	Delayed
Dacarbazine	Nausea and vomiting, diarrhea, pain along the injected vein, anaphylaxis	**Bone marrow depression,** impaired renal function, flulike syndrome, hepatic necrosis, photosensitivity, facial flushing and paresthesia
Procarbazine	Mild nausea and vomiting; disulfiram-like effect with alcohol; CNS depression	**Bone marrow depression,** peripheral neuropathy, pulmonary infiltration, azoospermia, anovulation, leukemia

Anaphylaxis has also occurred rarely. Some patients have experienced photosensitivity reactions.[296] Mice injected intradermally with dacarbazine experience skin toxicity when exposed to light,[288] and the syndrome is thought to reflect photodecomposition of the drug. Patients receiving dacarbazine should probably avoid intense light exposure after drug injection. There have been a few reports of alopecia, facial flushing, and facial paresthesia, and, like other methylating agents, dacarbazine is mutagenic and carcinogenic.

Procarbazine

When a series of hydrazine compounds synthesized as potential monoamine oxidase inhibitors was tested for anticancer activity, 1-methyl-2-benzyl-hydrazine was found to be active against some transplanted animal tumors.

$$CH_3-NH-NH-CH_2- \hspace{-0.5em} \langle \hspace{-0.5em} \rangle \hspace{-0.5em} -CONH-CH \underset{CH_3}{\overset{CH_3}{<}}$$

Procarbazine

Since this compound had an unsatisfactory therapeutic index, additional derivatives were synthesized and a few were found to have more favorable biological properties.[297] Procarbazine [1-methyl-2-*p*-(isopropylcarbamoyl) benzylhydrazine hydrochloride] was shown to be active against a variety of animal tumors,[298] and it now has an established role in the treatment of cancer in man. The biological effects and pharmacology of procarbazine have been reviewed by Reed,[299] by Prough and Tweedie,[300] and by Averbuch.[301]

MECHANISM OF ACTION. Although procarbazine has been shown to have a number of biochemical effects, its mechanism of action is not yet clearly defined. The drug prolongs interphase and produces chromosome breaks in Ehrlich ascites tumor cells.[302] Strand scission occurs when procarbazine is incubated with DNA in the presence of oxygen.[303] If oxygen is replaced by an inert gas, or if peroxidase, or catalase, is added, the viscosity of the DNA does not change. The parent drug undergoes autooxidation at 37°C in aqueous solution, producing hydrogen peroxide, which can degrade DNA. It does not appear, however, that hydrogen peroxide generation contributes in any significant way to the cytotoxic action of procarbazine.[304]

Administration of procarbazine to mice bearing L5178Y lymphoma markedly decreases the rate of incorporation of precursors into tumor DNA and RNA within 3 hours; the rate returns to normal 12 to 24 hours later.[305] Protein synthesis also decreases, but to a lesser extent and somewhat later, which suggests that the effect may be secondary to nucleic acid synthesis inhibition.[305] The rate of loss of radioactivity from prelabeled DNA is not affected by the drug.[305] Although the mechanism of DNA synthesis inhibition has not been determined, it is clear that a metabolite of the drug is responsible. This can be inferred from the observation that procarbazine is much more toxic to tumor cells *in vitro* when the cells are cocultured with freshly isolated hepatocytes from phenobarbi-tal-treated rats.[306]

It has been shown that procarbazine acts as a methylating agent, and it is this property that is thought to be responsible for its cytotoxic activity.[307] The N-methyl group is partially oxidized *in vivo* in mice. It enters the one-carbon pool utilized in the *de novo* synthesis of purines, but trace amounts of the radiolabeled N-methyl groups are also used for nucleic acid methylation.[307] The major methylated base found in the cytoplasmic RNA of P815 ascites cells is 7-methyl guanine,[307] the methylation occurring through transfer of the intact N-methyl group. The exact process by which methylation occurs is unclear, but studies of procarbazine metabolism have led to the identification of its two principal routes of metabolic activation and to some postulated alkylating species (shown in Fig. 6–16).[300]

PHARMACOLOGY. In man, procarbazine is rapidly and completely absorbed from the gastrointestinal tract to yield plasma levels equivalent to those achieved with parenteral administration.[308] The drug is routinely administered orally. Indeed, intravenous administration appears to be counterproductive because most of the metabolic activation of the drug occurs during first-pass metabolism in the liver immediately after absorption from the gastrointestinal tract. On intravenous injection, the plasma half-life of the parent drug in patients is 7 minutes.[309] Procarbazine readily enters the cerebrospinal fluid of animals and man.[308] About 70% of a dose is recovered in the urine in 24 hours,[300] largely in the form of the metabolite N-isopropylterephthalamic acid.[308,309] Less than 5% of a dose is excreted as unchanged drug. Procarbazine is rapidly converted *in vivo* to azoprocarbazine, which is the major circulating

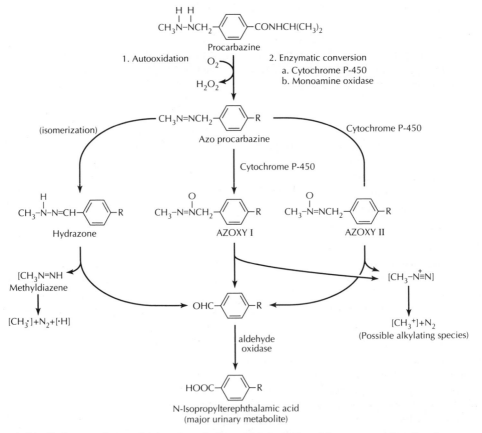

Figure 6–16 Pathways of procarbazine degradation and metabolism. The compounds in brackets are postulated but unidentified intermediates. For an extensive review of metabolic products, see Prough and Tweedie.[300]

metabolite. As shown in the scheme of Figure 6–16, azoprocarbazine can be produced through either chemical oxidation or by oxidative metabolism. In the former pathway, procarbazine is oxidized in aqueous solutions containing oxygen and metal ions, with the generation of peroxide. The azoprocarbazine produced under these conditions tautomerizes to hydrazone, a toxic compound. Under physiologic conditions, this pathway of decomposition is not important,[300] although it does account for the instability of procarbazine in aqueous solutions. In the body, procarbazine is converted to azoprocarbazine in an NADPH-dependent manner by cytochrome P-450 enzymes and in an NADPH-independent manner by monoamine oxidase.[309] Monoamine oxidase is responsible for about 40% of the total rate of procarbazine oxidation in hepatocytes from untreated rats and 25% in hepatocytes from phenobarbital-treated rats.[309]

Azoprocarbazine is further metabolized by cytochrome P-450 (but not by monoamine oxidase) to two isomeric derivatives, AZOXY I and AZOXY II (Fig. 6–16).[310] Again, this conversion is increased by phenobarbital pretreatment.[311,312] Consistent with the observations at the enzyme level, pretreatment of mice with phenobarbital or diphenylhydantoin increases the antitumor cytotoxicity of procarbazine.[313] Further microsomal metabolism of the azoxy metabolites yields the benzaldehyde derivatives and reactive species, such as the possible methyl diazonium ion, or possibly diazomethane, which can decompose to form a methyl carbonium ion (see Fig. 6–16). It has been shown that rat liver microsomal proteins catalyze the oxidation of procarbazine to unidentified carbon-centered radicals,[314] and in mice about 20% of the N-methyl moiety of procarbazine is ultimately eliminated as CO_2.[315] The benzaldehyde derivative is oxidized by aldehyde oxidase to the major urinary metabolite isopropylterephthalamic acid.

USE AND TOXICITY. Procarbazine is used in combination drug therapy of patients with advanced Hodgkin's disease as part of the MOPP (mechlorethamine, vincristine (Oncovin®), procarbazine, prednisone)[316] and CVPP (cyclophosphamide, vinblastine, procarbazine, prednisone)[317] regimens. It is also used in various drug

Table 6–11. Procarbazine Neurotoxicity

Disorders in consciousness
  Sedation
  Depression, lassitude
  Agitation, psychosis (rare)
Peripheral neuropathy
  Paresthesia of the extremities
  Hypoactive deep tendon reflexes
  Myalgia
Ataxia
Orthostatic hypotension
Side effects that result from enzyme inhibition
  Alcohol intolerance
  Increased CNS depression with phenothiazines, barbiturates, and narcotics
  Sensitivity to catecholamines and tyramine-containing foods

protocols to treat non-Hodgkin's lymphomas,[318] small-cell carcinomas of the lung,[319] and malignant melanoma.[320] Because of its activity against the intracerebral L1210 rat leukemia model and its good penetration into the cerebrospinal fluid, procarbazine has been used to treat malignant brain tumors.[321] Resistance to procarbazine can be demonstrated *in vitro*, but the mechanism is not clear.[322] Of importance clinically is the fact that cross-resistance with other alkylating agents does not occur.[323]

The major toxicity of procarbazine is a dose-related, reversible bone marrow depression, with leukopenia and thrombocytopenia.[318] Nausea and vomiting occur frequently after the initial administration of the drug but tend to be mild and to subside as therapy continues. Procarbazine is also neurotoxic, and may produce altered levels of consciousness or peripheral neuropathy (see Table 6–11).[324] Central nervous system depression ranges from mild drowsiness to profound stupor, and transient mental changes, including hallucinations, agitation, and manic psychosis, have also been reported,[324] though they are rare. Paresthesias of the extremities and hypoactive deep tendon reflexes can occur; they are reversible on cessation of therapy. Occasionally, patients may experience diffuse aching pains in proximal muscle groups, but these myalgias often subside despite continuation of therapy. Ataxia has been reported, but it is reversible and is not dose-limiting.[324] The reported incidence of neurotoxicity with oral therapy is between 10%

and 20%. Procarbazine lowers plasma pyridoxal phosphate levels in animals, and it has been suggested that this may play a role in its neurotoxic effect.[325] Administration of pyridoxine, however, has not been found to reverse this toxicity in man.

Several nervous system side effects can occur because of interactions of procarbazine with enzymes that metabolize other drugs or sympathomimetic compounds. Procarbazine has been shown to be a weak monoamine oxidase inhibitor,[326] and hypertension can occur if patients are concomitantly exposed to sympathomimetic agents, tricyclic antidepressants, or such tyramine-containing foods as cheese, red wine, beer, and yogurt. Procarbazine has been reported to cause orthostatic hypotension, which soon disappears on cessation of therapy.[327] The hypotension is not due to an inhibition of monoamine oxidase but to an action this class of compounds has on other functions in the sympathetic nervous system. Procarbazine potentiates the sedative effects of phenothiazines, barbiturates, and narcotics.[324] It has been shown that liver microsomes from mice treated with procarbazine have decreased cytochrome P-450 levels and a decreased ability to metabolize these drugs.[328] Potentiation of the depressive effects observed with other drugs is probably the result of a direct hypnotic effect of procarbazine, as well as the inhibition of mixed-function oxidase activity. After alcohol ingestion, some patients on procarbazine therapy experience a syndrome characterized by facial flushing, headache, and sweating.[324] This disulfiram-like effect is probably due to an inhibition of the alcohol-metabolizing enzymes. The physician should be cautious about administering medication that has a depressant effect on the central nervous system, and patients on procarbazine therapy should be told to avoid alcohol and foods with a high tyramine content.

Patients receiving procarbazine may develop stomatitis and diarrhea. Occasional instances of hypersensitivity reactions have been reported,[62] including urticaria, maculopapular rash, arthralgias, and pulmonary infiltration with eosinophilia.[329,330] Procarbazine is immunosuppressive,[331] it is teratogenic,[332] and it is carcinogenic.[333] Patients with Hodgkin's disease who undergo chemotherapy have a higher risk of developing acute myeloid leukemia[334] and solid tumors[335] after cure of their disease than those in an age-matched control population. Because virtually all of these patients receive combination drug therapy, it is impossible to separate out the effects of each drug, but procarbazine and other alkylating agents are clear candidates for being the carcinogens. Procarbazine is also associated with the azoospermia and anovulation observed in Hodgkin's disease patients undergoing chemotherapy.[336,337] *In vitro,* procarbazine causes oxidative damage to erythrocytes from glucose-6-phosphate dehydrogenase-deficient patients.[338] This has not been noted in its clinical use, however, probably because the drug is rapidly metabolized instead of being converted to the hydrazone, which is a potent oxidant.[338]

REFERENCES

1. C. C. Price: "Chemistry of alkylation," in *Antineoplastic and Immunosuppressive Agents,* Part II, ed. by A. C. Sartorelli and D. G. Johns. Berlin: Springer-Verlag, 1975, pp. 1–5.

2. D. R. Krieg: Ethyl methanesulfonate-induced reversion of bacteriophage T₄rII mutants. *Genetics* 48:561 (1963).

3. T. A. Connors: "Mechanism of action of 2-chloroethylamine derivatives, sulfur mustards, epoxides, and aziridines," in *Antineoplastic and Immunosuppressive Agents,* Part II, ed. by A. C. Sartorelli and D. G. Johns. Berlin: Springer-Verlag, 1975, pp. 18–34.

4. H. B. Brewer, J. P. Comstock, and L. Aronow: Effects of nitrogen mustard on protein and nucleic and synthesis in mouse fibroblasts growing *in vitro. Biochem. Pharmacol.* 8:281 (1961).

5. B. A. Booth, W. A. Creasey, and A. C. Sartorelli: Alterations in cellular metabolism associated with cell death induced by uracil mustard and 6-thioguanine. *Proc. Natl. Acad. Sci. USA* 52:1396 (1964).

6. P. D. Lawley and P. Brookes: Molecular mechanisms of the cytotoxic action of difunctional alkylating agents and of resistance to this action. *Nature* 206:480 (1965).

7. R. W. Ruddon and J. M. Johnson: The effects of nitrogen mustard on DNA template activity in purified DNA and RNA polymerase systems. *Mol. Pharmacol.* 4:258 (1968).

8. J. J. Roberts, T. P. Brent, and A. R. Crathorn: Evidence for the inactivation and repair of the mammalian DNA template after alkylation by mustard gas and half mustard gas. *Eur. J. Cancer* 7:515 (1971).

9. E. P. Geiduschek: Reversible DNA. *Proc. Natl. Acad. Sci. USA* 47:950 (1961).

10. K. W. Kohn, C. L. Spears, and P. Doty: Interstrand

cross-linking of DNA by nitrogen mustard. *J. Mol. Biol.* 19:266 (1966).

11. P. D. Lawley and P. Brookes: Interstrand cross-linking of DNA by difunctional alkylating agents. *J. Mol. Biol.* 25:143 (1967).

12. P. D. Lawley, J. H. Lethbridge, P. A. Edwards, and K. V. Shooter: Inactivation of bacteriophage T_7 by mono- and difunctional sulfur mustards in relation to cross-linking and depurination of bacteriophage DNA. *J. Mol. Biol.* 39:181 (1969).

13. J. J. Roberts, T. P. Brent, and A. R. Crathorn: "The mechanism of the cytotoxic action of alkylating agents on mammalian cells," in *The Interaction of Drugs and Subcellular Components in Animal Cells,* ed. by P. M. Campbell. London: Churchill, 1968, pp. 5–27.

14. L. C. Erickson, M. O. Bradley, J. M. Ducore, R. A. G. Ewig, and K. W. Kohn: DNA crosslinking and cytotoxicity in normal and transformed human cells treated with antitumor nitrosoureas. *Proc. Natl. Acad. Sci. USA* 77:467 (1980).

15. S. T. Garcia, A. McQuillan, and L. Panasci: Correlation between the cytotoxicity of melphalan and DNA crosslinks as detected by the ethidium bromide fluorescence assay in the F_1 variant of B_{16} melanoma cells. *Biochem. Pharmacol.* 37:3189 (1988).

16. C. B. Thomas, R. Osieka, and K. W. Kohn: DNA cross-linking by *in vivo* treatment with 1-(2-chloroethyl)-3-(4-methylcyclohexyl)-1-nitrosourea of sensitive and resistant human colon carcinoma xenografts in nude mice. *Cancer Res.* 38:2448 (1978).

17. M. Fox: "Drug resistance and DNA repair," in *Antitumor Drug Resistance,* ed. by B. W. Fox and M. Fox. Berlin: Springer-Verlag, 1984, pp. 335–369.

18. J. D. Regan and R. B. Setlow: Two forms of repair in the DNA of human cells damaged by chemical carcinogens and mutagens. *Cancer Res.* 34:3318 (1974).

19. S. Venitt: Interstrand cross-links in the DNA of *Escherichia coli* B/r and B_{s-1} and their removal by the resistant strain. *Biochem. Biophys. Res. Commun.* 31:355 (1968).

20. R. A. G. Ewig and K. W. Kohn: DNA damage and repair in mouse leukemia L1210 cells treated with nitrogen mustard, 1,3-bis (2-chloroethyl)-1-nitrosourea, and other nitrosoureas. *Cancer Res.* 37:2114 (1977).

21. K. W. Kohn, N. H. Steigbigel, and C. L. Spears: Cross-linking and repair of DNA in sensitive and resistant strains of *E. coli* treated with nitrogen mustards. *Proc. Natl. Acad. Sci. USA* 53:1154 (1965).

22. V. M. Maher and J. J. McCormick: "Relationship between excision repair and the cytotoxic and mutagenic action of chemicals and UV radiation," in *Induced Mutagenesis,* ed. by W. Lawrence. New York: Plenum, 1983, pp. 271–284.

23. A. Meister: "Novel drugs that affect glutathione metabolism," in *Mechanisms of Drug Resistance in Neoplastic Cells,* ed. by P. W. Woolley and K. D. Tew. New York: Academic Press, 1988, pp. 99–126.

24. K. D. Tew and M. L. Clapper: "Glutathione S-transferase and anticancer drug resistance," in *Mechanisms of Drug Resistance in Neoplastic Cells,* ed by P. W. Woolley and K. D. Tew. New York: Academic Press, 1988, pp. 141–159.

25. O. W. Griffith and A. Meister: Potent and specific inhibition of glutathione synthesis by butathionine sulfoximine (S-n-butyl homocysteine sulfoximine). *J. Biol Chem.* 254:7558 (1979).

26. C. N. Coleman, E. A. Bump, and R. A. Kramer: Chemical modifiers of cancer treatment. *J. Clin. Oncol.* 6:709 (1988).

27. J. A. Green, D. T. Vistica, R. C. Young, T. C. Hamilton, A. M. Rogan, and R. F. Ozols: Potentiation of melphalan cytotoxicity in human ovarian cancer cell lines by glutathione depletion. *Cancer Res.* 44:5427 (1984).

28. R. F. Ozols, K. G. Louie, J. Plowman, B. C. Behrens, R. L. Fine, D. Dykes, and T. C. Hamilton: Enhanced melphalan cytotoxicity in human ovarian cancer *in vitro* and in tumor-bearing nude mice by butathione sulfoximine depletion of glutathione. *Biochem. Pharmacol.* 36:147 (1987).

29. G. J. Goldenberg and A. Begleiter: "Alterations of drug transport," in *Antitumor Drug Resistance,* ed. by B. W. Fox and M. Fox. Berlin: Springer-Verlag, 1984, pp. 241–298.

30. M. K. Wolpert and R. W. Ruddon: A study on the mechanism of resistance to nitrogen mustard (HN_2) in Ehrlich ascites tumor cells: Comparison of uptake of HN_2-^{14}C into sensitive and resistant cells. *Cancer Res.* 29:873 (1969).

31. R. M. Lyons and G. J. Goldenberg: Active transport of nitrogen mustard and choline by normal and leukemic human lymphoid cells. *Cancer Res.* 32:1679 (1972).

32. G. J. Goldenberg: The role of drug transport in resistance to nitrogen mustard and other alkylating agents in L5178Y lymphoblasts. *Cancer Res.* 35:1687 (1975).

33. F. M. Schabel, M. W. Trader, W. R. Laster, G. P. Wheeler, and M. H. Witt: Patterns of resistance and therapeutic synergism among alkylating agents. *Antibiot. Chemother.* 23:200 (1978).

34. E. Frei, C. A. Cucchi, A. Rosowsky, R. Tantravahi, S. Bernal, T. J. Ervin, R. M. Ruprecht, and W. A. Haseltine: Alkylating agent resistance. *In vitro* studies with human cell lines. *Proc. Natl. Acad. Sci. USA* 82:2158 (1985).

35. E. Frei, B. A. Teicher, C. A. Cucchi, A. Rosowsky, J. L. Flatlow, M. J. Kelley, and P. Genereux: "Resistance to alkylating agents: Basic studies and therapeutic implications," in *Mechanisms of Drug Resistance in Neoplastic Cells,* ed. by P. V. Woolley and K. D. Tew. New York: Academic Press, 1988, pp. 69–86.

36. K. Antman, J. P. Eder, A. Elias, T. Shea, W. P. Peters, J. Andersen, S. Schryber, W. D. Henner, R. Finberg, D. Wilmore, W. Kaplan, M. Lew, M. S. Kruskall, K. Anderson, B. Gorgone, R. Bast, L. Schnipper, E. Frei, and the Solid Tumor Autologous Bone Marrow Team: High-dose combination alkylating agent preparative regimen with autologous bone marrow support: The Dana-Farber Cancer Institute/Beth Israel Hospital experience. *Cancer Treat. Rep.* 71:119 (1987).

37. L. M. Van Putten and P. Lelieveld: Factors determining cell killing by chemotherapeutic agents *in vivo*—II. Melphalan, chlorambucil and nitrogen mustard. *Eur. J. Cancer* 7:11 (1971).

38. V. T. Oliverio and C. G. Zubrod: Clinical pharmacology of the effective antitumor drugs. *Ann. Rev. Pharmacol.* 5:335 (1965).

39. D. S. Alberts, S. Y. Chang, H. S. G. Chen, B. J. Larcom, and S. E. Jones: Pharmacokinetics and metabolism of

chlorambucil in man: A preliminary report. *Cancer Treat. Rev. 6 (Suppl.):9* (1979).

40. A. McLean: Pharmacokinetics and metabolism of chlorambucil in patients with malignant disease. *Cancer Treat. Rev. 6 (Suppl.):33* (1979).

41. D. S. Alberts, S. Y. Chang, H. S. G. Chen, B. J. Larcom, and T. L. Evans: Comparative pharmacokinetics of chlorambucil and melphalan in man. *Recent Results Cancer Res. 74:124* (1980).

42. U. Loos, E. Musch, M. Engel, J. H. Hartlapp, E. Hügl, and H. J. Dengler: The pharmacokinetics of melphalan during intermittent therapy of multiple myeloma. *Eur. J. Clin. Pharmacol. 35:187* (1985).

43. D. T. Vistica, J. N. Toal, and M. Rabinovitz: Amino acid conferred protection against melphalan: Interference with leucine protection of melphalan cytotoxicity by the basic amino acids in cultured murine L1210 leukemia cells. *Mol. Pharmacol. 14:1136* (1978).

44. G. J. Goldenberg and E. K. Froese: Antagonism of the cytocidal activity and uptake of melphalan by tamoxifen in human breast cancer cells *in vitro. Biochem. Pharmacol. 34:763* (1985).

45. G. E. Foley, O. M. Friedman, and B. P. Drolet: Studies on the mechanism of action of cytoxan: Evidence of activation *in vivo* and *in vitro. Cancer Res. 21:57* (1961).

46. T. A. Connors, P. J. Cox, P. B. Farmer, A. B. Foster, and M. Jarman: Some studies of the active intermediates formed in the microsomal metabolism of cyclophosphamide and isophosphamide. *Biochem. Pharmacol. 23:115* (1974).

47. R. F. Struck, M. C. Kirk, L. B. Mellet, S. El Dareer, and D. L. Hill: Urinary metabolites of the antitumor agent cyclophosphamide. *Mol. Pharmacol. 7:519* (1971).

48. R. A. Deitrich: Tissue and subcellular distribution of mammalian aldehyde-oxidizing capacity. *Biochem. Pharmacol. 15:1911* (1966).

49. P. J. Cox, B. J. Phillips, and P. Thomas: The enzymatic basis of the selective action of cyclophosphamide. *Cancer Res. 35:3755* (1975).

50. C. M. Bagley, F. W. Bostick, V. T. De Vita: Clinical pharmacology of cyclophosphamide. *Cancer Res. 33:226* (1973).

51. N. E. Sladek, D. Doeden, J. F. Powers, and W. Krivit: Plasma concentrations of 4-hydroxycyclophosphamide and phosphoramide mustard in patients repeatedly given high doses of cyclophosphamide in preparation for bone marrow transplantation. *Canc. Treat. Rev. 68:1247* (1984).

52. M. J. Moore, R. W. Hardy, J. J. Thiessen, S. J. Soldin, and C. Erlichman: Rapid development of enhanced clearance after high-dose cyclophosphamide. *Clin. Pharmacol. Ther. 44:622* (1988).

53. N. E. Sladek: Therapeutic efficacy of cyclophosphamide as a function of its metabolism. *Cancer Res. 32:535* (1972).

54. E. S. Vesell, G. T. Passanti, and F. E. Greene: Impairment of drug metabolism in man by allopurinol and nortryptaline. *New Engl. J. Med. 283:1484* (1970).

55. R. F. Struck, D. S. Alberts, K. Horne, J. G. Phillips, Y. M. Peng, and D. J. Roe: Plasma pharmacokinetics of cyclophosphamide and its cytotoxic metabolites after intravenous versus oral administration in a randomized, crossover trial. *Cancer Res. 47:2723* (1987).

56. L. B. Grochow and M. Colvin: Clinical pharmacokinetics of cyclophosphamide. *Clin. Pharmacokin. 4:380* (1979).

57. F. D. Juma, H. J. Rodgers, and J. R. Trounce: Pharmacokinetics of cyclophosphamide and alkylating activity in man after intravenous and oral administration. *Br. J. Clin. Pharmacol. 8:209* (1979).

58. M. Colvin and B. A. Chabner: "Alkylating agents" in *Cancer Chemotherapy,* ed by B. A. Chabner and J. M. Collins. Philadelphia: J.B. Lippincott, 1990, pp. 276–313.

59. J. E. Low, R. F. Borch, and N. E. Sladek: Further studies on the conversion of 4-hydroxyoxazaphosphorines to reactive mustards and aerolein in inorganic buffers. *Cancer Res. 43:5815* (1983).

60. W. P. Brade, K. Herdrich, and M. Varini: Ifosfamide-pharmacology, safety and therapeutic potential. *Canc. Treat. Rev. 12:1* (1985).

61. V. T. DeVita, G. P. Canellos, and J. H. Moxley: A decade of combination chemotherapy of advanced Hodgkin's disease. *Cancer 30:1495* (1972).

62. R. B. Weiss and S. Bruno: Hypersensitivity reactions to cancer chemotherapeutic agents. *Ann. Int. Med. 94:66* (1981).

63. C. C. Harris: The carcinogenicity of anticancer drugs: A hazard in man. *Cancer 37:1014* (1976).

64. I. Penn: Second malignant neoplasms associated with immunosuppressive medications. *Cancer 37:1024* (1976).

65. M. A. Tucker, C. N. Coleman, R. S. Cox, A. Yarghese, and S. A. Rosenberg: Risk of second cancers after treatment for Hodgkin's disease. *New Engl. J. Med. 318:76* (1988).

66. W. H. Knospe, V. Loeb, and C. M. Huguley: Biweekly chlorambucil treatment of chronic lymphocytic leukemia. *Cancer 33:555* (1974).

67. C. S. Portlock, D. S. Fischer, E. Cadman, W. B. Lundberg, A. Levy, S. Bobrow, J. R. Bertino, and L. Farber: High-dose pulse chlorambucil in advanced, low-grade non-Hodgkin's lymphoma. *Cancer Treat. Rep. 71:1029* (1987).

68. D. G. Miller: Alkylating agents and human spermatogenesis. *JAMA 217:1662* (1971).

69. H. J. Lerner: Acute myelogenous leukemia in patients receiving chlorambucil as long-term adjuvant chemotherapy for stage II breast cancer. *Cancer Treat. Rep. 62:1135* (1978).

70. R. P. George, J. L. Poth, D. Gordon, and S. L. Schrier: Multiple myeloma—intermittent combination chemotherapy compared to continuous therapy. *Cancer 29:1665* (1972).

71. S. B. Howell, G. E. Pfeifle, and R. A. Olshen: Intraperitoneal chemotherapy with melphalan. *Ann. Int. Med. 101:14* (1984).

72. B. Fisher, B. Sherman, H. Rockette, C. Redmond, R. Margolese, and E. R. Fisher: L-Phenylalamine mustard (L-PAM) in the management of premenopausal patients with primary breast cancer. *Cancer 44:847* (1979).

73. M. H. Greene, E. L. Harris, D. M. Gershenson, G. D. Malksian, L. J. Melton, A. J. Dembo, J. M. Bennett, W. C. Moloney, and J. D. Boice: Melphalan may be a more potent leukemogen than cyclophosphamide. *Ann. Int. Med. 105:360* (1986).

74. A. S. Townes, J. M. Sowa, and L. E. S. Schulman:

Controlled trial of cyclophosphamide in rheumatoid arthritis (RA): An 11-month double-blind crossover study. *Arthritis Rheum. 15:*129 (1972).

75. T. E. Starzl, C. G. Groth, C. W. Putnam, J. Corman, C. G. Halgrimson, I. Penn, B. Husberg, A. Gustafsson, S. Cascardo, P. Geis, and S. Iwatsuki: Cyclophosphamide for clinical renal and hepatic transplantation. *Transplant. Proc. 5:*511 (1973).

76. E. D. Thomas, C. D. Buckner, M. A. Cheever, R. A. Clift, A. B. Einstein, A. Fefer, P. E. Neiman, J. Sanders, R. Storb, and P. L. Weiden: Marrow transplantation for leukemia and aplastic anemia. *Transplant. Proc. 8:*603 (1976).

77. S. R. Kaplan and P. Calabresi: Immunosuppressive agents [first of two parts]. *New Engl. J. Med. 289:*952 (1973).

78. M. E. Gershwin, E. J. Goetzl, and A. D. Steinberg: Cyclophosphamide: Use in practice. *Ann. Int. Med. 80:*531 (1974).

79. E. R. Hurd: The effect of cyclophosphamide treatment on B- and T-lymphocytes in patients with connective tissue diseases. *Arthritis Rheum. 16:*554 (1973).

80. G. M. Mullins and M. Colvin: Intensive cyclophosphamide (NSC-26271) therapy for solid tumors. *Cancer Chemother. Rep. 59:*411 (1975).

81. L. Ganci and B. Serrou: Changes in hair pigmentation associated with cancer chemotherapy. *Cancer Treat. Rep. 64:*193 (1980).

82. H. Koyama, T. Wada, Y. Nishizawa, T. Iwanaga, Y. Aoki, T. Terasawa, G. Kosaki, T. Yamamoto, and A. Wada: Cyclophosphamide-induced ovarian failure and its therapeutic significance in patients with breast cancer. *Cancer 39:*1403 (1977).

83. K. F. Fairley, J. U. Barrie, and W. Johnson: Sterility and testicular atrophy related to cyclophosphamide therapy. *Lancet 1:*568 (1972).

84. G. J. Mark, A. Lehimgar-Zadeh, and B. D. Ragsdale: Cyclophosphamide pneumonitis. *Thorax 33:*89 (1978).

85. W. W. Johnson and D. C. Meadows: Urinary-bladder fibrosis and telangiectasia associated with long term cyclophosphamide therapy. *New Engl. J. Med. 284:*290 (1971).

86. P. J. Cox: Cyclophosphamide cystitis—identification of acrolein as the causative agent. *Biochem. Pharmacol. 28:*2045 (1979).

87. W. Brade, S. Seeber, and K. Herdrich: Comparative activity of ifosfamide and cyclophosphamide. *Cancer Chemother. Pharmacol. 18 (Suppl. 2):*S1 (1986).

88. M. R. Habs and D. Schmähl: Prevention of urinary bladder tumors in cyclophosphamide-treated rats by additional medication with the uroprotectors sodium 2-mercaptoethane sulfonate (mesna) and disodium 2,2'-dithio-bis-ethane sulfonate (dimesna). *Cancer 51:*606 (1983).

89. R. A. DeFronzo, H. Braine, O. M. Colvin, and P. J. Davis: Water intoxication in man after cyclophosphamide therapy. Time course and relation to drug action. *Ann. Int. Med. 78:*861 (1973).

90. T. P. Green and B. L. Mirkin: Prevention of cyclophosphamide-induced antidiuresis by furosamide infusion. *Clin. Pharmacol. Ther. 29:*634 (1981).

91. Symposium: Proceedings of a symposium on ifosfamide (Mitoxana®; Holoxan®) and Mesna (Uromitexan®). *Cancer Treat. Rev. 10 (Suppl. A):*1–192 (1983).

92. M. Colvin: The comparative pharmacology of cyclophosphamide and ifosfamide. *Semin. Oncol. 9:*2 (1982).

93. G. Teufel and A. Pfleiderer: Ifosfamid im Vergleich zu Endoxan bei forgeschrittenen Ovarialkarzinomen. *Geburtschilfe Frauenheilkund. 36:*274 (1976).

94. B. M. Bryant, M. Jarman, H. T. Ford, and I. E. Smith: Prevention of isophosphamide-induced urothelial toxicity with 2-mercaptoethane sulfonate sodium (mesnum) in patients with advanced carcinoma. *Lancet 2:*658 (1980).

95. G. L. Andriole, J. T. Sandlund, J. S. Miser, V. Arasi, M. Linehan, and I. T. Magrath: The efficacy of mesna (2-mercaptoethane sodium sulfonate) as a uroprotectant in patients with hemorrhagic cystitis receiving further oxazaphosphorine chemotherapy. *J. Clin. Oncol. 5:*799 (1987).

96. N. Brock and J. Pohl: The development of mesna for regional detoxification. *Cancer Treat. Rev. 10 (Suppl. A):*33 (1983).

97. M. Moncrieff and A. Foot: Fanconi syndrome after ifosfamide. *Cancer Chemother. Pharmacol. 23:*121 (1989).

98. C. A. Meanwell, K. A. Kelly, G. Blacklodge: Avoiding ifosfamide/mesna encephalopathy. *Lancet 2:*406 (1986).

99. M. P. Goren, R. K. Wright, C. B. Pratt, and F. E. Pell: Dechloroethylation of ifosfamide and neurotoxicity. *Lancet 2:*1219 (1986).

100. P. B. Farmer: Metabolism and reactions of alkylating agents. *Pharmac. Ther. 35:*301 (1987).

101. L. B. Mellett, P. E. Hodgson, and L. A. Woods: Absorption and fate of C^{14}-labeled N,N'N''-triethylenthiophosphoramide (thio-TEPA) in humans and dogs. *J. Lab. Clin. Med. 60:*818 (1962).

102. M. S. Soloway and K. S. Ford: Thiotepa-induced myelosuppression: Review of 670 bladder installations. *J. Urol. 130:*889 (1983).

103. I. Nissenkorn, C. Servadio, E. Vilikowski, and I. Glanz: Long-term intravesicle thiotepa treatment in patients with superficial bladder tumors and vesicoureteral reflux. *J. Urol. 133:*198 (1985).

104. C. J. Rutty and T. A. Connors: *In vitro* studies with hexamethylmelamine. *Biochem. Pharmacol. 26:*2385 (1977).

105. M. D'Incalci: Metabolism of triazine anticancer agents. *Pharmac. Ther. 35:*291 (1987).

106. M. M. Ames, M. E. Sanders, and W. S. Tiede: Role of N-methylopentamethylmelamine in the metabolic activation of hexamethylmelamine. *Cancer Res. 43:*500 (1983).

107. M. D'Incalci, E. Erba, G. Balconi, L. Morasca, and S. Garattini: Time dependence of the *in vitro* cytotoxicity of hexamethylmelamine and its metabolites. *Br. J. Cancer 41:*630 (1980).

108. K. J. Miller, R. M. McGovern, and M. M. Ames: Effect of a hepatic activation system on the antiproliferative activity of hexamethylmelamine against human tumor cell lines. *Cancer Chemother. Pharmacol. 15:*49 (1985).

109. D. Ross, S. P. Langdon, A. Gescher, and M. F. G. Stevens: Studies of the mode of action of antitumor triazenes and triazines—V. The correlation of the *in vitro* cytotoxicity and *in vivo* antitumor activity of hexamethyl-

melamine analogues with their metabolism. *Biochem. Pharmacol.* 33:1131 (1984).

110. J. Dubois, R. Arnould, F. Abikhalil, M. Hanocq, G. Atassi, G. Ghanem, A. Libert, and F. J. Lejeune: *In vitro* cytotoxicity of hexamethylmelamine (HMM) and its derivatives. *Anticancer Res.* 10:827 (1990).

111. M. M. Ames, R. L. Richardson, J. S. Kovach, C. G. Moertel, and M. J. O'Connell: Phase I and clinical pharmacological evaluation of a parenteral hexamethylmelamine formulation. *Cancer Res.* 50:206 (1990).

112. B. J. Foster, B. J. Harding, B. Leyland-Jones, and D. Hoth: Hexamethylmelamine: A critical review of an active drug. *Cancer Treat. Rev.* 13:197 (1986).

113. P. J. M. Klippert, A. Hulshoff, M. J. Mingels, G. Hofman, and J. Noordhoek: Low bioavailability of hexamethylmelamine in the rat due to simultaneous hepatic and intestinal metabolism. *Cancer Res.* 43:3160 (1983).

114. J. F. Worzalla, B. D. Kaiman, B. M. Johnson, G. Ramirez, and G. T. Bryan: Metabolism of hexamethylmelamine-ring-^{14}C in rats and man. *Cancer Res.* 34:2669 (1974).

115. G. T. Bryan, J. F. Worzalla, A. L. Gorske, and G. Ramirez: Plasma levels and urinary excretion of hexamethylmelamine following oral administration to human subjects with cancer. *Clin. Pharm. Ther.* 9:777 (1968).

116. J. F. Worzalla, B. M. Johnson, G. Ramirez, and G. T. Bryan: N-Demethylation of the antineoplastic agent hexamethylmelamine by rats and man. *Cancer Res.* 33:2810 (1973).

117. E. Grattini, J. Colombo, M. G. Donelli, P. Catalani, M. Bianchi, M. D'Incalci, and C. Pantarotto: Distribution, metabolism, and irreversible binding of hexamethylmelamine in mice bearing ovarian carcinoma. *Cancer Chemother. Pharmacol.* 11:51 (1983).

118. A. Paolini and M. D'Incalci: Effect of phenobarbital pretreatment on the metabolism and antitumor activity of hexamethylmelamine. *Cancer Treat. Rep.* 70:513 (1986).

119. K. Hande, G. Combs, R. Swingle, L. Combs, and L. Anthony: Effect of cimetidine and ranitidine on the metabolism and toxicity of hexamethylmelamine. *Cancer Treat. Rep.* 70:1443 (1986).

120. S. S. Legha, M. Slavik, and S. K. Carter: Hexamethylmelamine: An evaluation of its role in the therapy of cancer. *Cancer* 38:27 (1976).

121. S. E. Vogel, M. Pagano, T. E. Davis, N. Einhorn, J. C. Tunca, B. H. Kaplan, and J. C. Arseneau: Hexamethylmelamine and cisplatin in advanced ovarian cancer after failure of alkylating-agent therapy. *Cancer Treat. Rep.* 66:1285 (1982).

122. H. Kersten: "Mechanism of action of mitomycins," in *Antineoplastic and Immunosuppressive Agents,* Part II, ed. by A. C. Sartorelli and D. G. Johns. Berlin: Springer-Verlag, 1975, pp. 47–64.

123. V. N. Iyer and W. Szybalski: A molecular mechanism of mitomycin action: Linking of complementary DNA strands. *Proc. Natl. Acad Sci. USA* 50:355 (1963).

124. M. Tomasz, R. Lipman, D. Chowdary, J. Pawlak, G. L. Verdine and K. Nakanishi: Isolation and structure of a covalent cross-link adduct between mitomycin C and DNA. *Science* 235:1204 (1987).

125. V. N. Iyer and W. Szybalski: Mitomycins and porfiromycin: Chemical mechanism of activation and cross-linking of DNA. *Science* 145:55 (1964).

126. M. Tomasz, A. K. Chawla, and R. Lipman: Mechanism of monofunctional and bifunctional alkylation of DNA by mitomycin C. *Biochemistry* 27:3182 (1988).

127. H. W. Moore: Bioactivation as a model for drug design bioreductive alkylation. *Science* 197:527 (1977).

128. M. Egbertson and S. J. Danishefsky: Modeling of the electrophilic activation of mitomycins: Chemical evidence for the intermediacy of a mitosene semiquinone as the active electrophile. *J. Am. Chem. Soc.* 109:2204 (1987).

129. A. C. Sartorelli: The role of mitomycin antibiotics in the chemotherapy of solid tumors. *Biochem. Pharmacol.* 35:67 (1986).

130. S. R. Keyes, P. M. Fracasso, D. C. Heimbrook, S. Rockwell, S. G. Sligar, and A. C. Sartorelli: Role of NADPH-cytochrome c reductase and DT-diaphorase in the biotransformation of mitomycin C. *Cancer Res.* 44:5638 (1984).

131. S. S. Tan, P. A. Andrews, C. J. Glover, and N. R. Bachur: Reductive activation of mitomycin C and mitomycin C metabolites catalyzed by NADPH-cytochrome P-450 reductase and xanthine oxidase. *J. Biol. Chem.* 259:959 (1984).

132. N. R. Bachur, S. L. Gordon, and M. V. Gee: A general mechanism for microsomal activation of quinone anticancer agents to free radicals. *Cancer Res.* 38:1745 (1978).

133. P. M. Fracasso and A. C. Sartorelli: Cytotoxicity and DNA lesions produced by mitomycin C and porfiromycin in hypoxic and aerobic EMT6 and Chinese hamster ovary cells. *Cancer Res.* 46:3939 (1986).

134. S. Rockwell, S. R. Keys, and A. C. Sartorelli: Modulation of the cytotoxicity of mitomycin C to EMT6 mouse mammary tumor cells by dicoumarol *in vitro. Cancer Res.* 48:5471 (1988).

135. M. Tomasz, R. Lipman, M. S. Lee, G. L. Verdine, and K. Nakanishi: Reaction of acid-activated mitomycin C with calf thymus DNA and model guanines: Elucidation of the base-catalyzed degradation of N7-alkylguanine nucleosides. *Biochemistry* 26:2010 (1987).

136. H. Borowy-Borowski, R. Lipman, and M. Tomasz: Recognition between mitomycin C and specific DNA sequences for cross-link formation. *Biochemistry* 29:2999 (1990).

137. P. R. Hoban, M. I. Walton, C. N. Robson, J. Godden, I. J. Stratford, P. Workman, A. L. Harris, and I. D. Hickson: Decreased NADPH:cytochrome P-450 reductase activity and impaired drug activation in a mammalian cell line resistant to mitomycin C under aerobic but not hypoxic conditions. *Cancer Res.* 50:4692 (1990).

138. A. M. Dulhanty, M. Li, and G. F. Whitmore: Isolation of Chinese hamster ovary cell mutants deficient in excision repair and mitomycin C bioactivation. *Cancer Res.* 49:117 (1989).

139. R. T. Dorr, J. D. Liddil, J. M. Trent, and W. S. Dalton: Mitomycin C resistant L1210 leukemia cells: Association with pleotropic drug resistance. *Biochem. Pharmacol.* 36:3115 (1987).

140. S. T. Crooke, M. Henderson, M. Samson, and L. H. Baker: Phase I study of oral mitomycin C. *Cancer Treat. Rep.* 60:1633 (1976).

141. J. den Hartigh, J. G. Mc Vie, W. J. van Oort, and H. M. Pinedo: Pharmacokinetics of mitomycin C in humans. *Cancer Res.* 43:5017 (1983).

142. R. T. Dorr: New findings in the pharmacokinetic,

metabolic and drug-resistance aspects of mitomycin C. *Semin. Oncol. 15 (Suppl. 4):*32 (1988).

143. J. Lankelma, M. Stuurman, J. van Hoogenhuijze, A. van Bochove, J. B. Vermorken, J. Verweij, and H. M. Pinedo: The pharmacokinetic plasma profile of mitomycin C, measured after sequential intermittent intravenous administration. *Eur. J. Cancer Clin. Oncol. 24:*175 (1988).

144. J. Verweij, M. Stuurman, J. de Vries, and H. M. Pinedo: The difference in pharmacokinetics of mitomycin C, given either as a single agent or as part of combination chemotherapy. *J. Cancer Res. Clin. Oncol. 112:*283 (1986).

145. S. T. Crooke and W. T. Bradner: Mitomycin C: A review. *Canc. Treatment Rev. 3:*121 (1976).

146. Z. Wajsman, R. A. Dhafir, M. Pfeffer, S. MacDonald, A. Block, N. Dragone, and J. E. Pontes: Studies of mitomycin C absorption after intravesical treatment of superficial bladder tumors. *J. Urol. 132:*30 (1984).

147. L. C. Argenta and E. K. Manders: Mitomycin C extravasation injuries. *Cancer 51:*1080 (1983).

148. J. Verweij, T. van Zanten, T. Souren, R. Golding, and H. M. Pinedo: Prospective study on the dose relationship of mitomycin C-induced interstitial pneumonitis. *Cancer 60:*756 (1987).

149. J. Verweij, M. E. L. van der Burg, and H. M. Pinedo: Mitomycin C-induced hemolytic uremic syndrome. Six case reports and review of the literature on renal, pulmonary and cardiac side effects of the drug. *Radiother. Oncol. 8:*33 (1987).

150. R. Valavaara and E. Nordman: Renal complications of mitomycin C therapy with special reference to the total dose. *Cancer 55:*47 (1985).

151. H. M. Lazarus, M. R. Gottfried, R. H. Herzig, G. L. Phillips, R. S. Weiner, G. P. Sarna, J. Fay, S. N. Wolff, O. Sudilovsky, R. P. Gale, and G. P. Herzig: Veno-occlusive disease of the liver after high-dose mitomycin C therapy and autologous bone marrow transplantation. *Cancer 49:*1789 (1982).

152. W. P. Tong and D. B. Ludlum: Crosslinking of DNA by busulfan formation of diguanyl derivatives. *Biochim. Biophys. Acta. 608:*174 (1980).

153. P. Bedford and B. W. Fox: DNA-DNA interstrand crosslinking by dimethanesulphonic acid esters. Correlation with cytotoxicity and antitumor activity in the Yoshida lymphosarcoma model and relationship to chain length. *Biochem. Pharmacol. 32:*2297 (1983).

154. B. A. Bridges and R. J. Munson: Excision-repair of DNA damage in an auxotrophic strain of *Escherichia coli. Biophys. Res. Commun. 22:*268 (1966).

155. M. Fox and B. W. Fox: The establishment of cloned cell lines from Yoshida sarcomas having differential sensitivities to methylene dimethane sulfonate *in vivo* and their cross-sensitivity to X-rays, UV and other alkylating agents. *Chem.-Biol. Interactions 4:*363 (1972).

156. P. Bedford and B. W. Fox: Repair of DNA interstrand crosslinks after busulphan. A possible mode of resistance. *Cancer Chemother. Pharmacol. 8:*3 (1982).

157. W. Fried, A. Kedo, and J. Barone: Effects of cyclophosphamide and of busulfan on spleen colony-forming units and on hematopoietic stroma. *Cancer Res. 37:*1205 (1977).

158. D. A. Galton: Chemotherapy of chronic myelocytic leukemia. *Semin. Hematol. 6:*323 (1969).

159. P. J. Tutschka, E. A. Copelan, and J. P. Klein: Bone marrow transplantation for leukemia following a new busulfan and cyclophosphamide regimen. *Blood 70:*1382 (1987).

160. H. Ehrsson, M. Hassan, M. Ehrnebo, and M. Beran: Busulfan kinetics. *Clin. Pharmacol. Ther. 34:*86 (1983).

161. H. Vodopick, H. E. Hamilton, H. L. Jackson, C. T. Peng, and R. F. Sheets: Metabolic fate of tritiated busulfan in man. *J. Lab. Clin. Med. 73:*266 (1969).

162. M. V. Nadkarni, E. G. Trams, and P. K. Smith: Preliminary studies on the distribution and fate of TEM, TEPA, and myeran in the human. *Cancer Res. 19:*713 (1959).

163. H. D. Sostman, R. A. Matthay, C. E. Putman: Cytotoxic drug-induced lung disease. *Am. J. Med. 62:*608 (1977).

164. J. K. V. Wilson: Pulmonary toxicity of antineoplastic drugs. *Cancer Treat. Rep. 62:*2003 (1978).

165. E. G. Trams, M. V. Nadkarni, V. deQuattro, G. D. Maengwyn-Davies, and P. K. Smith: Dimethanesulphonoxybutane (Myleran): Preliminary studies on distribution and metabolic fate in the rat. *Biochem. Pharmacol. 2:*7 (1959).

166. H. Stott, W. Fox, D. J. Girling, R. J. Stephens, and D. A. Galton: Acute leukemia after busulfan. *Br. Med. J. 2:*1513 (1977).

167. D. J. Reed, H. E. May, R. B. Boose, K. M. Gregory, and M. A. Beilstein: 2-Chloroethanol formation as evidence for a 2-chloroethyl alkylating intermediate during chemical degradation of 1-(2-chloroethyl)-3-cyclohexyl-1-nitrosourea and 1-(2-chloroethyl)-3-(trans-4-methylcyclohexyl)-1-nitrosourea. *Cancer Res. 35:*568 (1975).

168. J. A. Montgomery, R. James, G. S. McCaleb, M. C. Kirk, and T. P. Johnston: Decomposition of N-(2-chloroethyl)-N-nitrosoureas in aqueous media. *J. Med. Chem. 18:*568 (1975).

169. J. A. Montgomery, R. James, G. S. McCaleb, and T. P. Johnston: The modes of decomposition of 1,3-*bis*(2-chloroethyl)-1-nitrosourea and related compounds. *J. Med Chem. 10:*668 (1967).

170. M. Colvin, R. B. Brundrett, W. Cowens, I. Jardine, and D. B. Ludlum: A chemical basis for the antitumor activity of chloroethylnitrosoureas. *Biochem. Pharmacol. 25:*695 (1976).

171. K. W. Kohn: Interstrand cross-linking of DNA by 1,3-*bis*(2-chloroethyl)-1-nitrosourea and other 1-(2-haloethyl)-1-nitrosoureas. *Cancer Res. 37:*1450 (1977).

172. R. A. G. Ewig and K. W. Kohn: DNA damage and repair in mouse leukemia L1210 cells treated with nitrogen mustard, 1,3-*bis*(2-chloroethyl)-1-nitrosourea, and other nitrosoureas. *Cancer Res. 37:*2114 (1977).

173. W. T. Briscoe, S. P. Anderson, and H. E. May: Base sequence specificity of three 2-chloroethylnitrosoureas. *Biochem. Pharmacol. 40:*1201 (1990).

174. T. P. Brent, S. O. Lestrud, D. G. Smith, and J. S. Remack: Formation of DNA interstrand cross-links by the novel chloroethylating agent 2-chloroethyl(methanesulfonyl)methanesulfonate: Suppression by O⁶-alkylguanine-DNA alkyltransferase purified from human leukemic lymphoblasts. *Cancer Res. 47:*3384 (1987).

175. F. Ali-Osman: Quenching of DNA cross-link precursors of chloroethylnitrosoureas and attenuation of

DNA interstrand cross-linking by glutathione. *Cancer Res.* 49:5258 (1989).

176. M. D'Incalci, L. Citti, P. Taverna, and C. V. Catapano: Importance of the DNA repair enzyme O^6-alkyl guanine alkyltransferase (AT) in cancer chemotherapy. *Cancer Treat. Rev.* 15:279 (1988).

177. T. Aida and W. J. Bodell: Cellular resistance to chloroethylnitrosoureas, nitrogen mustard, and *cis*-diamminedichloroplatinum (II) in human glial-derived cell lines. *Cancer Res.* 47:1361 (1987).

178. T. P. Brent, P. J. Houghton, and J. A. Houghton: O^6-alkylguanine-DNA alkyltransferase activity correlates with the therapeutic response of human rhabdomyosarcoma xenografts to 1-(chloroethyl)-3-(trans-4-methylcyclohexyl)-1-nitrosourea. *Proc. Natl. Acad. Sci. USA* 82:2985 (1985).

179. H. Fox, J. Brennand, and G. P. Margison: Protection of Chinese hamster cells against the cytotoxic and mutagenic effects of alkylating agents by transfection of the *Escherichia coli* alkyltransferase gene and a truncated derivative. *Mutagenesis* 2:491 (1987).

180. C. J. Cheng, S. Fujimura, D. Grunberger, and I. B. Weinstein: Interaction of 1-(2-chloroethyl)-4-cyclohexyl-1-nitrosourea (NSC 79037) with nucleic acids and proteins *in vivo* and *in vitro*. *Cancer Res.* 32:22 (1972).

181. B. Schmall, C. J. Cheng, S. Fujimura, N. Gersten, D. Grunberger, and I. B. Weinstein: Modification of proteins by 1-(2-chloroethyl)-3-cyclohexyl-2-nitrosourea (NSC-79037) *in vitro*. *Cancer Res.* 33:1921 (1973).

182. H. E. Kann: Comparison of biochemical and biological effects of four nitrosoureas with differing carbamoylating activities. *Cancer Res.* 38:2363 (1978).

183. L. C. Panasci, D. Green, R. Nagourney, P. Fox, and P. S. Schein: A structure-activity analysis of chemical and biological parameters of chloroethylnitrosoureas in mice. *Cancer Res.* 37:2615 (1977).

184. N. Rakieten, M. L. Rakieten, and M. Nadkarni: Studies on the diabetogenic action of streptozotocin (NSC-37917). *Cancer Chemother. Rep.* 29:91 (1963).

185. L. E. Broder and S. K. Carter: Pancreatic islet cell carcinoma. II. Results of therapy with streptozotocin in 52 patients. *Ann. Int. Med.* 79:108 (1973).

186. R. J. Gralla, C. T. C. Tan, and C. W. Young: Phase I trial of chlorozotocin. *Cancer Treat. Rep.* 63:17 (1979).

187. D. Green, K. D. Tew, T. Hisamatsu, and P. S. Schein: Correlation of nitrosourea murine bone marrow toxicity with deoxyribonucleic acid alkylation and chromatin binding sites. *Biochem. Pharmacol.* 31:1671 (1982).

188. V. T. De Vita, C. Denham, J. D. Davidson, and V. T. Oliverio: The physiological disposition of the carcinostatic 1-3-*bis*(2-chloroethyl)-1-nitrosourea (BCNU) in man and animals. *Clin. Pharm. Ther.* 8:566 (1967).

189. B. R. Freed, R. L. McQuinn, R. S. Tilbury, and G. A. Digenis: Distribution of ^{13}N in rat tissues following intravenous administration of nitroso-labeled BCNU. *Cancer Chemother. Pharmacol.* 10:16 (1982).

190. W. D. Henner, W. P. Peters, J. P. Eder, K. Antman, L. Schnipper, and E. Frei: Pharmacokinetics and immediate effects of high-dose carmustine in man. *Cancer Treat. Rep.* 70:877 (1986).

191. V. A. Levin, W. Hoffman, and R. J. Weinkam: Pharmacokinetics of BCNU in man: A preliminary study of 20 patients. *Cancer Treat. Rep.* 62:1305 (1978).

192. R. J. Weinkam, A. Finn, V. A. Levin, and J. P. Kane: Lipophilic drugs and lipoproteins: Partitioning effects on chloroethylnitrosourea reaction rates in serum. *J. Pharm. Exptl. Ther.* 214:318 (1980).

193. R. W. Sponzo, V. T. DeVita, and V. T. Oliverio: Physiologic disposition of 1-(2-chloroethyl)-3-cyclohexyl-1-nitrosourea (CCNU) and 1-(2-chloroethyl)-3-(4-methyl-cyclohexyl)-1-nitrosourea (MeCCNU) in man. *Cancer* 31:1154 (1973).

194. M. D. Walker and J. Hilton: Nitrosourea pharmacodynamics in relation to the central nervous system. *Cancer Treat. Rep.* 60:725 (1976).

195. M. Diksic, K. Sako, W. Feindel, A. Kato, Y. L. Yamamoto, S. Farrokhzad, and C. Thompson: Pharmacokinetics of positron-labeled 1,3-*bis*(2-chloroethyl)nitrosourea in human brain tumors using positron emission tomography. *Cancer Res.* 44:3120 (1984).

196. D. L. Hill, M. C. Kirk, and R. F. Struck: Microsomal metabolism of nitrosoureas. *Cancer Res.* 35:296 (1975).

197. V. A. Levin, J. Stearns, A. Byrd, A. Finn, and R. J. Weinkam: The effect of phenobarbital pretreatment on the antitumor activity of 1,3-*bis*(2-chloroethyl)-1-nitrosourea (BCNU), 1-(2-chloroethyl)-3-cyclohexyl-1-nitrosourea (CCNU) and 1-(2-chloroethyl)-3-(2,6-dioxo)-3-piperidyl-1-nitrosourea (PCNU), and on the plasma pharmacokinetics and biotransformation of BCNU. *J. Pharm. Exptl. Ther.* 208:1 (1979).

198. J. Hilton and M. D. Walker: Hydroxylation of 1-(2-chloroethyl)-3-cyclohexyl-1-nitrosourea. *Biochem. Pharmacol.* 24:2153 (1975).

199. G. P. Wheeler, T. P. Johnston, B. J. Bowdon, G. S. McCaleb, D. L. Hill, and J. A. Montgomery: Comparison of the properties of metabolites of CCNU. *Biochem. Pharmacol.* 26:2331 (1977).

200. F. Y. F. Lee, P. Workman, J. T. Roberts, and N. M. Bleehen: Clinical pharmacokinetics of oral CCNU (lomustine). *Cancer Chemother. Pharmacol.* 14:125 (1985).

201. P. Schein, R. Kahn, P. Gorden, S. Wells, and V. T. DeVita: Streptozotocin for malignant insulinomas and carcinoid tumor. *Arch. Int. Med.* 132:555 91973).

202. E. H. Karunanayake, J. R. J. Baker, R. A. Christian, D. J. Hearse, and G. Mellows: Autoradiographic study of the distribution and cellular uptake of (^{14}C)-streptozotocin in the rat. *Diabetologia* 12:123 (1976).

203. T. H. Wasserman, M. Slavik, and S. K. Carter: Clinical comparison of the nitrosoureas. *Cancer* 36:1258 (1975).

204. EORTC Brain Tumor Group: Effect of CCNU on survival, rate of objective remission and duration of free interval in patients with malignant brain glioma—First evaluation. *Eur. J. Cancer* 12:41 (1976).

205. Proceedings of the seventh New Drug Seminar on the Nitrosoureas: *Cancer Treatment Rep.* 60: Issue No. 6 (1976).

206. C. G. Moertel, J. A. Hanley, and L. A. Johnson: Streptozocin alone compared with streptozocin plus fluorouracil in the treatment of advanced islet-cell carcinoma. *New Engl. J. Med.* 303:1189 (1980).

207. T. H. Wasserman, M. Slavik, and S. K. Carter: Review of CCNU in clinical cancer therapy. *Cancer Treatment Rev.* 1:131 (1974).

208. W. E. Harmon, H. J. Cohen, E. E. Schneeberger, and W. E. Grupe: Chronic renal failure in children treated

with methyl CCNU. *New Engl. J. Med.* 300:1200 (1979).

209. A. C. Smith: The pulmonary toxicity of nitrosoureas. *Pharmac. Ther.* 41:443 (1989).

210. G. Ramirez, W. Wilson, T. Grage, and G. Hill: Phase II evaluation of 1,3-*bis*(2-chloroethyl)-1-nitrosourea (BCNU; NSC-409962) in patients with solid tumors. *Canc. Chemother. Rep.* 56:787 (1972).

211. A. J. Tomson: The interactions of platinum compounds with biological molecules. *Rec. Res. Cancer Res.* 48:38 (1974).

212. B. Rosenberg, L. Van Camp, and T. Krigas: Inhibition of cell division in *Escherichia coli* by electrolysis products from a platinum electrode. *Nature* 205:698 (1965).

213. B. Rosenberg, E. Renshaw, L. Van Camp, J. Hartwick, and J. Drobnik: Platinum-induced filamentous growth in *Escherichia coli*. *J. Bacteriol.* 93:716 (1967).

214. B. Rosenberg, L. Van Camp, E. B. Grimley, and A. J. Tomson: The inhibition of growth and cell division in *Escherichia coli* by different ionic species of platinum (IV) complexes. *J. Biol. Chem.* 242:1347 (1967).

215. A. Eastman: Glutathione-mediated activation of anticancer platinum (IV) complexes. *Biochem. Pharmacol.* 36:4177 (1987).

216. B. Rosenberg, L. Van Camp, J. E. Trosko, and V. H. Mansour: Platinum compounds: A new class of potent antitumor agents. *Nature* 222:385 (1969).

217. M. Nicolini (ed.): *Platinum and Other Coordination Compounds in Cancer Chemotherapy.* Boston: Martinus Nijhoff, 1988, 775 pp.

218. E. Reed and K. W. Kohn: "Platinum analogues," in *Cancer Chemotherapy: Principles and Practice*, ed. by B. A. Chabner and J. M. Collins. Philadelphia: J.B. Lippincott, 1990, pp. 465–490.

219. Symposium: Carboplatin (JM-8, CBDCA). A new platinum compound. *Semin. Oncol.* 16 *(Suppl. 5)*:1–48 (1989).

220. F. K. V. Leh and W. Wolf: Platinum complexes: A new class of antineoplastic agents. *J. Pharmaceutical Sci.* 65:315 (1976).

221. P. D. Braddock, T. A. Connors, M. Jones, A. R. Khokhar, D. H. Melzack, and M. L. Tobe: Structure and activity relationships of platinum complexes with anti-tumour activity. *Chem.-Biol. Interactions* 11:145 (1975).

222. A. L. Pinto and S. J. Lippard: Binding of the antitumor drug *cis*-diamminedichloroplatinum(II) (cisplatin) to DNA. *Biochim. Biophys. Acta.* 780:167 (1985).

223. A. Eastman: Reevaluation of interaction of *cis*-dichloro(ethylenediamine) platinum(II) with DNA. *Biochemistry* 25:3912 (1986).

224. A. C. M. Plooy, A. M. J. Fichtinger-Schepman, H. H. Schutte, M. van Dijk, and P. H. M. Lohman: The quantitative detection of various Pt-DNA adducts in Chinese hamster ovary cells treated with cisplatin: Application of immunochemical techniques. *Carcinogenesis* 6:561 (1985).

225. A. M. J. Fichtinger-Schepman, A. T. van Oosterom, P. H. M. Lohman, and F. Berends: *cis*-Diamminedichloroplatinum(II)-induced DNA adducts in peripheral leukocytes from seven cancer patients: Quantitative immunochemical detection of the adduct induction and removal after a single dose of *cis*-diamminedichloroplatinum (II). *Cancer Res.* 47:3000 (1987).

226. A. Eastman: Interstrand cross-links and sequence specificity in the reaction of *cis*-dichloro(ethylenediamine)platinum(II) with DNA. *Biochemistry* 24:5027 (1985).

227. L. A. Zwelling, J. Filipski, and K. W. Kohn: Effect of thiourea on survival and DNA cross-link formation in cells treated with platinum(II) complexes, L-phenylalanine mustard and *bis*(2-chloroethyl)methylamine. *Cancer Res.* 39:4989 (1979).

228. R. J. Knox, F. Friedlos, D. A. Lydall, and J. J. Roberts: Mechanism of cytotoxicity of anticancer platinum drugs: Evidence that *cis*-diamminedichloroplatinum(II) and *cis*-diammine(1,1-cyclobutanedicarboxylato)platinum(II) differ only in the kinetics of their interaction with DNA. *Cancer Res.* 46:1972 (1986).

229. J. A. Rice, D. M. Crothers, A. L. Pinto, and S. J. Lippard: The major adduct of the antitumor drug *cis*-diamminedichloroplatinum(II) with DNA bends the duplex by ≈40° toward the major groove. *Proc. Natl. Acad. Sci. USA* 85:4158 (1988).

230. A. L. Pinto and S. J. Lippard: Sequence-dependent termination of *in vitro* DNA synthesis by *cis*- and *trans*-diamminedichloroplatinum(II). *Proc. Natl. Acad. Sci. USA* 82:4616 (1985).

231. J. D. Gralla, S. Sasse-Dwight, and L. G. Poljack: Formation of blocking lesions at identical DNA sequences by the nitrosourea and platinum classes of anticancer drugs. *Cancer Res.* 47:5092 (1987).

232. E. Reed, S. H. Yuspa, L. A. Zwelling, R. F. Ozols, and M. C. Poirier: Quantitation of *cis*-diamminedichloroplatinum II (cisplatin)-DNA-intrastrand adducts in testicular and ovarian cancer patients receiving cisplatin chemotherapy. *J. Clin. Invest.* 77:545 (1986).

233. L. A. Zwelling, T. Anderson, and K. W. Kohn: DNA-protein and DNA interstrand cross-linking by *cis*- and *trans*-platinum (II) diamminedichloride in L1210 mouse leukemia cells and relation to cytotoxicity. *Cancer Res.* 39:365 (1979).

234. A. Eastman and N. Schulte: Enhanced DNA repair as a mechanism of resistance to *cis*-diamminedichloroplatinum(II). *Biochemistry* 27:4730 (1988).

235. R. E. Meyn, S. F. Jenkins, and L. H. Thompson: Defective removal of DNA cross-links in a repair-deficient mutant of Chinese hamster cells. *Cancer Res.* 42:3106 (1982).

236. P. Bedford, A. M. J. Fichtinger-Schepman, S. A. Shellard, M. C. Walker, J. R. W. Masters, and B. T. Hill: Differential repair of platinum-DNA adducts in human bladder and testicular tumor continuous cell lines. *Cancer Res.* 48:3019 (1988).

237. B. C. Behrens, T. C. Hamilton, H. Masuda, K. R. Grotzinger, J. Whang-Peng, K. G. Lovie, T. Knutsen, W. M. KcKoy, R. C. Young, and R. F. Ozols: Characterization of a *cis*-diamminedichloroplatinum(II)-resistant human ovarian cancer cell line and its use in evaluation of platinum analogues. *Cancer Res.* 47:414 (1987).

238. R. A. Hromas, P. A. Andrews, M. P. Murphy, and C. P. Burns: Glutathione depletion reverses cisplatin resistance in murine L1210 leukemia cells. *Cancer Lett.* 34:9 (1987).

239. B. A. Arrick and C. F. Nathan: Glutathione metabolism as a determinant of therapeutic efficacy: A review. *Cancer Res.* 44:4224 (1984).

240. K. Micetich, L. A. Zwelling, and K. W. Kohn:

Quenching of DNA:platinum(II) monoadducts as a possible mechanism of resistance to cis-diamminedichloroplatinum (II) in L1210 cells. *Cancer Res. 43:*3609 (1983).

241. L. Endresen, L. Schjerven, and H. E. Rugstad: Tumours from a cell strain with a high content of metallothionein show enhanced resistance against *cis*-dichlorodiammineplatinum. *Acta Pharmacol. Toxicol. 55:*183 (1984).

242. P. A. Andrews, M. P. Murphy, and S. B. Howell: Metallothionein-mediated cisplatin resistance in human ovarian carcinoma cells. *Cancer Chemother. Pharmacol. 19:*149 (1987).

243. S. L. Kelley, A. Basu, B. A. Teicher, M. P. Hacker, D. H. Hamer, and J. S. Lazo: Overexpression of metallothionein confers resistance to anticancer drugs. *Science 241:*1813 (1988).

244. M. Rozencweig, D. D. Von Hoff, M. Slavik, and F. M. Muggia: *Cis*-diamminedichloroplatinum(II): A new anticancer drug. *Ann. Int. Med. 86:*803 (1977).

245. R. H. Earhart: Instability of *cis*-dichlorodiammine platinum in dextrose solution. *Cancer Treat. Rep. 62:*1105 (1978).

246. M. J. Cleare: Some aspects of platinum complex chemistry and their relation to antitumor activity. *J. Clin. Hematol. Oncol. 7:*1 (1977).

247. D. F. Bajorin, G. J. Bosl, N. W. Alcock, D. Niedzwiecki, E. Gallina, and B. Shurgot: Pharmacokinetics of *cis*-diamminedichloroplatinum (II) after administration in hypertonic saline. *Cancer Res. 46:*5969 (1986).

248. K. J. Himmelstein, T. F. Patton, R. J. Belt, S. Taylor, A. J. Repta, and L. A. Sternson: Clinical kinetics of intact cisplatin and some related species. *Clin. Pharmacol. Ther. 29:*658 (1981).

249. J. B. Vermorken, W. J. F. van der Vijgh, I. Klein, A. A. M. Hart, H. E. Gall, and H. M. Pinedo: Pharmacokinetics of free and total platinum species after short-term infusion of cisplatin. *Cancer Treat. Rep. 68:*505 (1984).

250. B. J. Corden, R. L. Fine, R. F. Ozols, and J. M. Collins: Clinical pharmacology of high dose cisplatin. *Cancer Chemother. Pharmacol. 14:*38 (1985).

251. R. C. DeConti, B. R. Toftness, R. C. Lange, and W. A. Creasey: Clinical and pharmacological studies with *cis*-diamminedichloroplatinum (II). *Cancer Res. 33:*1310 (1973).

252. L. Hegedus, W. J. F. van der Vijgh, I. Klein, S. Kerpel-Fronius, and H. M Pinedo: Chemical reactivity of cisplatin bound to plasma proteins. *Cancer Chemother. Pharmacol. 20:*211 (1987).

253. C. Jacobs, S. M. Kalman, M. Tretton, and M. W. Weiner: Renal handling of *cis*-diamminedichloroplatinum(II). *Cancer Treat. Rep. 64:*1223 (1980).

254. P. A. Reece, J. F. Bishop, I. N. Olver, I. Stafford, B. L. Hillcoat, and G. Morstyn: Pharmacokinetics of unchanged carboplatin (CBDCA) in patients with small cell lung carcinoma. *Cancer Chemother. Pharmacol. 19:*326 (1987).

255. S. Oguri, T. Sakakibara, H. Mase, T. Shimizu, K. Ishikawa, K. Kimura, and R. D. Smyth: Clinical pharmacokinetics of carboplatin. *J. Clin. Pharmacol. 28:*208 (1988).

256. M. J. Egorin, D. A. Van Echo, S. J. Tipping, E. A. Olman, M. Y. Whitacre, B. W. Thompson, and J. Aisner: Pharmacokinetics and dosage reduction of *cis*-diammine (1,1-cyclobutanedicarboxylato) platinum in patients with impaired renal function. *Cancer Res. 44:*5432 (1984).

257. Symposium: Cisplatin: contemporary treatment approaches. *Semin. Oncol 16 (Suppl. 6):*1–128 (1989).

258. L. H. Einhorn: Have new aggressive chemotherapy regimens improved results in advanced germ cell tumors? *Eur. J. Cancer Clin. Oncol. 22:*1289 (1986).

259. R. F. Ozols and R. C. Young: Chemotherapy of ovarian cancer. *Semin. Oncol. 18:*222 (1991).

260. D. D. Von Hoff: Whither carboplatin?—A replacement for or an alternative to cisplatin? *J. Clin. Oncol. 5:*169 (1987).

261. G. Daugaard and V. Abildgaard: Cisplatin toxicity: A review. *Cancer Chemother. Pharmacol. 25:*1 (1989).

262. R. Safirstein, J. Winston, M. Goldstein, D. Moel, S. Dickman, and J. Guttenplan: Cisplatin nephrotoxicity. *Am. J. Kidney Dis. 8:*356 (1986).

263. M. Dentino, F. C. Luft, M. N. Yum, S. D. Williams, and L. H. Einhorn: Long term effect of *cis*-diamminedichloroplatinum (CDDP) on renal function and structure in man. *Cancer 41:*1274 (1978).

264. B. J. Leonard, E. Eccleston, D. Jones, P. Todd, and A. Walpole: Antileukemic and nephrotoxic properties of platinum compounds. *Nature 234:*43 (1971).

265. J. M. Ward, M. E. Grabin, E. Berlin, and D. M. Young: Prevention of renal failure in rats receiving *cis*-diamminedichloroplatinum (II) by administration of furosamide. *Cancer Res. 37:*1238 (1977).

266. E. Cvitkovic, J. Spaulding, V. Bethune, J. Martin, and W. F. Whitmore: Improvement of *cis*-dichlorodiammineplatinum (NSC 119875) therapeutic index in an animal model. *Cancer 39:*1357 (1977).

267. D. M. Hayes, E. Cvitkovic, R. B. Golbey, E. Scheiner, L. Helson, and I. H. Krakoff: High dose *cis*-platinum diammine dichloride: Amelioration of renal toxicity by mannitol diuresis. *Cancer 39:*1372 (1977).

268. R. F. Ozols, B. J. Corden, J. Jacob, M. N. Wesley, Y. Ostchega, and R. C. Young: High-dose cisplatin in hypertonic saline. *Ann. Int. Med. 100:*19 (1984).

269. C. E. Pfeifle, S. B. Howell, R. D. Felthouse, T. B. S. Woliver, P. A. Andrews, M. Markman, and M. P. Murphy: High-dose cisplatin with sodium thiosulfate protection. *J. Clin. Oncol. 3:*237 (1985).

270. R. F. Borch, J. C. Katz, P. H. Lieder, and M. E. Pleasants: Effect of diethyldithiocarbamate rescue on tumor response to *cis*-platinum in a rat model. *Proc. Natl. Acad. Sci. USA. 77:*5441 (1980).

271. D. Golver, J. H. Glick, C. Weiler, K. Fox, and D. Guerry: WR-2721 and high-dose cisplatin: An active combination in the treatment of metastatic melanoma. *J. Clin. Oncol. 5:*574 (1987).

272. M. Markman: Intraperitoneal chemotherapy. *Semin. Oncol. 18:*248 (1991).

273. E. F. McClay and S. B. Howell: A review: Intraperitoneal cisplatin in the management of patients with ovarian cancer. *Gynecol. Oncol. 36:*1 (1990).

274. I. J. Piel, D. Meyer, C. P. Perlia, and V. I. Wolfe: Effects of *cis*-diamminedichloroplatinum (NSC-119875) on hearing function in man. *Cancer Chemother. Rep. 58:*871 (1974).

275. A. J. Lippman, C. Helson, L. Helson, and I. H. Krakoff: Clinical trials of *cis*-diamminedichloroplatinum (NSC-119875). *Cancer Chemother. Rep. 57:*191 (1973).

276. S. W. Stadnicki, R. W. Fleischmann, U. Schaeppi, and P. Merriam: *Cis*-dichlorodiammineplatinum (II) (NSC-

119875): Hearing loss and other toxic effects in rhesus monkeys. *Cancer Chemother. Rep.* 59:467 (1975).

277. R. W. Fleischmann, S. W. Stadnicki, M. F. Ethier, and U. Schaeppi: Ototoxicity of *cis*-dichlorodiammine platinum (II) in the guinea pig. *Toxicol. Appl. Pharmacol.* 33:320 (1975).

278. S. D. Comis, P. H. Rhys-Evans, M. P. Osborne, J. O. Pickles, D. J. R. Jeffries, and H. A. C. Pearse: Early morphological and chemical changes induced by cisplatin in the guinea pig organ of Corti. *J. Laryngol. Otol.* 100:1375 (1986).

279. V. G. Schweitzer, D. F. Dolan; G. E. Abrams, T. Davidson, and R. Snyder: Amelioration of cisplatin-induced ototoxicity by fosfomycin. *Laryngoscope* 96:948 (1986).

280. A. Khan, J. M. Hill, W. Grater, E. Loeb, A. MacLellan, and N. Hill: Atopic hypersensitivity to *cis*-dichlorodiammineplatinum (II) and other platinum complexes. *Cancer Res.* 35:2766 (1975).

281. R. J. Cersosimo: Cisplatin neurotoxicity. *Cancer Treat. Rev.* 16:195 (1989).

282. J. A. Montgomery: Experimental studies at Southern Research Institute with DTIC (NSC-45388). *Cancer Treat. Rep.* 60:125 (1976).

283. T. A. Connors, P. M. Goddard, K. Merai, W. C. J. Ross, and D. E. V. Wilman: Tumour inhibitory triazenes: Structural requirements for an active metabolite. *Biochem. Pharmacol.* 25:241.(1976).

284. L. Meer, R. C. Janzer, P. Kleihues, and G. F. Kolar: In vivo metabolism and reaction with DNA of the cytostatic agent, 5-(3,3-dimethyl-1-triazeno)-imidazole-4-carboxamide (DTIC). *Biochem. Pharmacol.* 35:3243 (1986).

285. U. Lonn and S. Lonn: Prevention of dacarbazine damage of human neoplastic cell DNA by aphidicolin. *Cancer Res.* 47:26 (1987).

286. U. Lonn and S. Lonn: Inhibition of poly(ADP-ribase) synthetase potentiates cell dacarbazine cytotoxicity. *Biochem. Biophys. Res. Commun.* 142:1089 (1987).

287. T. L. Loo, J. K. Luce, J. H. Jardine, and E. Frei: Pharmacologic studies of the antitumor agent 5-(dimethyl-triazeno)imidazole-4-carboximide. *Cancer Res.* 28:2448 (1968).

288. R. T. Dorr, D. S. Alberts, J. Einspahr, N. Mason-Liddil, and M. Soble: Experimental dacarbazine antitumor activity and skin toxicity in relation to light exposure and pharmacologic antidotes. *Cancer Treat. Rep.* 71:267 (1987).

289. H. Breithaupt, A. Dammann, and K. Aigner: Pharmacokinetics of dacarbazine (DTIC) and its metabolite 5-aminoimidazole-4-carboxamide (AIC) following different dose schedules. *Cancer Chemother. Pharmacol.* 9:103 (1982).

290. T. L. Loo, G. E. Housholder, A. H. Gerulath, P. H. Saunders, and D. Farquhar: Mechanism of action and pharmacology studies with DTIC (NSC-45388). *Cancer Treat. Rep.* 60:149 (1976).

291. J. L. Skibba and G. T. Bryan: Methylation of nucleic acids and urinary excretion of ^{14}C-labeled 7-methylguanine by rats and man after administration of 4(5)-(3,3-dimethyl-1-triazeno)-imidazole 5(4)-carboxamide. *Toxicol. Appl. Pharmacol.* 18:707 (1971).

292. L. E. Flaherty, B. G. Redman, G. G. Chabot, S. Martino, S. M. Gualdoni, L. K. Heilbrun, M. Valdivieso,

and E. C. Bradley: A phase I-II study of dacarbazine in combination with outpatient interleukin-2 in metastatic malignant melanoma. *Cancer* 65:2471 (1990).

293. Symposium: Proceedings of the 6th new drug seminar: DTIC. *Cancer Treat. Rep.* 60:123 (1976).

294. E. McClay, C. J. Lusch, and M. J. Mastrangelo: Allergy-induced toxicity associated with dacarbazine. *Cancer Treat. Rep.* 71:219 (1987).

295. W. Feaux de Lacroix, U. Runne, H. Hauk, K. Doepfmer, W. Groth, and D. Wacker: Acute liver dystophy with thrombosis of hepatic veins: A fatal complication of dacarbazine treatment. *Cancer Treat. Rep.* 67:779 (1983).

296. J. M. Buesa, M. Gracia, M. Valle, E. Estrada, O. F. Hidalgo, and A. J. Lacave: Phase I trial of intermittent high-dose dacarbazine. *Cancer Treat. Rep.* 68:499 (1984).

297. P. Zeller, H. Gutmann, B. Hegedüs, A. Kaiser, A. Langemann, and M. Müller: Methylhydrazine derivatives, a new class of cytotoxic agents. *Experientia* 19:129 (1963).

298. W. Bollag and E. Grunberg: Tumour inhibitory effects of a new class of cytotoxic agents: Methylhydrazine derivatives. *Experientia* 19:130 (1963).

299. D. J. Reed: "Procarbazine," in *Antineoplastic and Immunosuppressive Agents,* Part II, ed. by A. C. Sartorelli and D. G. Johns. Berlin: Springer-Verlag, 1975, pp. 747–765.

300. R. A. Prough and D. J. Tweedie: "Procarbazine," in *Metabolism and Action of Anticancer Drugs,* ed by G. Powis and R. H. Prough. London: Taylor & Francis, 1987, pp. 29–47.

301. S. D. Averbuch: "Nonclassic alkylating agents," in *Cancer Chemotherapy: Principles and Practice,* ed by B. A. Chabner and J. M. Collins. Philadelphia: J.B. Lippincott, 1990, pp. 314–340.

302. A. Rutishauser and W. Bolag: Cytological investigations with a new class of cytotoxic agents: Methylhydrazine derivatives. *Experientia* 19:131 (1963).

303. K. Bernies, M. Kofler, W. Bolag, A. Kaiser, and A. Langemann: The degradation of deoxyribonucleic acid by new tumor inhibiting compounds: The intermediate formation of hydrogen peroxide. *Experientia* 19:132 (1963).

304. G. R. Gale, J. G. Simpson, and A. B. Smith: Studies on the mode of action of N-isopropyl-α(2-methylhydrazino)-p-toluamide. *Cancer Res.* 27:1186 (1967).

305. A. C. Sartorelli and S. Tsunamura: Studies on the biochemical mode of action of a cytotoxic methylhydrazine derivative, N-isopropyl-α(2-methylhydrazine)-p-toluamide. *Mol. Pharmacol.* 2:275 (1966).

306. M. C. Alley, G. Powis, P. L. Appel, K. L. Kooistra, and M. M. Lieber: Activation and inactivation of cancer chemotherapeutic agents by rat hepatocytes cocultured with human tumor cell lines. *Cancer Res.* 44:549 (1984).

307. V. T. Oliverio, C. Denham, V. T. De Vita, and M. G. Kelley: Some pharmacologic properties of a new antitumor agent, N-isopropyl-α(2-methylhydrazino)-p-toluamide hydrochloride (NSC-77213). *Cancer Chemother. Rep.* 42:1 (1964).

308. J. Raaflaub and D. E. Schwartz: Über den Metabolismus eines cytostatisch wirksamen Methylhydrazin-Derivates (Natulan). *Experientia* 21:44 (1965).

309. M. W. Coomes and R. A. Prough: The mitochondrial metabolism of 1,2-disubstituted hydrazines, procar-

bazine and 1,2-dimethylhydrazine. *Drug Metab. Disp.* 11:550 (1983).

310. P. Wiebkin and R. A. Prough: Oxidative metabolism of N-isopropyl-α-(2-methylazo)-p-toluamide (azoprocarbazine) by rodent liver microsomes. *Cancer Res.* 40:3524 (1980).

311. S. W. Cummings, F. P. Guengerich, and R. A. Prough: The characterization of N-isopropyl-p-hydroxymethylbenzamide formed during the oxidative metabolism of azo-procarbazine. *Drug. Metab. Disp.* 10:459 (1982).

312. R. A. Prough, M. I. Brown, G. A. Dannan, and F. P. Guengerich: Major isozymes of rat liver microsomal cytochrome P-450 involved in the N-oxidation of N-isopropyl-α-(2-methylazo)-p-toluamide, the azo derivative of procarbazine. *Cancer Res.* 44:543 (1984).

313. D. A. Shiba and R. J. Weinkam: The in vivo cytotoxic activity of procarbazine and procarbazine metabolites against L1210 ascites leukemia cells in CDF$_1$ mice and the effects of pretreatment with procarbazine, phenobarbital, diphenylhydantoin, and methylprednisolone upon in vivo procarbazine activity. *Cancer Chemother. Pharmacol.* 11:124 (1983).

314. B. K. Sinha: Metabolic activation of procarbazine: Evidence for carbon-centered free-radical intermediates. *Biochem. Pharmacol.* 33:2777 (1984).

315. A. Gescher and C. Raymont: Studies of the metabolism of N-methyl containing antitumour agents. *Biochem. Pharmacol.* 30:1245 (1981).

316. V. T. De Vita, G. P. Canellos, and J. H. Moxley: A decade of combination chemotherapy of advanced Hodgkin's disease. *Cancer* 30:1495 (1972).

317. C. D. Bloomfield, R. B. Weiss, I. Fortuny, G. Vosika, and B. J. Kennedy: Combined chemotherapy with cyclophosphamide, vinblastine, procarbazine, and prednisone (CVPP) for patients with advanced Hodgkin's disease: An alternative program to MOPP. *Cancer* 38:42 (1976).

318. S. D. Spivack: Procarbazine. *Ann. Int. Med.* 81:795 (1974).

319. D. W. Nixon, R. W. Carey, H. D. Suit, and A. C. Aisenberg: Combination chemotherapy in oat cell carcinoma of the lung. *Cancer* 36:867 (1975).

320. R. L. Comis and S. K. Carter: Integration of chemotherapy into combined modality therapy of solid tumors. IV. Malignant melanoma. *Cancer Treatment Rev.* 1:285 (1974).

321. P. H. Gutin, C. B. Wilson, A. R. Vansantha, E. B. Boldrey, V. Levin, M. Powell and K. J. Enot: Phase II study of procarbazine, CCNU, and vincristine combination chemotherapy in the treatment of malignant brain tumors. *Cancer* 35:1398 (1975).

322. J. Gutterman, A. T. Huang, and P. Hochstein: Studies on the mode of action of N-isopropyl-α-(2-methylhydrazino)-p-toluamide (MIH). *Proc. Soc. Exptl. Biol. Med.* 130:797 (1969).

323. H. E. Skipper, D. J. Hutchison, F. M. Schabel, L. H. Schmidt, A. Goldin, R. W. Brockman, J. M. Venditti, and I. Wodinsky: A quick reference chart on cross-resistance

between anticancer agents. *Cancer Chemother. Rep.* 56:493 (1972).

324. H. D. Weiss, M. D. Walker, and P. Weirnik: Neurotoxicity of commonly used antineoplastic agents (second of two parts). *New Engl. J. Med.* 291:127 (1974).

325. B. A. Chabner, V. T. De Vita, N. Considine, and V. T. Oliverio: Plasma pyridoxal phosphate depletion by the carcinostatic procarbazine. *Proc. Soc. Exptl. Biol. Med.* 132:1119 (1969).

326. V. T. DeVita, M. A. Hahn, and V. T. Oliverio: Monoamine oxidase inhibition by a new carcinostatic agent, N-isopropyl-α-(2-methylhydrazino)-p-toluamide (MIH). *Proc. Soc. Exptl. Biol. Med.* 120:51 (1965).

327. M. L. Samuels, W. B. Leary, and R. Alexanian: Clinical trials with N-isopropyl-α-(2-methylhydrazino)-p-toluamide hydrochloride in malignant lymphoma and other disseminated neoplasia. *Cancer* 20:1187 (1967).

328. I. P. Lee and G. W. Lucier: The potentiation of barbiturate-induced narcosis by procarbazine. *J. Pharmacol. Exptl. Ther.* 196:586 (1976).

329. S. E. Jones, M. Moore, N. Blank, and R. A. Castellino: Hypersensitivity to procarbazine (Matulane) manifested by fever and pleuropulmonary reaction. *Cancer* 29:498 (1972).

330. J. J. Lokich and W. C. Moloney: Allergic reaction to procarbazine. *Clin. Pharmacol. Ther.* 13:575 (1972).

331. R. Liske: A comparative study of the action of cyclophosphamide and procarbazine on the antibody production in mice. *Clin. Exptl. Immunol.* 15:271 (1973).

332. S. Chaube and M. L. Murphy: Fetal malformations produced in rats by N-isopropyl-α-(2-methylhydrazino)-p-toluamide hydrochloride (procarbazine). *Teratology* 2:23 (1969).

333. M. G. Kelley, R. W. O'Gara, S. T. Yancey, K. Gadekar, C. Botkin, and V. T. Oliverio: Comparative carcinogenicity of N-isopropyl-α-(2-methylhydrazino)-p-toluamide HCl (procarbazine hydrochloride), its degradation products, other hydrazines, and isonicotinic acid hydrazide. *J. Natl. Cancer Inst.* 42:337 (1969).

334. H. W. Grunwald and F. Rosner: Acute myeloid leukemia following treatment of Hodgkin's disease. A review. *Cancer* 50:677 (1982).

335. M. A. Tucker, C. N. Coleman, R. S. Cox, A. Varghese, and S. A. Rosenberg: Risk of second cancers after treatment for Hodgkin's disease. *New Engl. J. Med.* 318:76 (1988).

336. J. H. X. Waxman, Y. A. Terry, P. F. M. Wrigley, J. S. Malpas, L. H. Rees, G. M. Besser, and T. A. Lister: Gonadal function in Hodgkin's disease: Long-term follow up of chemotherapy. *Br. Med. J.* 285:1612 (1982).

337. R. L. Schilsky, R. J. Sherins, S. M. Hubbard, M. N. Wesley, R. C. Young, and V. T. DeVita: Long-term follow up of ovarian function in women treated with MOPP chemotherapy for Hodgkin's disease. *Am. J. Med.* 71:552 (1981).

338. R. W. Sponzo, J. C. Arseneau, and G. P. Canellos: Procarbazine induced oxidative heamolysis: Relationship to *in vitro* red cell survival. *Br. J. Haematol.* 27:587 (1974).

Noncovalent DNA-Binding Drugs

ANTHRACYCLINES
  Daunorubicin
  Doxorubicin
  Idarubicin
MITOXANTRONE

DACTINOMYCIN
BLEOMYCIN
PLICAMYCIN

The intercalating drugs all have planar regions that stack between the paired bases in DNA, forming a tight drug–DNA interaction that is critical for their cytotoxic, mutagenic, and carcinogenic effects. Many of the intercalating compounds used in cancer chemotherapy were originally discovered in screening programs that tested antibiotics for cytotoxic activity. The intercalators in routine clinical use are the anthracycline antibiotics, mitoxantrone, and dactinomycin.

Anthracyclines

Doxorubicin (Adriamycin®) and daunorubicin (daunomycin, rubidomycin) are anthracycline antibiotics isolated from different species of *Streptomyces*. They both have a characteristic four-ring structure that is linked, via a glycosidic bond, to daunosamine, an amino sugar (Fig. 7–1). The antibiotics are identical, except for the presence of a hydroxyl or a hydrogen at the 14 position of the anthracycline ring. Doxorubicin is used to treat a broad spectrum of solid tumors, whereas the clinical use of daunorubicin is limited to the treatment of acute nonlymphocytic leukemia. Another clinically

useful anthracycline is idarubicin, which is 4-demethoxy-daunorubicin. This minor structural alteration at position 4 of the chromophore ring makes the drug more lipophilic and alters the metabolism to yield a longer bioactive half-life. The chemistry and biological effects of these anthracyclines and their many analogs have been reviewed extensively.[1-3]

Mechanism of Action of the Anthracycline Antibiotics

BINDING TO DNA. The anthracycline drugs bind tightly to DNA, and their cytotoxicity is largely the result of this binding. These drugs bind to double-stranded DNA, both in its purified form in solution and in its natural form in chromatin. In human chromosome preparations treated with anthracyclines, the bound drug can be observed as well-defined, orange-red fluorescent bands.[4] The interaction of doxorubicin and daunorubicin with DNA by intercalation has been demonstrated by several methods. One method that is used to identify a number of intercalating compounds exploits the effect of such compounds on the supercoiling of closed circular duplex DNA.[5] As shown diagrammatically in Figure 7–2, when inter-

155

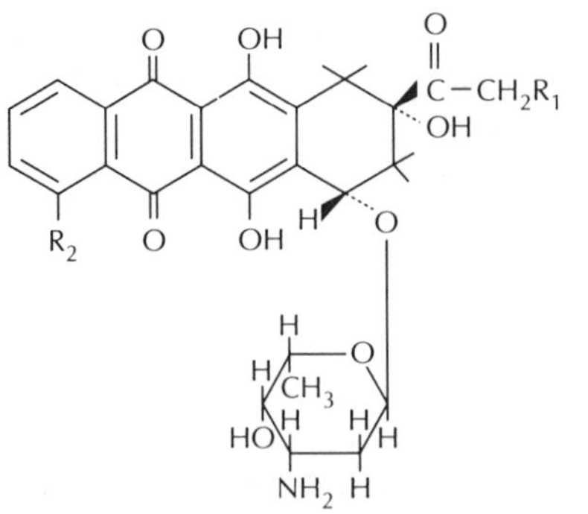

	R_1	R_2
Doxorubicin	OH	OCH_3
Daunorubicin	H	OCH_3
Idarubicin	H	H

Figure 7–1   Structures of the anthracyclines in clinical use.

calating compounds become associated with DNA, there is a local uncoiling of the double helix as a result of the separation of the stacked bases by the intercalated moiety. Because of the topological restrictions inherent in the structure of closed circular duplex DNA, the supercoiled double helix is changed greatly by the cumulative effects of these local uncoiling events. As shown in Figure 7–3, when the replicative form of ϕX174 DNA is exposed to increasing concentrations of daunorubicin, the right-handed supercoil uncoils to form untwisted open circles, which have a slower sedimentation rate. At even higher concentrations of bound drug, left-handed supercoils are formed, and since these supercoiled circles are more compact, they sediment more rapidly. Thus, one can rather quickly determine whether or not a drug intercalates by following the changes in sedimentation coefficient of the closed circular duplex DNA.[5] X-ray diffraction analysis of the DNA-daunorubicin complex shows that the hydrophobic faces of the base pairs interact extensively with the planar rings of the drug, and the amino sugar of the antibiotic is located in the minor groove without directly interacting with the DNA.[6,7] In contrast to another intercalating drug, dactinomycin, there is no base specificity for the interaction of anthracycline antibiotics and DNA.[7]

CONSEQUENCES OF INTERCALATION. Modifications of anthracycline structure that yield reduced DNA binding are usually accompanied by a reduction or loss of antitumor activity.[7] Thus, DNA binding seems to be critical for the drug action, but the pathway leading to cytotoxicity is not at all clear. Although DNA and

RNA synthesis are inhibited in intact cells and in cell-free systems directed by purified polymerases,[8,9] these effects require high drug concentrations and they are not thought to be critical for cytotoxicity.[10]

Many intercalating antitumor drugs have been shown to induce protein-linked double-strand DNA breaks in cultured mammalian cells.[11] Although the mechanism is not completely understood, the DNA breaks are caused by topoisomerase II. This enzyme controls the degree of DNA supercoiling by cleaving and reannealing DNA such that the coil is relaxed by one turn. Topoisomerase II is directly inhibited by several drugs, such as the epipodophyllotoxins, which are discussed in Chapter 8, and the mechanism of DNA unwinding by topoisomerases is presented in more detail in the beginning of that chapter. The intercalators somehow interfere with the DNA strand breakage-reunion reaction of topoisomerase II.[12] The topoisomerase II–associated DNA breaks occur in an appropriately low anthracycline concentration range to account for the cytotoxicity.[10] A direct relationship between topoisomerase II inhibition and cytotoxicity was indicated when a cell line selected for resistance to epipodophyllotoxin was found to be cross-resistant to doxorubicin.[13] As the levels of both drugs were the same in the resistant cells, it is clear this multidrug resistance was not due to the increased drug efflux mechanism discussed in Chapter 4. The demonstration of a direct correlation between topoisomerase II activity and anthracycline resistance in several cell lines strongly supports the involvement of topoisomerase II in the cytotoxicity pathway.[14,15]

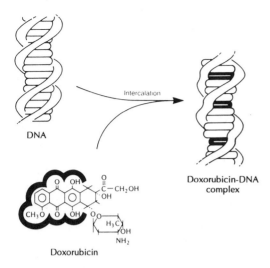

Doxorubicin

Doxorubicin-DNA complex

Intercalation

DNA

Figure 7–2 Diagrammatic model of the intercalation of doxorubicin into DNA showing that local unwinding of the helical structure must occur as the base pairs are moved apart by intercalation. The open, wafer-shaped units on the right represent doxorubicin (viewed in the plane of the anthracycline portion of the molecule) intercalated between base pairs. In a more detailed model, the amino sugar moiety of the drug would be seen to be located in the minor groove of the DNA.

The topoisomerase II mechanism is not the only way in which anthracyclines cleave DNA. Anthracyclines can precipitate the formation of active oxygen species that then cause predominantly single-strand breakage. The anthracycline chromophore contains a hydroxyquinone, which is a well-described iron-chelating structure.[16] The doxorubicin·Fe complex forms a ternary complex with DNA that is different from the intercalated drug–DNA complex.[17] The drug·Fe·DNA complex, like the free drug·Fe complex, catalyzes the transfer of electrons from glutathione to oxygen, resulting in the formation of active oxygen species. The drug·Fe·DNA complex also generates hydroxyl radicals from hydrogen peroxide, which results in DNA cleavage (see Fig. 7–6).[18] In most cells, the contribution of this type of free radical damage to the antitumor effect of Adriamycin is probably minor; however, as discussed later, free radical generation by the drug·Fe complex is critical for anthracycline-induced cardiotoxicity. It has been shown in Ehrlich ascites carcinoma that the cy-

totoxicity of doxorubicin can be reduced by antioxidant enzymes, hydroxyl radical scavengers, and iron chelators.[19] However, tumor cell killing by 5-iminodaunorubicin, a doxorubicin analog with a modified quinone function that prohibits oxidation-reduction cycling, was not ameliorated by any of the free radical scavengers.[19] These observations are consistent with the proposal that free radical generation contributes to but does not account for the antitumor effect. Free radical generation may be more important in certain cell types, such as

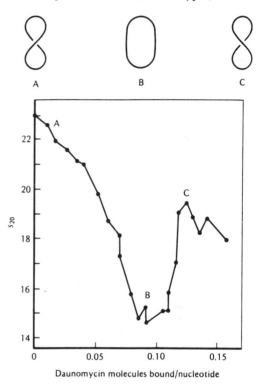

Figure 7–3 The effect of daunorubicin on the sedimentation coefficient (S_{20}) of ϕX174 replicative form DNA. Phage DNA was prepared from infected *Escherichia coli* and the sedimentation rate was determined by ultracentrifugation in the presence of the drug. As the amount of drug intercalated between bases in the closed circular duplex DNA increases, the right-handed supercoils (A) uncoil to form untwisted open circles (B), which are less compact and have a slower sedimentation rate. At higher drug-to-DNA ratios, left-handed supercoils (C) are formed and the sedimentation rate increases. This assay has been used to demonstrate that a variety of drugs, such as the anthracycline antibiotics and dactinomycin, are intercalating agents. (Data from Waring[5])

human breast tumor cells, where some resistant sublines have been found to have elevated glutathione peroxidase activity (see Fig. 7–7).[20] The glutathione peroxidase would detoxify reactive oxygen intermediates, implying their importance in the cytotoxic mechanism.

Adriamycin and daunorubicin are cytotoxic to both exponentially growing cells and plateau phase cells, but the latter are less sensitive.[21] Although these drugs are active throughout the cell cycle, studies in synchronized cell populations have shown that cells in the S and G_2 phases are more sensitive than cells in the G_1 phase.[21]

Anthracycline Resistance

The most common resistance mechanism in cells selected for anthracycline resistance *in vitro* is increased drug efflux due to amplification of the gene for P-glycoprotein, the multidrug transporter discussed in detail in Chapter 4. Cells selected for resistance to an anthracycline are usually resistant to the vinca alkaloids and to other antibiotics, such as actinomycin D. As illustrated in Table 4-4, the relative degree of cross-resistance to different drugs may vary from one cell line to another and can also vary according to the selecting agent. The basis for this variation in resistance pattern has never been adequately explained, but in all cases, the cells are multidrug resistant. The reader is referred to the section on multidrug resistance in Chapter 4 for a comprehensive discussion of this critical anthracycline resistance mechanism.

Two other mechanisms of resistance have been cited above to support the arguments that topoisomerase II inhibition and free radical generation are involved in the cytotoxicity pathway. Thus, in some cell lines decreased topoisomerase II activity has been found to correlate with anthracycline resistance,[13–15] and other cell lines have been found to have increased glutathione peroxidase activity.[20] As described in Chapter 4, reduced glutathione reacts with drug-generated reactive oxygen compounds such as peroxides (see Fig. 4–6)[22] and increased levels of glutathione or glutathione S-transferase have been found in some anthracycline-resistant cell lines.[23] In such cell lines, butathione sulfoximine (BSO), the inhibitor of γ-

glutamyl synthetase (Fig. 4–6), reduces glutathione levels and partially reverses doxorubicin resistance[24] (see discussion of BSO effects in Chapter 4). Interestingly, multidrug-resistant cell lines have been selected that have both decreased anthracycline accumulation due to an increase in the P-glycoprotein transporter and increased detoxification of reactive oxygen due to an increase in glutathione-dependent peroxidase activity. In these cells, combined treatment with the efflux blocker verapamil (see Fig. 4–5) and the glutathione lowering agent butathione sulfoximine led to impressive reversal of doxorubicin resistance.[24]

Pharmacology of the Anthracyclines

Doxorubicin and daunorubicin are given parenterally, since the glycosidic bond joining the daunosamine and the anthracycline nucleus is split in the gastrointestinal tract, rendering the drugs inactive by the oral roue.[25] The anthracycline antibiotics are very irritating to tissue, and care should be taken to avoid extravasation. They are usually injected into the tubing of a rapidly flowing intravenous infusion. Doxorubicin is administered as single dose of 60 mg/m^2 that is repeated after 21 days. Daunorubicin is administered at doses of 30 to 45 mg/m^2 daily for 3 days, and idarubicin is administered at a dose of 12 mg/m^2 daily for 3 days.

The metabolic pathways of doxorubicin and daunorubicin are similar[26,27] and the major reactions involved in the metabolism of doxorubicin in humans are presented in Figure 7–4.[26] A major metabolic step for both drugs is their reduction to doxorubicinol and daunorubicinol, which are active cytotoxic agents.[28] This reduction is catalyzed by cytoplasmic NADPH-dependent aldoketo reductases that have been found in all the tissues analyzed,[25] and these enzymes probably play a major role in determining the overall pharmacokinetics of the drugs. Daunorubicin is a better reductase substrate than doxorubicin. Thus, after a few hours, the principal circulating form of daunorubicin is daunorubicinol, whereas the principal circulating form of doxorubicin is the unmetabolized drug.[29] The drugs and their reduced forms, doxorubicinol and daunorubicinol, are substrates for microsomal glycosi-

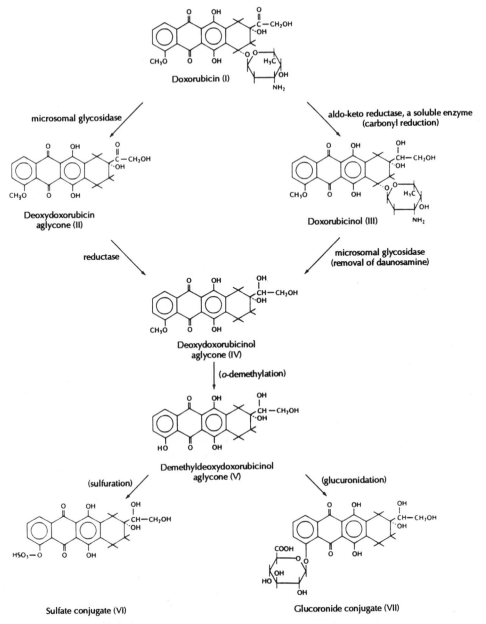

Figure 7–4 Major metabolic pathway for doxorubicin in humans. The fluorescence assay employed identified metabolites with an intact ring system. Other fluorescent metabolites are produced in small amounts.

dases that are present in most tissues. These enzymes split the drugs into inactive aglycones (e.g., compounds II and IV, Fig. 7–4) and the free amino sugar. Again, daunorubicin is a better glycosidase substrate than doxorubicin. Like the -ol compounds, the aglycones are cytotoxic but less active than the parent drugs.[30] The aglycones are demethylated, conjugated to

the sulfate (VI) and glucuronide (VII) esters, and excreted principally in the bile.

The pharmacology of the anthracyclines is summarized in Table 7–1. Doxorubicin has a two-phase pharmacokinetic profile with half-lives of approximately 10 minutes and 30 hours.[31,32] The slow β phase appears to reflect the release of the drug from tissue depots where

Table 7-1   Pharmacology of the Anthracyclines

Drug	Pharmacokinetics	Characteristics
Doxorubicin	$t1/2\alpha \sim 10$ minutes $t1/2\beta \sim 30$ hours	Principal circulating form is the unmetabolized drug
Daunorubicin	$t1/2\alpha \sim 40$ minutes $t1/2\beta \sim 50$ hours	Principal circulating form is daunorubicinol, which is less active than the parent drug
Idarubicin	$t1/2\alpha \sim 20$ minutes $t1/2\beta \sim 15$ hours for the parent drug and ~ 55 hours for idarubicinol	Cytotoxicity primarily due to long-lived idarubicinol metabolite

it is largely intercalated in the DNA. The extensive tissue binding accounts for the large apparent volume of distribution of about 25 L/kg for doxorubicin.[31] Daunorubicin has an initial half-life of 40 minutes, followed by a slow decline over about 50 hours. Idarubicin is rapidly metabolized to idarubicinol,[33] which is nearly as cytotoxic as the parent compound[34] and accounts for most of the plasma AUC[35] and cytotoxicity.[36] In addition to intravenous administration, idarubicin can be given orally and has an average bioavailability of 29% with a wide variability between individuals.[33]

Doxorubicin is eliminated primarily in the bile,[37] but mild to moderate hepatic dysfunction does not alter the plasma pharmacokinetics.[38,39] Clearly, caution is advised when administering the anthracyclines to patients with severely compromised hepatic function.

Use and Toxicity of the Anthracyclines

Doxorubicin has a very broad range of clinical usefulness; it is active against carcinomas of the breast, bladder, endometrium, lung, ovaries, stomach, and thyroid, as well as sarcomas of the bone and soft tissue, pediatric solid tumors, and lymphoid and myelogenous tumors.[40] Daunorubicin has a much more limited clinical application, being used almost solely to treat acute myelogenous leukemia. Idarubicin appears to be as effective as daunorubicin in combination treatment (with cytosine arabinoside) of acute myelogenous leukemia,[41] with perhaps more efficacy than daunorubicin in patients less than 60 years of age.[42]

The anthracyclines frequently cause nausea and vomiting, and patients may experience anorexia and diarrhea. The drugs and their metabolites may color the urine red for 1 or 2 days after administration. Local necrosis at the site of injection can be a serious complication if care is not taken to avoid extravasation.[43]

Myelosuppression is dose related and occurs in 60% to 80% of patients.[44] It is manifested primarily as leukopenia, which reaches a low point at 10 to 14 days, with recovery usually occurring by the 21st day. Thrombocytopenia and anemia may occur at the same time, but they are not as severe. Stomatitis is dose-related and may be severe. Alopecia involving the scalp, axillary, and pubic hair occurs in most patients and reverses when therapy is stopped. Hyperpigmentation and hypersensitivity phenomena (including fever, urticaria, and anaphylaxis) have been reported. The anthracyclines potentiate the effects of irradiation, and enhancement of radiation reactions and "recall" of radiation effects on normal tissues (particularly the esophagus and the skin) have been observed.[45,46] The anthracycline antibiotics are immunosuppressive and are mutagenic and carcinogenic agents.[47,48]

CARDIOTOXICITY. The anthracyclines produce unique cardiotoxic reactions in both adults and children.[49,50] The cardiotoxicity of doxorubicin has been the most thoroughly studied, and two types of reactions are observed: 1) early, transient electrocardiographic changes, and 2) a delayed progressive cardiomyopathy.[49] Acute changes in the electrocardiogram, including tachycardia, extrasystolic contractions, and ST-T wave alterations, may occur in the week following drug administration. Arrhythmias generally reverse within a few hours, and the S-T segment and T-wave abnormalities usually reverse in 1 or 2 weeks after a single dose. Electrocardiographic changes are observed in about 11% of patients receiving doxorubicin.[49]

The drug-induced cardiomyopathy presents as a severe, rapidly progressive congestive heart failure, with the classical signs of tachycardia, tachypnea, hepatomegaly, cardiomegaly, peripheral or pulmonary edema, venous congestion, and pleural effusion. Antecedent symptoms are uncommon and the condition develops late, up to 6 months after administration of the last dose to an adult.[51] There are reports of children developing congestive heart failure several years after doxorubicin treatment,[52,53] and subclinical myocardial damage can be detected in a substantial fraction (23%) of children who received moderate doses of the drug.[54]

As shown in Table 7–2, this cardiomyopathy is a cumulative dose-dependent effect.[55] The risk of congestive heart failure is considerable at total doses of doxorubicin higher than 550 mg/m², and this dosage should not be exceeded in most cases. The dose limit for daunorubicin is 900 mg/m². When patients who developed congestive failure were compared to those who received the same total dose of doxorubicin without developing congestive failure, several risk factors were identified.[56] The early, transient electrocardiographic changes are not predictive of congestive failure. Both radiotherapy to the heart region and high doses of cyclophosphamide have been reported to be potentially cardiotoxic,[49] and concurrent cyclophosphamide treatment or prior radiotherapy to the mediastinum lowers the total doxorubicin dose that predisposes to cardiotoxicity.[56] In patients who have already received mediastinal

irradiation or alkylating agents, the cumulative doxorubicin dose is usually limited to 400 mg/m². Additional risk factors may include uncontrolled hypertension and other conditions, such as aortic stenosis, which increase ventricular stress.[56]

Pathological studies of patients who have died of congestive heart failure show a decrease in the number of cardiac muscle cells and signs of degeneration in the remaining myocardial cells.[57] Loss of myofibrils, distortion of the Z-line substance, and swollen mitochondria with dense inclusion bodies are observed on electron microscopic examination.[57] It is thought that the critical site of anthracycline-induced damage within the myocardial cell is the sarcoplasmic reticulum.[3] A substantial body of evidence has accrued in support of the proposal that the myocardial injury is due to drug-induced production of reactive oxygen species,[58] in particular the hydroxyl radical ($\cdot OH$).[10]

Oxygen-derived free radicals are generated from redox cycling of the anthracycline quinone, which can undergo one electron reduction to the semiquinone or two electron reduction to the corresponding dihydroquinone derivative (see Fig. 7–5).[10] One electron reduction is carried out by a number of enzymes, including xanthine oxidase, P-450 reductase, cytochrome b5 reductase, and NADH dehydrogenase. Xanthine oxidase and ferridoxin reductase can catalyze 2-electron reduction.[10] The semiquinone reacts rapidly with oxygen to generate superoxide anion $O_2^{\cdot-}$. Superoxide anion can dismutate to peroxide, which reacts with a number of species to produce $\cdot OH$. The most important pathways of $\cdot OH$ generation

Table 7–2 Relationship Between Cardiomyopathy and Total Doxorubicin Dose. (From Blum and Carter.[55])

Total Dose (mg/m² Body-Surface Area)	Number of Patients at Risk	Number of Patients Who Developed Congestive Heart Failure		
		Nonfatal	Fatal	Frequency (%)
<450	663	0	0	0
451–500	23	0	0	0
501–550	31	0	1	3
551–600	14	1	2	21
>600	27	2	6	30
Total	758	3	9	1.6

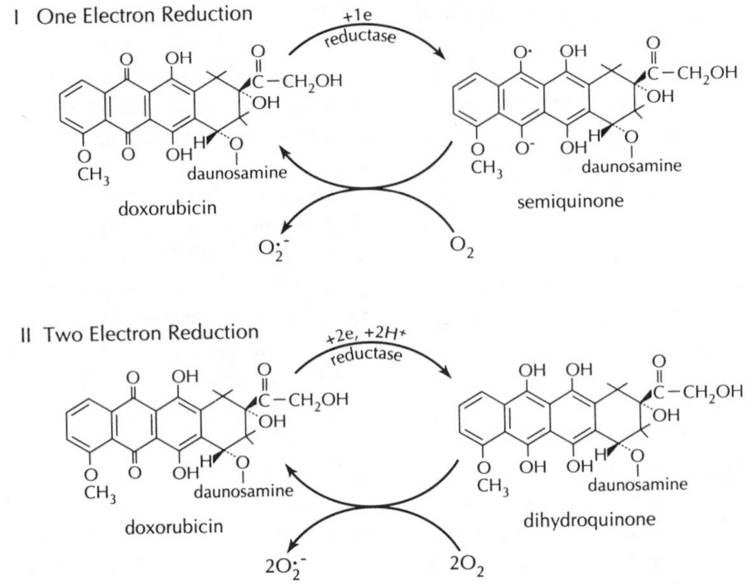

Figure 7–5 One-electron and two-electron reduction of doxorubicin. The anthracyclines are reduced by a variety of quinone reductases. (I) The product of one electron reduction is the semiquinone, which reacts rapidly with oxygen to produce superoxide anion $O_2^{\cdot -}$. (II) Similarly, two-electron reduction yields the dihydroquinone derivative, which reacts with oxygen to produce $2O_2^{\cdot -}$ or H_2O_2.

with respect to the cardiotoxicity appear to be the two metal ion-dependent pathways shown in Figure 7–6.[10] One of these involves reduction of Fe(III) to Fe(II) by either $O_2^{\cdot -}$ or the drug semiquinone, followed by a reaction between the reduced metal ion and H_2O_2. The second mechanism involves a direct reaction between the anthracycline Fe(III) complex and H_2O_2.[59]

In the heart, a major pathway for detoxification of reactive oxygen metabolites is likely via the concerted action of superoxide dismutase and selenium-dependent glutathione peroxidase (Fig. 7–7).[60,61] The heart may be especially prone to adriamycin toxicity because it contains lower levels of critical detoxifying enzyme activities (e.g., catalase and superoxide dismutase) than other organs, such as the

I

$$O_2^{\cdot -} + \text{Fe(III)} \longrightarrow O_2 + \text{Fe(II)}$$

$$\text{doxorubicin semiquinone} + \text{Fe(III)} \longrightarrow \text{doxorubicin} + \text{Fe(II)}$$

$$\text{Fe(II)} + H_2O_2 \longrightarrow \text{Fe(III)} + \cdot OH + {}^{-}OH$$

II

$$H_2O_2 + 2GSH \xrightarrow{\text{doxorubicin}\cdot\text{Fe(III)}} GSSG + \cdot OH + {}^{-}OH$$

Figure 7–6 Iron-dependent generation of hydroxyl radical from doxorubicin. Hydroxyl radical ($\cdot$OH) can be produced from anthracyclines in several ways. It appears that iron-dependent pathways for generating $\cdot$OH are of particular importance with regard to the cardiac toxicity. In pathway I, either superoxide anion or the drug semiquinone derivative reduces Fe(III) to Fe(II), which, in turn, reacts with H_2O_2 to produce $\cdot$OH. In pathway II, the doxorubicin·Fe(III) complex mediates peroxide-dependent hydroxyl radical formation as suggested by Myers *et al.*[59]

$$2O_2^{\cdot-} + 2H^+ \xrightarrow{\text{superoxide dismutase}} H_2O_2 + O_2$$

$$H_2O_2 + GSH \xrightarrow{\text{glutathione peroxidase}} GSSG + H_2O$$

Figure 7–7 Detoxification of superoxide anion. Superoxide anion produced from reaction of the reduced quinone derivative of the anthracycline with molecular oxygen (see Fig. 7–5) dismutates to H_2O_2, which may react with a number of species to produce $\cdot OH$. Reaction of peroxide with reduced glutathione (GSH) protects cells against the toxic species.

liver.[60] It has been shown that doxorubicin administration leads to lipid peroxidation in cardiac tissue (see Fig. 7–8 for a scheme of lipid peroxidation), and that this peroxidative process can be blocked by the free radical scavenger α-tocopherol.[62,63] As shown in Figure 7–9, when mice were injected with 85 units of α-tocopherol 24 hours before a lethal dose of doxorubicin, survival was significantly affected during the 17-day period of observation. Since there is neither extensive bone marrow depression nor gastrointestinal toxicity with this dose, it is thought that improved survival pri-

marily represents diminished cardiac toxicity. Pretreatment with α-tocopherol was shown to prevent the loss of ventricular mass[62] and the production of cardiac lipid peroxides[63] that occur a few days after doxorubicin administration in mice. A marked reduction in the drug-induced cardiomyopathy is observed on histological examination of hearts obtained from α-tocopherol-pretreated animals 5 days after doxorubicin administration.[63] Treatment of mice with the free radical scavenger, however, does not affect the ability of doxorubicin to inhibit DNA synthesis in P388 ascites tumor tissue, nor does it impair the responsiveness of the tumor to doxorubicin.[63] These observations support the hypothesis that the animal model cardiomyopathy involves a free radical mechanism, which may be selectively inhibited without diminishing the antitumor effect that depends upon DNA binding.

REDUCTION OF CARDIOTOXICITY WITH DEXRAZOXANE. Because free radical scavengers were not successful at controlling the cardiac toxicity in humans[64] and because it was shown that doxorubicin-induced lipid peroxidation required iron,[65] efforts to reduce cardio-

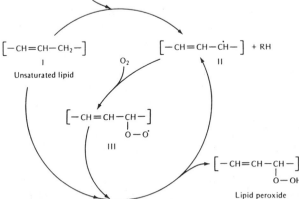

Figure 7–8 Cycle of lipid peroxidation. Reactive species of oxygen ($R\cdot$), such as $\cdot OH$ and $O_2^{\cdot-}$, can remove hydrogen from unsaturated fatty acid (I) to yield the fatty acid free radical (II), which reacts with oxygen to produce a fatty acid peroxy radical (III). A cycle is set up in which III can abstract a proton from another molecule of I to yield an unsaturated fatty-acid hydroperoxide and another molecule of II, which can continue the autocatalytic chain reaction of lipid peroxidation. Continued lipid peroxidation destroys membranes, impairing the function of cell organelles (e.g., sarcoplasmic reticulum) and producing the degenerative changes noted on electron microscopic examination of the myocardia. (Adapted from a lipid peroxidation scheme of Slater.[61])

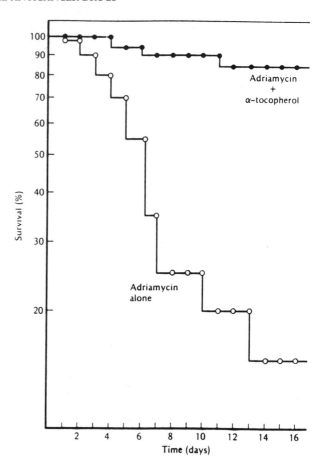

Figure 7–9 Effect of α-tocopherol (vitamin E) on the lethality of doxorubicin. Twenty CDF$_1$ male mice were injected with 15 mg of doxorubicin/kg at time 0. The survival of these mice (O—O) was compared to a matched group of animals who received 85 units of α-tocopherol by intraperitoneal injection 24 hours before receiving 15 mg of doxorubicin/kg (●—●). The difference in survival at 14 days is significant (p < 0.01). (From Myers *et al.*[62])

toxicity focused iron chelators. Early studies showed that razoxane, a piperazine derivative of the metal-chelating agent ethylenediaminetetraacetic acid (EDTA), protected mice against anthracycline toxicity.[66] Later studies extended the observation to a variety of experimental animal models of anthracycline-induced cardiotoxicity.[67] The more soluble (+) enantiomer of razoxane, dexrazoxane (ICRF-187), was shown to yield long-lasting protection against doxorubicin cardiotoxicity[67] without blocking the antitumor effect.[68] Dexrazoxane is hydrolyzed in cells to an opened ring product (Fig. 7–10), which has an EDTA-type of structure and is a strong chelator of iron and copper.[69] Adriamycin forms a very stable complex with iron, but the open-ring hydrolysis product of dexrazoxane removes the iron from the drug quickly and completely,[69] thus reducing oxygen-free-radical generation and cardiotoxicity.

Dexrazoxane is administered by intravenous infusion once weekly for a total of four weeks. The drug has biphasic pharmacokinetics with half-lives of 1 hour and 3.2 hours for the α and β phases, respectively.[70] The apparent volume of distribution in adults is 1.3 L/kg and about 34% of the drug is excreted in the urine in 24 hours.[70] Some of the excreted drug must be the Fe(III)•dexrazoxane complex, because dexrazoxane stimulates the urinary clearance of iron in man by 10-fold.[71] Children have a larger volume of distribution and a more rapid total body clearance than adults,[72] which may in part explain the increased tolerance of children to the drug.

In randomized prospective clinical trial in patients with advanced breast cancer receiving fluorouracil, doxorubicin, and cyclophosphamide, pretreatment with dexrazoxane was shown to protect against cardiotoxicity (incidence 6% with dexrazoxane included in the drug regimen, 47% without).[73,74] In phase I

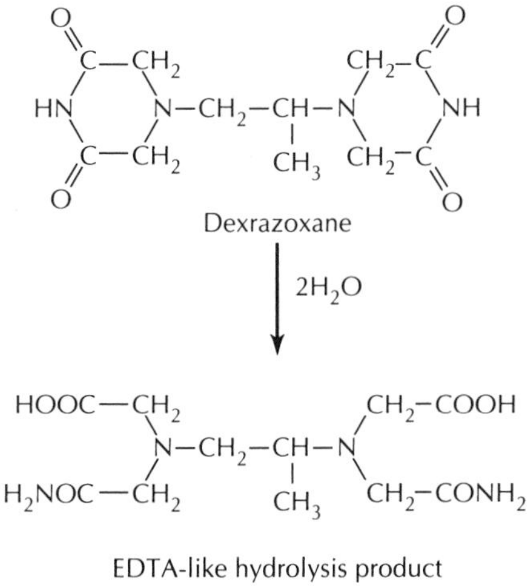

Dexrazoxane

2H₂O

EDTA-like hydrolysis product

Figure 7–10   Dexrazoxane is hydrolyzed in cells to a ring-opened product with an EDTA-like structure that has a high affinity for binding iron.

clinical trials it was found that dexrazoxane produces a dose-limiting myelosuppression in adults who have been heavily pretreated with anticancer drugs.[70] Such patients also experience mild reversible hepatotoxicity manifested by transient SGOT elevation. As might be expected with a drug that promotes the urinary clearance of iron, some patients develop anemia.[70] In general, other adverse effects have been mild.

Mitoxantrone

Mitoxantrone is a member of the anthracenedione class of synthetic antitumor compounds. It lacks the sugar moiety of the anthracycline

Mitoxantrone

drugs but retains the planar polycyclic aromatic ring structure that permits its intercalation into DNA. Importantly, mitoxantrone does not have the ability to produce quinone-type free radicals and thus it does not have the cardiotoxicity of the anthracyclines. Mitoxantrone has been the subject of detailed review.[75]

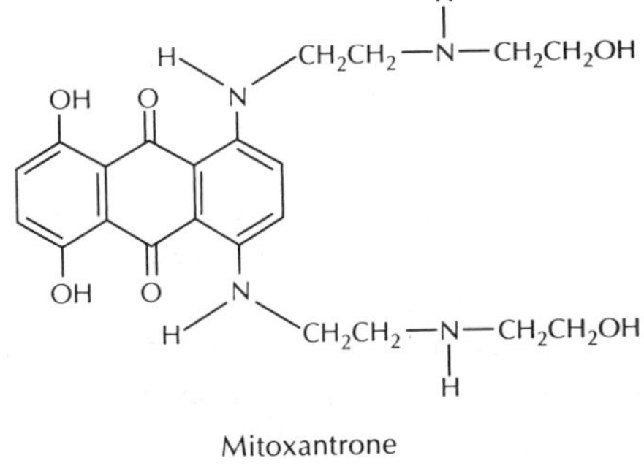

MECHANISM OF ACTION. Mitoxantrone interacts with DNA in two ways: the highest-affinity interaction is by intercalation[76] and the lower-affinity binding represents electrostatic interactions, which may account for the observation that in cells the drug causes compaction of the chromatin structure.[77] The intercalation of the chromaphore seems to occur preferentially at G-C base pairs, with the portion of the molecule containing the side chains lying in the minor groove of the DNA.[78] As discussed for the anthracyclines, intercalation of mitoxantrone into DNA interferes with the strand-reunion reaction of topoisomerase II, resulting in production of protein-linked double-strand DNA breaks. The fact that cells selected for resistance to mitoxantrone have shown cross-resistance to both topoisomerase inhibitors, like etoposide, and other intercalators, like anthracyclines and dactinomycin, in the absence of P-glycoprotein overexpression, strongly supports a central role for intercalation-mediated topoisomerase II inhibition in mitoxantrone cytotoxicity.[79] As with the anthracyclines, mitoxantrone causes some non-protein-linked single-strand breakage[76,77] but this appears to be a minor contribution to the cytotoxicity. In contrast to the anthracyclines, this type of DNA damage is not due to the generation of active species of oxygen, but is apparently due to oxidative activation of mitoxantrone itself, which reacts with DNA.[80]

Although mitoxantrone is cytotoxic to cells throughout the cell cycle, cells in late S phase are more sensitive.[75] Tumor cells selected for resistance to mitoxantrone may show cross-resistance to other natural products. Presumably some of the multidrug resistance reflects amplification of the P-glycoprotein drug efflux transporter; but changes in topoisomerase II and DNA-repair activities contribute to varying degrees to the resistance and in some cell lines there is clearly no P-glycoprotein amplification.[75]

PHARMACOLOGY. Mitoxantrone is administered by intravenous infusion. The plasma disappearance curve is triphasic, with initial α and β distribution phases being followed by a very slow γ elimination phase, which has ranged from 23 to 43 hours, depending on the study.[81,82] Extensive binding of mitoxantrone in the tissues is reflected in a very high volume of distribution, and slow release from this reservoir accounts for a long γ phase of elimination. Only about 10% of a radiolabeled dose of mitoxantrone is recovered in the urine within 5 days,[82] mostly as unchanged drug, but with some in the form of mono- and dicarboxylic acid derivatives which are not cytotoxic.[75] About 20% of a dose of mitoxantrone is excreted in the bile and recovered in stool over 5 days, and the drug has been detected in tissues of patients who died several weeks to several months after receiving their last dose.[75]

USE AND TOXICITY. Mitoxantrone has a much narrower range of clinically useful activity than doxorubicin, being used primarily for the treatment of leukemias and lymphomas,[83,84] as well as advanced breast cancer.

Patients receiving mitoxantrone should be warned that there may be a blue-green coloration of the sclerae and nails as well as the urine. The primary acute adverse effect is nausea and vomiting, which occurs in about 40% of patients and is usually mild to moderate.[84] The major delayed toxicity is myelosuppression, with the leukocyte nadir occurring at 8 to 14 days.[84] Stomatitis and alopecia occur in some patients. The extent of inherent cardiotoxicity of mitoxantrone is difficult to evaluate. The incidence of congestive heart failure has been low (less than 3%) and it has usually occurred in patients who had received prior treatment with doxorubicin. Because mitoxantrone does not induce free-radical formation, does not stimulate lipid peroxidation, and actually inhibits doxorubicin-stimulated lipid peroxidation,[85] any inherent cardiotoxicity must have a different mechanism than that of the anthracyclines.

Dactinomycin (Actinomycin D)

The first actinomycin was isolated from a culture of a *Streptomyces* species in 1940.[86] Sub-

sequently, numerous other actinomycins have been isolated from natural sources or developed by chemical modification. Actinomycin D, the only one used clinically, has the generic name of dactinomycin. The drug has a phenoxazone ring system, to which two identical cyclic poly-

Dactinomycin
(actinomycin D)

peptides are attached. The phenoxazone ring is the chromophore moiety, which imparts a red color to the drug. The synthesis, biological action, and use of this antibiotic have been extensively reviewed.[87,88]

Mechanism of Action of Dactinomycin

INHIBITION OF NUCLEIC ACID SYNTHESIS. At low concentrations, dactinomycin inhibits DNA-directed RNA synthesis;[89] at higher concentrations, DNA synthesis is also inhibited. All types of RNA are affected, with ribosomal RNA formation being more sensitive to drug inhibition. Dactinomycin binds to double-stranded DNA, permitting RNA chain initiation but blocking chain elongation.[90] Its effect is specific for DNA-directed functions. Thus, at concentrations that completely inhibit host-cell RNA synthesis, viral RNA-directed RNA synthesis is unaffected.[89] In contrast, the RNA viruses that replicate by producing a DNA intermediate (e.g., the Rous sarcoma virus) and the

DNA viruses are inhibited by the drug. The cytotoxicity of dactinomycin is primarily a consequence of the drug interaction with DNA.

Early studies of the association of the drug with synthetic DNA duplexes demonstrated that binding depends on the presence of guanine.[91] The tight binding of dactinomycin to DNA has been demonstrated by spectroscopy, by DNA density and melting experiments, and by kinetic studies.[92] It is clear that the phenoxazone chromophore region of the antibiotic intercalates between bases in the DNA[5,92] and that the 2-amino group of guanine is important for the formation of a stable drug–DNA complex.[93] Detailed X-ray crystallography and nuclear magnetic resonance and electron spin resonance studies of drug-nucleotide and drug–DNA complexes have established the following model of the interaction.

DACTINOMYCIN INTERACTION WITH DNA. The spectral changes that accompany the addition of deoxyguanosine to dactinomycin in solution are similar to those that accompany the binding of the drug to DNA,[94] and it is possible to study the nature of the drug–DNA interaction by X-ray diffraction analysis of cocrystallized complexes of dactinomycin and deoxyguanosine.[95] These studies show that dactinomycin is a symmetrical molecule stabilized by two hydrogen bonds between the two valine residues in the cyclic pentapeptide side chains,[95] with the two polypeptide side chains in one axis and the planar chromophore region protruding on an axis almost perpendicular to them (Fig. 7–11A). In the dactinomycin-deoxyguanosine complex (Fig. 7–11B), the phenoxazone ring lies between the two deoxyguanosine molecules. Strong hydrogen bonds connect the 2-amino group of guanine and the carbonyl oxygen of the threonine residues in the polypeptide side chains.[96] Several studies suggest that stacking forces are primarily responsible for the recognition and preferential binding of a guanine base when dactinomycin intercalates into DNA.[92,97]

A   Dactinomycin

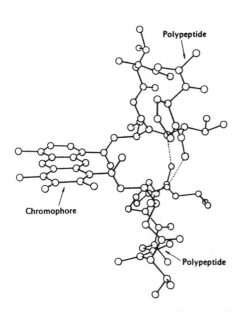

B   Dactinomycin-deoxyguanosine complex

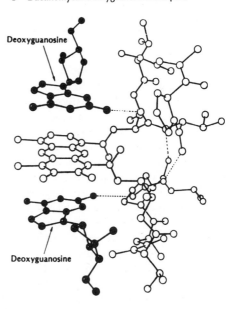

Figure 7–11 The structure of dactinomycin (A) and an illustration of the dactinomycin-deoxyguanosine complex (B). The twofold symmetry of the drug and the stabilizing hydrogen bonds (- - - - -) between the peptide side chains may be noted. In the dactinomycin-deoxyguanosine complex, the two deoxyguanosine molecules (●—●) stack on alternate sides of the chromophore ring. Strong hydrogen bonds (- - - - -) connect the 2-amino group of each guanosine with the carbonyl oxygen of the L-threonine residues in the polypeptide side chain. (Redrawn from Sobell *et al.*[95])

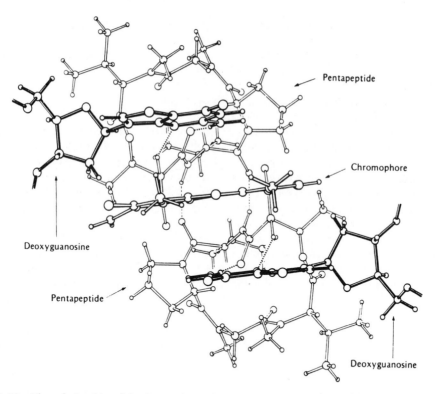

Figure 7–12   The relationship of dactinomycin to doxyguanosine residues as they are oriented in opposite strands of the DNA double helix. Deoxyguanosine moieties are defined by the structures with the solid bonds; the dactinomycin by the structure with the open bonds. The region of dactinomycin defined by the bolder lines is the chromophore ring system protruding toward the observer. (From Sobell and Jain[98])

In Figure 7–12, the dactinomycin-deoxyguanosine complex shown from a different angle demonstrates the spatial relationship between the chromophore ring system and the two guanine residues oriented as they would occur in opposite strands of the DNA double helix.[98] In this model, the chromophore ring is intercalated between two G-C pairs, and the polypeptide units lie in the narrow groove of the DNA helix. This general binding model has been confirmed in studies of the interaction of dactinomycin with synthetic oligonucleotides that assume a double-helix structure.[99,100]

One physical characteristic that distinguishes dactinomycin from its biologically inactive analogs is the very slow rate of DNA–drug dissociation. This tight binding reflects the intermolecular hydrogen bonds shown as dotted lines in Figure 7–12, the planar interactions between the purine rings and the chromophore, and the numerous van der Waals' bonds between the pentapeptide side chains and the DNA backbone. Presumably the tight binding of the drug prevents unwinding of the DNA to facilitate its interaction with RNA polymerase. Given the importance of interactions between RNA polymerase and single-stranded segments of DNA, it is perhaps notable that dactinomycin also binds to single-stranded DNA, where it apparently forms somewhat weaker stacking complexes.[101] In any event, this complex of the drug with the DNA template prevents the synthesis of RNA by DNA-dependent RNA polymerase, and this blockade is responsible for the cytotoxic effect. The exact mechanism of the cytotoxicity is not clear, but in some cells the dactinomycin insult initiates the phenomenon of programmed cell death (apoptosis) that was discussed in Chapter 5.[102] Dactinomycin is cytotoxic to cells in any phase of the cell cycle, and it is probably nearly equally toxic to exponentially growing cells and stationary cells.[103]

DACTINOMYCIN RESISTANCE. Several early studies suggested that dactinomycin resistance was associated with decreased levels of drug in resistant versus sensitive cells.[104,105] Subsequently, it became clear that selection of cells for resistance to dactinomycin could yield cross-resistance to anthracyclines and vinca alkaloids as a result of amplification of the gene for P-glycoprotein[106,107] (see Chapter 4). As diagrammed in Figure 4–4, dactinomycin resistance in these cells can be reversed by competition with verapamil[108] or a variety of other lipophilic compounds.[109] In some multidrug-resistant cell lines there is cross-resistance of dactinomycin with other intercalators and with topoisomerase II inhibitors without amplification of P-glycoprotein expression.[79] This supports the proposal that intercalation-mediated topoisomerase II inhibition with production of protein-linked double-strand DNA breaks may play an important role in dactinomycin cytotoxicity in some cell types.

Pharmacology of Dactinomycin

Dactinomycin is routinely given intravenously. Extravasation is accompanied by a severe local reaction, which can be avoided by injecting the drug into the tubing of a rapidly flowing intravenous infusion. Although dactinomycin is usually given in fractionated doses of 15 μg/kg per day for 5 days, several studies suggest that it can be given as a single 60 μg/kg dose with similar therapeutic efficacy and no increase in toxicity.[110] Most of the information available on the pharmacology of dactinomycin has been obtained from animal studies.[111] Upon intravenous injection in animals, the drug is rapidly removed from the plasma and accumulates in the tissues. The drug does not accumulate in the brain. The tissue half-life of the drug is long, with a mean half-life of 47 hours calculated for various tissues in the dog.[111] Dactinomycin is not metabolized by the rat, dog, or monkey, and it is excreted by both the biliary and the urinary routes.[111] A limited study of the human pharmacology is in essential agreement with the observations made in animals.[112] The drug is not retained in erythrocytes, but it is concentrated in the nucleated cells of the blood. Dactinomycin does not enter the cerebrospinal fluid in humans. In patients, a very small amount of the drug was found to be metabolized to monolactones.[112] Urinary and fecal excretion is prolonged and only about 30% of

a dose of radioactive dactinomycin is recovered in 9 days. The slow phase of the plasma disappearance curve in man has a half-life of about 36 hours.[112]

Use and Toxicity of Dactinomycin

Dactinomycin is used primarily to treat pediatric solid tumors, including Wilms' tumor, Ewing's sarcoma, and embryonal rhabdomyosarcoma, where it may be curative.[113] Dactinomycin is effective in the treatment of methotrexate-resistant gestational choriocarcinoma,[114] and objective responses have been demonstrated in patients with Hodgkin's and non-Hodgkin's lymphomas, metastatic testicular cancer, and Kaposi's sarcoma.[113,115]

The regimen for several solid tumors (e.g., Wilms' tumor, Ewing's sarcoma) may include the combination of radiotherapy and dactinomycin (usually in combination drug therapy). In addition to an improved antitumor effect, accelerated skin and gastrointestinal reactions as well as an increased incidence of late radiation tissue changes in the lung and liver are encountered in patients receiving the combined modality therapy. Dactinomycin apparently potentiates the radiation effect by inhibiting repair of radiation-induced DNA damage.[116] A "recall" effect is observed in some patients who are treated with dactinomycin after X-irradiation.[117] During dactinomycin therapy, a reaction may develop in normal-appearing skin that has been previously irradiated. The response is restricted to the previously irradiated areas, and the severity of the reaction ranges from mild erythema to pronounced desquamation.[117]

Dactinomycin causes nausea, vomiting, and malaise, which begin several hours after treatment and last for as long as 1 day.[113] The major and dose-limiting toxicity is myelosuppression. The leukocyte count and usually the platelet count are depressed, with a low at 8 to 15 days.[113] Ulceration of the oral mucosa and the gastrointestinal tract, with pain and diarrhea, is common, and alopecia and severe acneiform skin lesions occur in some patients. About 1% of patients with Wilm's tumor treated with regimens containing actinomycin D experience hepatomegaly with abnormal liver function tests and severe thrombocytopenia.[118] The syndrome lasts for about 12 days and resolves with supportive therapy. Dactinomycin is immuno-suppressive and it has been used clinically for this purpose. The drug has been shown to be carcinogenic in animals.[119]

Bleomycin

The bleomycins are water-soluble glycopeptide antibiotics isolated from cultures of *Strepto-myces verticillus*. These compounds differ only in their terminal amine moieties. "Bleomycin" refers to the commercial preparation, which is a mixture, the predominant component (ap-proximately 70%) being bleomycin A_2, with the remainder being largely bleomycin B_2. Bleo-

	R
Bleomycin A_2	$NHCH_2CH_2CH_2\overset{+}{S}<^{CH_3}_{CH_3}$
Bleomycin B_2	$NHCH_2CH_2CH_2CH_2NHC\overset{NH}{\underset{NH_2}{\diagdown}}$

mycin is unique among the commercially avail-able antitumor antibiotics in that it produces very little bone-marrow depression. It has been found to be particularly useful in the treatment of testicular carcinoma, squamous cell carci-nomas, and lymphomas. The chemistry and bi-ological effects and mechanism of action of bleomycin have been reviewed in detail.[120,121]

Mechanism of Action of Bleomycin

Bleomycin inhibits prokaryotic and eukaryotic cell proliferation[122] and prevents DNA virus replication.[123] In intact cells, the drug has been found to profoundly inhibit DNA synthesis; RNA and protein synthesis are much less af-fected.[124] In most cell types, bleomycin pro-

duces a block in the early G_2 phase of the cell cycle.[125] Bleomycin causes DNA fragmenta-tion, with predominantly single-strand but also some double-strand breakage occurring.[122,123] Bleomycin-induced DNA damage can be re-paired, and the extent of breakage is correlated with the cytotoxic effect of the drug (assayed by the colony-forming ability of L1210 leuke-mic cells).[126] The ability of bleomycin analogs to damage DNA *in vitro* is in general agree-ment with their cellular cytotoxicity.[125]

Bleomycin has a complex glycopeptide structure[127] with two major domains—a bith-iazole ring moiety that interacts with DNA by intercalalation,[128,129] and a large portion con-taining primary amine, pyrimidine, and imid-azole nitrogens that function as ligands to form a metal coordination site. Both iron and oxy-gen are required for the degradation of DNA by bleomycin.[130,131] When Fe^{2+}, bleomycin, O_2, and DNA are mixed, an activated complex containing dioxygen and two molecules of DNA-bound Fe•bleomycin is formed.[132] The DNA-bound, activated complex of O_2^{2-}–Fe(III)bleomycin generates active oxygen spe-cies, such as superoxide and hydroxyl radicals, that cause DNA-strand breakage.[121]

In the overall reaction bleomycin essentially acts as a ferrous oxidase, catalyzing the oxida-tion of Fe(II) to Fe(III) and the reduction of ox-ygen.[133] Fe(II) bleomycin can be regenerated from Fe(III) bleomycin by an NADH-depen-dent enzyme system in the nucleus, and this redox recycling of the iron-coordinated drug is accompanied by increased DNA damage.[134] Similar redox cycling can be effected by thiols, such as cysteine or glutathione. Such redox cy-cling may be important in the intact cell be-cause very little drug enters tumor cells and it may be the oxidized form, Fe(III)bleomycin, that first binds to DNA in cells.[121]

DNA cleavage is not random. Strand cleav-age preferentially occurs between the bases of 5'-purine-pyrimidine-3' sequences, with GC and GT sequences preferred.[135] Interestingly, the metal-binding domain (rather than the bith-iazole ring moiety that intercalates into the DNA) may be the primary determinant of se-quence specificity of DNA cleavage.[136] The base on the 5' side of the intercalation site may exert some influence on sequence specificity as well.[121] Single-strand cleavage of DNA results in formation of free nucleic bases and free base propenals (Base$-$CH$=$CH$-$CHO). This is consistent with a reaction mechanism initiated by free radical abstraction of the C-4 proton of deoxyribose leading to oxidative cleavage of the (C-3')$-$(C-4') bond.[137] The reader is referred to a review by Stubble and Kozarich[138] for details of the organic chemistry involved in DNA breakage. The base propenals are themselves reactive species, and it is possible they contribute to both the antitumor and toxic effects of bleomycin.[139]

The mechanisms by which initially susceptible human tumors become resistant to bleomycin have not been defined. From studies on animal cells, several mechanisms may be considered, including increased bleomycin inactivating activity,[140] altered levels of glutathione or glutathione S-transferase,[141] decreased drug entry,[142] possibly increased outward transport of the drug,[106] and, at least theoretically, increased DNA repair.[143]

Pharmacology of Bleomycin

Bleomycin can be given by a number of parenteral routes but is most commonly injected intravenously or intramuscularly. The volume of distribution of bleomycin is 17.5 L/m^2 or 0.35 L/kg.[144,145] After intravenous bolus administration, the plasma decay curve is biphasic, with a half-life for the β phase of 2 to 4 hours.[144,145] Peak serum levels are attained 1 to 2 hours after intramuscular injection and the half-life is 2.5 hours.[146] Bleomycin is administered by intracavitary injection for treating malignant effusions of lung, breast, and ovarian carcinoma and pharmacokinetic data for the intrapleural and intraperitoneal routes of administration are available.[147,148]

Half to two-thirds of a dose of bleomycin is excreted in the urine within 24 hours.[144] Elimination is predominantly by glomerular filtration, and in patients with a creatinine clearance of less than 35 ml/minute the elimination

half-life increases exponentially,[149] with consequent increased risk of developing pulmonary toxicity.[150]

The cellular pharmacology of bleomycin is particularly important with regard to understanding the toxic effects of the drug. Because very little bleomycin is taken up by cultured human cells and the interaction with DNA is reversible,[151] the drug-inactivating activity of cells can have a profound effect on drug toxicity. When the distribution of biologically active drug was determined by a microbiological assay, very low levels were found in all tissues except skin and lung.[152] This is very important, since these two organs are very susceptible to bleomycin toxicity. Assay of bleomycin-inactivating activity in extracts of a number of different mouse tissues revealed high levels of inactivating activity in liver, intestine, testis, spleen, and plasma and somewhat lower levels in lung and brain; the skin had almost no inactivating activity. Subsequent analysis of bleomycin-inactivating activity using a specific chemical assay showed a correlation between low levels of activity in extracts of lung tissue and susceptibility to bleomycin-induced pulmonary toxicity.[155]

The bleomycin-inactivating enzyme, which has been purified from several sources,[156,157] acts like an aminopeptidase to convert the β-aminoalanine moiety in bleomycin to the corresponding desamidobleomycin.[158] This changes the pKa of the α amino group of the β aminoalanine moiety, and it is thought that at physiological pH the free carboxylic acid of the aminoalanine moiety rather than the protonated α amino group occupies the fifth coordination site of the iron. This would result in a marked decrease in formation of the activated terniary iron-oxygen-bleomycin complex, with a resulting decrease in free radical generation.[159] The deaminated bleomycin is considerably less potent than the parent compound at causing DNA fragmentation and inhibiting tumor growth.[160] Also, the metabolite has much less pulmonary toxicity than the parent drug.[155]

A number of early studies suggested that this bleomycin hydrolase activity may be a major determinant of tumor responsiveness. For example, Umezawa and colleagues[152] found a correlation between the level of drug-inactivating activity and the therapeutic response of different types of methylcholanthrene-induced mouse tumors. When mouse skin is painted with 20-methylcholanthrene, squamous cell carcinomas are produced that are responsive to bleomycin therapy. After subcutaneous injection of the carcinogen, however, skin sarcomas are produced that are not responsive to treatment with bleomycin. After injection of bleomycin in tumor-bearing mice, most of the drug recovered in carcinomas was found to be biologically active, whereas most of the drug in sarcomas was inactive.[152] Other studies, however, have not found a correlation between bleomycin hydrolase activity and the responsiveness of human tumor cells in culture to bleomycin treatment.[161] It seems fair to conclude that bleomycin hydrolase activity contributes to the unique toxicity spectrum of bleomycin but that other factors contribute to intrinsic tumor responsiveness to the drug.

Use and Toxicity of Bleomycin

Bleomycin is used in combination protocols to treat squamous-cell carcinomas of the head and neck, the skin and the genitalia (including the cervix and vulvo-vaginal area),[162] and also has activity against Hodgkin's and non-Hodgkin's lymphomas. The principal curative use is in the treatment of testicular carcinomas, where the overall response rate is about 30% with bleomycin alone and 90% with bleomycin plus vinblastine.[162] With the triple-drug regimen of bleomycin, vinblastine (or etoposide), and cisplatin the initial response rate for testicular cancer is nearly 100%, with the majority of patients being cured (see Table 1–6).[163,164]

Bleomycin has a unique spectrum of toxicities compared with most anticancer drugs. The drug rarely causes myelosuppression;[162,165] therefore, it is a particularly useful compound to include in drug-combination protocols. In the usual dose regimens, the gastrointestinal tract, liver, kidneys, and central nervous system are not affected[165] (damage to the liver and kidney is unusual, although it has been reported). The drug is not immunosuppressive in man.[166] Despite these advantages, bleomycin is quite toxic. As shown in Table 7–3, the most common toxic effects involve the skin and mucous membranes.[167] Oral mucositis is dose related and common in the more aggressive regimens. Alopecia occurs in 10% to 20% of patients. Some patients experience Raynaud's phenomenon. Toxic reactions in the skin include hyperpigmentation, edema, and erythema of the hands and feet, thickening of the nail beds, and hyperkeratosis.[162] Hyperpigmentation may occur over the elbows, knees, and the small joints of the hands, or as linear streaks on the trunk.[168] Sclerotic changes may also be seen in the skin of the hands and fingers. These cutaneous effects are reversible on discontinuation of the drug.[168] It is not surprising that bleomycin is toxic to the skin. As noted in the preceding section, this tissue has almost no ability to inactivate bleomycin,[152] and the highest levels of biologically active drug are found in the skin and the lungs.[153]

The most severe, dose-limiting bleomycin toxicity is pulmonary. Clinically, the syndrome presents with dyspnea, tachypnea, and a nonproductive cough. Fine rales may be heard at the base of the lungs and radiography may show patchy basilar infiltrates and, in some cases, a diffuse interstitial pattern of fibrosis.[162] The pathological picture is that of interstitial edema and fibrosis, with alveolar squamous metaplasia and hyalinization.[165,169] The overall incidence of pulmonary toxicity is about 10%, with fatalities occurring in about 1% of

Table 7–3   Approximate Incidence of Untoward Effects of Bleomycin. (Modified from Gottlieb[167])

Untoward Effect	Incidence (%)
Skin toxicity	44
Fever and chills	31
Nausea and vomiting	26
Stomatitis	16
Alopecia	11
Pulmonary toxicity	10
Fatal pulmonary toxicity	1
Anaphylactoid reactions	<1

patients with this dose-related syndrome. Although the incidence is relatively constant at lower doses, there is a marked rise above a total dosage of 400 units, and in the unusual case in which more than 400 units of bleomycin are given, extreme caution must be used. Patients over 70 years of age are much more prone to pulmonary toxicity than younger patients are.[163]

Pulmonary toxicity occurs more commonly in patients with compromised renal function,[150] and when the drug is used with cisplatin, which itself is nephrotoxic, the risk of pulmonary toxicity is increased.[170,171] Prior radiotherapy to the chest predisposes to the development of pulmonary toxicity.[172,173] At the cellular level, bleomycin and X-irradiation cause similar damage, but the DNA lesions appear to be produced and repaired independently,[174] and their effects on cell survival are generally additive.[175] The risk of pulmonary toxicity is also potentiated in patients who are exposed to elevated but nontoxic concentrations of oxygen.[176] Although it is still somewhat controversial,[170] pulmonary function testing (including carbon monoxide diffusion capacity) has not been particularly helpful in predicting the toxicity,[177] and patients should be monitored by respiratory symptoms (cough, dyspnea), physical examination, and periodic chest X ray. Obviously, extreme caution should be employed in patients with preexisting pulmonary disease.

The pathogenesis of the pulmonary toxicity has been reviewed by Lazo and colleagues.[178] Initially, there is damage to the pulmonary capillary bed with edema and infiltration of neutrophils, macrophages, and lymphocytes. Within 1 to 2 weeks, there is proliferation of both type II endothelial cells and fibroblasts, and within 4 weeks, the alveolar walls begin to thicken and there is increased production of extracellular matrix. The initial changes may be reversible, but the last stage of interstitial pulmonary fibrosis is not. The fibrosis is a late response common to a variety of lung injuries, including toxicity by other anticancer drugs (e.g., cyclophosphamide, nitrosoureas). As mentioned above, the pulmonary toxicity of bleomycin is thought to reflect the low levels of bleomycin hydrolase activity found in lung tissue.[155,179]

Most of the other toxic effects of bleomycin are acute in nature (Table 7–3). Nausea, vomiting, and anorexia occasionally occur, most commonly during the initial injections, and are often self-limited and mild.[162] Diarrhea is rare. Drug-induced chills and fever occur in about 30% of patients, most commonly during the first few hours following bleomycin administration.[162] For unknown reasons, many lymphoma patients experience fever with the initial doses.[180] Bleomycin is also hyperpyrexic in rabbits, and during the fever peak, a circulating pyrogen that can be transferred to other rabbits is present.[181] When rabbit or human leukocytes are incubated with bleomycin, a rapid-acting pyrogen is produced. The pyrogen does not show cross-tolerance with endotoxin, and it has been suggested that the drug causes fever by liberating an endogenous pyrogen from the host cells.[181] Other possible causes, such as contaminants or trace metabolites, have not been ruled out.

A few bleomycin-treated patients develop an acute fulminating reaction, with high fever, hypotension, varying degrees of respiratory distress, and, in some cases, sustained cardiorespiratory collapse.[162,182] The overall incidence of this reaction is under 1%, but most cases have involved lymphoma patients and the incidence in this group is 1–6%.[183] Its mechanism is not known. Several features are not consistent with classic anaphylaxis, so it has been called an anaphylactoid response.[183] The reaction may occur immediately or several hours after treatment with bleomycin. Because of the possibility of anaphylactoid reaction, some experts advise that lymphoma patients be given a test dose of 1 unit of drug 24 hours prior to initiating the regular dosage schedule.

Plicamycin (Mithramycin)

Plicamycin is an antibiotic derived from *Streptomyces plicatus*. Although plicamycin is the proper generic name, the drug is more generally recognized by its common name mithramycin, which will be the one used here. Mithramycin is similar in structure and mechanism of action to chromomycin and olivomycin, but it is the only one of the chromomycin antibiotic group used clinically in the United States. Its use now is limited largely to the treatment

Mithramycin

DNA to thermal denaturation and failure to remove supercoils from closed circular duplex DNA.[5] Mithramycin is thought to bind tightly in the minor groove of the DNA[192,193] as a drug dimer.[193,194] Binding of the drug is accompanied by widening of the minor groove and structural alterations in the DNA that are propagated beyond the drug-binding site itself.[195] The presence of the drug and the accompanying distortion of DNA structure prevents binding of transcriptional activating proteins to DNA, thus blocking transcriptional initiation.[196,197]

Cells selected for multidrug resistance have shown cross-resistance with mithramycin, which suggests that the drug is carried by the P-glycoprotein multidrug transporter.[198]

of hypercalcemia associated with malignancy. The chromomycin antibiotics have been reviewed by Slavik and Carter.[184]

Mechanism of Action of Mithramycin

Mithramycin inhibits nucleic acid synthesis in intact cells, with RNA synthesis being more severely affected than DNA synthesis.[185,186] It reversibly inhibits DNA virus replication in tissue culture but not RNA virus replication.[187] This is probably due to the fact that synthesis of RNA by purified RNA polymerase is inhibited only when the template is a DNA preparation containing guanine.[188] The drug binds reversibly to DNA as an antibiotic-Mg^{2+} complex.[188,189] Studies with an analog, chromomycin, show that the number of drug-binding sites depends on the source of DNA, increasing with increasing guanine content.[190] Binding of the chromomycin antibiotics, like the binding of dactinomycin discussed earlier, appears to require the 2-amino group of guanine, since the template function of poly dI–poly dC is not affected.[188] Indeed, mithramycin can displace dactinomycin from its strong binding site on DNA.[191] The drug binds with highest affinity to GpG, especially when this base duplex is located within a GC-rich environment.[192] Although the data are somewhat controversial, mithramycin apparently does not intercalate between base pairs. This is inferred from several observations, including failure to stabilize

Pharmacology of Mithramycin

Very little is known about the pharmacology of mithramycin. A study of the distribution of tritium-labeled drug after intraperitoneal injection in mice showed the greatest concentration of isotope in the liver and the kidney, particularly the Kupffer cells in the liver and the cells of the renal tubules.[199] Concentrations of the drug in the brain were low, but levels in the cerebrospinal fluid equaled those in the blood at 4 hours postinjection. The drug was largely cleared from the blood of mice in the first 2 hours. Excretion was rapid, with 67% of the measured excretion (urine and feces) occurring in the first 4 hours after injection and total recovery of isotope ranging from 41% to 57% of the dose.[199] The nature of any metabolism is not known. The only human pharmacological data were obtained from a patient with glioblastoma who was injected intravenously with tritium-labeled mithramycin.[200] In this patient, the level of radioactivity in the blood fell by 85% in 3 hours, with 27% of the total radioactivity accounted for in the urine during the first 2 hours. In this patient, radioactivity was found in the intratumoral cyst fluid at a concentration about twice that in the blood and cerebrospinal fluid at 4 hours after the intravenous injection.[200] Mithramycin is inactive by the oral route and is routinely administered by slow intravenous infusion. The drug is usually infused over a period of 4 to 6 hours to reduce the severity of the gastrointestinal side effects.

Phlebitis can occur on administration, as can local tissue irritation when extravasation occurs.

Use and Toxicity of Mithramycin

Because of its toxicity and limited clinical spectrum, mithramycin is used only rarely in cancer chemotherapy. It was originally used to treat metastatic testicular tumors, the best responses being obtained in patients with embryonal cell carcinoma.[201,202] Mithramycin is now used only to treat patients with testicular tumors that have become resistant to other forms of therapy. Interestingly, mithramycin has been reported to reverse the myeloid blast crisis in patients with chronic granulocytic leukemia,[203] and it is used in combination therapy for this purpose. Mithramycin is used at lower doses to treat the hypercalcemia associated with advanced malignancy. Mithramycin was found to lower serum calcium values in patients with hypercalcemia secondary to neoplastic osteolysis, as well as in patients with hypercalcemia of non-neoplastic origin and in normocalcemic subjects.[204,205] The effect varies somewhat from patient to patient, and lasts only a few days. Mithramycin acts by preventing osteoclastic bone resorption.[206,207]

Mithramycin is very toxic, and nausea and vomiting commonly accompany its administration. Diarrhea and stomatitis, skin rashes, and fever occur occasionally. A number of central nervous system symptoms, including irritability, weakness, lethargy, and headache, have been observed;[208] severe facial flushing occurs in 3% of patients. There is a high incidence of hepatotoxicity manifested by elevated liver enzyme activities, and appreciable renal toxicity with increased blood urea nitrogen and serum creatinine levels.[201] Electrolyte abnormalities, including hypocalcemia, hypophosphatemia, and hypokalemia, occur. Leukopenia is not often a major problem, but thrombocytopenia occurs and may be severe. The most important toxicity of mithramycin is a hemorrhagic diathesis that presents with epistaxis or ecchymoses and progresses to generalized bleeding. Deaths have resulted from uncontrolled gastrointestinal hemorrhage. The incidence depends upon drug dosage, being 5.4% for patients receiving 10 to 30 μg/kg daily for four to ten doses.[208] Hemorrhage apparently is the result of a number of effects, including thrombocytopenia, platelet dysfunction,[209,210] increased prothrombin time and fibrinolytic activity, and depression of clotting factors II, V, VII, and X.[211]

The severe toxicity of mithramycin has limited its clinical usefulness in cancer chemotherapy, and a number of drug-related deaths have occurred. Toxicity is reduced by administering the drug every other day. Much less toxicity is observed at the lower dosage employed for the treatment of hypercalcemia. Mithramycin may be contraindicated in patients with preexisting thrombocytopenia or hemorrhagic tendencies. Platelet counts, prothrombin times, and bleeding times should be obtained frequently, and liver and renal function should be rigorously monitored during therapy.

REFERENCES

1. Symposium: Proceedings of the fifth new drug seminar on adriamycin (Washington, D.C., Dec. 16–17, 1974) and the adriamycin new drug seminar (San Francisco, Jan. 15–16, 1975). *Cancer Chemother. Rep.* (Part 3) 6:83–419 (1975).

2. J. W. Lowan (ed.) *Anthracycline and Anthracenedione-based Anticancer Agents*. Amsterdam: Elsevier, 1988, 753 pp.

3. C. E. Myers, and B. A. Chabner: "Anthracyclines," in *Cancer Chemotherapy: Principles & Practice*, ed. by B. A. Chabner and J. M. Collins. Philadelphia: J.B. Lippincott Co., 1990, pp. 356–381.

4. C. C. Lin and J. H. van de Sande: Differential fluorescent staining of human chromosomes with daunomycin and adriamycin—the D-bands. *Science* 190:61 (1975).

5. M. Waring: Variation of the supercoils in closed circular DNA by binding of antibiotics and drugs: Evidence for molecular models involving intercalation. *J. Mol. Biol.* 54:247 (1970).

6. A. H. J. Wang, G. Ughetto, G. J. Quigley, and A. Rich: Interactions between an anthracycline antibiotic and DNA: Molecular structure of daunomycin complexed to d(CpGpTpApCpG) at 1.2-Å resolution. *Biochemistry* 26:1152 (1987).

7. G. Ughetto: "X-Ray diffraction analysis of anthracycline-oligonucleotide complexes," in *Anthracycline and Anthracenedione-Based Anticancer Agents,* ed. by J. W. Lown. Amsterdam: Elsevier, 1988, pp. 295–333.

8. R. L. Momparler, M. Karon, S. E. Siegel, and F. Avila: Effect of adriamycin on DNA, RNA and protein synthesis in cell-free systems and intact cells. *Cancer Res.* 36:2891 (1976).

9. N. S. Mizuno, B. Zakis, and R. W. Decker: Binding of daunomycin to DNA and the inhibition of RNA and DNA synthesis. *Cancer Res.* 35:1542 (1975).

10. C. E. Myers, E. G. Mimnaugh, G. C. Yeh, and B. K. Sinha: "Biochemical mechanisms of tumor cell kill by the anthracyclines," in *Anthracycline and Anthracene-dione-Based Anticancer Agents*, ed. by J. W. Lown. Amsterdam: Elsevier, 1988, pp. 527–569.

11. E. M. Nelson, K. M. Tewey, and L. F. Liu: Mechanism of antitumor drug action: Poisoning of mammalian DNA topoisomerase II on DNA by 4'-(9-acridinylamino)-methanesulfon-*m*-anisidide. *Proc. Natl. Acad. Sci. USA* 81:1361 (1984).

12. K. M. Tewey, G. L. Chen, E. M. Nelson, and L. F. Liu: Intercalative antitumor drugs interfere with the breakage-reunion reaction of mammalian DNA topoisomerase II. *J. Biol. Chem.* 259:9182 (1984).

13. B. Glisson, R. Gupta, P. Hodges, and W. Ross: Cross-resistance to intercalating agents in an epipodophyllotoxin-resistant Chinese hamster ovary cell line: Evidence for a common intracellular target. *Cancer Res.* 46:1939 (1986).

14. Y. Pommier, D. Kerrigan, R. E. Schwartz, J. A. Swack, and A. McCurdy: Altered DNA topoisomerase II activity in Chinese hamster cells resistant to topoisomerase II inhibitors. *Cancer Res.* 46:3075 (1986).

15. A. M. Deffie, J. K. Batra, and G. J. Goldenberg: Direct correlation between DNA topoisomerase II activity and cytotoxicity in adriamycin-sensitive and resistant P388 leukemia cell lines. *Cancer Res.* 49:58 (1989).

16. C. Myers, L. Gianni, J. Zweier, J. Muindi, B. K. Sinha, and H. Eliot: Role of iron in adriamycin biochemistry. *Fed. Proc.* 45:2792 (1986).

17. H. Eliot, L. Gianni, and C. Myers: Oxidative destruction of DNA by the adriamycin-iron complex. *Biochemistry* 23:928 (1984).

18. J. Muindi, B. K. Sinha, L. Gianni, and C. Myers: Thiol-dependent DNA damage produced by anthracycline-iron complexes: The structure-activity relationships and molecular mechanisms. *Mol. Pharmacol.* 27:356 (1985).

19. J. H. Doroshow: Role of hydrogen peroxide and hydroxyl radical formation in the killing of Ehrlich tumor cells by anticancer quinones. *Proc. Natl. Acad. Sci. USA* 83:4514 (1986).

20. B. K. Sinha, E. G. Mimnaugh, S. Rajagopakin, and C. E. Myers: Adriamycin activation and oxygen free radical formation in human breast tumor cells: Protective role of glutathione peroxidase in adriamycin resistance. *Cancer Res.* 49:3844 (1989).

21. A. Krishan and E. Frei III: Effect of adriamycin on the cell cycle traverse and kinetics of cultured human lymphoblasts. *Cancer Res.* 36:143 (1976).

22. K. D. Tew and M. L. Clapper: "Glutathione S-transferase and anticancer drug resistance," in *Mechanisms of Drug Resistance in Neoplastic Cells*, ed. by P. W. Woolley and K. D. Tew. New York: Academic Press, 1988, pp. 141–159.

23. G. Batist, A. Tulpule, B. K. Sinha, A. G. Katki, C. E. Myers, and K. H. Cowan: Overexpression of a novel anionic glutathione transferase in multidrug-resistant human breast cancer cells. *J. Biol. Chem.* 261:15544 (1986).

24. R. A. Kramer, J. Zakher, and G. Kim: Role of the glutathione redox cycle in acquired and de novo multidrug resistance. *Science* 241:694 (1988).

25. N. R. Bachur: "Biochemical pharmacology of the anthracycline antibiotics," in *Cancer Chemotherapy*, ed. by A. C. Sartorelli. Am. Chem. Soc. Symposium Series: Washington D.C., 1976, pp. 58–70.

26. S. Takanashi and N. R. Bachur: Adriamycin metabolism in man. Evidence from urinary metabolites. *Drug Metab. Disp.* 4:79 (1976).

27. S. Takanashi and N. R. Bachur: Daunorubicin metabolites in human urine. *J. Pharmacol. Exptl. Ther.* 195:41 (1975).

28. R. S. Benjamin, C. E. Riggs, and N. R. Bachur: Plasma pharmacokinetics of adriamycin and its metabolites in humans with normal hepatic and renal function. *Cancer Res.* 37:1416 (1977).

29. P. Gill, R. Favre, A. Durand, A. Iliadis, J. P. Cano, and Y. Carcassone: Time dependency of adriamycin and adriamycinol kinetics. *Cancer Chemother. Pharmacol.* 10:120 (1983).

30. R. F. Ozols, J. K. V. Willson, M. D. Weltz, K. R. Grotzinger, C. E. Myers, and R. C. Young: Inhibition of human ovarian cancer colony formation by adriamycin and its major metabolites. *Cancer Res.* 40:4109 (1980).

31. R. F. Greene, J. M. Collins, J. F. Jenkins, J. L. Speyer, and C. E. Myers: Plasma pharmacokinetics of adriamycin and adriamycinol: Implications for the design of *in vitro* experiments and treatment protocols. *Cancer Res.* 43:3417 (1983).

32. P. A. J. Speth, Q. G. C. M. van Hoesel, and C. Haanen: Clinical pharmacokinetics of doxorubicin. *Clin. Pharmacokin.* 15:15 (1988).

33. H. C. Gillies, D. Herriott, R. Liang, K. Ohashi, H. J. Rogers, and P. G. Harper: Pharmacokinetics of idarubicin (4-demethoxydaunorubicin; IMI-30; NSC 256439) following intravenous and oral administration in patients with advanced cancer. *Br. J. Clin. Pharmacol.* 23:303 (1987).

34. P. Dodion, C. Sanders, W. Rombaut, M. A. Mattelaer, M. Rozencweig, P. Stryckmans, and Y. Kenis: Effect of daunorubicin, carminomycin, idarubicin and 4-demethoxydaunorubicinol against human normal myeloid stem cells and human malignant cells *in vitro*. *Eur. J. Cancer Clin. Oncol.* 23:1909 (1987).

35. P. A. Speth, H. Minderman, and C. Haanen: Idarubicin *v* daunorubicin: Preclinical and clinical pharmacokinetic studies. *Semin. Oncol.* 16 (*Suppl.* 2):2 (1989).

36. M. A. LeBot, J. M. Begue, D. Kernaleguen, J. Robert, D. Ratanasavanh, J. Airiau, C. Riche, and A. Guillouzo: Different cytotoxicity and metabolism of doxorubicin, daunorubicin, epirubicin, esorubicin and idarubicin in cultured human and rat hepatocytes. *Biochem. Pharmacol.* 37:3877 (1988).

37. C. E. Riggs, R. S. Benjamin, A. A. Serpick, and N. R. Bachur: Biliary disposition of adriamycin. *Clin. Pharmacol. Ther.* 22:234 (1977).

38. K. K. Chan, R. T. Chlebowski, M. Tong, H. S. G. Chen, J. F. Gross and J. R. Bateman: Clinical pharmacokinetics of adriamycin in hepatoma patients with cirrhosis. *Cancer Res.* 40:1263 (1980).

39. D. E. Brenner, P. H. Wiernik, M. Wesley and N. R. Bachur: Acute doxorubicin toxicity: Relationship to

pretreatment liver function, response and pharmacokinetics in patients with acute normocytic leukemia. *Cancer* 53:1042 (1984).

40. S. K. Carter: Adriamycin—a review. *J. Natl. Cancer Inst.* 55:1265 (1975).

41. P. Wiernik (ed.): Idarubicin: A New Presence in Leukemias. *Semin. Oncol.* 16 (Suppl. 2):36 pp. (1989).

42. E. Berman, G. Heller, J. Santorso, S. McKenzie, et al.: Results of a randomized trial comparing idarubicin and cytosine arabinoside with daunorubicin and cytosine arabinoside in adult patients with newly diagnosed acute myelogenous leukemia. *Blood* 77:1666 (1991).

43. R. Rudolph, R. S. Stein and R. A. Pattillo: Skin ulcers due to adriamycin. *Cancer* 38:1087 (1976).

44. R. M. O'Bryan, L. H. Baker, J. E. Gottlieb, S. E. Rivkin, S. P. Balcerzak, G. N. Grummet, S. E. Salmon, T. E. Moon, and B. Hoogstraten: Dose response evaluation of adriamycin in human neoplasia. *Cancer* 39:1940 (1977).

45. J. R. Cassady, M. P. Richter, A. J. Piro, and N. Jaffe: Radiation-adriamycin interactions: Preliminary clinical observations. *Cancer* 36:946 (1975).

46. F. A. Greco, H. D. Brereton, H. Kent, H. Zimbler, J. Merrill, and R. E. Johnson: Adriamycin and enhanced radiation reaction in normal esophagus and skin. *Ann. Int. Med.* 85:294 (1976).

47. A. Vecchi, A. Mantovani, A. Tagliabue, and F. Spreafico: A characterization of the immunosuppressive activity of adriamycin and daunomycin on humoral antibody production and tumor allograft rejection. *Cancer Res.* 36:1222 (1976).

48. H. Marquardt, F. S. Philips, and S. Sternberg: Tumorigenicity *in vivo* and induction of malignant transformation and mutagenesis in cell cultures by adriamycin and daunomycin. *Cancer Res.* 36:2065 (1976).

49. L. Lenaz and J. A. Page: Cardiotoxicity of adriamycin and related anthracyclines. *Cancer Treatment Rev.* 3:111 (1976).

50. A. C. Gilladoga, C. Manuel, C. T. C. Tan, N. Wollner, S. S. Sternberg, and M. L. Murphy: The cardiotoxicity of adriamycin and daunomycin in children. *Cancer* 37:1072 (1976).

51. R. A. Minow, R. S. Benjamin, and J. A. Gottlieb: Adriamycin (NSC-123127) cardiomyopathy—an overview with determination of risk factors. *Cancer Chemother. Rep.* (Part 3) 6:195 (1975).

52. A. M. Goorin, A. R. Chauvenet, A. R. Perez-Atayde, J. Cruz, R. McKone, and S. E. Lipshultz: Initial congestive heart failure, six to ten years after doxorubicin chemotherapy for childhood cancer. *J. Pediat.* 116:144 (1990).

53. S. E. Lipshultz, S. D. Colan, R. D. Gelber, A. R. Perez-Atayde, S. E. Sallan, and S. P. Sanders: Late cardiac effects of doxorubicin therapy for acute lymphoblastic leukemia in childhood. *New Engl. J. Med.* 324:808 (1991).

54. S. T. Yeung, C. Yoong, J. Spink, A. Galbraith, and P. J. Smith: Functional myocardial impairment in children treated with anthracyclines for cancer. *Lancet* 337:816 (1991).

55. R. H. Blum and S. K. Carter: Adriamycin. A new antitumor drug with significant clinical activity. *Ann. Int. Med.* 80:249 (1974).

56. R. A. Minow, R. S. Benjamin, E. T. Lee, and J. A. Gottlieb: Adriamycin cardiomyopathy—risk factors. *Cancer* 39:1397 (1977).

57. E. A. Lefrak, J. Pitha, S. Rosenheim, and J. A. Gottlieb: A clinicopathologic analysis of adriamycin cardiotoxicity. *Cancer* 32:302 (1973).

58. J. H. Doroshow: "Role of reactive oxygen production in doxorubicin cardiac toxicity," in *Organ Directed Toxicities of Anticancer Drugs,* ed. by M. P. Hacker, J. S. Lazo, and T. R. Tritton. Boston: Martinus Nijhoff Pub., 1988, pp. 31–40.

59. C. E. Myers, L. Gianni, C. B. Simone, R. Klecker, and R. Greene: Oxidative destruction of erythrocyte ghost membranes catalyzed by the doxorubicin-iron complex. *Biochemistry* 21:1707 (1982).

60. J. H. Doroshow, G. Y. Locker, and C. E. Myers: Enzymatic defenses of the mouse heart against reactive oxygen metabolites. *J. Clin. Invest.* 65:128 (1980).

61. T. F. Slater: *Free Radical Mechanisms in Tissue Injury.* London: Pion Ltd., 1972, p. 30.

62. C. E. Myers, W. M. McGuire, and R. Young: Adriamycin: Amelioration of toxicity by α-tocopherol. *Cancer Treat. Rep.* 60:961 (1976).

63. C. E. Myers, W. P. McGuire, R. H. Liss, I. Ifrim, K. Grotzinger, and R. C. Young: Adriamycin: The role of lipid peroxidation in cardiac toxicity and tumor response. *Science* 197:165 (1977).

64. C. Myers, R. Bonow, S. Palmeri, J. Jenkins, B. Corden, G. Locker, J. Dorashow, and S. Epstein: A randomized controlled trial assessing the prevention of doxorubicin cardiomyopathy by N-acetylcysteine. *Semin. Oncol.* 10 (Suppl. 1):53 (1983).

65. J. H. Doroshow: Effect of anthracycline antibiotics on oxygen radical formation in rat heart. *Cancer Res.* 43:4543 (1983).

66. E. H. Herman, R. Mhatre, and D. Chadwick: Modification of some of the toxic effects of daunomycin (NSC-82151) by pretreatment with the antineoplastic agent ICRF-159 (NSC-129943). *Toxicol. Appl. Pharmacol.* 27:517 (1974).

67. E. H. Herman, D. T. Witiak, K. Hellman, and V. S. Waravdekar: Biological properties of ICRF-159 and related bis(dioxopiperazine) compounds. *Adv. Pharmacol. Chemother.* 19:249 (1982).

68. S. Wadler, M. D. Green, and F. M. Muggia: Synergistic activity of doxorubicin and the bisdioxopiperazine (+)-1,2-bis(3,5-dioxopiperazinyl-1-yl)propane (ICRF-187) against the murine sarcoma S180 cell line. *Cancer Res.* 46:1176 (1986).

69. B. B. Hasinoff: The interaction of the cardioprotective agent ICRF-187 ((+)-1,2-bis(3,5-dioxopiperazinyl-1-yl)propane); its hydrolysis product (ICRF-198); and other chelating agents with the Fe(III) and Cu(II) complexes of adriamycin. *Agents Actions* 26:378 (1989).

70. C. L. Vogel, E. Gorowski, E. Davila, M. Eisenberger, J. Kosinski, R. P. Agarwal, and N. Savaraj: Phase I clinical trial and pharmacokinetics of weekly ICRF-187 (NSC 169780) infusion in patients with solid tumors. *Invest. New Drugs* 5:187 (1987).

71. J. Koning, P. Palmer, C. R. Franks, D. E. Mulder, J. L. Speyer, M. D. Green, and K. Hellmann: Cardioxane—ICRF-187: Towards anticancer drug specificity through selective toxicity reduction. *Cancer Treat. Rev.* 18:1 (1991).

72. J. S. Holcenberg, K. D. Tutsch, R. H. Earhart, R. S. Ungerleider, B. A. Kamen, C. B. Pratt, T. J. Gribble, and D. L. Glaubiger: Phase I study of ICRF-187 in pediatric cancer patients and comparison of its pharmacokinetics in children and adults. *Cancer Treat. Rep.* 70:703 (1986).

73. J. L. Speyer, et al.: Protective effect of the bispiperazinedione ICRF-187 against doxorubicin-induced cardiac toxicity in women with adanced breast cancer. *New Engl. J. Med.* 319:745 (1988).

74. J. L. Speyer, M. D. Green, J. Sanger, A. Zeleniuch-Jacquotte, E. Kramer, M. Rey, J. C. Wernz, R. H. Blum, H. Hochster, M. Meyers, and F. M. Muggia: A prospective randomized trial of ICRF-187 for prevention of cumulative doxorubicin-induced cardiac toxicity in women with breast cancer. *Cancer Treat. Rev.* 17:161 (1990).

75. D. Faulds, J. A. Balfour, P. Chrisp, and H. D. Langtry: Mitoxantrone: A review of its pharmacodynamic and pharmacokinetic properties, and therapeutic potential in the chemotherapy of cancer. *Drugs* 41:400 (1991).

76. J. W. Lown, C. C. Hanstock, R. D. Bradley, and D. C. Scraba: Interactions of the antitumor agents mitoxantrone and bisantrene with deoxyribonucleic acids studied by electron microscopy. *Mol. Pharmacol.* 25:178 (1984).

77. G. T. Bowden, R. Roberts, D. S. Alberts, Y.-M. Peng, and D. Garcia: Comparative molecular pharmacology in leukemic L1210 cells of the anthracene anticancer drugs mitoxantrone and bisantrene. *Cancer Res.* 45:4915 (1985).

78. J. W. Lown, A. R. Morgan, S.-F. Yen, Y.-H. Wang, and W. D. Wilson: Characteristics of the binding of the anticancer agents mitoxantrone and ametantrone and ametantrone and related structures to deoxyribonucleic acid. *Biochemistry* 24:4028 (1985).

79. W. G. Harker, D. L. Slade, W. S. Dalton, P. S. Meltzer, and J. M. Trent: Multidrug resistance in mitoxantrone-selected HL-60 leukemia cells in the absence of P-glycoprotein overexpression. *Cancer Res.* 49:4542 (1989).

80. K. Reszka, J. A. Hartley, P. Kolodziejczyk, and J. W. Lown: Interaction of the peroxidase-derived metabolite of mitoxantrone with nucleic acids. Evidence for covalent binding of ^{14}C-labeled drug. *Biochem. Pharmacol.* 38:4253 (1989).

81. J. F. Smyth, J. S. Macpherson, P. S. Warrington, R. C. R. Leonard, and C. R. Wolf: The clinical pharmacology of mitoxantrone. *Cancer Chemother. Pharmacol.* 17:149 (1986).

82. D. S. Alberts, Y.-M. Peng, S. Leigh, T. P. Davis, and D. L. Woodward: Disposition of mitoxantrone in cancer patients. *Cancer Res.* 45:1879 (1985).

83. Symposium (multiple authors): Clinical evaluation of mitoxantrone in lymphoma therapy. *Semin. Oncol.* 17 *(Suppl. 10)*:44 pp. (1990).

84. R. T. Silver, D. C. Case, R. H. Wheeler, T. P. Miller, R. S. Stein, J. J. Stuart, B. A. Peterson, S. E. Rivkin, H. M. Golomb, J. J. Costanzi, A. J. Erslev, A. Reisman, and M. Dugan: Multicenter clinical trial of mitoxantrone in non-Hodgkin's lymphoma and Hodgkin's disease. *J. Clin. Oncol.* 9:754 (1991).

85. F. E. Durr: "Biochemical pharmacology and tumor biology of mitoxantrone and ametantrone," in *Anthracycline and Anthracenedione-based Anticancer Agents,* ed. by J. W. Lown. Amsterdam: Elsevier, 1988, pp. 163–200.

86. S. A. Waksman and H. B. Woodruff: Bacteriostatic and bactericidal substances produced by a soil actinomyces. *Proc. Soc. Exptl. Biol. Med.* 45:609 (1940).

87. Selman A. Waksman Conference on Actinomycins: Their Potential for Cancer Chemotherapy. *Cancer Chemother. Rep. 58 (No. 1)* (1974).

88. I. H. Goldberg: "Actinomycin D," in *Antineoplastic and Immunosuppressive Agents,* Part II, ed. by A. C. Sartorelli and D. G. Johns. Berlin: Springer-Verlag, 1975, pp. 582–592.

89. E. Reich, R. M. Franklin, A. J. Shatkin, and E. L. Tatum: Action of actinomycin D on animal cells and viruses. *Proc. Natl. Acad. Sci. USA* 48:1238 (1962).

90. J. P. Richardson: The binding of RNA polymerase to DNA. *J. Mol. Biol.* 21:83 (1966).

91. I. H. Goldberg, M. Rabinowitz, and E. Reich: Basis of actinomycin D action. I. DNA binding and inhibition of RNA-polymerase synthetic reactions by actinomycin. *Proc. Natl. Acad. Sci. USA* 48:2094 (1962).

92. W. Müller and D. M. Crothers: Studies of the binding of actinomycin and related compounds to DNA. *J. Mol. Biol.* 35:251 (1968).

93. A. Cerami, E. Reich, D. C. Ward, and I. H. Goldberg: The interaction of actinomycin with DNA. Requirement for the 2-amino group of purines. *Proc. Natl. Acad. Sci. USA* 57:1036 (1967).

94. T. R. Krugh: Association of actinomycin D and deoxyribonucleotides as a model for binding of the drug to DNA. *Proc. Natl. Acad. Sci. USA* 69:1911 (1972).

95. H. M. Sobell, S. C. Jain, T. D. Sakore, and C. E. Nordman: Stereochemistry of actinomycin-DNA binding. *Nature New Biol.* 231:200 (1971).

96. S. C. Jain and H. M. Sobell: Stereochemistry of actinomycin binding to DNA. I. Refinement and further structural details of the actinomycin-deoxyguanosine crystalline complex. *J. Mol. Biol.* 68:1 (1972).

97. Y.-C. C. Chiao and T. R. Krugh: Actinomycin D complexes with oligonucleotides as models for the binding of the drug to DNA. Paramagnetic induced relaxation experiments on drug-nucleic acid complexes. *Biochemistry* 16:747 (1977).

98. H. M. Sobel and S. C. Jain: Stereochemistry of actinomycin binding to DNA. II. Detailed molecular model of actinomycin-DNA complex and its implications. *J. Mol. Biol.* 68:21 (1972).

99. F. Takusagawa, B. M. Goldstein, S. Youngster, R. A. Jones, and H. M. Berman: Crystallization and preliminary X-ray study of a complex between d(ATGCAT) and actinomycin D. *J. Biol. Chem.* 259:4214 (1984).

100. S. C. Brown, K. Mullis, C. Levenson, and R. H. Shafer: Aqueous solution structure of an intercalated actinomycin D-dATGCAT complex by two-dimensional and one-dimensional proton NMR. *Biochemistry* 23:403 (1984).

101. R. M. Wadkins and T. M. Jovin: Actinomycin D and 7-aminoactinomycin D binding to single-stranded DNA. *Biochemistry* 30:9469 (1991).

102. S. J. Martin, S. V. Lennon, A. M. Bonham, and T. G. Cotter: Induction of apoptosis (programmed cell death) in human leukemic HL-60 cells by inhibition of RNA or protein synthesis. *J. Immunol.* 145:1859 (1990).

103. B. K. Bhuyan, T. J. Fraser, and K. J. Day: Cell pro-

liferation kinetics and drug sensitivity of exponential and stationary populations of cultered L1210 cells. *Cancer Res.* 37:1057 (1977).

104. D. Kessel and I. Wodinsky: Uptake *in vivo* of actinomycin D by mouse leukemias as factors in survival. *Biochem. Pharmacol.* 17:161 (1968).

105. R. H. F. Peterson, J. A. O'Neil, and J. L. Biedler: Some biochemical properties of Chinese hamster cells sensitive and resistant to actinomycin D. *J. Cell. Biol.* 63:773 (1974).

106. H. Diddens, V. Gekeler, M. Neumann, and D. Niethammer: Characterization of actinomycin-D-resistant CHO cell lines exhibiting a multidrug-resistance phenotype and amplified DNA sequences. *Int. J. Cancer* 40:635 (1987).

107. Y. Sugimoto and T. Tsuruo: "Development of multidrug resistance in rodent cell lines," in *Molecular and Cellular Biology of Multidrug Resistance in Tumor Cells,* ed. by I. B. Roninson. New York: Plenum Press, 1991, pp. 57–70.

108. J. Okabe-Kado, M. Hayashi, Y. Honma, M. Hozumi, and T. Tsuruo: Effects of inducers of erythroid differentiation of human leukemia K562 cells on vincristine-resistant K562/VCR cells. *Leukemia Res.* 7:481 (1983).

109. E. Hofsli and J. Nissen-Meyer: Reversal of multidrug resistance by lipophilic drugs. *Cancer Res.* 50:3997 (1990).

110. B. de Camargo, E. L. Franco, and the Brazilian Wilm's Tumor Study Group: Single-dose versus fractionated-dose dactinomycin in the treatment of Wilm's tumor. *Cancer* 65:2990 (1991).

111. W. M. Galbraith and L. B. Mellett: Tissue disposition of ^{3}H-actinomycin D (NSC-3053) in the rat, monkey, and dog. *Cancer Chemother. Rep.* 59:1061 (1975).

112. M. H. N. Tattersall, J. E. Sodergren, S. K. Sengupta, D. H. Trites, E. J. Modest, and E. Frei III: Pharmacokinetics of actinomycin D in patients with malignant malanoma. *Clin. Pharmacol. Ther.* 17:701 (1975).

113. E. Frei III: The clinical use of actinomycin. *Cancer Chemother. Rep.* 58:49 (1974).

114. J. L. Lewis: Chemotherapy of gestational choriocarcinoma. *Cancer* 30:1517 (1972).

115. R. B. Livingston and S. K. Carter: *Single Agents in Cancer Chemotherapy.* New York: IFI/Plenum, 1970.

116. A. J. Piro, C. C. Taylor, and J. A. Belli: Interaction between radiation and drug damage in mammalian cells. II. The effect of actinomycin D on the repair of sublethal radiation damage in plateau phase cells. *Cancer* 37:2697 (1976).

117. G. J. D'Angio, S. Farber, and C. L. Maddock: Potentiation of X-ray effects by actinomycin D. *Radiology* 73:175 (1959).

118. J. Raine, A. Bowman, K. Wallendszus, and J. Pritchard: Hepatopathy–thrombocytopenia syndrome—a complication of dactinomycin therapy for Wilm's tumor: A report from the United Kingdom Children's Cancer Study Group. *J. Clin. Oncol.* 9:268 (1991).

119. D. Svoboda, J. Reddy, and C. Harris: Invasive tumors induced in rats with actinomycin D. *Cancer Res.* 30:2271 (1970).

120. B. A. Chabner: "Bleomycin," in *Cancer Chemotherapy: Principles and Practice,* ed. by B. A. Chabner and J. M. Collins. Philadelphia: J.B. Lippincott Co., 1990, pp. 341–355.

121. D. H. Petering, R. W. Byrnes, and W. E. Antholine: The role of redox-active metals in the mechanism of action of bleomycin. *Chem.-Biol. Interactions* 73:133 (1990).

122. W. E. G. Müller and R. K. Zahn: "Bleomycin, an antibiotic that removes thymine from double-stranded DNA," in *Progress in Nucleic Acid Research and Molecular Biology,* ed. by W. E. Cohn. New York: Academic Press, 1977, pp. 21–57.

123. M. Takeshita, S. B. Horwitz, and A. P. Grollman: Bleomycin, an inhibitor of vaccinia virus replication. *Virology* 60:455 (1974).

124. W. E. G. Müller, A. Totsuka, I. Nusser, R. K. Zahn, and H. Umezawa: Bleomycin inhibition of DNA synthesis in isolated enzyme systems and in intact cell systems. *Biochem. Pharmacol.* 24:911 (1975).

125. P. R. Twentyman: Bleomycin—mode of action with particular reference to the cell cycle. *Pharmac. Ther.* 23:417 (1984).

126. K. W. Kohn and R. A. G. Ewig: Effect of pH on the bleomycin-induced DNA single-strand scission in L1210 cells and the relation to cell survival. *Cancer Res.* 36:3839 (1976).

127. N. J. Oppenheimer, L. O. Rodriguez, and S. M. Hecht: Proton nuclear magnetic resonance study of the structure of bleomycin and the zinc-bleomycin complex. *Biochemistry* 18:3439 (1979).

128. L. F. Povirk, M. Hogan, and N. Dattagupta: Binding of bleomycin to DNA: Intercalation of the bithiazole rings. *Biochemistry* 18:96 (1979).

129. S. Y. Lin and A. P. Grollman: Interactions of a fragment of bleomycin with deoxyribonucleotides: Nuclear magnetic resonance studies. *Biochemistry* 20:7589 (1981).

130. E. A. Sausville, J. Peisach, and S. B. Horwitz: A role for ferrous ion and oxygen in the degradation of DNA by bleomycin. *Biochem. Biophys. Res. Commun.* 73:814 (1976).

131. E. A. Sausville, J. Peisach, and S. B. Horwitz: Effect of chelating agents and metal ions on the degradation of DNA by bleomycin. *Biochemistry* 17:2740 (1978).

132. R. M. Burger, J. Peisach, and S. B. Horwitz: Activated bleomycin: A transient complex of drug, iron, and oxygen that degrades DNA. *J. Biol. Chem.* 256:11636 (1981).

133. W. J. Caspary, C. Niziak, D. A. Lanzo, R. Friedman, and N. R. Bachur: Bleomycin A_2: A ferrous oxidase. *Mol. Pharmacol.* 16:256 (1979).

134. I. Mahmutoglu and H. Kappus: Redox cycling of bleomycin-Fe(III) by an NADPH-dependent enzyme, and DNA damage in isolated rat liver nuclei. *Biochem. Pharmacol.* 36:3677 (1987).

135. M. Takeshita, L. S. Kappen, A. P. Grollman, M. Eisenberg, and I. H. Goldberg: Strand scission of deoxyribonucleic acid by neocarzinostatin, auromomycin, and bleomycin: Studies on base release and nucleotide sequence specificity. *Biochemistry* 20:7599 (1981).

136. B. J. Carter, V. S. Murty, K. S. Reddy, S. N. Wang, and S. M. Hecht: A role for the metal binding domain in determining the DNA sequence selectivity of Fe-bleomycin. *J. Biol. Chem.* 265:4193 (1990).

137. L. Giloni, M. Takeshita, F. Johnson, C. Iden, and A. P. Grollman: Bleomycin-induced strand-scission of

DNA. Mechanism of deoxyribose cleavage. *J. Biol. Chem.* 256:8608 (1981).

138. J. Stubble and J. W. Kozarich: Mechanisms of bleomycin-induced DNA degradation. *Chem. Rev.* 87:1107 (1987).

139. A. P. Grollman: "Base propenals and the toxicity of bleomycin," in *Organ Directed Toxicities of Anticancer Drugs*, ed. by M. P. Hacker, J. S. Lazo, and T. R. Tritton. Boston: Martinus Nijhoff Pub., 1987, pp. 79–90.

140. S. M. Sebti, J. P. Jani, J. S. Mistry, E. Gorelik, and J. S. Lazo: Metabolic inactivation: A mechanism of human tumor resistance to bleomycin. *Cancer Res.* 51:227 (1991).

141. A. J. Giaccia, A. D. Lewis, N. C. Denko, A. Cholon, J. W. Evans, C. A. Waldren, T. D. Stamato, and J. M. Brown: The hypersensitivity of the Chinese hamster ovary variant BL-10 to bleomycin killing is due to a lack of glutathione S-transferase-α activity. *Cancer Res.* 51:4463 (1991).

142. S. Brabbs and J. R. Warr: Isolation and characterization of bleomycin-resistant clones of CHO cells. *Genet. Res.* 34:269 (1979).

143. M. Miyaki, S. Morohashi, and T. Ono: Single strand scission and repair of DNA in bleomycin sensitive and resistant rat ascites hepatoma cells. *J. Antibiot.* 26:369 (1973).

144. D. S. Alberts, H.-S. Chen, R. Liu, K. J. Himmelstein, M. Mayersohn, D. Perrier, J. Gross, T. Moon, A. Broughton, and S. E. Salmon: Bleomycin pharmacokinetics in man. I. Intravenous administration. *Cancer Chemother. Pharmacol.* 1:177 (1978).

145. W. G. Kramer, S. Feldman, A. Broughton, J. E. Strong, S. W. Hall, and P. Y. Holoye: The pharmacokinetics of bleomycin in man. *J. Clin. Pharmacol.* 18:346 (1978).

146. M. M. Oken, S. T. Crooke, M. K. Elson, J. E. Strong, and R. B. Shafer: Pharmacokinetics of bleomycin after im administration in man. *Cancer Treat. Rep.* 65:485 (1981).

147. D. S. Alberts, H-S. G. Chen, M. Mayersohn, D. Perrier, T. E. Moon, and J. F. Gross: Bleomycin pharmacokinetics in man, II. Intracavitary administration. *Cancer Chemother. Pharmacol.* 2:127 (1979).

148. S. B. Howell, M. Schiefer, P. A. Andrews, M. Markman, and I. Abramson: The pharmacology of intraperitoneally administered bleomycin. *J. Clin. Oncol.* 5:2009 (1987).

149. S. T. Crooke, R. L. Comis, L. H. Einhorn, J. E. Strong, A. Broughton, and A. W. Prestayko: Effects of variations in renal function on the clinical pharmacology of bleomycin administered as an iv bolus. *Cancer Treat. Rep.* 61:1631 (1977).

150. A. G. Dalgleish, R. L. Woods, and J. A. Levi: Bleomycin pulmonary toxicity: Its relationship to renal dysfunction. *Med. Pediat. Oncol.* 12:313 (1984).

151. S. N. Roy and S. B. Horwitz: Characterization of the association of radiolabeled bleomycin A$_2$ with He La cells. *Cancer Res.* 44:1541 (1984).

152. H. Umezawa, T. Takeuchi, S. Hori, T. Sawa, and M. Ishizuka: Studies on the mechanism of antitumor effect of bleomycin on squamous cell carcinoma. *J. Antibiot.* 25:409 (1972).

153. T. Ohnuma, J. F. Holland, H. Masuda, J. A. Waligunda, and G. A. Goldberg: Microbiological assay of bleo-

mycin: Inactivation, tissue distribution, and clearance. *Cancer* 33:1230 (1974).

154. W. E. G. Müller, A. Totsuka, R. K. Zahn, and H. Umezawa: Methode zur Bestimmung der Bleomycin-inaktivierenden Enzymaktivität in Geweben. *Z. Krebsforsch.* 83:151 (1975).

155. J. S. Lazo and C. J. Humphreys: Lack of metabolism as the biochemical basis of bleomycin-induced pulmonary toxicity. *Proc. Natl. Acad. Sci. USA* 80:3064 (1983).

156. C. Nishimura, N. Tanaka, H. Suzuki, and N. Tanaka: Purification of bleomycin hydrolase with a monoclonal antibody and its characterization. *Biochemistry* 26:1574 (1987).

157. S. M. Sebti, J. C. DeLeon, and J. S. Lazo: Purification, characterization, and amino acid composition of rabbit pulmonary bleomycin hydrolase. *Biochemistry* 26:4213 (1987).

158. S. M. Sebti and J. S. Lazo: Separation of the protective enzyme bleomycin hydrolase from rabbit pulmonary aminopeptidases. *Biochemistry* 26:432 (1987).

159. J. S. Lazo, J. E. Mignano, and S. M. Sebti: "Pulmonary metabolic inactivation of bleomycin and protection from drug-induced lung injury," in *Organ Directed Toxicities of Anticancer Drugs,* ed. by M. P. Hacker, J. S. Lazo, and T. R. Tritton. Boston: Martinus Nijhoff Pub., 1987, pp. 128–139.

160. S. M. Sebti, J. C. DeLeon, L. T. Ma, S. M. Hecht, and J. S. Lazo: Substrate specificity of bleomycin hydrolase. *Biochem. Pharmacol.* 38:141 (1989).

161. J. S. Lazo, C. J. Boland, and P. E. Schwartz: Bleomycin hydrolase activity and cytotoxicity in human tumors. *Cancer Res.* 42:4026 (1982).

162. R. H. Blum, S. K. Carter, and K. Agre: A clinical review of bleomycin—a new antineoplastic agent. *Cancer* 31:903 (1973).

163. L. H. Einhorn and J. Donohue: Cis-diamminedichloroplatinum, vinblastine, and bleomycin combination chemotherapy in disseminated testicular cancer. *Ann. Int. Med.* 87:293 (1977).

164. S. D. Williams, R. Birch, L. H. Einhorn, L. Irwin, F. A. Greco, and P. J. Loehrer: Treatment of disseminated germ-cell tumors with cisplatin, bleomycin, and either vinblastine or etoposide. *New Engl. J. Med.* 316:1435 (1987).

165. A. Yagoda, B. Mukherji, C. Young, E. Etcubanas, C. Lamonte, J. R. Smith, C. T. C. Tan, and I. R. Krakoff: Bleomycin, an antitumor antibiotic. Clinical experience in 274 patients. *Ann. Int. Med.* 77:861 (1972).

166. D. E. Lehane, E. Hurd, and M. Lane: The effects of bleomycin on immunocompetence in man. *Cancer Res.* 35:2724 (1975).

167. J. A. Gottlieb: "New drugs introduced into clinical trials," in *Cancer Chemotherapy. Fundamental Concepts and Recent Advances.* Chicago: Year Book Med. Pub., 1975, pp. 79–98.

168. I. S. Cohen, M. B. Mosher, E. J. O'Keefe, S. N. Klaus, and R. C. DeConti: Cutaneous toxicity of bleomycin therapy. *Arch. Dermatol.* 107:553 (1973).

169. G. Bonadonna, M. De Lena, S. Monfardini, C. Bartoli, E. Bajetta, G. Beretta, and F. Fossati-Bellani: Clinical trials with bleomycin in lymphomas and in solid tumors. *Europ. J. Cancer* 8:205 (1972).

170. P. W. C. van Barneveld, D. T. Sleifer, T. W. van der

Mark, N. H. Mulder, A. J. M. Donker, S. Meijer, H. Schraffordt Koops, H. J. Sluiter, and R. Peset: Influence of platinum-induced renal toxicity on bleomycin-induced pulmonary toxicity in patients with disseminated testicular carcinoma. *Oncology* 41:4 (1984).

171. W. M. Bennett, L. Pastore, and D. C. Houghton: Fatal pulmonary bleomycin toxicity in cisplatin-induced acute renal failure. *Cancer Treat. Rep.* 64:921 (1980).

172. L. Einhorn, M. Krause, N. Hornback, and B. Furnas: Enhanced pulmonary toxicity with bleomycin and radiotherapy in oat cell lung cancer. *Cancer* 37:2414 (1976).

173. M. L. Samuels, D. E. Johnson, P. Y. Holoye, and V. J. Lanzotti: Large-dose bleomycin therapy and pulmonary toxicity. A possible role of prior radiotherapy. *J. Am. Med. Assoc.* 235:1117 (1976).

174. J. E. Byfield, Y. C. Lee, L. Tu, and F. Kulhanian: Molecular interactions of the combined effects of bleomycin and X-rays on mammalian cell survival. *Cancer Res.* 36:1138 (1976).

175. N. M. Bleehan, N. E. Gillies, and P. R. Twentyman: The effect of bleomycin and radiation in combination on bacteria and mammalian cells in culture. *Br. J. Radiol.* 47:346 (1974).

176. C. H. Toledo, W. E. Ross, C. I. Hood, and E. R. Block: Potentiation of bleomycin toxicity by oxygen. *Cancer Treat. Rep* 66:359 (1982).

177. M. J. McKeage, B. D. Evans, C. Atkinson, D. Perez, G. V. Forgeson, and P. J. Dady: Carbon monoxide diffusing capacity is a poor predictor of clinically significant bleomycin lung. *J. Clin. Oncol.* 8:779 (1990).

178. J. S. Lazo, D. G. Hoyt, S. M. Sebti, and B. R. Pitt: Bleomycin: A pharmacologic tool of the pathogenesis of interstitial pulmonary fibrosis. *Pharmac. Ther.* 47:347 (1990).

179. S. M. Sebti and J. S. Lazo: Metabolic inactivation of bleomycin analogs by bleomycin hydrolase. *Pharmac. Ther.* 38:321 (1988).

180. M. B. Mosher, R. C. DeConti, and J. R. Bertino: Bleomycin therapy in advanced Hodgkin's disease and epidermoid cancers. *Cancer* 30:56 (1972).

181. C. A. Dinarello, S. B. Ward, and S. M. Wolff: Pyrogenic properties of bleomycin (NSC-125066). *Cancer Chemother. Rep.* 57:393 (1973).

182. W. H. Leung, J. Y. N. Lau, T. K. Chan, and C. R. Kumana: Fulminant hyperpyrexia induced by bleomycin. *Postgrad. Med. J.* 65:417 (1989).

183. R. B. Weiss and S. Bruno: Hypersensitivity reactions to cancer chemotherapeutic agents. *Ann. Int. Med.* 94:66 (1981).

184. M. Slavik and S. K. Carter: Chromomycin A$_3$, mithramycin, and olivomycin: Antitumor antibiotics of related structure. *Adv. Pharmacol. Chemother.* 12:1 (1975).

185. W. Kersten, H. Kersten, F. E. Steiner, and B. Emmerich: The effect of chromomycin and mithramycin on the synthesis of deoxyribonucleic acid and ribonucleic acids. *Hoppe Seyler's Z. Physiol. Chem.* 348:1415 (1967).

186. G. Northrop, S. G. Taylor, and R. L. Northrop: Biochemical effects of mithramycin on cultured cells. *Cancer Res.* 29:1916 (1969).

187. R. D. Smith, D. Henson, J. Gehrke, and J. R. Barton: Reversible inhibition of DNA virus replication with mithramycin. *Proc. Soc. Exptl. Biol. Med.* 121:209 (1966).

188. D. C. Ward, E. Reich, and I. H. Goldberg: Base specificity in the interaction of polynucleotides with antibiotic drugs. *Science* 149:1259 (1965).

189. B. M. G. Cons and K. R. Fox: Interaction of mithramycin with metal ions and DNA. *Biochem. Biophys. Res. Commun.* 160:517 (1989).

190. W. Behr, K. Honikel, and G. Hartmann: Interaction of the RNA polymerase inhibitor chromomycin with DNA. *Eur. J. Biochem.* 9:82 (1969).

191. L. Blau and R. Bittman: Equilibrium and kinetic measurements of actinomycin binding to deoxyribonucleic acid in the presence of competing drugs. *Mol. Pharmacol.* 11:716 (1975).

192. B. M. G. Cons and K. R. Fox: Footprinting studies of sequence recognition by mithramycin. *Anti-Cancer Drug Design* 5:93 (1990).

193. D. L. Banville, M. A. Keniry, and R. H. Shafer: NMR investigation of mithramycin A binding to d(ATGCAT)$_2$: A comparative study with chromomycin A$_3$. *Biochemistry* 29:9294 (1990).

194. C. Demicheli, J. P. Albertini, and A. Garnier-Suillerot: Interaction of mithramycin with DNA. Evidence that mithramycin binds to DNA as a dimer in a right-handed screw conformation. *Eur. J. Biochem.* 198:333 (1991).

195. B. M. G. Cons and K. R. Fox: Effects of the antitumor antibiotic mithramycin on the structure of repetitive DNA regions adjacent to its GC-rich binding site. *Biochemistry* 30:6314 (1991).

196. R. Ray, R. C. Snyder, S. Thomas, C. A. Koller, and D. M. Miller: Mithraymcin blocks protein binding and function of the SV40 early promoter. *J. Clin. Invest.* 83:2003 (1989).

197. R. C. Snyder, R. Ray, S. Blume, and D. M. Miller: Mithramycin blocks transcriptional initiation of the c-myc P1 and P2 promoters. *Biochemistry* 30:4290 (1991).

198. R. S. Gupta: Cross-resistance of vinblastine- and taxol-resistant mutants of Chinese hamster ovary cells to other anticancer drugs. *Cancer Treat. Rep.* 69:515 (1985).

199. B. J. Kennedy, M. Sandberg-Wollheim, M. Loken, and J. W. Yarbro: Studies with tritiated mithramycin in C3H mice. *Cancer Res.* 27:1534 (1967).

200. J. Ransohoff, B. C. Martin, T. J. Medrek, M. N. Harris, F. M. Golomb, and J. C. Wright: Preliminary clinical study of mithramycin (NSC-24559) in primary tumors of the central nervous system. *Cancer Chemother. Rep.* 49:51 (1965).

201. B. J. Kennedy: Mithramycin therapy in advanced testicular neoplasms. *Cancer* 26:755 (1970).

202. G. J. Hill, N. Sedransk, D. Rochlin, H. Bisel, N. C. Andrews, W. Fletcher, J. M. Schroeder, and W. L. Wilson: Mithramycin (NSC 24559) therapy of testicular tumors. *Cancer* 30:900 (1972).

203. C. A. Koller and D. M. Miller: Preliminary observations on the therapy of the myeloid blast phase of chronic granulocytic leukemia with plicamycin and hydroxyurea. *New Engl. J. Med.* 315:1433 (1986).

204. C. P. Perlia, N. J. Gubisch, J. Wolter, D. Edelberg, M. M. Dederick, and S. G. Taylor: Mithramycin treatment of hypercalcemia. *Cancer* 25:389 (1970).

205. R. E. Slayton, B. I. Shnider, E. Elias, J. Horton, and C. P. Perlia: New approach to the treatment of hypercal-

cemia. The effect of short-term treatment with mithramy-cin. *Clin. Pharmacol. Ther.* 12:833 (1971).

206. P. R. Robins and J. Jowsey: Effect of mithramycin on normal and abnormal bone turnover. *J. Lab. Clin. Med.* 82:576 (1973).

207. D. T. Kiang, M. K. Loken, and B. J. Kennedy: Mechanism of the hypocalcemic effect of mithramycin. *J. Clin. Endocrinol. Metab.* 48:341 (1979).

208. N. Pitts: "Clinical data accumulated by Pfizer for NDA for mithramycin," in *Proceedings of the Chemotherapy Conference on Mithramycin,* ed. by S. K. Carter and M. A. Friedman. Cancer Chemotherapy Evaluation Branch, National Cancer Institute, 1970, pp. 33–43.

209. D. J. Ahr, S. J. Scialla, and D. B. Kimball: Acquired platelet dysfunction following mithramycin therapy. *Cancer* 41:448 (1978).

210. P. Kubisz, P. Klener, and S. Cronberg: Influence of mithramycin on some platelet functions in vitro. *Acta Haematol.* 63:101 (1980).

211. R. W. Monto, R. W. Talley, M. J. Caldwell, W. C. Levin, and M. M. Guest: Observations on the mechanism of hemorrhagic toxicity in mithramycin (NSC 24559) therapy. *Cancer Res.* 29:697 (1969).

CHAPTER 8

Inhibitors of Chromatin Function

TOPOISOMERASE INHIBITORS
  Epipodophyllotoxins
    Etoposide (VP-16)
    Teniposide (VM-26)
  Amsacrine (m-AMSA)
  Camptothecin, CPT-11

MICROTUBULE INHIBITORS
  Vinca alkaloids
    Vinblastine
    Vincristine
    Vindesine
  Taxol

Eukaryotic chromosomes are complex structures which undergo many changes in conformation and intracellular position during the cell cycle. Such changes are necessary for cells to carry out DNA replication and mitosis, and it has been found that agents that interfere with the proteins responsible for these changes are selectively toxic to proliferating cells. The two groups of drugs discussed in this chapter, topoisomerase inhibitors and microtubule antagonists, each are thought to owe their antitumor effects to disruption of chromosomal dynamics.

Topoisomerase Inhibitors

DNA in eukaryotic cells must be packed very efficiently to be able to fit into the nucleus. This packing takes place at several levels, including the wrapping of DNA helices around histone octamers to form nucleosomes, coiling of nucleosomes to form solenoids, and organization of solenoids into looped domains.[1] As a result, chromosomal DNA is twisted extensively and the activities of enzymes called *topoisomerases* are needed to permit selected regions of DNA

to become sufficiently untangled and relaxed to allow transcription, replication, and other essential functions to proceed. The key property of topoisomerases that allows them to perform this function is their ability to temporarily break DNA strands and, after the necessary topological changes have taken place, to reseal these breaks.[2] Topoisomerases are divided into two groups, based on whether they transiently break only one DNA strand (type-I enzymes) or both strands (type-II enzymes). At the present time, only inhibitors of topoisomerase II have approved clinical indications, and these drugs will be discussed first. Some topoisomerase-I inhibitors have shown impressive activity in early clinical trials, and these drugs will be discussed briefly at the end of this section.

Etoposide (VP-16)

BIOCHEMICAL ACTIONS AND CYTOTOXIC MECHANISM. Etoposide is a semisynthetic derivative of podophyllotoxin, a microtubule inhibitor found in extracts of the mandrake plant. Although it was initially thought that etoposide, too, might inhibit microtubule function, further investigation indicated that topo-

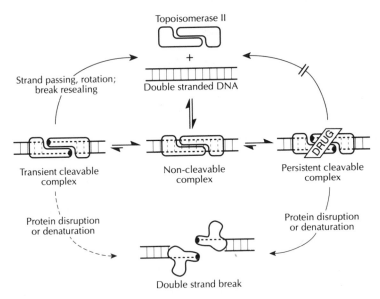

Etoposide (VP-16)

isomerase II is the major target of this drug in eukaryotic cells.[3]

Topoisomerase II first interacts with DNA by reversibly forming a noncovalent complex (Fig. 8-1). At this stage no DNA strand breaks have been made and, because abrupt removal of the enzyme would leave no residual damage, this initial complex is termed "noncleavable." The enzyme then cuts both DNA strands, forming a covalent bond between each protein subunit and one of the newly formed 5'-phosphate ends of the DNA. This complex is considered "cleavable," since removal or disruption of the protein would result in a permanent double-strand break. In the absence of inhibitors the cleavable complex is either rapidly converted back to the noncleavable complex or, after accomplishing a topological change by strand passage or rotation, the breaks are resealed and the enzyme dissociates from the DNA. Inhibitors such as etoposide stabilize the cleavable complex, preventing it from going back to the noncleavable complex or from completing strand passage or rotation.

Although stabilization of the cleavable complex persists while the inhibitory drug is present, removal of the drug results in a rapid return of apparently normal topoisomerase function, including resealing of the great majority of DNA strand breaks.[4] It is unclear what lesions are produced while the cleavable complex is trapped, which ultimately lead to cell death. One possibility is that a small number of topoisomerase molecules are rendered nonfunctional during drug treatment (e.g., by pro-

Figure 8–1   DNA damage induced by inhibition of topoisomerase II. Temporary double-strand breaks are induced by topoisomerase II in the course of its normal catalytic cycle, by formation of a cleavable complex. Disruption of this complex, which results in a permanent double-strand break, occurs infrequently in the absence of drugs. Inhibitors of topoisomerase II cause the cleavable complex to persist, thereby increasing the probability that the cleavable complex will be converted to an irreversible double strand break.

teolysis or spontaneous denaturation), leading to the generation of unrepairable double-strand breaks at critical sites.[5,6] It has also been observed[7] that etoposide treatment prevents activation of the protein kinase, p34[cdc2]. This kinase, which ordinarily becomes activated at the end of the G_2 phase of the cell cycle, is thought to have a critical role in allowing cells to begin mitosis. It is therefore possible that the arrest of cells in the G_2 phase of the cell cycle observed after treatment with etoposide (and perhaps other DNA damaging agents) is due to interference with p34[cdc2] function.

Resistance to etoposide or the related drug, teniposide, is commonly accompanied by cross-resistance to several other drugs.[8] To some extent this is due to the "classical" multidrug-resistance phenomenon discussed in Chapter 4, characterized by overexpression of P-glycoprotein, which pumps lipophilic drugs out of the cell. Evidence for this mechanism of resistance to topoisomerase-II inhibitors includes decreased intracellular drug accumulation,[9] reduced flux of drugs across cellular membranes,[10,11] and the ability of resistance to be conferred by transfection of sensitive cells with DNA coding for the MDR gene.[12] In addition, an "atypical" multidrug-resistance phenotype has been identified in which cells that are resistant to topoisomerase-II inhibitors retain normal sensitivity to vinca alkaloids and normal drug-transport characteristics.[13] This phenotype appears to arise from expression of forms of topoisomerase II with altered catalytic activities,[14,15] including one that has been found to contain a mutation in the part of the gene coding for the ATP binding domain.[16] Another form of resistance has been traced to a mutation that resulted in underexpression of topoisomerase-II protein with otherwise normal catalytic properties.[17]

PHARMACOLOGY. Etoposide is usually given orally or intravenously, although intraperitoneal, intrapleural, and intracarotid routes have also been tested.[18] The two main oral formulations are a solution and a soft gelatin capsule.[19] Bioavailability of etoposide after oral administration varies considerably within and among individuals, but averages about 50% overall.[18] The volume of distribution is typically 10–15 L/m^2 in adults and slightly lower in children.[18]

Elimination most often follows biphasic kinetics with a terminal half-life of 4–8 hours.[20] Approximately 30–50% of etoposide is recovered as unchanged drug. Virtually all of this is found in urine, with only a few percent excreted in the bile.[20] As much as 20% of the dose has been recovered as metabolites, including hydroxy acids[21,22] and glucuronide and sulfate conjugates.[23,24] A significant portion of administered drug is frequently unaccounted for (20–30%), possibly due to tight binding to tissue proteins.[25]

CLINICAL USE AND TOXICITY. Etoposide has shown activity against a variety of tumor types in both preclinical[26] and clinical studies.[26,27] Its greatest impact has come in the treatment of testicular cancers (Table 8–1), in which it was found to be effective in patients whose tumors were resistant to prior treatment.[28,29] Preclinical studies suggesting that etoposide might be synergistic with cisplatinum[30] were validated in clinical trials.[31] Further investigation demonstrated that the combination of etoposide with

Table 8–1   *Pharmacology of Topoisomerase Inhibitors.* Dose-limiting lesions are shown in bold type

Drug	Principal Indications	Toxicities
Etoposide	Testicular cancer, small cell lung cancer	**Bone marrow depression,** nausea, diarrhea, mucositis, hypotension
Teniposide	Acute lymphocytic leukemia, neuroblastoma	**Bone marrow depression,** nausea, vomiting, hypotension
Amsacrine	Acute nonlymphocytic leukemia	**Bone marrow depression,** stomatitis, cardiac arrhythmias
CPT-11	Non-small cell lung cancer (investigational)	**Bone marrow depression,** diarrhea, nausea, vomiting

bleomycin and cisplatinum was superior to vinblastine with bleomycin and cisplatinum,[32,33] and the former combination has replaced the latter as standard therapy for this disease.

Small-cell lung cancer is another disease in which etoposide has an important therapeutic role. Studies in which etoposide was given as a single agent, either orally or intravenously, showed that it produced response rates of 10% to 84% in patients who had not received previous therapy.[34] The variability of these results appears to be due to differences in administration schedules, with more protracted regimens (e.g., daily treatments for 2–4 weeks) being more effective than single, more intensive treatments at 2–3-week intervals.[34,35] Substitution of etoposide for vincristine[36] or doxorubicin[37] yields a significant improvement in median survival time in patients with extensive disease, although the prognosis for such patients is still poor.

The major toxicity attributable to etoposide is myelosuppression, primarily leukopenia with some thrombocytopenia.[26] Nausea and diarrhea are common but are usually not severe. Mucositis can be dose-limiting at higher doses, in which marrow is rescued by transplantation.[38] Rapid drug infusions occasionally cause hypotension.[39]

Teniposide (VM-26)

Teniposide, like etoposide, is an epipodophyllotoxin. The structure of teniposide differs from that of etoposide by having a sulfur-containing (thenylidine) substituent on its sugar ring, rather than a methyl group.[20]

Teniposide (VM-26)

Most evidence indicates that teniposide and etoposide have the same mechanisms of cytotoxicity and resistance.[20,40] However, teniposide is taken up into cells more rapidly and retained more avidly than is etoposide,[41] possibly because teniposide is more lipophilic than etoposide. Because both drugs are extensively bound to plasma proteins (etoposide 94%, teniposide 99%), their pharmacokinetics and pharmacodynamics are sensitive to factors that alter protein binding.[20,42] Protein binding may also contribute to the longer half-life and reduced renal clearance of teniposide as compared to etoposide.[20]

Although teniposide was brought into clinical use before etoposide, it has been studied much less extensively. The choice to pursue development of etoposide, rather than teniposide, was based on a limited number of early clinical and preclinical studies, and it is not clear that etoposide is necessarily better than or equivalent to teniposide in all cases.[40,43] Teniposide appears to be an effective agent for treatment of acute lymphocytic leukemia and neuroblastoma in children and brain tumors in adults.[43] Toxicity caused by teniposide is similar to that of etoposide (i.e., primarily myelosuppression), although acute allergic reactions to teniposide were observed in some patients who did not subsequently react to etoposide.[44]

Amsacrine (m-AMSA)

In contrast to etoposide and teniposide, amsacrine contains a planar aromatic domain (an acridine ring system) that can become intercalated into DNA. Although it was initially thought that such intercalation was responsible for amsacrine-induced DNA damage and cytotoxicity, this hypothesis was refuted by experiments showing that the ability to intercalate did not, by itself, dictate the formation of DNA breaks and DNA-protein cross-links.[45] These and subsequent studies[46,47] led to the conclusion that the critical effect of amsacrine treatment is stabilization of topoisomerase-II cleavable complexes. However, even though toposiomerase II is the common target of amsacrine and of the epipodophyllotoxins, these agents do not all inhibit that enzyme in the same way, as evidenced by data showing that a mutant form of topoisomerase II was resistant

Amsacrine (m-AMSA)

to inhibition by amsacrine but was normally sensitive to etoposide.[48-50] More recent studies suggest that intercalating topoisomerase-II inhibitors, including amsacrine, interact with a different structural domain of the enzyme than do nonintercalating inhibitors.[51-53]

Amsacrine is effective in the treatment of acute nonlymphocytic leukemia. Its primary use is in patients who are refractory to standard induction therapy.[54,55] Although it is not significantly better than daunorubicin as part of a combination regimen for treating newly diagnosed patients with acute nonlymphocytic leukemia,[56] amsacrine produces much less cardiotoxicity than daunorubicin and may therefore be more appropriate in patients who also have compromised myocardial function.[57] Amsacrine is poorly absorbed after oral administration and is usually given intravenously.[58] The drug is primarily cleared by hepatic metabolism, resulting in the formation in a metabolite (probably a glutathione, based on studies in rodents[59]) that is excreted in the bile.[60] Disappearance of the drug from plasma follows biphasic kinetics with a terminal half-life of 7-9 hours in patients with normal hepatic function and about 17 hours in patients with severe liver dysfunction.[60,61] Amsacrine distributes into a volume exceeding total body water, and has been found to accumulate in the liver.[58,60] Myelosuppression is usually the dose-limiting toxicity, although stomatitis can be severe at higher doses.[58] Cardiac arrhythmias attributable to amsacrine treatment are rare, but can be fatal.[62]

Camptothecin, CPT-11

Camptothecin and its derivatives are the only drugs currently identified as inhibitors of topoisomerase I.[63] The parent compound, camptothecin, was isolated from the bark of a Chinese tree (*Camptotheca acuminata*) and was found to be very active against experimental tumors.[64] Initial clinical studies of camptothecin were discouraging, producing little response while causing severe cystitis.[65] However, it was later determined that camptothecin's activity requires that the lactone ring be intact, and that this ring was being opened by preparation of the sodium salt of the drug for injection. Furthermore, it was found that the acidic environment of the bladder catalyzed reclosure of the lactone ring, thus reactivating excreted drug and accounting for its toxicity to that organ.[65] The realization that camptothecin's poor solubility could not be overcome by sodium salt formulation led to the development of more soluble analogs, one of which, CPT-11,[66] is now in Phase II clinical trials.

The hypothesis that topoisomerase I is the major cellular target for camptothecin is supported by several pieces of evidence,[63] including specific inhibition of topoisomerase-I activity in experiments with isolated DNA,[67] immunoprecipitation of camptothecin-induced DNA-protein cross-links by anti-topoisomerase-I antibodies,[68] and elution studies demonstrating a one-to-one relationship between DNA single-strand-break formation and DNA-protein cross-links in camptothecin-treated cells.[69] As is the case with topoisomerase-II inhibitors, the "breaks" induced by camptothecin are readily reversible unless the drug-stabilized topoisomerase-I cleavable complex is denatured,[67,69] raising the question of how transient breaks become lethal events. Because the DNA polymerase inhibitor, aphidicolin, was found to prevent

Camptothecin: $R_1 = H$, $R_2 = H$

CPT-11: $R_1 = CH_2CH_3$, $R_2 =$

camptothecin-induced cytotoxicity and DNA damage[70] it has been proposed that permanent lesions may result from the interaction of immobile cleavable complexes with moving replication forks.[70] Resistance to camptothecin has been primarily attributed to changes in the target enzyme. This can be due to reduced expression of normal topoisomerase I[71,72] or to expression of mutant forms of the enzyme.[73,74] Unlike the topoisomerase-II inhibitors, camptothecin has not yet been shown to be subject to multiple-drug-resistance phenomena.[63]

Because of the difficulties noted above, clinical development of CPT-11 has superseded that of its parent, camptothecin. Studies in rodents indicate that the disposition of CPT-11 is dose-dependent.[75,76] At lower doses (2–10 mg/kg), intravenously administered CPT-11 disappears from plasma with a half-life of 1–2 hours, largely due to conversion to 7-ethyl-10-hydroxycamptothecin (referred to as SN-38). This metabolite, which is about 1,000 times more potent than CPT-11 *in vitro,* is inactivated by glucuronidation. At higher doses (10–40 mg/kg), CPT-11 is mostly excreted as unchanged drug into the urine, bile, and feces. Initial results from studies with human subjects are consistent with the rodent data, indicating dose-dependent conversion of CPT-11 to SN-38, with elimination half-lives of 2–4 hours for the parent drug and 3–18 hours for the metabolite.[77]

In a phase II clinical study of patients with inoperable non-small-cell lung cancer, CPT-11 was shown to be more effective than any previously tested single-agent therapy, producing a response rate of 31.9%.[78] CPT-11 also produced responses in patients with refractory leukemia and lymphomas.[79] Leukopenia and diarrhea were the most severe toxicities in these studies. Nausea and vomiting were common, but manageable.

Microtubule Inhibitors

Microtubules are protein polymers that are responsible for various aspects of cellular morphology and movement.[80] The major component of microtubules is tubulin, a protein containing two nonidentical (α and β) 50-kDa subunits, arranged head-to-tail in linear protofilaments. A single microtubule is composed of thirteen parallel protofilaments, forming a hollow structure with a "minus" end, which is usually stabilized by attachment to an organizing center, and a "plus" end, at which growth or shrinkage of the microtubule takes place (Fig. 8–2). Although some microtubules appear to be relatively stable (e.g., in cilia and neuronal axons), others, such as those involved in chromosome segregation, are very labile. Individual microtubules can oscillate between polymerization and depolymerization, and the net status of the microtubule population is very sensitive to factors affecting the equilibrium between

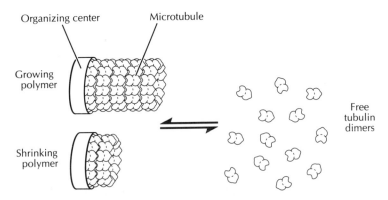

Figure 8–2 Microtubule dynamics. Microtubules are formed by the reversible aggregation of tubulin dimers into parallel protofilaments. Individual microtubules oscillate between states of growth and shrinkage, depending upon the availability of numerous factors including tubulin, GTP, magnesium ions, and nontubulin proteins.

Vincristine (VCR): R=CHO
Vinblastine (VBL): R=CH₃

Vindesine

free tubulin dimers and assembled polymers. The drugs discussed here act by disrupting this equilibrium.

Vinca Alkaloids

The microtubule antagonists that are currently administered as part of standard chemotherapeutic regimens are two closely related alkaloids, vincristine and vinblastine, which were isolated from the periwinkle plant *Catharanthus rosea* (also called *Vinca rosea.*)[81] A third, synthetic vinca alkaloid, vindesine, has also been shown to have some activity against human tumors and is under evaluation in experimental protocols. Although each of these agents has distinctive characteristics, especially with regard to their toxicology, most evidence indicates that they share common biochemical properties.

BIOCHEMICAL ACTIONS AND CYTOTOXIC MECHANISM. The vinca alkaloids are part of a structurally diverse group of compounds (including colchicine, podophyllotoxin, and maytansine) that bind specifically to free tubulin dimers. Although these agents do not all share the same binding site, their interactions with tubulin have the common effect of disrupting the balance between microtubule polymerization and depolymerization, resulting in the net dissolution of microtubules (Fig. 8–3), destruction of the mitotic spindle, and arrest of cells in metaphase.[82-84] Vinca alkaloids are unique in that, upon binding to tubulin, they cause the formation of paracrystalline aggregates containing equimolar amounts of drug and tubulin dimers.[85,86] Binding of vinca alkaloids to tubulin is kinetically complex[87] and depends on many factors, including ionic strength,[88] magnesium-ion concentration,[89] interaction with

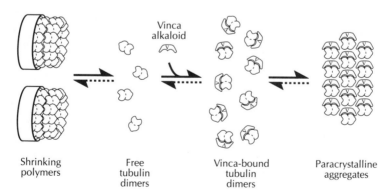

| Shrinking polymers | Free tubulin dimers | Vinca-bound tubulin dimers | Paracrystalline aggregates |

Figure 8–3 Disruption of tubulin/microtubule equilibrium by vinca alkaloids. Upon binding to vinca alkaloids, tubulin dimers are unable to aggregate to form microtubules. This effectively decreases the pool of free tubulin dimers available for microtubule assembly, resulting in a shift of the equilibrium toward disassembly. Formation of paracrystalline aggregates by vinca-bound tubulin dimers shifts the equilibrium even further toward disassembly and microtubule shrinkage.

nontubulin proteins,[90] and nucleotide concentrations.[91] The level of GTP has been found to be of particular importance in the interaction between vinca alkaloids and tubulin,[92] and it has been proposed that observed variations of vincristine retention among tumors and normal tissues[93] may be related to differences in GTP hydrolysis.[91,94]

Acquired resistance to vinca alkaloids usually results from overexpression of the P-glycoprotein described in Chapter 4. Although this overexpression usually produces parallel increases in resistance to all of the drugs subject to multidrug resistance, mutant forms of the glycoprotein can cause preferential resistance to the agent responsible for selective pressure.[95]

Multidrug resistance can be overcome *in vitro* by incubation of cells with compounds that compete with vinca alkaloids for binding to P-glycoprotein,[96] and studies with one such agent, verapamil, indicate that this strategy may also be practical *in vivo*.[97,98] Application of this approach has been limited by the calcium-channel-blocking actions of racemic preparations of verapamil. However, the D isomer of verapamil has been found to be as effective at potentiating vinca accumulation in human leukemic cells as the L isomer, even though the L isomer is an order of magnitude more effective as a calcium-channel blocker,[99] suggesting that it may be possible to deliver high enough concentrations of D isomer to overcome resistance without causing cardiovascular complications.

Resistance to drugs that cause microtubule depolymerization can also be due to alterations in tubulin structure. In some instances these mutations affect drug binding to tubulin.[100] Many other mutants have been isolated, however, in which tubulin has been altered so as to affect its intrinsic ability to form microtubules.[101] These mutants have several common characteristics, including relatively low levels of resistance (two- to threefold), cross-resistance to other microtubule-assembly inhibitors, and collateral sensitivity to microtubule-stabilizing drugs (e.g., taxol, discussed in the next section).[101,102] These properties have led to the hypothesis that in such mutants the equilibrium between free tubulin and microtubules is shifted in the direction of polymerization.[103] It has been speculated that mutation of the GTP-binding domain of tubulin may be the structural basis for changes in this equilibrium.[102]

PHARMACOLOGY. The vinca alkaloids are usually given by bolus intravenous injection, although protocols using continuous infusions are under investigation.[104] Analysis of the distribution and elimination of these drugs is limited by the methodology available to measure them at pharmacologic concentrations. Most of the current data were obtained using immunoassay techniques that are more sensitive than the chromatographic assays they replaced, but which do not distinguish parent drug from some metabolites.[105] All three vinca alkaloids appear to leave the general circulation with triexponential kinetics, having similar alpha and beta half-lives (2–5 minutes and 50–150 minutes, respectively).[105] Vindesine and vinblastine each have a terminal half-life of about 24 hours. Vincristine is eliminated much more slowly, with a terminal half-life of about 85 hours.[105] The volumes of distribution of these drugs are quite high (8–27 L/kg),[105–107] indicating a substantial degree of tissue binding. Penetration of the blood-brain barrier by vincristine is minimal.[108]

Studies using radiolabeled drugs show that vinca alkaloids are primarily eliminated by a combination of hepatic metabolism and biliary excretion, with only a small amount of parent drug and metabolites being recovered in the urine (5–25%).[106,107,109–112] Many vinca metabolites are produced in humans and animals, not all of which have been characterized.[81] It is likely, however, that a number of these metabolites are active cytotoxic agents (e.g., vindesine is a metabolite of vinblastine[106]) and that the pharmacologic effects of vinca administration are felt long after the parent drug is gone.

CLINICAL USE AND TOXICITY. Vincristine, together with prednisone, is the nucleus of combination chemotherapy for induction of remission of acute leukemias in adults and children (Table 8–2). Complete remissions are obtained in 80–90% of such patients.[81,113,114] Similar success is achieved in treating Hodgkin's lymphoma[115,116] and aggressive non-Hodgkin's lymphoma[117] with vincristine-containing combinations. In each of these cases the long-term survival rate (≥10 years) is 50–65%. Vincris-

Table 8–2   *Pharmacology of Microtubule Inhibitors.* Dose-limiting lesions are shown in bold type

Drug	Principal Indications	Toxicities
Vincristine	Acute leukemias, Hodgkin's and non-Hodgkin's lymphoma, small-cell lung cancer, breast cancer, Wilm's tumor, neuroblastoma, rhabdomyosarcoma, Ewing's sarcoma	**Peripheral neuropathy,** autonomic neuropathy (abdominal pain, constipation, paralytic ileus, urinary retention, orthostatic hypotension), other neurological symptoms, cardiac ischemia
Vinblastine	Hodgkin's and non-Hodgkin's lymphoma, testicular cancer, ovarian cancer	**Bone marrow depression,** neurotoxicities as for vincristine (less common, less severe), cardiac ischemia
Vindesine	Acute lymphocytic leukemia, blast crisis of chronic myelogenous leukemia, Hodgkin's and non-Hodgkin's lymphoma (investigational)	**Bone marrow depression,** neurotoxicities as for vincristine (less common, less severe), cardiac ischemia
Taxol	Ovarian and breast cancer (investigational)	**Bone marrow depression,** hypersensitivity reaction, mucositis, peripheral neuropathies, cardiac arrhythmias and conduction blocks

tine is also included in combinations for treating various solid tumors, such as small-cell lung carcinoma and breast carcinoma in adults, and Wilm's tumor, neuroblastoma, rhabdomyosarcoma, and Ewing's sarcoma in children.[81,118,119]

The dose-limiting toxicity for vincristine is almost always peripheral neuropathy, the most common symptom of which is a depressed Achilles tendon reflex.[120] This symptom is usually followed by paresthesias in the extremities. Although the paresthesias will typically resolve upon discontinuation of the drug, loss of the tendon reflex may be permanent.[121] Autonomic neuropathy often occurs early in the course of vincristine administration, resulting in abdominal pain, constipation, paralytic ileus, urinary retention, and orthostatic hypotension.[121,122] Preliminary studies indicate that it may be possible to reduce some of these symptoms by coadministration of glutamic acid,[123,124] which has been shown to stabilize microtubules *in vitro*.[125] Other toxicities associated with vincristine treatment include cranial nerve palsies, transient cortical blindness, confusion, delirium, and depression.[121,122,126] Unlike the great majority of antineoplastic agents, vincristine usually does not cause significant myelosuppression.

Vinblastine is an important drug in the treatment of Hodgkin's lymphoma, where it has been used in place of vincristine, providing similar antitumor activity with less neurotoxic-ity,[127,128] and as part of an alternating combination protocol in which both vinca drugs are used.[129] Vinblastine is also effective against non-Hodgkin's lymphoma[130] and has produced responses in patients who had become resistant to vincristine, indicating that there is not always cross-resistance between these two drugs.[131] Vinblastine also has been used extensively in combination with cisplatinum and bleomycin to treat testicular and ovarian cancers, although several studies suggest that replacement of vinblastine by etoposide in this combination produces similar or superior antitumor effect with less severe toxicity.[33,132-134] Other uses for vinblastine include transitional cell carcinoma of the urinary tract, breast cancer, and Kaposi's sarcoma.[81] Myelosuppression (primarily neutropenia) is the major toxicity caused by vinblastine.[81] The neurotoxic symptoms caused by vinblastine are similar to (although less common and less severe than) those resulting from vincristine administration. Gastrointestinal symptoms are more common with vincristine than vinblastine.

Vindesine has significant activity, comparable to that of vincristine, in treatment of acute lymphocytic leukemia, blast crisis of chronic myelogenous leukemia, Hodgkin's lymphoma, and non-Hodgkin's lymphoma.[135] In some cases, especially in patients with acute lymphocytic leukemia, responses to vindesine were obtained after vincristine treatment had failed, indicating a lack of cross-resistance between the two drugs.[136] Vindesine produces some responses in patients with non-small-cell lung cancer, although it is not clear if these are sufficiently beneficial to warrant the accompanying toxicities.[137,138] Leukopenia is usually the dose-limiting toxicity for vindesine.[81,135] Neurotoxicity, like that caused by vincristine, also occurs frequently in patients receiving vindesine.[135] All three vinca drugs share a variety of less common side effects, including severe damage to subcutaneous tissues (upon extravasation), cardiac ischemia (sometimes leading to myocardial infarction), and alopecia.[81]

Taxol

BIOCHEMICAL ACTIONS AND RESISTANCE. The importance of microtubules as a target for taxol was suggested by its ability to induce G_2/M cell-cycle arrest under conditions that had minimal effect on RNA, DNA, or protein synthesis.[139] However, in contrast to the other known microtubule antagonists, taxol disrupts the equilibrium between free tubulin and microtubules by shifting it in the direction of assembly, rather than disassembly. As a result, taxol treatment causes both the stabilization of ordinary cytoplasmic microtubules and the formation of abnormal bundles of microtubules.[140,141] In a study of human leukemic cell lines, the reversibility of bundle formation was correlated with resistance to taxol cytotoxicity.[142]

In studies using purified tubulin it was found that taxol binds reversibly to formed microtubules with a stoichiometry of about one drug molecule per molecule of polymerized tubulin dimer, and an apparent binding constant of 8.7

$\times$ 10^{-7} M.[143] Competitive binding experiments demonstrated that the taxol binding site is distinct from those used by colchicine, vinblastine, podophyllotoxin, and GTP.[144,145] The stabilization of microtubules by taxol binding is manifested in various ways, including a reduction of the critical tubulin concentration required for polymerization,[141] loss of the requirement for GTP or microtubule-associated proteins to initiate microtubule formation, and enhanced stability of microtubules in conditions that normally cause disaggregation, such as cold temperatures or high concentrations of calcium.[144–146]

Resistance to taxol arises through the same two mechanisms involved in resistance to vinca alkaloids—i.e., multidrug resistance[147,148] and mutation of the gene coding for one of the tubulin subunits.[149] In the latter case it has been hypothesized that, in the absence of drugs, the equilibrium between free tubulin and microtubules is shifted toward disaggregation,[101] thereby endowing the mutant cells with slightly greater tolerance for taxol-induced stabilization than that of the parent cells. Some mutants were not only resistant to taxol, they required it for growth, presumably as a result of an extreme shift toward disaggregation. It was also observed that taxol-resistant tubulin mutants were more sensitive to colchicine or vinblastine than wild-type cells, consistent with the concept that the microtubules in these mutants are inherently unstable.

PHARMACOLOGY, CLINICAL USE, AND TOXICITY. The clinical development of taxol has been impeded by its scarcity and by the lack of a route for chemical synthesis. The major source of taxol is the bark of a slow-growing yew, *Taxus brevifolia*.[150] Unfortunately, the process of stripping bark for drug extraction of taxol kills the tree, and the yield of drug is relatively low. Although an alternative source has not been found for taxol, an analogous compound containing the same complex ring structure as taxol has been isolated from a more easily renewable source (needles of a related plant).[146] This analog (10-deacetyl baccatin III) can be used as starting material for the semisynthetic production of taxol and other, more water-soluble taxol analogs such as taxotere,[151]

Taxol

which has recently entered Phase I clinical trials.[81]

Taxol has been administered in both short (1–6-hour) and long (24-hour) infusions,[152] at doses of 200–300 mg/m². Because administration of these doses over the shorter time periods has been associated with severe hypersensitivity reactions (see below), it is currently recommended that 24-hour infusions be used.[81] Taxol binds extensively to plasma proteins (95–98%) and has an apparent volume of distribution far in excess of total body volume (55–182 L/m²).[81] Most studies have shown that taxol elimination follows biphasic kinetics, with a terminal half-life of about 5 hours.[81,153] Because very little taxol is recovered from urine as intact drug, it is presumed that its clearance is primarily metabolic.[81] Studies in rats indicate that hepatic conversion of taxol to hydroxylated metabolites may be a major mechanism of elimination.[154]

Although taxol is still in a relatively early stage of clinical development, it has been shown to be very active in the treatment of refractory ovarian cancer.[152,155] In one phase II study, taxol produced objective responses in 30% of patients who had received prior treatment.[155] Encouraging results have also been obtained in patients with metastatic breast cancer.[156] Neutropenia is the most common dose-limiting toxicity for taxol.[81] White-blood-cell counts typically reached a nadir at about 10–11 days and returned to normal levels at about 18 days posttreatment.[153] Another major toxicity in early studies was a hypersensitivity reaction characterized by dyspnea, urticaria, and hypotension.[157] It is not clear if these reactions were due to taxol or to the vehicle used to formulate the drug (polyoxyethylated castor oil, Cremophor EL). A number of measures have been recommended to minimize this toxicity, including avoidance of bolus injections or short infusions and premedication with antihistamines.[157] Severe mucositis, manifested as ulcerations of the mouth and throat, seems to be a cumulative effect of taxol administration.[152] Taxol causes some reversible neurotoxicities, most often numbness and paresthesias in the hands and feet.[152] A variety of cardiac abnormalities have also been associated with taxol treatment, including ventricular arrhythmias, bradycardia, and conduction blocks.[158] As with the hypersensitivity reactions, it is not clear whether these cardiac effects are caused by taxol or the vehicle used to solubilize it.

REFERENCES

1. L. Manuelidis and T. L. Chen: A unified model of eukaryotic chromosomes. *Cytometry* 11:8 (1990).

2. E. Schneider, Y. H. Hsiang, and L. F. Liu: DNA topoisomerases as anticancer drug targets. *Adv. Pharmacol.* 21:149 (1990).

3. W. Ross, T. Rowe, B. Glisson, J. Yalowich, and L. Liu: Role of topoisomerase II in mediating epipodophyllotoxin-induced DNA cleavage. *Cancer Res.* 44:5857 (1984).

4. B. H. Long, S. T. Musial, and M. G. Brattain: Single- and double-strand DNA breakage and repair in human lung adenocarcinoma cells exposed to etoposide and teniposide. *Cancer Res.* 45:3106 (1985).

5. P. J. Smith: DNA topoisomerase dysfunction: A new goal for antitumor chemotherapy. *Bioessays* 12:167 (1990).

6. D. A. Gewirtz: Does bulk damage to DNA explain the cytostatic and cytotoxic effects of topoisomerase II inhibitors? *Biochem. Pharmacol.* 42:2253 (1991).

7. R. B. Lock and W. E. Ross: Inhibition of p34^cdc2 kinase activity by etoposide or irradiation as a mechanism of G2 arrest in Chinese hamster ovary cells. *Cancer Res.* 50:3761 (1990).

8. R. S. Gupta: Genetic, biochemical, and cross-resistance studies with mutants of Chinese hamster ovary cells resistant to the anticancer drugs, VM-26 and VP16-213. *Cancer Res.* 43:1568 (1983).

9. B. K. Sinha, N. Haim, L. Dusre, D. Kerrigan, and Y. Pommier: DNA strand breaks produced by etoposide (VP-16,213) in sensitive and resistant human breast tumor cells: Implications for the mechanism of action. *Cancer Res.* 48:5096 (1988).

10. T. Lee and D. Roberts: Flux of teniposide (VM-26) across the plasma membrane of teniposide-resistant sublines of L1210 cells. *Cancer Res.* 44:2986 (1984).

11. P. M. Politi and B. K. Sinha: Role of differential drug uptake, efflux, and binding of etoposide in sensitive and resistant human tumor cell lines: Implications for the mechanisms of drug resistance. *Mol. Pharmacol.* 35:271 (1989).

12. E. Schurr, M. Raymond, J. C. Bell, and P. Gros: Characterization of the multidrug resistance protein expressed in cell clones stably transfected with the mouse mdr1 cDNA. *Cancer Res.* 49:2729 (1989).

13. M. K. Danks, J. C. Yalowich, and W. T. Beck: Atypical multiple drug resistance in a human leukemic cell line selected for resistance to teniposide (VM-26). *Cancer Res.* 47:1297 (1987).

14. D. M. Sullivan, M. D. Latham, T. C. Rowe, and W. E. Ross: Purification and characterization of an altered topoisomerase II from a drug-resistant Chinese hamster ovary cell line. *Biochemistry* 28:5680 (1989).

15. B. Glisson, R. Gupta, S. Smallwood-Kentro, and W. Ross: Characterization of acquired epipodophyllotoxin resistance in a Chinese hamster ovary cell line: Loss of drug-

stimulated DNA cleavage activity. *Cancer Res. 46:*1934 (1986).

16. B. Y. Bugg, M. K. Danks, W. T. Beck, and D. P. Suttle: Expression of a mutant DNA topoisomerase II in CCRF-CEM human leukemic cells selected for resistance to teniposide. *Proc. Natl. Acad. Sci. USA 88:*7654 (1991).

17. A. M. Deffie, D. J. Bosman, and G. J. Goldenberg: Evidence for a mutant allele of the gene for DNA topoisomerase II in adriamycin-resistant P388 murine leukemia cells. *Cancer Res. 49:*6879 (1989).

18. M. L. Slevin: The clinical pharmacology of etoposide. *Cancer 67:*319 (1991).

19. D. N. Carney: The pharmacology of intravenous and oral etoposide. *Cancer 67:*299 (1991).

20. P. I. Clark and M. L. Slevin: The clinical pharmacology of etoposide and teniposide. *Clin. Pharmacokinet.* 12:223 (1987).

21. L. M. Allen, C. Marks, and P. J. Creaven: 4'-Demethyl-epipodophyllic acid-9-(4,6-O-ethylidene-beta-D-glucopyranoside), the major urinary metabolite of VP 16-213 in man. *Proc. Am. Assoc. Cancer Res.* 17:6 (1976).

22. F. R. Pelsor, L. M. Allen, and P. J. Creaven: Multicompartment pharmacokinetic model of 4'-demethylepipodophyllotoxin 9-(4,6-O-ethylidene-beta-D-glucopyranoside) in humans. *J. Pharm. Sci.* 67:1106 (1978).

23. M. D'Incalci, C. Sessa, C. Rossi, G. Roviaro, and C. Mangioni: Pharmacokinetics of etoposide in gestochoriocarcinoma. *Cancer Treat. Rep.* 69:69 (1985).

24. J. Holthuis, M. Brouwer, P. Postmus, W. van Oort, A. Hulshoff, D. Sleijfer, H. Verleun and N. Mulder: Pharmacokinetics of high dose etoposide (VP-16). *Proc. Am. Soc. Clin. Oncol.* 5:29 (1986).

25. F. A. Greco: Future directions for etoposide therapy. *Cancer 67:*315 (1991).

26. B. F. Issell and S. T. Crooke: Etoposide (VP-16-213). *Cancer Treat. Rev.* 6:107 (1979).

27. J. Aisner and E. J. Lee: Etoposide. Current and future status. *Cancer 67*215 (1991).

28. P. J. Loehrer: Etoposide therapy for testicular cancer. *Cancer 67:*220 (1991).

29. E. S. Newlands and K. D. Bagshawe: Epipodophylin derivative (VP 16-23) in malignant teratomas and chonocarcinomas. *Lancet* 2:87 (1977).

30. F. M. Schabel, Jr., M. W. Trader, W. R. Laster, Jr., T. H. Corbett, and D. P. Griswold, Jr.: cis-Dichlorodiammineplatinum(II): Combination chemotherapy and cross-resistance studies with tumors of mice. *Cancer Treat. Rep.* 63:1459 (1979).

31. J. D. Hainsworth, S. D. Williams, L. H. Einhorn, R. Birch, and F. A. Greco: Successful treatment of resistant germinal neoplasms with VP-16 and cisplatin: Results of a Southeastern Cancer Study Group trial. *J. Clin. Oncol.* 3:666 (1985).

32. M. J. Peckham, A. Barrett, K. H. Liew, A. Horwich, B. Robinson, H. J. Dobbs, T. J. McElwain, and W. F. Hendry: The treatment of metastatic germ-cell testicular tumours with bleomycin, etoposide and cis-platin (BEP). *Br. J. Cancer* 47:613 (1983).

33. S. D. Williams, R. Birch, L. H. Einhorn, L. Irwin, F. A. Greco, and P. J. Loehrer: Treatment of disseminated germ-cell tumors with cisplatin, bleomycin, and either vinblastine or etoposide. *New Engl. J. Med.* 316:1435 (1987).

34. D. H. Johnson, J. D. Hainsworth, K. R. Hande, and F. A. Greco: Current status of etoposide in the management of small cell lung cancer. *Cancer 67:*231 (1991).

35. M. L. Slevin, P. I. Clark, S. P. Joel, S. Malik, R. J. Osborne, W. M. Gregory, D. G. Lowe, R. H. Reznek, and P. F. Wrigley: A randomized trial to evaluate the effect of schedule on the activity of etoposide in small-cell lung cancer. *J. Clin. Oncol.* 7:1333 (1989).

36. L. H. Einhorn, F. A. Greco, G. Wampler, J. Randolph, and Bristol-Myers Lung Cancer Study Group: Cytoxan (C), adriamycin (A), etoposide (E) versus cytoxan, adriamycin, vincristine (V) in the treatment of small cell lung cancer. *Proc. Am. Soc. Clin. Oncol.* 6:168 (1987).

37. W. K. Hong, C. Nicaise, R. Lawson, J. A. Maroun, R. Comis, J. Speer, D. Luedke, M. Hurtubise, V. Lanzotti, and J. Goodlow: Etoposide combined with cyclophosphamide plus vincristine compared with doxorubicin plus cyclophosphamide plus vincristine and with high-dose cyclophosphamide plus vincristine in the treatment of small-cell carcinoma of the lung: A randomized trial of the Bristol Lung Cancer Study Group: *J. Clin. Oncol.* 7:450 (1989).

38. R. H. Herzig: High-dose etoposide and marrow transplantation. *Cancer 67:*292 (1991).

39. M. H. Cohen, L. E. Broder, B. E. Fossieck, D. C. Ihde, and J. D. Minna: Phase II clinical trial of weekly administration of VP-16-213 in small cell bronchogenic carcinoma. *Cancer Treat. Rep.* 61:489 (1977).

40. M. Rozencweig, D. D. Von Hoff, J. E. Henney, and F. M. Muggia: VM 26 and VP 16-213: A comparative analysis. *Cancer* 40:334 (1977).

41. L. M. Allen: Comparison of uptake and binding of two epipodophyllotoxin glucopyranosides, 4'-demethyl epipodophyllotoxin thenylidene-beta-D- glucoside and 4'-demethyl epipodophyllotoxin ethylidene-beta-D- glucoside, in the L1210 leukemia cell. *Cancer Res.* 38:2549 (1978).

42. L. M. Allen, F. Tejada, A. D. Okonmah, and S. Nordqvist: Combination chemotherapy of the epipodophyllotoxin derivatives, teniposide and etoposide. A pharmacodynamic rationale? *Cancer Chemother. Pharmacol.* 7:151 (1982).

43. P. J. O'Dwyer, M. T. Alonso, B. Leyland-Jones, and S. Marsoni: Teniposide: A review of 12 years of experience. *Cancer Treat. Rep.* 68:1455 (1984).

44. F. A. Hayes, M. Abromowitch, and A. A. Green: Allergic reactions to teniposide in patients with neuroblastoma and lymphoid malignancies. *Cancer Treat. Rep.* 69:439 (1985).

45. L. A. Zwelling, S. Michaels, L. C. Erickson, R. S. Ungerleider, M. Nichols, and K. W. Kohn: Protein-associated deoxyribonucleic acid strand breaks in L1210 cells treated with the deoxyribonucleic acid intercalating agents 4'-(9-acridinylamino) methanesulfon-m-anisidide and adriamycin. *Biochemistry* 20:6553 (1981).

46. E. M. Nelson, K. M. Tewey, and L. F. Liu: Mechanism of antitumor drug action: Poisoning of mammalian DNA topoisomerase II on DNA by 4'-(9-acridinylamino)-methanesulfon-m-anisidide. *Proc. Natl. Acad. Sci. USA.* 81:1361 (1984).

47. J. Minford, Y. Pommier, J. Filipski, K. W. Kohn, D. Kerrigan, M. Mattern, S. Michaels, R. Schwartz, and L. A. Zwelling: Isolation of intercalator-dependent protein-

linked DNA strand cleavage activity from cell nuclei and identification as topoisomerase II. *Biochemistry 25:9* (1986).

48. M. Beran and B. S. Andersson: Development and characterization of a human myelogenous leukemia cell line resistant to 4'-(9-acridinylamino)—methanesulfon-m-anisidide. *Cancer Res. 47:1897* (1987).

49. L. A. Zwelling, M. Hinds, D. Chan, J. Mayes, K. L. Sie, E. Parker, L. Silberman, A. Radcliffe, M. Beran, and M. Blick: Characterization of an amsacrine-resistant line of human leukemia cells. Evidence for a drug-resistant form of topoisomerase II. *J. Biol. Chem. 264:16411* (1989).

50. M. Hinds, K. Deisseroth, J. Mayes, E. Altschuler, R. Jansen, F. D. Ledley, and L. A. Zwelling: Identification of a point mutation in the topoisomerase II gene from a human leukemia cell line containing an amsacrine-resistant form of topoisomerase II. *Cancer Res. 51:4729* (1991).

51. L. A. Zwelling: Topoisomerase II as a target of antileukemia drugs: A review of controversial areas. *Hematol. Pathol. 3:101* (1989).

52. L. A. Zwelling, J. Mayes, M. Hinds, D. Chan, E. Altschuler, B. Carroll, E. Parker, K. Deisseroth, A. Radcliffe, and M. Seligman: Cross-resistance of an amsacrine-resistant human leukemia line to topoisomerase II reactive DNA intercalating agents. Evidence for two topoisomerase II directed drug actions. *Biochemistry 30:4048* (1991).

53. L. A. Zwelling, M. J. Mitchell, P. Satitpunwaycha, J. Mayes, E. Altschuler, M. Hinds, and B. C. Baguley: Relative activity of structural analogues of amsacrine against human leukemia cell lines containing amsacrine-sensitive or -resistant forms of topoisomerase II: Use of computer simulations in new drug development. *Cancer Res. 52:209* (1992).

54. P. A. Cassileth and R. P. Gale: Amsacrine: A review. *Leuk. Res. 10:1257* (1986).

55. A. W. Dekker, H. K. Nieuwenhuis, and L. F. Verdonck: Intermediate-dose cytosine arabinoside and amsacrine. An effective regimen with low toxicity in refractory acute nonlymphocytic leukemia. *Cancer 65:1891* (1990).

56. R. S. Stein, W. R. Vogler, E. F. Winton, H. J. Cohen, M. R. Raney, and A. Bartolucci: Therapy of acute myelogenous leukemia in patients over the age of 50: A randomized Southeastern Cancer Study Group trial. *Leuk. Res. 14:895* (1990).

57. Z. A. Arlin, E. J. Feldman, A. Mittelman, T. Ahmed, C. Puccio, H. G. Chun, P. Cook, P. Baskind, C. Marboe, and R. Mehta: Amsacrine is safe and effective therapy for patients with myocardial dysfunction and acute leukemia. *Cancer 68:1198* (1991).

58. J. Hornedo and D. A. Van Echo: Amsacrine (m-AMSA): A new antineoplastic agent. Pharmacology, clinical activity and toxicity. *Pharmacotherapy 5:78* (1985).

59. R. L. Cysyk, D. Shoemaker, and R. H. Adamson: The pharmacologic disposition of 4'-(9-acridinylamino)methanesulfon-m-anisidide in mice and rats. *Drug Metab. Dispos. 5:579* (1977).

60. S. W. Hall, J. Friedman, S. S. Legha, R. S. Benjamin, J. U. Gutterman, and T. L. Loo: Human pharmacokinetics of a new acridine derivative, 4'-(9-acridinylamino)methanesulfon-m-anisidide (NSC 249992). *Cancer Res. 43:3422* (1983).

61. D. A. Van Echo, D. F. Chiuten, P. E. Gormley, J. L. Lichtenfeld, M. Scoltock, and P. H. Wiernik: Phase I clinical and pharmacological study of 4'-(9-acridinylamino)-methanesulfon-m-anisidide using an intermittent biweekly schedule. *Cancer Res. 39:3881* (1979).

62. D. D. Von Hoff, D. Elson, G. Polk, and C. Coltman, Jr.: Acute ventricular fibrillation and death during infusion of 4'-(9-acridinylamino)methanesulfon-m-anisidide (AMSA). *Cancer Treat. Rep. 64:356* (1980).

63. L. F. Liu and P. D'Arpa: Topoisomerase-targeting antitumor drugs: Mechanisms of cytotoxicity and resistance. *Important Adv. Oncol. 79* (1992).

64. M. E. Wall, M. C. Wani, C. E. Cook, K. H. Palmer, A. T. McPhail, and G. A. Sim: Plant antitumor agents. I. The isolation and structure of camptothecin, a novel alkaloidal and tumor inhibitor from *Camptotheca acuminata*. *J. Am. Chem. Soc. 88:3888* (1966).

65. B. A. Chabner: Camptothecins. *J. Clin. Oncol. 10:3* (1992).

66. T. Kunimoto, K. Nitta, T. Tanaka, N. Uehara, H. Baba, M. Takeuchi, T. Yokokura, S. Sawada, T. Miyasaka, and M. Mutai: Antitumor activity of 7-ethyl-10-[4-(1-piperidino)-1-piperidino]carbonyloxy-camptothecin, a novel water-soluble derivative of camptothecin, against murine tumors. *Cancer Res. 47:5944* (1987).

67. Y. H. Hsiang, R. Hertzberg, S. Hecht, and L. F. Liu: Camptothecin induces protein-linked DNA breaks via mammalian DNA topoisomerase I. *J. Biol. Chem. 260:14873* (1985).

68. Y. H. Hsiang and L. F. Liu: Identification of mammalian DNA topoisomerase I as an intracellular target of the anticancer drug camptothecin. *Cancer Res. 48:1722* (1988).

69. J. M. Covey, C. Jaxel, K. W. Kohn, and Y. Pommier: Protein-linked DNA strand breaks induced in mammalian cells by camptothecin, an inhibitor of topoisomerase I. *Cancer Res. 49:5016* (1989).

70. Y. H. Hsiang, M. G. Lihou, and L. F. Liu: Arrest of replication forks by drug-stabilized topoisomerase I-DNA cleavable complexes as a mechanism of cell killing by camptothecin. *Cancer Res. 49:5077* (1989).

71. Y. Sugimoto, S. Tsukahara, T. Oh-hara, T. Isoe, and T. Tsuruo: Decreased expression of DNA topoisomerase I in camptothecin-resistant tumor cell lines as determined by a monoclonal antibody. *Cancer Res. 50:6925* (1990).

72. W. K. Eng, F. L. McCabe, K. B. Tan, M. R. Mattern, G. A. Hofmann, R. D. Woessner, R. P. Hertzberg, and R. K. Johnson: Development of a stable camptothecin-resistant subline of P388 leukemia with reduced topoisomerase I content. *Mol. Pharmacol. 38:471* (1990).

73. T. Andoh, K. Ishii, Y. Suzuki, Y. Ikegami, Y. Kusunoki, Y. Takemoto, and K. Okada: Characterization of a mammalian mutant with a camptothecin-resistant DNA topoisomerase I. *Proc. Natl. Acad. Sci. USA 84:5565* (1987).

74. R. S. Gupta, R. Gupta, B. Eng, R. B. Lock, W. E. Ross, R. P. Hertzberg, M. J. Caranfa, and R. K. Johnson: Camptothecin-resistant mutants of Chinese hamster ovary cells containing a resistant form of topoisomerase I. *Cancer Res. 48:6404* (1988).

75. N. Kaneda and T. Yokokura: Nonlinear pharmacokinetics of CPT-11 in rats. *Cancer Res. 50:1721* (1990).

76. N. Kaneda, H. Nagata, T. Furuta, and T. Yokokura: Metabolism and pharmacokinetics of the camptothecin analogue CPT-11 in the mouse. *Cancer Res. 50:1715* (1990).

77. S. Negoro, M. Fukuoka, N. Masuda, M. Takada, Y. Kusunoki, K. Matsui, N. Takifuji, S. Kudoh, H. Niitani, and T. Taguchi: Phase I study of weekly intravenous infusions of CPT-11, a new derivative of camptothecin, in the treatment of advanced non-small-cell lung cancer. *J. Natl. Cancer Inst.* 83:1164 (1991).

78. M. Fukuoka, H. Niitani, A. Suzuki, M. Motomiya, K. Hasegawa, Y. Nishiwaki, T. Kuriyama, Y. Ariyoshi, S. Negoro, and N. Masuda: A phase II study of CPT-11, a new derivative of camptothecin, for previously untreated non-small-cell lung cancer. *J. Clin. Oncol.* 10:16 (1992).

79. R. Ohno, K. Okada, T. Masaoka, A. Kuramoto, T. Arima, Y. Yoshida, H. Ariyoshi, M. Ichimaru, Y. Sakai, and M. Oguro: An early phase II study of CPT-11: A new derivative of camptothecin, for the treatment of leukemia and lymphoma. *J. Clin. Oncol.* 8:1907 (1990).

80. B. Alberts, D. Bray, J., Lewis, M. Raff, K. Roberts, and J. D. Watson: *Molecular Biology of the Cell,* 2nd ed. New York: Garland Publishing, 1989, pp. 652–661.

81. E. K. Rowinsky and R. C. Donehower: The clinical pharmacology and use of antimicrotubule agents in cancer chemotherapeutics. *Pharmacol. Ther.* 52:35 (1991).

82. L. Margulis: Colchicine-sensitive microtubules. *Int. Rev. Cytol.* 34:333 (1973).

83. L. Wilson, K. M. Creswell, and D. Chin: The mechanism of action of vinblastine. Binding of [acetyl-3H]vinblastine to embryonic chick brain tubulin and tubulin from sea urchin sperm tail outer doublet microtubules. *Biochemistry* 14:5586 (1975).

84. F. Mandelbaum-Shavit, M. K. Wolpert-DeFilippes, and D. G. Johns: Binding of maytansine to rat brain tubulin. *Biochem. Biophys. Res. Commun.* 72:47 (1976).

85. K. G. Bensch and S. E. Malawista: Microtubular crystals in mammalian cells. *J. Cell Biol.* 40:95 (1969).

86. J. Bryan: Vinblastine and microtubules. II. Characterization of two protein subunits from the isolated crystals. *J. Mol. Biol.* 66:157 (1972).

87. G. C. Na and S. N. Timasheff: Interaction of vinblastine with calf brain tubulin: Multiple equilibria. *Biochemistry* 25:6214 (1986).

88. W. D. Singer, R. T. Hersh, and R. H. Himes: Effect of solution variables on the binding of vinblastine to tubulin. *Biochem. Pharmacol.* 37:2691 (1988).

89. G. C. Na and S. N. Timasheff: Interaction of vinblastine with calf brain tubulin: Effects of magnesium ions. *Biochemistry* 25:6222 (1986).

90. J. A. Donoso, K. M. Haskins, and R. H. Himes: Effect of microtubule-associated proteins on the interaction of vincristine with microtubules and tubulin. *Cancer Res.* 39:1604 (1979).

91. L. C. Bowman, J. A. Houghton, and P. J. Houghton: Formation and stability of vincristine-tubulin complex in kidney cytosols. Role of GTP and GTP hydrolysis. *Biochem. Pharmacol.* 37:1251 (1988).

92. L. C. Bowman, J. A. Houghton, and P. J. Houghton: GTP influences the binding of vincristine in human tumor cytosols. *Biochem. Biophys. Res. Commun.* 135:695 (1986).

93. J. A. Houghton, L. G. Williams, and P. J. Houghton: Stability of vincristine complexes in cytosols derived from xenografts of human rhabdomyosarcoma and normal tissues of the mouse. *Cancer Res.* 45:3761 (1985).

94. P. J. Houghton, J. A. Houghton, L. C. Bowman, and B. J. Hazelton: Therapeutic selectivity of vinca alkaloids: A

role for guanosine 5′-triphosphate? *Anticancer Drug Des.* 2:165 (1987).

95. K. H. Choi, C. J. Chen, M. Kriegler, and I. B. Roninson: An altered pattern of cross-resistance in multidrug-resistant human cells results from spontaneous mutations in the mdr1 (P-glycoprotein) gene. *Cell* 53:519 (1988).

96. S. Akiyama, M. M. Cornwell, M. Kuwano, I. Pastan, and M. M. Gottesman: Most drugs that reverse multidrug resistance also inhibit photoaffinity labeling of P-glycoprotein by a vinblastine analog. *Mol. Pharmacol.* 33:144 (1988).

97. T. Tsuruo, H. Iida, K. Naganuma, S. Tsukagoshi, and Y. Sakurai: Promotion by verapamil of vincristine responsiveness in tumor cell lines inherently resistant to the drug. *Cancer Res.* 43:808 (1983).

98. W. S. Dalton, T. M. Grogan, P. S. Meltzer, R. J. Scheper, B. G. Durie, C. W. Taylor, T. P. Miller, and S. E. Salmon: Drug-resistance in multiple myeloma and non-Hodgkin's lymphoma: Detection of P-glycoprotein and potential circumvention by addition of verapamil to chemotherapy. *J. Clin. Oncol.* 7:415 (1989).

99. A. Gruber, C. Peterson, and P. Reizenstein: D-verapamil and L-verapamil are equally effective in increasing vincristine accumulation in leukemic cells in vitro. *Int. J. Cancer* 41:224 (1988).

100. V. Ling, J. E. Aubin, A. Chase, and F. Sarangi: Mutants of Chinese hamster ovary (CHO) cells with altered colcemid-binding affinity. *Cell* 18:423 (1979).

101. F. R. Cabral, R. C. Brady, and M. J. Schibler: A mechanism of cellular resistance to drugs that interfere with microtubule assembly. *Ann. N.Y. Acad. Sci.* 466:745 (1986).

102. F. Cabral and S. B. Barlow: Resistance to antimitotic agents as genetic probes of microtubule structure and function. *Pharmacol. Ther.* 52:159 (1991).

103. F. Cabral and S. B. Barlow: Mechanisms by which mammalian cells acquire resistance to drugs that affect microtubule assembly. *FASEB J.* 3:1593 (1989).

104. D. V. Jackson, Jr.: "The Periwinkle Alkaloids," in *Cancer Chemotherapy by Infusion,* ed. by J. J. Lokich. Chicago: Precept Press, 1990, pp. 155–175.

105. R. L. Nelson: The comparative clinical pharmacology and pharmacokinetics of vindesine, vincristine, and vinblastine in human patients with cancer. *Med. Pediatr. Oncol.* 10:115 (1982).

106. R. J. Owellen, C. A. Hartke, and F. O. Hains: Pharmacokinetics and metabolism of vinblastine in humans. *Cancer Res.* 37:2597 (1977).

107. R. J. Owellen, M. A. Root, and F. O. Hains: Pharmacokinetics of vindesine and vincristine in humans. *Cancer Res.* 37:2603 (1977).

108. D. V. Jackson, Jr., V. S. Sethi, C. L. Spurr, and J. M. McWhorter: Pharmacokinetics of vincristine in the cerebrospinal fluid of humans. *Cancer Res.* 41:1466 (1981).

109. R. A. Bender, M. C. Castle, D. A. Margileth, and V. T. Oliverio: The pharmacokinetics of [3H]-vincristine in man. *Clin. Pharmacol. Ther.* 22:430 (1977).

110. D. V. Jackson, Jr., M. C. Castle, and R. A. Bender: Biliary excretion of vincristine. *Clin. Pharmacol. Ther.* 24:101 (1978).

111. R. Rahmani, J. P. Kleisbauer, J. P. Cano, M. Martin, and J. Barbet: Clinical pharmacokinetics of vindesine infusion. *Cancer Treat. Rep.* 69:839 (1985).

112. K. Hande, J. Gay, J. Gober, and F. A. Greco: Toxicity and pharmacology of bolus vindesine injection and prolonged vindesine infusion. *Cancer Treat. Rev.* 7 (Suppl. 1):25 (1980).

113. R. Willemze, A. M. Drenthe-Schonke, J. van Rossum, and C. Haanen: Treatment of acute lymphoblastic leukaemia in adolescents and adults. *Scand. J. Haematol.* 24:421 (1980).

114. J. A. Ortega, M. E. Nesbit, Jr., M. H. Donaldson, R. E. Hittle, J. Weiner, M. Karon, and D. Hammond: L-Asparaginase, vincristine, and prednisone for induction of first remission in acute lymphocytic leukemia. *Cancer Res.* 37:535 (1977).

115. D. L. Longo, R. C. Young, M. Wesley, S. M. Hubbard, P. L. Duffey, E. S. Jaffe, and V. T. DeVita, Jr.: Twenty years of MOPP therapy for Hodgkin's disease. *J. Clin. Oncol.* 4:1295 (1986).

116. G. Bonadonna, P. Valagussa, and A. Santoro: Alternating non-cross-resistant combination chemotherapy or MOPP in stage IV Hodgkin's disease. A report of 8-year results. *Ann. Intern. Med.* 104:739 (1986).

117. D. L. Longo, V. T. DeVita, Jr., P. L. Duffey, M. N. Wesley, D. C. Ihde, S. M. Hubbard, M. Gilliom, E. S. Jaffe, J. Cossman, and R. I. Fisher: Superiority of ProMACE-CytaBOM over ProMACE-MOPP in the treatment of advanced diffuse aggressive lymphoma: Results of a prospective randomized trial. *J. Clin. Oncol.* 9:25 (1991).

118. D. H. Johnson, L. H. Einhorn, R. Birch, R. Vollmer, C. Perez, S. Krauss, G. Omura, and F. A. Greco: A randomized comparison of high-dose versus conventional-dose cyclophosphamide, doxorubicin, and vincristine for extensive-stage small-cell lung cancer: A phase III trial of the Southeastern Cancer Study Group. *J. Clin. Oncol.* 5:1731 (1987).

119. *Handbook of Cancer Chemotherapy*, ed. by R. T. Skeel. Boston: Little, Brown and Company, 1991, pp. 136–138.

120. S. G. Sandler, W. Tobin, and E. S. Henderson: Vincristine-induced neuropathy. A clinical study of fifty leukemic patients. *Neurology* 19:367 (1969).

121. S. Rosenthal and S. Kaufman: Vincristine neurotoxicity. *Ann. Intern. Med.* 80:733 (1974).

122. R. S. Kaplan and P. H. Wiernik: Neurotoxicity of antineoplastic drugs. *Semin. Oncol.* 9:103 (1982).

123. D. V. Jackson, H. B. Wells, J. N. Atkins, P. J. Zekan, D. R. White, F. Richards, J. M. Cruz, and H. B. Muss: Amelioration of vincristine neurotoxicity by glutamic acid. *Am. J. Med.* 84:1016 (1988).

124. D. V. Jackson, Jr., D. L. Rosenbaum, L. J. Carlisle, T. R. Long, H. B. Wells, and C. L. Spurr: Glutamic acid modification of vincristine toxicity. *Cancer Biochem. Biophys.* 7:245 (1984).

125. E. Hamel and C. M. Lin: Glutamate-induced polymerization of tubulin: Characteristics of the reaction and application to the large-scale purification of tubulin. *Arch. Biochem. Biophys.* 209:29 (1981).

126. R. L. Byrd, T. M. Rohrbaugh, R. B. Raney, Jr., and D. G. Norris: Transient cortical blindness secondary to vincristine therapy in childhood malignancies. *Cancer* 47:37 (1981).

127. S. B. Sutcliffe, P. F. Wrigley, J. Peto, T. A. Lister, A. G. Stansfeld, J. M. Whitehouse, D. Crowther, and J. S. Malpas: MVPP chemotherapy regimen for advanced Hodgkin's disease. *Br. Med. J.* 1:679 (1978).

128. C. H. Diggs, P. H. Wiernik, J. A. Levi, and L. K. Kvols: Cyclophosphamide, vinblastine, procarbazine and prednisone with CCNU and vinblastine maintenance for advanced Hodgkin's disease. *Cancer* 39:1949 (1977).

129. A. Santoro, G. Bonadonna, V. Bonfante, and P. Valagussa: Alternating drug combinations in the treatment of advanced Hodgkin's disease. *New Engl. J. Med.* 306:770 (1982).

130. G. Palmieri, R. Lauria, F. Caponigro, C. Pagliarulo, V. Montesarchio, F. Nuzzo, C. Gridelli, and A. R. Bianco: Salvage chemotherapy for non Hodgkin's lymphoma of unfavourable histology with a combination of CCNU and vinblastine. *Hematol. Oncol.* 8:179 (1990).

131. D. V. Jackson, Jr., C. L. Spurr, M. E. Caponera, D. R. White, H. B. Muss, M. D. Pavy, G. P. Sartiano, P. J. Zekan, and E. A. Hire: Vinblastine infusion in non-Hodgkin's lymphomas: Lack of total cross-resistance with vincristine. *Cancer Invest.* 5:535 (1987).

132. G. C. Garrow and D. H. Johnson: Treatment of "good risk" metastatic testicular cancer. *Semin. Oncol.* 19:159 (1992).

133. S. D. Williams, J. A. Blessing, D. H. Moore, H. D. Homesley, and L. Adcock: Cisplatin, vinblastine, and bleomycin in advanced and recurrent ovarian germ-cell tumors. A trial of the Gynecologic Oncology Group. *Ann. Intern. Med.* 111:22 (1989).

134. M. H. Taylor, A. D. Depetrillo, and A. R. Turner: Vinblastine, bleomycin, and cisplatin in malignant germ cell tumors of the ovary. *Cancer* 56:1341 (1985).

135. R. J. Cersosimo, R. Bromer, J. T. Licciardello, and W. K. Hong: Pharmacology, clinical efficacy and adverse effects of vindesine sulfate, a new vinca alkaloid. *Pharmacotherapy* 3:259 (1983).

136. G. Mathe, J. L. Misset, F. De Vassal, J. Gouveia, M. Hayat, D. Machover, D. Belpomme, J. L. Pico, L. Schwarzenberg, P. Ribaud, M. Musset, C. Jasmin, and L. De Luca: Phase II clinical trial with vindesine for remission induction in acute leukemia, blastic crisis of chronic myeloid leukemia, lymphosarcoma, and Hodgkin's disease: Absence of cross-resistance with vincristine. *Cancer Treat. Rep.* 62:805 (1978).

137. R. L. Woods, C. J. Williams, J. Levi, J. Page, D. Bell, M. Byrne, and Z. L. Kerestes: A randomised trial of cisplatin and vindesine versus supportive care only in advanced non-small cell lung cancer. *Br. J. Cancer* 61:608 (1990).

138. S. Niitamo-Korhonen, P. Holsti, L. R. Holsti, S. Pyrhonen, and K. Mattson: A comparison of cis-platinum-vindesine and cis-platinum-etoposide combined with radiotherapy for previously untreated localized inoperable non-small cell lung cancer. *Eur. J. Cancer Clin. Oncol.* 25:1039 (1989).

139. P. B. Schiff, J. Fant, L. A. Auster and S. B. Horwitz: Effects of taxol on cell growth and in vitro microtubule assembly. *J. Supramolec. Struct.* 8 (Suppl. 2):328 (1978).

140. P. B. Schiff and S. B. Horwitz: Taxol stabilizes microtubules in mouse fibroblast cells. *Proc. Natl. Acad. Sci. USA* 77:1561 (1980).

141. P. B. Schiff, J. Fant, and S. B. Horwitz: Promotion of microtubule assembly in vitro by taxol. *Nature* 277:665 (1979).

142. E. K. Rowinsky, R. C. Donehower, R. J. Jones, and R. W. Tucker: Microtubule changes and cytotoxicity in leukemic cell lines treated with taxol. *Cancer Res. 48:*4093 (1988).

143. J. Parness and S. B. Horwitz: Taxol binds to polymerized tubulin in vitro. *J. Cell Biol. 91:*479 (1981).

144. N. Kumar: Taxol-induced polymerization of purified tubulin. Mechanism of action. *J. Biol. Chem. 256:*10435 (1981).

145. P. B. Schiff and S. B. Horwitz: Taxol assembles tubulin in the absence of exogenous guanosine 5'-triphosphate or microtubule-associated proteins. *Biochemistry 20:*3247 (1981).

146. S. B. Horwitz: Mechanisms of action of taxol. *Trends. Pharmacol. Sci. 13:*134 (1992).

147. S. N. Roy and S. B. Horwitz: A phosphoglycoprotein associated with taxol resistance in J774.2 cells. *Cancer Res. 45:*3856 (1985).

148. L. M. Greenberger, S. S. Williams, and S. B. Horwitz: Biosynthesis of heterogeneous forms of multidrug resistance-associated glycoproteins. *J. Biol. Chem. 262:*13685 (1987).

149. M. J. Schibler and F. Cabral: Taxol-dependent mutants of Chinese hamster ovary cells with alterations in alpha- and beta-tubulin. *J. Cell Biol. 102:*1522 (1986).

150. M. C. Wani, H. L. Taylor, M. E. Wall, P. Coggon, and A. T. McPhail: Plant antitumor agents VI. The isolation and structure of taxol, a novel antileukemic and antitumor agent from *taxus brevifolia. J. Am. Chem. Soc. 93:*2325 (1971).

151. I. Ringel and S. B. Horwitz: Studies with RP 56976 (taxotere): A semisynthetic analogue of taxol. *J. Natl. Cancer Inst. 83:*288 (1991).

152. E. K. Rowinsky, L. A. Cazenave, and R. C. Donehower: Taxol: A novel investigational antimicrotubule agent. *J. Natl. Cancer Inst. 82:*1247 (1990).

153. P. H. Wiernik, E. L. Schwartz, J. J. Strauman, J. P. Dutcher, R. B. Lipton, and E. Paietta: Phase I clinical and pharmacokinetic study of taxol. *Cancer Res. 47:*2486 (1987).

154. B. Monsarrat, E. Mariel, S. Cros, M. Gares, D. Guenard, F. Gueritte-Voegelein, and M. Wright: Taxol metabolism. Isolation and identification of three major metabolites of taxol in rat bile. *Drug Metab. Dispos. 18:*895 (1990).

155. W. P. McGuire, E. K. Rowinsky, N. B. Rosenshein, F. C. Grumbine, D. S. Ettinger, D. K. Armstrong, and R. C. Donehower: Taxol: A unique antineoplastic agent with significant activity in advanced ovarian epithelial neoplasms. *Ann. Intern. Med. 111:*273 (1989).

156. F. A. Holmes, R. S. Walters, R. L. Theriault, A. D. Forman, L. K. Newton, M. N. Raber, A. U. Buzdar, D. K. Frye, and G. N. Hortobagyi: Phase II trial of taxol, an active drug in the treatment of metastatic breast cancer. *J. Natl. Cancer Inst. 83:*1797 (1991).

157. R. B. Weiss, R. C. Donehower, P. H. Wiernik, T. Ohnuma, R. J. Gralla, D. L. Trump, J. R. Baker, Jr., D. A. Van Echo, D. D. Von Hoff, and B. Leyland-Jones: Hypersensitivity reactions from taxol. *J. Clin. Oncol. 8:*1263 (1990).

158. E. K. Rowinsky, W. P. McGuire, T. Guarnieri, J. S. Fisherman, M. C. Christian, and R. C. Donehower: Cardiac disturbances during the administration of taxol. *J. Clin. Oncol. 9:*1704 (1991).

CHAPTER 9

Drugs Affecting Endocrine Function

GLUCOCORTICOIDS
  Prednisone
  Prednisolone
ESTROGENS
  Diethylstilbestrol (DES)
  Ethinyl Estradiol
ANTIESTROGENS
  Tamoxifen
PROGESTINS
  Medroxyprogesterone
  Megestrol

ANDROGENS
  Fluoxymestrone
  Testosterone
ANTIANDROGENS
  Cyproterone Acetate
  Flutamide
LHRH (GnRH) AGONISTS
  Goserelin
  Leuprolide
AROMATASE INHIBITORS
  Aminoglutethimide
ADRENOCORTICAL SUPPRESSORS
  Mitotane (o, p′-DDD)

Rationale for Steroid Therapy

The growth of several types of tumors can be modified by treatment with steroid hormones or their antagonists. In the case of the sex steroids (estrogens, progestins, androgens), the responding tumors arise from sexually differentiated tissues (breast, endometrium, prostate) that normally contain hormone receptors and respond physiologically to hormone. In some cases, tumors are hormone-responsive in the sense that treatment with a cognate hormone for that tissue inhibits the rate of tumor growth. Examples are the use of estrogens to treat some tumors of the breast and progestins to treat tumors of the endometrium. In other cases, tumors may be hormone-dependent, and therapy focuses on removing the major hormone-producing organ (ovariectomy or orchiectomy), on preventing hormone synthesis at other sites (e.g., by administering aromatase inhibitors), and on blocking endogenous hormone action on the tumor cell by treatment with antihormones.

Another class of steroid hormones, the glucocorticoids, have a lymphocytolytic effect that makes them very useful in the combined drug treatment of acute and chronic lymphocytic leukemias, Hodgkin's disease, and non-Hodgkin's lymphoma. The lymphocyte killing effect of glucocorticoids occurs when they are administered at doses that are higher than those required to achieve normal physiologic plasma concentrations of hormone—so-called *pharmacologic* as opposed to *physiologic* doses.

Carcinoma of the Prostate

The use of endocrine therapy in the treatment of prostate cancer was largely the result of the observation, by Huggins and Clark[1] in 1940, that castration or estrogen administration shrank the hyperplastic prostate gland in the dog. In a series of papers published in 1941, Huggins and his coworkers demonstrated the effectiveness of these procedures in the treatment of prostatic cancer in man.[2,3,4] The observation that castration and estrogen administration was effective in the treatment of prostatic carcinoma was preceded by the demonstration of the importance of the androgenic steroids in maintaining normal prostate size and function. Thus, it had been shown, again by Huggins and his coworkers,[5] that castration is followed by marked involution of the normal prostate gland and that this can be reversed by androgen administration.

Today, the principal hormonal approach to prostatic cancer is to decrease androgen production by the administration of an estrogen or an LHRH (GnRH) analog (e.g., leuprolide or goserelin) and simultaneously to block androgen stimulation of growth by administering an antiandrogen (e.g., flutamide). Estrogens (primarily diethylstilbestrol) are administered because they have been shown to markedly decrease plasma testosterone levels.[6] Administration of estrogens to males inhibits the production of luteinizing hormone (LH) by the anterior pituitary,[6,7] and since LH promotes testosterone production by the Leydig cells of the testis, estrogens indirectly prevent the synthesis of androgens, thus eliminating androgen stimulation of prostatic growth. The relationships between LHRH (GnRH), LH, and sex hormone secretion are illustrated in Figure 9–1. Hormone therapy in patients with cancer of the prostate is never curative, but 40–70% of patients with disseminated disease experience at least relief from symptoms with androgen-suppressive therapy.[8]

Carcinoma of the Breast

The use of hormones in cancer therapy is largely empirical. This is certainly the case for hormone treatment of cancer of the breast, where estrogens can both promote and inhibit tissue growth. Adenocarcinoma of the breast, the most common cancer of women in North America and Europe (see Fig. 1–1), was the first tumor to be treated by manipulating steroid

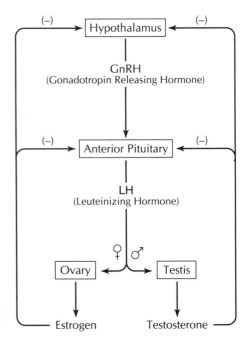

Figure 9–1 Regulation of sex hormone production. GnRH (gonadotropin releasing hormone; also called LHRH for luteinizing hormone releasing hormone) released from the hypothalamus stimulates the release of LH (luteinizing hormone) from the anterior pituitary. In the male, LH stimulates the production of testosterone by the Leydig cells of the testis. In the female, LH stimulates the thecal cells of the ovary to produce androgens, which diffuse into the granulosa cells where they are converted to estrogen under the influence of FSH (follicle stimulating hormone). Both testosterone and estrogen that are secreted into the general circulation, as well as these hormones when administered to the patient as drugs, inhibit the production of GnRH (LHRH) and LH by the hypothalamus and anterior pituitary, respectively (negative feedback effect denoted by negative signs in parentheses).

hormone levels. The initial report by Beatson[9] in 1896 describes the clinical courses of three breast cancer patients who benefited from removal of the ovaries. Removal of a hormone source, as in ovariectomy, is often called "ablative" therapy, whereas the administration of hormones, as in steroid therapy in breast cancer patients, is called "additive" therapy.

The association between estrogens and mammary tumorigenesis was first established in 1932 by Lacassagne, who produced breast tumors in male mice by injecting them with estrone.[10] The effect of estrogens on tumor growth has been examined in considerable detail in experimental animal systems, but therapy of human breast cancer developed in an essentially empirical manner after Haddow *et al.*[11] demonstrated in 1944 that administration of high doses of estrogen benefits some patients with breast cancer. Estrogens were subsequently shown to have a palliative effect in postmenopausal patients with breast cancer, but they are not effective in premenopausal patients. Because of their toxicity, estrogens are used only rarely in modern therapy, which focuses largely on efforts to combat the tumor-growth-promoting effects of the patient's endogenous estrogens.[12]

The most commonly used drug in the hormonal therapy of breast cancer is tamoxifen, which has a direct antiestrogenic effect on the tumor cell. Tamoxifen is used both in adjuvant therapy of early breast cancer and for treatment of metastatic disease in postmenopausal women. In a secondary approach, either progestins or the aromatase inhibitor aminoglutethimide may be administered in order to block the patient's endogenous estrogen production. Progestins, such as megestrol acetate, and medroxyprogesterone acetate, are as active in metastatic breast cancer as tamoxifen,[13] but they are generally employed as second- or third-line treatment. Because of their virilizing effects, androgens are now used only rarely.

Endometrial Cancer

Kelley and Baker[14] were the first to report (1961) the beneficial effects of progestins in patients with endometrial carcinoma. The relationship of sex hormones to the genesis of human endometrial cancer is not well defined, but on the basis of the coexistence of endometrial hyperplasia and endometrial carcinoma, it was suggested as early as 1949 that this tumor could be related to overstimulation by estrogens.[15] Subsequently, it was shown that the administration of large amounts of estrogen produces endometrial carcinoma in rabbits.[16] Endometrial carcinoma can also be induced in the rabbit by 3-methylcholanthrene. This tumor induction is estrogen-dependent, and it is prevented by progestins.[17] Progestins also

cause established carcinomas to regress.[17] Progesterone, which is normally produced by the corpus luteum after ovulation, causes the endometrium to mature into the secretory state. The action of progestins in treating endometrial cancer presumably reflects such a direct action in this normal target tissue. Progestins are used to treat advanced, progressing endometrial carcinoma that can no longer be treated by surgery or radiation therapy. About 35% of patients respond to progestin treatment and the responders survive an average of 27 months, four times longer than the nonresponders.[18] Patients with well-differentiated tumors are more apt to respond.

Leukemias and Lymphomas

Unlike the sex hormones, which act on a selected group of target tissues, corticosteroids of the glucocorticoid type act on a wide variety of tissues and organs.[19] Indeed, there is good reason to suggest that nearly all cells may be targets for the glucocorticoids *in vivo*. The physiological effects of the glucocorticoids vary widely according to cell type; in lymphoid tissues, they induce cell death.[20] In 1938, Ingle[21] noted that adrenocorticotrophin caused involution of the thymus in rats; this was followed by the observations of Dougherty and White,[22] in the early 1940s, that adrenocortical extracts caused degeneration of lymphocytes and involution of other lymphoid structures. Heilman and Kendall[23] were the first to report (1944) the antitumor effects of the glucocorticoids when they demonstrated that oral cortisone produced dramatic but temporary remission in mice bearing a transplantable lymphosarcoma. Subsequently, Pearson *et al.*[24] initiated cortisone therapy in several patients with lymphomatous tumors and short-term, partial remissions were observed. The effectiveness of glucocorticoid therapy in the treatment of acute lymphoblastic leukemia of childhood was definitively established in the early 1950s.[25]

Acute lymphoblastic leukemia is the cancer most responsive to glucocorticoid therapy, and prednisone has an established role in the induction of remission in this disease. Complete remission is induced in about 60% of patients receiving initial therapy,[26] and this increases to nearly 100% with the use of two or four drugs

Table 9–1   Percent of Patients With Acute Lymphocytic Leukemia or Hodgkin's Disease Achieving Complete Remissions With Single or Combination Drug Therapy. (Adapted from DeVita *et al.*[26])

Disease	Treatment	Percent of Patients Achieving Complete Remissions
Acute lymphocytic leukemia of childhood	Methotrexate	22
	6-Mercaptopurine	27
	Prednisone	63
	Cyclophosphamide	40
	Vincristine	57
	Daunorubicin	38
	Asparaginase	67
	Prednisone + vincristine	90
	Vincristine + prednisone + methotrexate + 6-mercaptopurine	94
	Prednisone + vincristine + daunorubicin	97
Hodgkin's disease	Prednisone	<5
	Nitrogen mustard	20
	Cyclophosphamide	20
	Vinblastine	27
	Vincristine	<10
	Procarbazine	<10
	Carmustine	<5
	Vinblastine + chlorambucil	40
	Mechlorethamine + vincristine + procarbazine + prednisone (MOPP)	81

in combination[27] (see Table 9–1 for comparative response rates).[26] Chronic lymphocytic leukemia may respond to glucocorticoid therapy, and prednisone is generally administered in addition to an alkylating agent. Prednisone is used in combination with an alkylating agent to treat patients with multiple myeloma, and some patients (under 10%) with acute myelogenous leukemia will respond to glucocorticoids. The effectiveness of glucocorticoid therapy in Hodgkin's disease (see Table 9–1) and non-Hodgkin's lymphoma is well established, and prednisone is usually included in the combination drug regimens used to treat these diseases.[28]

Mechanism of Steroid Hormone Action

Despite the different physiological effects that are produced by the steroid hormones in different cells and tissues, these drugs have a common mechanism of action at the molecular level. They all bind to receptors and permit the receptors to activate transcription from a limited number of genes. As a result, cells synthesize hormone-specific proteins that determine both the tumor growth response and the side effects of these drugs. The model presented in Figure 9–2 outlines in a very general manner the common steps leading to the physiological effects of the adrenocortical and sex steroids.

The steroid hormones are extremely lipophilic and they readily pass across cell membranes to rapidly establish an equilibrium between the concentration of free hormone in the cytosol and that in the cell environment (e.g., interstitial fluid, blood, culture medium). To have a physiological effect, the hormone must then bind to a receptor protein in the cytoplasm. There are only a few thousand (typically about 60,000) receptors present in each cell, and they bind the steroid in a very tight ($K_D < 10^{-9}$M) but noncovalent reversible manner.

The binding sites on the receptors are quite specific. A glucocorticoid receptor, for example, will bind the potent glucocorticoids very tightly, it will form weaker complexes with the less potent glucocorticoids, but it will not bind estrogens or androgens. Steroids are not chemically altered when they are bound by the receptors, although in some cases, natural steroids are modified prior to binding. In some androgen-sensitive tissues like the prostate, for example, testosterone is converted to dihydrotestosterone, which is the major bound form.

Unoccupied steroid receptors may be located in the cytoplasm or the nucleus, depending on the receptor, the cell type, and the metabolic state of the cell. Regardless of their location, after cell rupture, the adrenocorticoid and sex-steroid receptors are recovered as soluble complexes in the cytosolic fraction. These inactive receptors have sedimentation values of 8 to 9 S and molecular masses of about 300 kDa. They are heteroprotein complexes containing one molecule of the steroid-binding protein, a dimer of the 90 kDa heat shock protein, and undetermined amounts of two other heat shock proteins, hsp56 and hsp70.[29,30] When cells are exposed to steroid, the receptors dissociate from the hsp90 and become tightly bound to nuclear "acceptor" sites where the initial events in transcriptional activation occur. After cell rupture, these hormone-transformed receptors are recovered by salt extraction of nuclei as 4S receptor monomers, or in some cases homodimers.[29] The receptors appear to bind to the heat shock protein complex as they are being translated, and they remain docked to the complex (while they remain in the cytoplasm or while they make their journey to and within the nucleus) until such time as the hormone binding promotes undocking and progression to the appropriate response elements.[30]

The *hormone response elements* (HREs) are discrete genomic regions that are found upstream (5') of the transcriptional start sites of inducible genes. They are regulatory sequences that act independent of their orientation.[31,32] Thus, they act as *enhancer* elements that confer hormonal regulation on promoters, and they must be occupied by the steroid receptor for efficient transcription of certain genes. The response elements contain 13 to 15 base pairs arranged in a consensus sequence that is specific for a specific receptor. Thus, the glucocorticoid receptor binds to a glucocorticoid response element (a GRE) and the estrogen receptor to an estrogen response element (an ERE). The consensus sequences in the HREs are arranged in a pallindromic manner such that the receptors bind to them as dimers.[33] The precise way in which the binding of the receptors to HREs leads to transcriptional enhancement is not known, but it must involve direct interaction of the receptor with other nuclear proteins (called transcription factors) that are integral proteins in the transcription mechanism. The steroid receptors are thus *trans*-acting factors—that is, they are proteins produced from one gene that can regulate transcription from other (*trans*) genes.

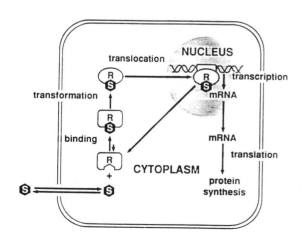

Figure 9–2 Model of the mechanism of steroid hormone action. After diffusing across the cell membrane, the steroid (S) binds to its receptor (R), which may be located in the cytoplasm (as shown) or in the nucleus. Binding of steroid promotes a transformation of the receptor into a state that moves into a high-affinity nuclear complex at the site of an appropriate hormone response element in the DNA where it enhances transcription of mRNA from neighboring genes regulated by that element. The resulting newly synthesized proteins mediate the growth-promoting, cytolytic, and physiological effects of these hormones.

Steroid Receptor Structure and Function

All of the human sex hormone and adrenocorticoid receptors have now been cloned and sequenced. The receptors contain common structural features that place them within a larger group of proteins called the *steroid/thyroid hormone receptor superfamily* or the *nuclear receptor family*.[34] Figure 9–3 shows the arrangement of different functional domains among some members of this nuclear receptor family. All of the receptors have a central 66 to 68 amino acid DNA-binding domain, which is highly conserved. This is the only portion of these receptors where the tertiary structure is known in detail, having been determined for the glucocorticoid receptor by crystallography.[35] The DNA-binding domain contains two cysteine-rich centers, each of which coordinates a molecule of zinc, forming two loops, called "zinc fingers," that are required for DNA binding.[36] The DNA-binding domain alone is sufficient for interaction with DNA, and it determines selective binding for the HRE specific for the receptor. In fact, the ability of the glucocorticoid receptor, for example, to discriminate between binding to the GRE versus the ERE is determined by the amino acid sequence of only a portion of the N-terminal zinc finger.[37]

Although the DNA-binding domain is required for transcriptional activation, a large portion of the N-terminal half of the receptor is required for any substantial enhancement of gene transcription.[34] This region required for maximal transcriptional activation is variable in both its length and amino acid sequence (see Fig. 9–3). Although specific functions for this domain have not been defined, this is likely the region that interacts with other nuclear proteins to increase the rate of gene transcription.

The hormone-binding domain contains the steroid binding pocket, a dimerization site, and a sequence of 20 amino acids that is highly conserved through all members of the nuclear receptor family. This 20 amino acid sequence is called the C_2 domain (for second conserved domain) to distinguish it from the highly conserved DNA-binding domain, C_1. The hormone-binding domain in general is not conserved, the diversity being important for determining specific binding pockets that are selective for the various hormone classes. The conserved segment C_2 within the hormone-binding domain must be responsible for determining some function common to all of the receptors. Thus, the C_2 region has been considered as a potential transducing domain.[38] That is, it determines a structure that is required for transducing the hormone binding into an acti-

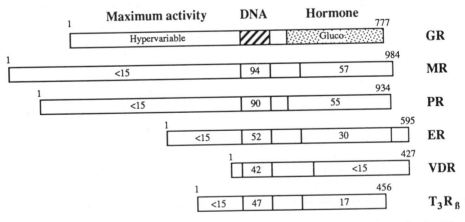

Figure 9–3 Diagram of the structures of some of the receptors in the nuclear receptor family. The amino acid sequences were aligned according to their DNA-binding domains (hatched lines), which have the highest similarity. The percentage of identity to the glucocorticoid receptor amino acid sequence is indicated within the boxes defining the major receptor domains. The C-terminus for the human receptor is indicated by the number above each structure on the right. GR, glucocorticoid receptor; MR, mineralocorticoid receptor; PR, progesterone receptor; ER, estrogen receptor; VDR, vitamin D receptor; T_3R_β, one form of the thyroid hormone receptor. (Adapted from Evans[34])

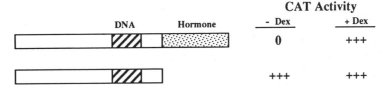

Figure 9–4 Demonstration that the hormone binding domain represses the transcriptional activating activity of the glucocorticoid receptors. In a cotransfection protocol that has been performed with several steroid receptors, the receptor cDNA is transfected into cells along with a reporter plasmid encoding the gene for chloramphenicol acetyl transferase (CAT) with several glucocorticoid response elements located 5′ to the promoter. After a period of time, the CAT activity is assayed in transfected cells that have been treated or not treated with the potent glucocorticoid dexamethasone (Dex). The + symbols indicate a normal hormone regulation when the intact receptor is present. However, when the hormone-binding domain (stippled region) is removed, the mutant receptor causes constitutive expression in the absence of hormone. Thus, the hormone-binding domain represses the transcriptional enhancer activity of the rest of the receptor and the binding of hormone relieves this repression.

vation of the receptor. The hormone-binding domain of the receptor also contains the site of receptor binding to hsp90.[38,39]

An intriguing aspect of receptor function that has emerged from the study of mutant receptors is that loss of the hormone-binding domain yields a receptor that is a constitutively active transcriptional enhancer (i.e., the mutant receptor enhances transcription in the absence of hormone).[40] This was shown in a cotransfunction system in which a receptor cDNA is cotransfected into monkey kidney cells along with a reporter plasmid containing the chloramphenicol acetyltransferase (CAT) gene located 3′ to several GREs. As illustrated in Figure 9–4, when the full length, human glucocorticoid receptor is present, it can bind the potent glucocorticoid dexamethasone, and by binding to the GREs, the hormone-transformed receptor stimulates CAT production. In the absence of the steroid, there is no expression from the CAT gene. When the cells are transfected with a mutant receptor cDNA that is deleted for the hormone-binding domain, then the CAT gene is transcribed and CAT activity is high in the absence of hormone. From this kind of observation with several steroid receptors, it became clear that the hormone-binding domain inhibits the activity of the rest of the receptor and that the binding of steroid relieves that inhibition.

Consistent with the observations in intact cells, it has been shown in cell-free systems that the 9 S glucocorticoid receptor–hsp90 complex is unable to bind to DNA. When the complex is bound by glucocorticoid, however, the receptor undergoes a temperature-dependent dissociation from hsp90 and concomitant conversion to the DNA-binding state (see Fig. 9–5).[41,42] Thus, in this cell-free model of the hormone action, the binding of steroid relieves an inhibition that is provided by the heat-shock protein. Consistent with this role for hsp90 in repression of receptor function, it has been shown that hormone-responsive human glucocorticoid receptors are recovered from cells in complex with hsp90, whereas constitutively active mutant receptors, such as the one shown in Figure 9–4, are not bound to hsp90.[38]

Another intriguing and unexpected observation is that the hormone-binding domain can act as a movable and transferable regulatory unit. If, for example, the hormone-binding domain is moved from the C-terminus to the N-terminus of the glucocorticoid receptor, as diagrammed in the top of Figure 9–6, transcriptional activating activity of the rearranged receptor is still repressed in the absence of hormone and binding of steroid relieves the inhibition. More striking is the demonstration that the hormone-binding domain of the receptor can be fused to other structurally very different proteins and confer hormone regulation on them. This is illustrated by the results of an experiment by Picard *et al.*,[43] shown at the bottom of Figure 9–6. In this case the hormone-binding domain of the glucocorticoid receptor was fused to the adenovirus E1A protein, which regulates expression from the adenovirus E3 promoter. In the absence of hormone, the function of E1A in the fusion protein is repressed, and in the presence of hormone, the fusion protein is hormone-responsive.

The hormone-binding domain thus acts as a regulatory unit that can confer hormone responsiveness onto other proteins. One of the more interesting examples of this transferable regulatory function is provided by formation of a chimera between the Myc oncoprotein and the hormone-binding domain of the human estrogen receptor.[44] The cell transforming activity of the resulting fusion protein is entirely dependent on the presence of estrogen. These observations can be explained by the *docking* model of steroid action,[45] in which a fusion protein is tightly bound to hsp90 at the hormone binding domain, as depicted for the glucocorticoid receptor in Figure 9–5. The fusion protein would remain docked to the heat shock

protein complex until the binding of steroid promotes its release, permitting it to progress to its ultimate site of action in the cell. Thus, proteins of widely different structure and function can be brought under hormonal control.

Steroid Receptors and Response to Therapy

Receptor Assay

It follows logically from the above discussion that hormone therapy should not be effective unless cells in the patient's tumor contain steroid receptors of the appropriate type. As receptor assays have proven to be an effective guide for hormonal therapy of breast and endometrial cancers,[46] it is appropriate here to review the procedure used to assay steroid recep-

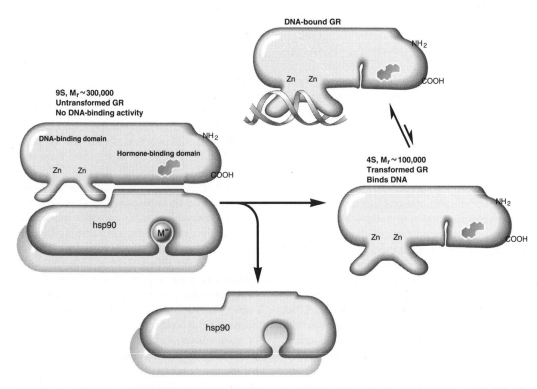

Figure 9–5   Model of the glucocorticoid receptor–hsp90 complex and the steroid effect in cytosol. Like the sex hormone receptors, the glucocorticoid receptor is recovered from hormone-free cells as a 9 S, hsp90-containing complex in which DNA binding function is repressed. Hsp90 binds to the receptor through the hormone-binding domain. Binding of steroid promotes temperature-dependent dissociation of the receptor from hsp90 and concomitant generation of the 4 S, DNA-binding form. The globe with the M= represents a binding site for transition metal oxyanions (e.g., molybdate) that stabilize the protein–protein interaction between the receptor and hsp90, preventing receptor transformation to the DNA-binding state.

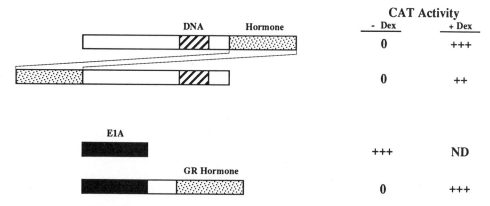

Figure 9–6 The steroid-binding domain of the glucocorticoid receptor functions as a movable hormone-regulated unit that can repress protein function in a manner that is relatively independent of protein structure. The above scheme summarizes some work published by Picard *et al.*[43] In the experiment of the top diagram, cells were transfected with a cDNA for the glucocorticoid receptor or with a mutant receptor in which the hormone-binding domain has been moved from the C-terminus to the N-terminus. CAT activity from a co-transfected reporter gene under the control of GREs was assayed in cells that were treated or not treated with dexamethasone (Dex). In both orientations the hormone-binding domain confers hormone regulation. In the experiment of the lower diagram, cells are transfected with the adenovirus E1A protein (solid black bar), which regulates expression from the adenovirus E3 promoter. Cells were also transfected with a cDNA for a chimeric protein consisting of E1A and the glucocorticoid receptor hormone-binding domain (stippled bar). The E1A constructions were cotransfected with a CAT reporter gene regulated by the E1A promoter/enhancer. The E1A-specific transcriptional activating activity of the chimeric protein is regulated by hormone.

tors as well as the correlations between receptor assay data and the therapeutic response of breast cancer to hormone manipulation.

Two types of receptor assays are performed—assays of steroid binding and direct immunoassay of receptor protein using monoclonal antireceptor antibodies.[47] Because steroid binding assays have been used since the early 1970s, virtually all of the data correlating receptor levels with tumor response have been obtained by this method. The procedure for receptor assay by steroid binding is straightforward. A sample of tumor tissue obtained by surgical resection is homogenized in buffer and centrifuged at high speed. The supernatant from this centrifugation, the cytosol fraction, contains the soluble receptor protein. Aliquots of the cytosol are usually incubated at low temperature with several different concentrations of a radiolabeled steroid in the presence and in the absence of a high concentration of a physiologically potent, nonradioactive steroid. After incubation for a sufficient time to allow the binding reaction to attain equilibrium, the bound steroid is separated from the unbound steroid by one of several techniques (dextran-coated charcoal absorption, protamine sulfate precipitation, gradient centrifugation, etc.) and the amount of bound radioactivity is determined.

The data plotted in Figure 9–7 present a typical assay for glucocorticoid receptor and demonstrate the principles of the procedure.[48] In this case, fibroblast cytosol was incubated with radiolabeled dexamethasone; the amount of binding is plotted on the ordinate and the concentration of free dexamethasone (note the logarithmic scale) on the abscissa (Fig. 9–7A). It can be seen that, as the concentration of radiolabeled dexamethasone increases, increasing amounts of the steroid can be recovered in the bound form (solid circles, total binding). When identical assays are carried out in the presence of a high concentration of another potent glucocorticoid (open circles), the nonradioactive steroid will occupy the receptor site and prevent radiolabeled drug binding. At high concentrations, some radiolabeled dexamethasone is bound to other proteins, even though the competing steroid is present; this is called nonspecific (i.e., not receptor-specific) binding. Spe-

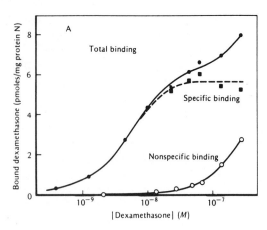

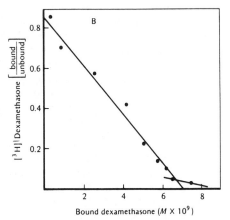

Figure 9–7   Receptor assay by steroid binding. Replicate aliquots of cytosol containing glucocorticoid receptors were incubated with different concentrations of radiolabeled dexamethasone in the presence or in the absence of a high concentration of competing nonradioactive triamcinolone acetonide. After incubation, the bound steroid was separated from the unbound steroid and the amount of bound radioactive steroid was determined. (A) The amount of bound steroid, expressed as picomoles bound per milligram of cytosol protein nitrogen, is plotted on the ordinate, the concentration of free dexamethasone on the abscissa. Key: ●, binding in the absence of competing triamcinolone acetonide (total binding); ○, binding in the presence of nonradioactive triamcinolone acetonide (nonspecific binding); ■, specific binding determined by subtracting nonspecific binding from total binding. (B) shows a Scatchard plot of the data for total binding. (From Pratt *et al.*[48])

cific receptor binding is obtained by subtracting nonspecific binding from the total binding obtained in the absence of competitor (dotted line, defined by solid squares). The specific binding curve plateaus at the concentration of dexamethasone that is required to occupy all the receptor sites. Since the receptor is half-saturated when the concentration of dexamethasone is only 8×10^{-9}M, the S-shaped specific binding curve clearly demonstrates high-affinity binding. The amount of receptor can be estimated simply by determining where the specific binding plateaus, or it can be more accurately calculated by plotting the data according to the method of Scatchard as shown in Figure 9–7B. The equilibrium dissociation constant for the binding reaction can be calculated from the slope of the Scatchard plot and the intercept on the abscissa gives the number of cytosol steroid binding sites.

The data from clinical tumor samples are expressed in a standardized fashion as fmole/mg cytosol protein. A broad range of receptor levels is detected in breast cancer using radioligand assay, with estrogen receptor ranging from 0 to higher than 1,000 fmole/mg and progesterone receptor between 0 and higher than 2,600 fmole/mg.[46]

Receptors and Response

BREAST CANCER About one in three unselected patients with breast cancer responds to endocrine therapy. If the patient population is selected according to the estrogen receptor status of the tumor, however, then patients who have cancers that are estrogen receptor positive (> 10 fmole/mg cytosol protein) have a response rate that is about twice the level of that of unselected patients.[49] Response rates for several forms of endocrine manipulation are summarized in Table 9–2.[50] It is important to note from the table that response to all the forms of endocrine therapy is correlated with the estrogen receptor status of the tumor. This supports the notion that the therapeutic effect for all endocrine manipulations is ultimately mediated through the estrogen receptor.

Several studies have demonstrated a direct quantitative relationship between response rate and estrogen binding activity of the tumor.[49] Higher receptor values appear to reflect a higher percentage of cells in the tumor that are expressing the receptor. It is important to realize that, like other tumors, breast tumors contain heterogeneous cell populations with some cells that express the estrogen receptor and some cells that do not. One would predict that if a tumor were receptor-negative, it should not respond to endocrine therapy at all. It has been shown, however, that administration of the antiestrogen tamoxifen in adjuvant therapy of estrogen receptor-negative breast cancer significantly prolongs the disease-free interval as compared to untreated controls.[51] Such a therapeutic effect in a tumor with estrogen binding activity so low that it is considered to be receptor-negative suggests that a very few estrogen-responsive cells may be able to affect the growth of other cells in the heterogeneous tumor population. In this respect, it is known that estrogen-stimulated breast cancer cells secrete paracrine growth factors.[52] Thus, it is possible that tamoxifen blockade of estrogen receptors in a few cells can affect the growth of estrogen receptor-negative tumor cells where growth depends upon estrogen-dependent secretion of growth factors from the few receptor-positive cells. Tumors that are no longer hormone-dependent may be composed of cells that have *dedifferentiated* to a state where they

produce the requisite autocrine and paracrine growth factors in a constitutive manner.[52]

About 40% of patients with estrogen receptor-positive breast cancers do not respond to endocrine therapy.[53] Thus, physicians have sought a rapid assay for determining whether tumors with estrogen receptors have an intact and functioning estrogen response pathway. The progesterone receptor is an estrogen-induced protein. Thus, the presence of progesterone binding activity in a tumor sample demonstrates that at least a portion of the cells respond to estrogens. The two steroid receptors can be measured in a single assay using a double-label approach with [^{125}I]estradiol in combination with [^{3}H]R5020 to measure the progesterone receptor.[47] Pooled data from several clinical studies show that about 75% of patients with tumors positive for both receptors have an objective response to endocrine therapy, whereas patients with tumors that are positive for estrogen receptor but negative for progesterone receptor have only one half that response rate.[53,54]

ENDOMETRIAL CANCER. There is a good correlation between the progesterone receptor content of tumor samples and response to progestin treatment in patients with advanced endometrial cancer. About 90% of patients with receptor-positive tumors respond, versus only 17% of those with receptor-negative tumors.[46] As in breast cancer, the presence of steroid receptors in endometrial cancer correlates with a more differentiated tumor state.[55] Despite the high correlation with response, steroid receptor assays do not play as prominent a role in the clinical management of endometrial cancer as they do in breast cancer.

PROSTATE CANCER. There appears to be a correlation between the presence of nuclear androgen receptor in biopsy specimens and the response of patients with prostate cancer to initial endocrine therapy.[56] However, such assays are not utilized routinely in guiding choice of therapy.

Table 9–2 Response Rates to Endocrine Therapy Among Breast Cancer Patients in General (Unselected) and Among Patients Whose Tumors Were Positive (ER+) or Negative (ER−) For Estrogen Binding. (Data from Henderson[50])

Endocrine Therapy	Response Rate (%)		
	Unselected	ER+	ER−
Tamoxifen	32	54	9
Ovariectomy	33	62	6
Aminoglutethimide	31	54	6
Estrogens	26	57	9

Glucocorticoid Resistance

Some children with acute lymphoblastic leukemia who initially respond to glucocorticoid therapy do not respond to subsequent courses of therapy,[57] and there is evidence that this resistance to therapy is associated with a decreased capacity to bind steroid. Blast cells isolated from a group of untreated patients with acute lymphoblastic leukemia, for example, were found to have much higher levels of glucocorticoid binding activity than those obtained from treated patients who had become resistant to therapy.[58] Lymphoblasts isolated from a few patients who had been on steroid therapy but who were still steroid responsive had the higher binding activity characteristic of the blast cells from the untreated group. The results of this study suggest that patients with acute lymphoblastic leukemia whose cells do not bind glucocorticoid will be resistant to therapy with these drugs. Patients whose cells have sufficient binding activity are more apt to respond to glucocorticoid therapy. A correlation between glucocorticoid binding activity of tumor cells and subsequent response to glucocorticoid therapy has also been demonstrated in adults with non-Hodgkin's lymphoma.[59]

In general, most of the resistance that develops to glucocorticoids reflects a decrease in steroid binding activity in the cell. This was first shown in mouse lymphoma cells selected for resistance to dexamethasone.[60] About 80% of the resistant cell lines were deficient in binding capacity and the rest were about equally divided between cell lines with normal cytosol binding, which were deficient in their ability to transfer the steroid-receptor complex to the nucleus, and cells with normal cytoplasmic binding and transfer, which were apparently deficient at some step subsequent to the nuclear localization of the steroid-receptor complex. Thus, moderate to high levels of glucocorticoid-receptor activity in lymphocyte cytosol do not guarantee that the cell will respond to the glucocorticoids, although cells with low levels of binding activity (or no activity) will not respond. Resistant human leukemic cell lines studied *in vitro* have been shown to be defective in some aspect of glucocorticoid receptor function.[61] In contrast to the mouse cell lines where loss of glucocorticoid binding activity reflects loss of receptor mRNA expression from the receptor gene,[62] loss of glucocorticoid binding activity in resistant cells selected from the human CEM-C7 leukemic T-cell line reflects muta-

tions in the receptor protein that affect the ability of the receptor to retain bound steroid.[63] There seems to be no question but that the majority of resistance that develops to glucocorticoid treatment in humans is related to mutation involving the receptor, but the mechanisms may be quite varied and the presence of normal glucocorticoid binding does not necessarily ensure a functional receptor.

Glucocorticoids

Physiological Effects

Cortisol (hydrocortisone), the principal endogenous glucocorticoid, is produced in the adrenal gland in circadian fashion under the stimulus of ACTH (adrenocorticotropic hormone) released from the pituitary. In a manner analogous to the regulation of sex hormone production shown in Figure 9–1, ACTH is secreted under the influence of corticotropin releasing factor, which is released from the hypothalamus, and both endogenous cortisol and the synthetic glucocorticoids are feedback inhibitors of the system at both the pituitary and hypothalamic levels.

Receptors for the glucocorticoids exist in every cell in the body with the exception of erythrocytes and platelets. The biochemical pathways affected and the physiological manifestations of glucocorticoid hormone action are protean. The use of glucocorticoids in medicine reflects these actions (e.g., antiinflammatory, immunosuppressive, gluconeogenic, antifibroproliferative, integrity of vascular permeability, lymphocytolytic, etc.). Indeed, the glucocorticoid hormones are administered to patients with a wide variety of diseases and clinical states for more separate physiological reasons than any other class of drugs. To appreciate their multiple effects and applications in medicine, the reader is referred to basic texts.[64,65]

The glucocorticoids are administered to cancer patients for three basic purposes: 1) in high dosage for a tumor cell killing effect; 2) in moderate dosage as adjunctive therapy for such purposes as reducing edema, treating hypercalcemia, managing thrombocytopenia, and symptomatic palliation of patients with severe hematopoietic depression; 3) in low (i.e., physiologic replacement) dosage as glucocorticoid replacement in patients receiving aminoglutethimide, which inhibits endogenous glucocorticoid synthesis. We are concerned here only with the first indication—tumor cell killing.

The use of glucocorticoids in the treatment of leukemias and lymphomas is an application of their lymphocytolytic effect. Thymus-derived lymphocytes (T cells) are the particularly vulnerable target. Within three hours after exposure to methylprednisolone, rat thymus cells undergo fragmentation of their DNA into 180 base pair units.[66] Fragmentation into such nucleosome-sized units is characteristic of the programmed cell death (apoptosis) discussed at the beginning of Chapter 5. Glucocorticoid-mediated cell killing and DNA fragmentation are inhibited by actinomycin and cycloheximide, demonstrating that new RNA and protein synthesis are required for the effects.[65] DNA fragmentation results from the action of an endonuclease that preferentially cleaves DNA in the linker regions between nucleosomes. Although several investigators have suggested that glucocorticoids cause apoptosis by directly inducing the endonuclease protein itself,[66] activation of endonuclease activity appears to result from induction of another protein (or proteins) that has not been identified.[67,68]

Prednisone is a component of some multidrug regimens used to treat breast cancer. Its use here does not exploit a well-defined physiologic effect and is entirely empirical. It should be noted, however, that glucocorticoids have a growth inhibitory (as opposed to cell killing) action on some cell types (e.g., fibroblasts[69]) that may be mechanistically related to any direct effort they may have on breast cancer cell growth.

Pharmacology

The glucocorticoid used most frequently for oral administration is prednisone. Prednisone itself is inactive until the ketone at carbon-11 is reduced to produce the 11β-hydroxyl compound prednisolone. The reduction is carried out by 11β-hydroxysteroid dehydrogenase,[70] primarily in the liver but also in other tissues. After oral administration, peak plasma levels of prednisolone (achieved in 1 to 2 hours) are about 4 to 10 times those of the parent com

Prednisolone

Prednisone

pound.[71] Because the plasma concentrations of predisolone achieved after administration of prednisone are nearly as high as those achieved with an equivalent oral dose of prednisolone, physicians have continued to administer prednisone. The pharmacology of prednisone and prednisolone has been reviewed in detail by Szefler.[72]

Prednisolone binds with low affinity to albumin and with high affinity to transcortin, which is present in limited amounts in the plasma. At low concentrations, prednisolone is 90% bound to plasma protein, but at higher concentrations, the transcortin binding sites become saturated and the free fraction of hormone increases.[71] The binding of prednisolone to transcortin is competed by cortisol.[73] When low doses of prednisone are administered, there is a circadian variation in plasma capacity to bind prednisolone, which reflects the circadian production of cortisol.[74] This effect is not seen at the high prednisone dosage administered in cancer chemotherapy. The plasma half-life of prednisolone is about 3.5 hours (see Table 9–3). The reduction reaction that produces prednisolone from prednisone is reversible, and if prednisolone is the administered drug, some prednisone will be present in the plasma. In urine, 2–5% of either administered drug is excreted as prednisone and 11–24% as prednisolone.[71] The primary route of elimination is via biotransformation in the liver. Reduction in the C-4,5 double bond in the A ring and reduction of

Table 9–3   Pharmacology of Prednisone and Prednisolone

Drug	Relative Glucocorticoid Potency	Plasma Half-Life	Half-Life of Biologic Activity	Pharmacological Characteristics
Cortisol (hydrocortisone)	1	1.5 hours	8–12 hours	The major endogenous human glucocorticoid
Prednisone	4	3.5 hours	12–36 hours	Rapidly converted to prednisolone by 11β-hydroxylation in the liver
Prednisolone	4	3.5 hours	12–36 hours	The active, reduced (11β-hydroxy) form of prednisone

the C-3 ketone yield the tetrahydro compound, which is conjugated primarily in the liver to water-soluble sulfate esters or glucuronides. Concomitant administration of phenobarbital and some other drugs that induce hepatic cytochrome P-450 increases the rate of prednisolone metabolism.[72,75]

Side Effects

Because they have so many physiological actions in the body, the glucocorticoids produce a wide variety of side effects. The adverse reactions to exogenous glucocorticoids can be divided into two general classes—those that re-

Table 9–4   Adverse Reactions to Glucocorticoids. (From Axelrod[76])

Ophthalmic
   Posterior subcapsular cataracts, increased intraocular pressure and glaucoma, exophthalmos
Cardiovascular
   Hypertension
   Congestive heart failure in predisposed patients
Gastrointestinal
   Peptic-ulcer disease, pancreatitis
Endocrine-metabolic
   Truncal obesity, moon facies, supraclavicular fat deposition, posterior cervical fat desposition (buffalo hump), mediastinal widening (lipomatosis), hepatomegaly due to fatty liver (rare)
   Acne, hirsutism or virilism, impotence, menstrual irregularities
   Suppression of growth in children
   Hyperglycemia; diabetic ketoacidosis; hyperosmolar, nonketotic diabetic coma; hyperlipoproteinemia
   Negative balance of nitrogen, potassium, and calcium
   Sodium retention, hypokalemia, metabolic alkalosis
   Secondary adrenal insufficiency
Musculoskeletal
   Myopathy
   Osteoporosis, vertebral compression fractures, spontaneous fractures
   Aseptic necrosis of femoral and humeral heads and other bones
Neuropsychiatric
   Convulsions
   Benign intracranial hypertension (pseudotumor cerebri)
   Alterations in mood or behavior, such as euphoria, insomnia, increased appetite, depression
   Psychosis
Dermatologic
   Facial erythema; thin, fragile skin; petechiae and ecchymoses; violaceous striae; impaired wound healing
   Panniculitis (following withdrawal)
Immune, infectious
   Suppression of delayed hypersensitivity
   Neutrophilia, monocytopenia, lymphocytopenia, decreased inflammatory responses
   Susceptibility to infections

sult from direct physiological actions and those that occur upon steroid withdrawal. The adverse reactions to these drugs are summarized in Table 9–4; the reader is referred to specialized texts and reviews for details.[76,77,78] With the exception of sodium retention and accompanying electrolyte and volume changes, all of the glucocorticoids produce all of the side effects. Prednisone has very little mineralocorticoid activity and sodium retention is not a major problem in anticancer therapy. Despite the variety of possible side effects, the glucocorticoids are not myelosuppressive; therefore, they are particularly useful compounds to include in combination drug protocols.

All of the synthetic glucocorticoids have a negative feedback effect on the hypothalamic-pituitary axis and suppress endogenous cortisol production.[78] Patients who are treated with more than a few doses of prednisone (as is always the case in cancer chemotherapy) require careful tapering of the dosage when the drug is withdrawn in order to permit return of normal adrenal function and avoid acute secondary adrenal insufficiency.[77]

Estrogens

As discussed earlier in this chapter, estrogens are now used primarily to treat carcinoma of the prostate—the rationale being to inhibit the production of luteinizing hormone (see Fig. 9–1) through negative effects at the level of the hypothalamus and pituitary, thereby markedly decreasing endogenous testosterone synthesis by the testis.[6,7] Estrogens are now used only rarely in the treatment of breast cancer (in postmenopausal patients only) and the basis for the beneficial effect of high-dose estrogen therapy here is simply not understood.

Pharmacology

Ethinyl estradiol, a derivative of estradiol, and diethylstilbestrol, a nonsteroidal estrogen, are the estrogens most commonly administered in cancer chemotherapy. Depending on the assay used to assess activity, diethylstilbestrol is 4 to 30 times more potent than estradiol and ethinyl estradiol is one hundred to several hundred times more potent than estradiol.[79] A major

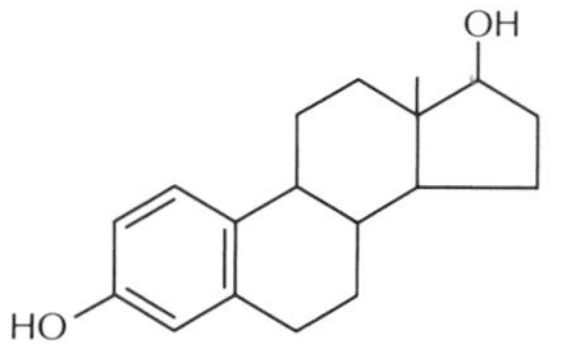

Estradiol

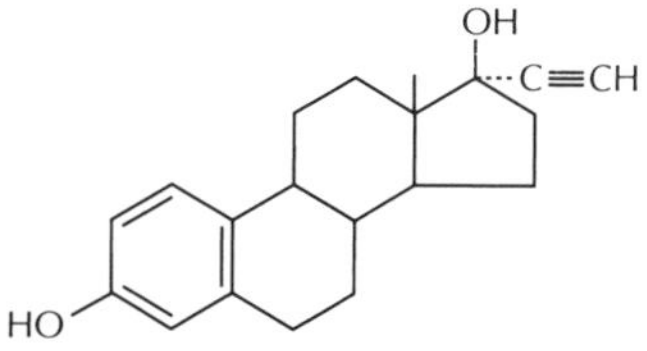

Ethinyl estradiol

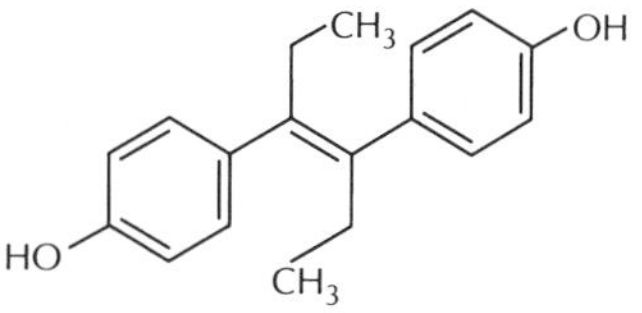

Diethylstilbestrol

portion of the high intrinsic potency reflects the very slow inactivation of both compounds in the liver and other tissues. Despite its lesser potency, diethylstilbestrol is more widely used than ethinyl estradiol.

Both compounds are well absorbed from the gastrointestinal tract. Diethylstilbestrol has a two-phase pharmacokinetic profile, with a half-life of 80 minutes for the first phase[80] followed by a very slow second phase.[80,81] The half-life of ethinyl estradiol is 28 hours.[82] Unlike the natural estrogens, these two synthetic compounds are not bound to sex hormone binding globulin in the plasma.[83] Metabolism of both compounds occurs principally in the liver, with ultimate excretion in the urine, principally as the glucuronide.[82] Diethylstilbestrol undergoes oxidative metabolism by three major pathways—aromatic hydroxylation to a catechol, aliphatic hydroxylation of the ethyl side chains, and dehydrogenation to Z,Z-dienestrol (Fig. 9–8).[84] The aromatic and aliphatic hydroxylations are thought to be cytochrome P-450-catalyzed processes, but the conversion to Z,Z-dienestrol is catalyzed by peroxidative enzymes, like horseradish peroxidase and prostaglandin synthase.[85] The postulated quinone intermediate in the peroxidative pathway (Fig.

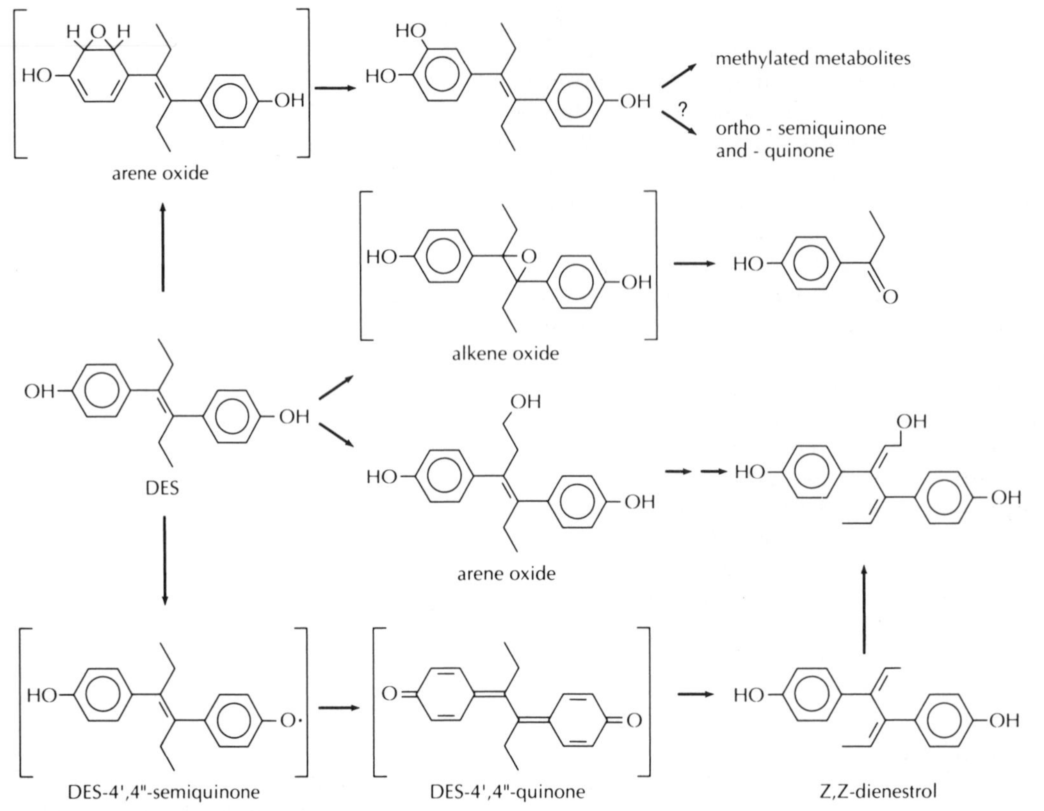

Figure 9–8   Oxidative metabolism of diethylstilbestrol (DES). Postulated reactive semiquinone and quinone intermediates are in brackets. (From Metzler[84])

9–8) has been synthesized and shown to bind to DNA.[86] It is thought that the quinone is the major carcinogenic intermediate derived from diethylstilbestrol.

In the 1940s and 1950s a number of women were treated with diethylstilbestrol to prevent miscarriage; subsequently, the daughters of these women developed adenocarcinoma of the vagina when they were in their late teens or early twenties.[87] Studies in animal models indicate that this transplacental carcinogenic action of diethylstilbestrol is a consequence of oxidative metabolism. Experiments in the rat show that radioactive diethylstilbestrol injected into pregnant animals readily distributes into the fetus.[88] The neonatal mouse has the capacity to oxidatively metabolize diethylstilbestrol,[89] and in cultures of mouse genital tract tissue, peroxidative metabolism to Z,Z-dienestrol appears to be the sole biotransformation pathway for the drug.[90] It has been shown that di-

ethylstilbestrol under peroxidative conditions causes the formation of superoxide radicals and the induction of DNA strand breaks in hamster embryo cells *in vitro*.[91] Also, hamster embryo fibroblasts exposed to the drug *in vitro* were rendered tumorigenic when injected into newborn hamsters.[92] Although diethylstilbestrol does not induce mutations in prokaryotes (negative in the Ames test with microsomes), it clearly causes damage to chromosomes (e.g., sister chromosome exchange and chromosome aberrations) in eukaryotic cells.[93,94] From observations such as these, it seems reasonable to conclude that treatment of pregnant women with diethylstilbestrol resulted in carcinogenic events in fetal genital tract tissue by oxidative metabolites of the drug. After the hormonal changes of their early teenage years and under the influence of continued hormonal stimulation, their daughters developed adenocarcinoma of the vagina.

Side Effects

The side effects of estrogen therapy of relevance to the oncologist can be divided into three general classes—effects resulting from actions on tumor cells (tumor flare); general systemic side effects, including feminization; and carcinogenic effects.

TUMOR FLARE. Although the goal of hormone therapy is to induce tumor regression, initiation of endocrine therapy can be accompanied by a transient exacerbation of signs and symptoms that is called *tumor flare*.[95] Tumor flare is manifested in three ways: the first is by an increase in swelling, erythema, itching, or pain in breast cancer soft tissue metastases or by development of new lesions; the second is by an increase in skeletal pain in patients with bone metastases; the third is by development of hypercalcemia.[95] Tumor flare occurs with endocrine therapy of both breast cancer and prostatic cancer, and it has been reported following administration of estrogens, antiestrogens (tamoxifen), androgens, and, rarely, progestins and GnRH agonists.[95,96] Hypercalcemia occurs most often in patients with widespread bone metastases. The increase in extracellular fluid calcium is accompanied by neurological changes (confusion, apathy, coma), polyuria, and cardiac arrhythmias. Hypercalcemia requires cessation of hormonal therapy, forced hydration, and in some cases saline diuresis and treatment with corticosteroids or plicamycin (Chapter 7). Plasma concentrations of calcium should be determined routinely in patients receiving hormonal treatment. When the drug-induced hypercalcemia is corrected (1 to 3 weeks), hormonal treatment may be cautiously reinitiated. Patients who experience tumor flare have a greater likelihood of having an antitumor response on continued hormonal treatment than does the patient population in general.

GENERAL SIDE EFFECTS. The most frequent acute side effect of estrogen therapy is nausea and vomiting,[97] often occurring like the "morning sickness" of early pregnancy (Table 9–5). The nausea usually disappears after one or two weeks with continued treatment, but rarely it is distressful enough to require cessation of therapy. Both the incidence and severity of the nausea are dose-related and the problem is usually avoided by initiating therapy with a small dose and increasing it gradually. Anorexia and diarrhea (usually mild) are also acute side effects.

Important delayed and dose-related effects on the cardiovascular system include hypertension and congestive failure resulting from estrogen-induced fluid retention, exacerbation of atherosclerosis, venous thrombosis, pulmonary embolus, and cerebral ischemia. Vaginal bleeding (usually mild), stress incontinence, and pigmentation of the nipples or areolae occur with moderate frequency.[97] Women may complain of pain or venous dilatation of the breast and dysmenorrhea. Gallbladder disease and dermatitis have been reported rarely. Men develop

Table 9–5 *Some Major Untoward Effects of Estrogens and Antiestrogens*

| Drug | Principal Toxicities | |
	Acute	Delayed
Estrogens Diethylstilbestrol Ethinyl estradiol	Nausea and vomiting, diarrhea, bone pain, hypercalcemia	Vaginal bleeding, edema, stress incontinence, hypertension, venous thrombosis, corneal opacities and retinopathy, increased pigmentation of nipples or areolae, breast pain, dysmenorrhea, rashes. Gynecomastia and breast pain in males
Antiestrogens Tamoxifen	Hot flashes, nausea and vomiting, bone pain, hypercalcemia	Vaginal discharge and bleeding, thrombocytopenia, rash, peripheral edema, thrombophlebitis, change in corneal curvature, retinopathy, headache, dizziness, depression

various degrees of gynecomastia and may also experience pain in the breast. Some patients undergo a change in the curvature of the cornea such that contact lenses do not fit.

CARCINOGENIC EFFECTS. The association between diethylstilbestrol and the development of vaginal adenocarcinoma in young women whose mothers had been treated with the drug during pregnancy has been discussed above. In addition to a risk of developing adenocarcinoma, 67% of these young women (versus 4% of controls) were found to have vaginal adenosis.[98] The long-term use of low doses of estrogens in postmenopausal women increases their risk of developing endometrial carcinoma.[99] It is virtually certain that endogenous sex hormones play a role in the causation of breast cancer,[100] but whether or not long-term estrogen use for contraception or for prevention of osteoporosis in the postmenopausal state is associated with an increased risk of breast cancer is controversial.[101] If estrogen replacement therapy does increase the risk, as some studies indicate,[102] then it would seem to be a modest effect.[101] The risk of ovarian cancer is decreased by the use of oral contraceptives.[103]

Antiestrogens

Several antiestrogens, including clomiphene, nafoxidine, and tamoxifen, have been tested in clinical trials for hormonal therapy of breast

Tamoxifen

cancer. Because of its low incidence of side effects, only tamoxifen is used for cancer treatment in the United States. Tamoxifen is now the first choice endocrine therapy for treatment of advanced breast cancer and for adjuvant treatment of metastatic breast cancer following mastectomy.[104] Figure 9–9 presents a reason-able sequence for endocrine treatment in the patient with metastatic breast cancer.[13]

Tamoxifen Action

Tamoxifen binds to estrogen receptors, acting as a complete antagonist in some systems and as an antagonist with partial agonist activity in other systems. The profile of the activity is complicated by the fact that some of the metabolites have agonist activity whereas others do not. This has led to a large and often confusing literature regarding the antitumor effect, and the reader is referred to comprehensive reviews for details of tamoxifen action and pharmacology.[104,105]

By binding to the estrogen receptor, tamoxifen competes for the binding of endogenous estradiol, and its major therapeutic effect in breast cancer reflects this antiestrogenic mechanism. As illustrated in Table 9–2, the presence of estrogen receptors is predictive of response to tamoxifen. Although the tamoxifen-receptor complex can become tightly associated with nuclear components, the complex is not transcriptionally active in systems like the chick oviduct where the drug is a complete antagonist. In other systems, the tamoxifen-receptor complex (or a metabolite-receptor complex) is transcriptionally active. For example, after exposure of a hormone-dependent, cultured, human breast cancer cell line to a low tamoxifen concentration, progesterone receptors were induced,[106] indicating a completely intact response pathway. However, it seems unlikely that such partial agonist effects (if they occur in human tumors) contribute significantly to tamoxifen's effectiveness in treating breast cancer. In the same breast cancer cell line, a high concentration of tamoxifen inhibited cell growth and induction of progesterone receptor in a manner that was reversed by estrogen.[106]

Tamoxifen Pharmacology

Tamoxifen is administered orally and peak plasma levels are achieved in 3 to 6 hours.[107] The pharmacokinetics are biphasic, with a half-life of 7 to 14 hours for the initial phase and about 7 days for the second phase.[106] Continuous therapy with tamoxifen (10 mg bid) pro-

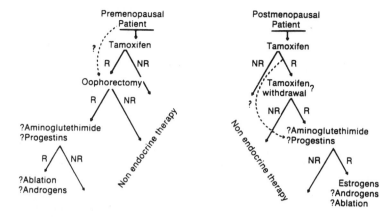

Figure 9–9   Optimal sequence of endocrine treatments of metastatic breast cancer based on relative toxicities and efficacy in premenopausal and postmenopausal women. R, response; NR, no response. (From Henderson[13])

duces steady-state levels (100–200 ng/ml serum) within 4 weeks. The drug is metabolized by the cytochrome P450 system to at least 6 metabolites. The major metabolite is N-desmethyltamoxifen, which is present in the plasma at levels that are generally twice those of the parent drug.[108] N-desmethyltamoxifen has the same affinity for the estrogen receptor as tamoxifen.[107] Another metabolite, monohydroxytamoxifen, is present at low levels in the serum (<10 ng) but has about 100-fold higher affinity for the estrogen receptor.[107] The action of tamoxifen *in vivo* reflects the net activity of the parent drug and its metabolites competing for the occupation of estrogen receptors in the tumor.

The tamoxifen metabolites are conjugated principally as glucuronides and excreted in the bile. After enterohepatic circulation, about 75% of the drug is eliminated in the feces and impaired renal function does not result in increased tamoxifen blood levels.[109] The metabolites have especially long half-lives (2 weeks) because of extensive protein binding in the plasma and efficient reuptake from the intestinal tract.

Untoward Effects

Tamoxifen is very well tolerated.[13] The most frequent side effect is mild nausea (9.5%), which is reduced by taking the drug after meals and usually disappears after a few weeks of therapy. Hot flashes are common (8.4%) but are rarely severe enough to require discontin-

uation of the drug. Tumor flare following initiation of therapy occurs in 4% to 6% of patients.[13] Mild, transient thrombocytopenia (4.6%) and leukopenia (1.6%) may also occur, but routine monitoring of leukocyte and platelet counts is probably not required. Other delayed effects listed in Table 9–5 occur at a frequency of less than 1%.[13]

Progestins

Progestins are used primarily to treat advanced endometrial carcinoma that cannot be treated by surgery or by radiation.[18,110] The normal physiologic role of progestins is to promote maturation of the secretory epithelium of the endometrium. Their therapeutic effect reflects a direct action on the endometrial tumor cells and correlates with the presence of progesterone receptors in the tumor.[46] Progestins are also used as a second-line drug to treat occasional patients with metastatic breast cancer (Fig. 9–9), where their therapeutic effect is equivalent to that of tamoxifen.[13,110] This therapeutic effect probably reflects both a direct action via progesterone receptors in the breast tumor cells[111] as well as an indirect action via a decrease in the serum levels of LH and estrone.[112,113]

Pharmacology

Medroxyprogesterone acetate and megestrol acetate are the most frequently used preparations. Megestrol acetate is administered orally (40 to 320 mg daily for treatment of endometrial carcinoma) and medroxyprogesterone acetate may be administered either orally or in-

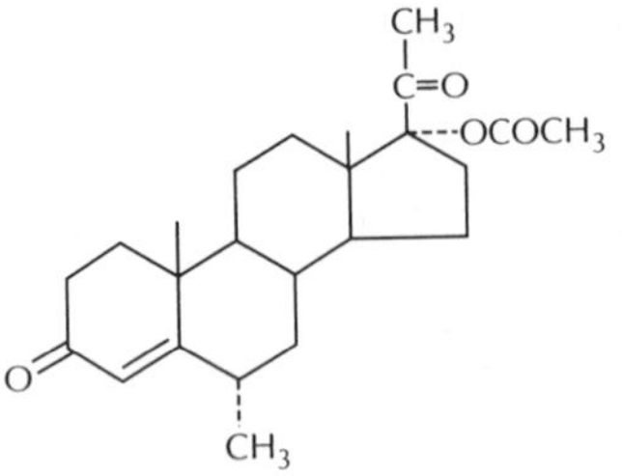

Medroxyprogesterone
Acetate

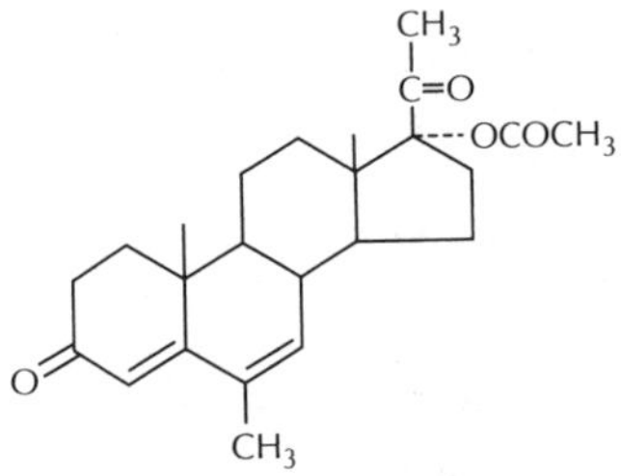

Megestrol Acetate

tramuscularly (weekly injection of 400 to 1,000 mg). Both drugs are well absorbed after oral administration, with peak plasma levels being achieved after 2–4 hours.[113,114] The plasma concentration present 12 hours after an oral dose of medroxyprogesterone acetate is about 5 times that achieved after intramuscular administration.[115] Both drugs are metabolized by hydroxylation and then glucoronidation.[82] Excretion is primarily renal with very little excretion of unchanged drug.[82]

Side Effects

The principal side effect is weight gain, which appears to be dose-related and results from increased appetite as well as some fluid retention.[13] Some patients may experience hot flashes, and as with other hormonal therapies, hypercalcemia and tumor flare can occur with initiation of therapy. Vaginal bleeding occurs in 5% to 10% of patients, either during treatment or upon discontinuation of therapy. There is a risk of thrombophlebitis and embolism, and the presence of preexisting thrombo-

phlebitis or thromboembolic disorders requires special caution, as do conditions that may be exacerbated by fluid retention. Infrequently, patients may experience neurologic symptoms.[13] Many patients report an improved sense of well-being when starting progestin therapy.[113]

Androgens

Some patients (about 10%) with metastatic breast cancer respond to androgen treatment.[13] The major part of the antitumor effect probably reflects suppression of LH production and consequent decrease in endogenous estrogen synthesis. The masculizing side effects lead to very poor patient acceptance, and androgens are now considered to be a fourth line of treatment after tamoxifen, progestins, and aminoglutethimide (Fig. 9–9).[13]

Pharmacology

Fluoxymestrone is the androgen most commonly employed in breast cancer treatment, being administered orally at 10–40 mg daily in divided doses. For parenteral treatment, testos-

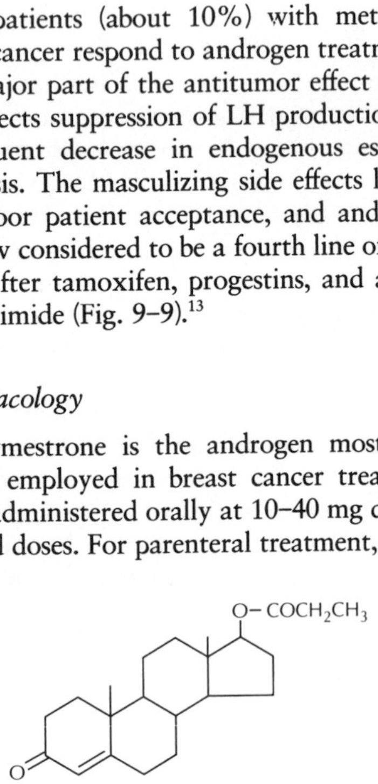

Testosterone propionate

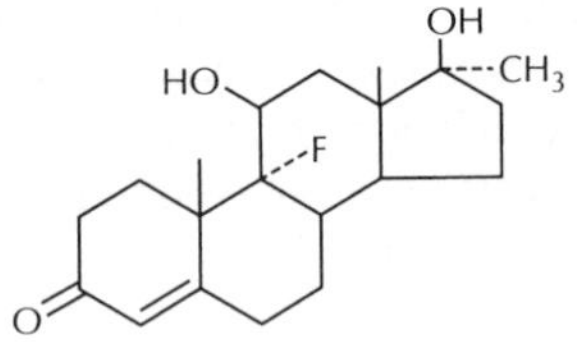

Fluoxymesterone

terone propionate may be administered intramuscularly (50–100 mg) three times weekly. Testosterone has a short half-life of less than 15 minutes as the unaltered drug. In the tissues, testosterone is reduced by 5α-reductase to dihydrotestosterone, which is the form that binds to the androgen receptor. Indeed, the absence or deficiency of 5α-reductase results in male pseudohermaphoditism.[116] Most of the administered testosterone is inactivated in the liver via conversion to androsterone and etiocholanolone, which are the major metabolites recovered in the urine.[82] These 3α-hydroxy products are excreted in the urine mainly as glucuronides. Fluoxymestrone is metabolized less rapidly than testosterone and has a longer half-life, about 2 to 3 hours.

Side Effects

The principal side effect is masculinization, including facial hair growth, acne, and deepening of the voice. After long-term treatment, male pattern baldness, body hair growth, and clitoral enlargement occur and the changes are irreversible. Water retention occurs and caution should be exercised in patients with pre-existing cardiac disease. Fluoxymestrone (and other 17α-methyl compounds) can cause cholestatic jaundice, which usually develops after several months of therapy and is reversible on discontinuation of treatment.[117] This is not seen with parenteral administration of testosterone propionate. Patients who have undergone long-term treatment with 17α-alkyl derivatives have developed hepatic adenocarcinoma.[117] As with other forms of hormonal therapy, initiation of androgen treatment may cause hypercalcemia and tumor flare, although the incidence is probably less than that with estrogen treatment.

Antiandrogens

Several antiandrogens have been tested for their effect on prostatic carcinoma. As mentioned early in this chapter, carcinoma of the prostate is an androgen-dependent tumor and hormonal chemotherapy focuses on decreasing androgen production by administration of an LHRH agonist or an estrogen. When an LHRH agonist, such as leuprolide is administered, the antiandrogenic drug flutamide is also administered to block the action of dihydrotestosterone in the cells of the carcinoma. Both steroidal and nonsteroidal antiandrogens have been synthesized. Cyproterone acetate, the most potent of the steroidal androgen antagonists, is an investigational drug in the United States. The drug has progestational activity and suppresses gonadotropin secretion.[118] Flutamide is the nonsteroidal antiandrogen that is

Cyproterone acetate

Flutamide

used in the United States. Both of these drugs directly compete for the binding of dihydrotestosterone to the androgen receptor.[119] Although flutamide itself does not have hormonal activity, when it is administered alone, it blocks the feedback inhibition of LH production by testosterone (Fig. 9–1) and plasma levels of LH and testosterone rise.[120,121] The rise in plasma testosterone would tend to counteract its antiandrogenic activity, and in the treatment of prostate cancer, flutamide is now always administered in combination with an LHRH agonist. Both cyproterone acetate and flutamide have been demonstrated to be effective therapy (roughly equivalent to an estrogen) when used alone in the treatment of carcinoma of the prostate.[122] Combined androgen blockade with an LHRH agonist and flutamide provides a modest increase in time to tumor progression over treatment with an LHRH agonist alone.[123]

PHARMACOLOGY. Flutamide is rapidly and completely absorbed from the gastrointestinal tract.[124] The parent drug is rapidly converted to a variety of metabolites, the major one being hydroxyflutamide.[124] The parent compound flutamide has a very low affinity for the androgen receptor, but the affinity of hydroxyflutamide is about 20 times higher,[125,126] making it the active form of the drug. Peak plasma levels of hydroxyflutamide are achieved 2 hours after a single oral administration of flutamide[127] and the plasma levels decline with a half-life of 2–4 hours as a result of renal excretion. In patients receiving flutamide at the usual dosage of 250 mg every 8 hours, the minimal plasma concentration of hydroxyflutamide is about 5 μM, which is 5,000 times the plasma concentration of testosterone (1 nM) in patients treated with an LHRH agonist.[127] As hydroxyflutamide is only one percent as potent as testosterone in competing for binding to the androgen receptor,[126] a plasma level of 5 μM hydroxyflutamide is required to ensure effective competition.[127]

Cyproterone acetate is also administered orally. After absorption from the gastrointestinal tract, it is converted by hydroxylation to a metabolite that is also antiandrogenic.

SIDE EFFECTS. Flutamide causes nausea, diarrhea, and dizziness in some (about 5%) patients,[128] but unlike GnRH agonists, it does not produce tumor flare. The principal side effect is gynecomastia, often associated with tenderness in the nipples and areolae.[129] In contrast to other hormonal therapies, flutamide causes impotence only infrequently, if at all (see Table 9–6). Transient rises in hepatic enzymes may occur. Cyproterone does cause impotence but has relatively few other side effects.[130]

LHRH (GnRH) Agonists

Mechanism of Action

LH is released from the anterior pituitary cells when they are stimulated by gonadotropin-releasing hormone (GnRH). A newer term for GnRH is luteinizing hormone-releasing hormone (LHRH). LHRH is a decapeptide that is cleaved from a 92 amino acid precursor in the hypothalamus, and under appropriate neuronal influences is released into the hypothalamohypophyseal portal venous system, which directly bathes the LH-producing cells of the anterior pituitary (Fig. 9–1). Because the portal venous system into which LHRH is released constitutes such a limited volume of distribution, release of only tiny amounts of hormone permits occupancy of LHRH receptors on the surface of the pituitary cells. Normally, the pituitary cells are exposed to pulsatile releases of LHRH, and through a mechanism involving the Ca^{2+}/diacylglycerol-mediated activation of protein kinase C, the gonadotropins LH and FSH are released.

In addition to LH release, occupancy of the pituitary cell receptors by LHRH leads to receptor internalization and desensitization.[131] It is this *downregulation* of the receptor that is responsible for the marked decrease in LH and FSH released during continuous exposure to LHRH agonists in therapy.[132] Because the required stimulus of LH is no longer present, plasma testosterone levels decline substantially in humans treated with LHRH agonists.[133] The plasma concentrations of testosterone in male patients treated with LHRH agonists are similar to those existing after castration; thus, such treatment constitutes a pharmacological orchiectomy that is reversible on discontinuation of the drug.[133,134] Treatment of women with LHRH agonists reduces plasma estradiol concentrations to those seen in oophorectomized or postmenopausal women.[135]

LHRH agonists are used to treat advanced

Table 9–6   Relative Incidence of Side Effects Accompanying Different Endocrine Manipulations in the Treatment of Prostatic Cancer. (Modified from Grayhack et al.[130])

	Orchiectomy	Estrogens	LHRH Agonists	Flutamide
Cardiovascular	−	+	−	−
Tumor flare	−	−	++	−
Gastrointestinal distress	−	+	−	+
Impotence	++	++	+++	−
Gynecomastia	−	++++	−	++
Hot flashes	+	±	++	−

prostate cancer. Although there is only a small increase in response to combined androgen blockade with an LHRH agonist and flutamide compared to LHRH agonist therapy alone,[123] the combined drug approach is usually employed. The results of treatment of prostate cancer with LHRH agonists are similar to those obtained with diethylstilbestrol[136] or with orchiectomy.[137] Both premenopausal and postmenopausal patients with metastatic breast cancer respond to treatment with LHRH agonists, but they are not considered to be standard therapies at present.[12]

Pharmacology

Leuprolide and goserelin are the two LHRH agonists available in the United States for treating prostatic carcinoma (Table 9–7). These compounds were prepared to specifically modify the pharmacology of natural LHRH in order to obtain a long-lasting occupancy of the LHRH receptor on pituitary cells and permit continuous suppression of LH production. Native LHRH (gonadorelin) is rapidly degraded by peptidases and excreted by the kidney, such that its half-life is too short to permit it to be useful in obtaining continuous suppression of LH production.[138] The major site of cleavage of native LHRH is at the sixth amino acid position (Table 9–7) and substitution of a dextrorotary for the levo-amino acid (Gly) at this position enhances biologic activity and substitution with a hydrophobic D-amino acid further enhances potency.[138] Substitution of the glycine in position 10 with N-ethylamide (leuprolide) or Azgly (goserelin) increases affinity for the receptor by markedly slowing the rate of dissociation.

Leuprolide is available in a form for daily injection or as a depot preparation that is administered once monthly. Leuprolide acetate, 1 mg administered by daily subcutaneous injection, produces a 95% decrease in testicular androgen production.[132] Initially, there is an elevation of plasma LH and testosterone, followed within three days to a week by continuous suppression for as long as treatment is continued.[132] Leuprolide acetate is also provided in a microsphere form containing 7.5 mg of drug that is released slowly from the intramuscular injection site over the course of several weeks. Once-monthly injection of the depot prepara-

Table 9–7   Structures of LHRH Agonists

pyroGlu-His-Trp-Ser-Tyr-Gly-Leu-Arg-Pro-Gly-NH₂
 1   2   3   4   5   6   7   8   9   10

LHRH (GnRH) Agonist	Substitution at Residue 6	Substitution at Residue 10
Leuprolide	D-Leu	ethylamide
Goserelin	D-(t-butyl) Ser	Azgly

tion reduces testosterone plasma levels by 95% and maintains these castrate levels for the duration of treatment. Leuprolide acetate has a plasma half-life of approximately 3 hours and bioavailability of either the short-acting subcutaneous or the depot intramuscular preparation is in the range of 90%.

Goserelin acetate is provided as a slow-release implant containing 3.6 mg of drug. The implant is a cylindrical rod prepared from a lactide-glycolide copolymer that is completely biodegradable, and no material is recoverable from the injection site after 5 weeks.[139] The goserelin is released continuously from the copolymer for up to 30 days, permitting administration of the drug every 28 days by implantation with a 16-gauge needle into the subcutaneous fat.[139] Administered in this manner, goserelin reduces plasma testosterone concentration by 95% and maintains it at castrate levels for the duration of therapy.[139]

Side Effects

LHRH agonists are generally well tolerated. The most common side effect is the experience of hot flashes, reported by more than 50% of patients in most studies.[136] Because the LHRH agonists initially cause LH release and increase plasma testosterone concentration prior to pituitary cell desensitization, patients with metastatic prostatic carcinoma may experience tumor flare with increase in bone pain and plasma acid phosphatase.[130] An advantage of total androgen blockade therapy is that flutamide ameliorates or blocks the flare by competing for the binding of the testosterone to the androgen receptor. Some patients may experience a temporary increase in urinary tract obstruction during the first week of treatment.

Gynecomastia and breast tenderness occur much less often than with diethylstilbestrol

Aromatase pathway

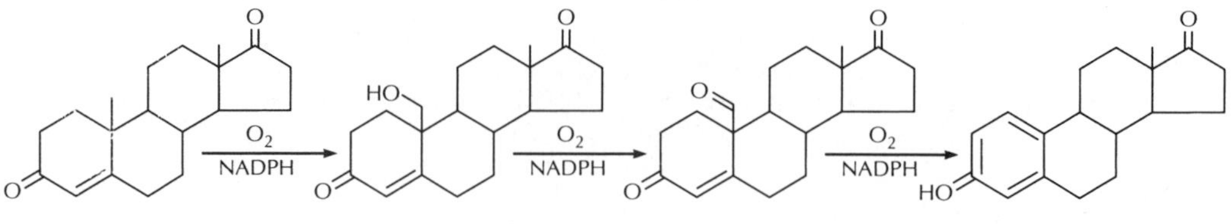

Androstenedione · Estrone

therapy and LHRH therapy is not associated with the cardiovascular risks of estrogen treatment (Table 9–6).[136] Side effects from decreased testosterone levels, including decreased libido and impotence, occur commonly. Sperm density and motility fall markedly, but in one study sperm density was shown to return to pretreatment levels after termination of therapy.[133]

Aromatase Inhibitors

Rationale

Estrogens are synthesized in the body from androgens via the action of an enzyme complex called aromatase. In premenopausal women, the major site of aromatization and estrogen synthesis is the ovary. In postmenopausal women, estrogens are synthesized from androstenedione that is synthesized in the adrenal gland and undergoes aromatization at extraglandular sites, in particular in adipose tissue.[140] Because aromatization is the final step in estrogen synthesis (see Fig. 9–10),[141] there has been a lot of interest in synthesizing selective aromatase inhibitors for treatment of metastatic breast cancer in postmenopausal women and in premenopausal women who have undergone ovariectomy. The aromatase inhibitors available for cancer treatment in the United States are the nonsteroidal compound aminoglutethimide and the steroidal compound testolactone.

Aminoglutethimide was initially introduced as an anticonvulsive drug in 1958, but it was withdrawn because of endocrine system side effects, including inhibition of adrenal steroidogenesis. The side effect on steroid synthesis was first exploited in the treatment of Cushing's syndrome[142] and then in the treatment of breast

cancer.[143] As outlined in Figure 9–10, aminoglutethimide inhibits cholesterol side chain cleavage as well as 11β-hydroxylase and 18-hydroxylase activities involved in the synthesis of aldosterone and hydrocortisone (cortisol).[141] When aminoglutethimide effects on steroid levels were measured in patients, it was found that plasma levels of estrone and estradiol were reduced markedly (95%) as a result of aromatase inhibition.[144] Aminoglutethimide appears to act by interacting directly with the aromatase P-450[145] and the peripheral aromatase appears to be more sensitive to inhibition than ovarian aromatase.[146] Although the major component of aminoglutethimide action reflects aromatase

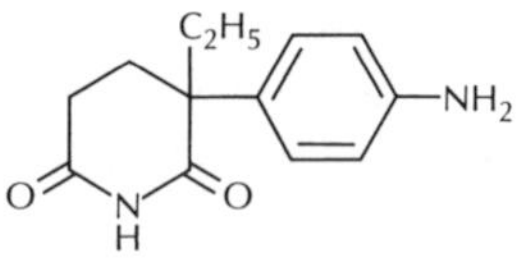

Aminoglutethimide

inhibition, some studies suggest that it also stimulates the rate of metabolism of estrone and estrone sulfate.[147]

Clinical Use

Clinical studies have shown that aminoglutethimide administered at the usual dosage of 1,000 mg daily is as effective as any other form of endocrine therapy in treating advanced breast carcinoma in postmenopausal women (see Table 9–2),[13] where an objective response rate of 32% is achieved in unselected patients and 52% in women with estrogen receptor-positive tumors.[148,149] Although the higher dosage is used routinely, an equivalent response can be achieved with 500 mg daily with less severe

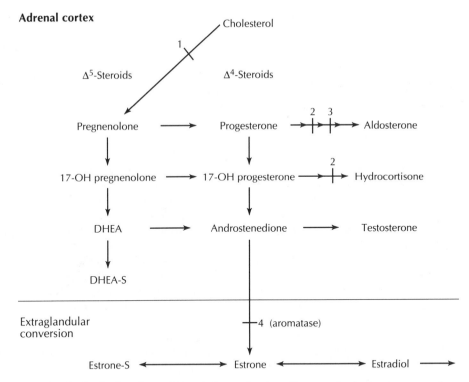

Figure 9–10 Synthesis of adrenal steroids and the production of estrone in the postmenopausal state. Inhibition of reactions 1, 2, and 3 by aminoglutethimide results in decreased plasmal levels of cortisol (hytrocortisone), an effect that is partially compensated by the action of increased levels of ACTH resulting from decreased feedback inhibition by cortisol at the hypothalamus and pituitary. Inhibition of estrone synthesis results from aminoglutethimide inhibition of peripheral aromatase. Bars across the arrows designate reactions inhibited by aminoglutethimide: 1) cholesterol side-chain cleavage enzyme (desmolase); 2) 11β-hydroxylase; 3) 18-hydroxylase; 4) aromatase (nonglandular). DHEA-S dehydroepiandrosterone sulfate. (Adapted from Lonning and Kvinnsland[141])

side effects.[150] Because adrenosteroidogenesis is inhibited, the plasma level of hydrocortisone declines, but the effect is transitory because, as a result of the interruption in negative feedback, ACTH secretion increases sufficiently to partially overcome the drug-induced adrenal blockade.[148] Hydrocortisone, 40 mg/day divided into 3 or 4 doses, is administered for replacement to prevent this reflex ACTH increase. Dexamethasone should not be administered because aminoglutethimide increases the rate of its metabolism, but the metabolism of hydrocortisone is not affected.[148]

Aminoglutethimide-plus-hydrocortisone treatment inhibits androgen production in the adrenal gland and decreases the plasma levels of most of the endogenous androgens in castrate males.[151] It is unclear, however, whether aminoglutethimide is effective in treating patients with prostate carcinoma who have become refractory to other treatments,[152] and the drug is not generally used for this purpose in the United States. Indeed, the androgen suppression that occurs can be caused by the hydrocortisone component alone inhibiting ACTH production.[153]

Several aromatase inhibitors are being developed for use in cancer treatment. One of these, 4-hydroxyandrostenedione, is undergoing clinical trial.[154] This compound acts as a suicide substrate that permanently inactivates the aromatase, and its action is more selective than aminoglutethimide in that it does not appear to inhibit adrenal steroidogenesis.[154] Testolactone is a testosterone derivative that is devoid of androgenic activity. Although it has a more selective antiaromatase action and is better tolerated than aminoglutethimide, its antitumor potency is less.[154]

Aminoglutethimide Pharmacology

Aminoglutethimide is usually administered as a 250-mg tablet taken four times daily. Absorption of an oral dose is good, with peak plasma levels occurring in about 1 hour.[155] After administration of a single dose, there is an initial rapid decline followed by a slower decline with a half-life of 10–15 hours (clearance 2.6 liters per hour).[155,156] The volume of distribution is 70–90 liters with a relatively low binding (20–24%) to plasma protein.[155] Aminoglutethimide induces its own metabolism and the half-life declines to about 7 hours (clearance 5.3 liters per hour) after a few weeks of treatment at 250 mg four times daily.[156] One study suggests that a change in distribution volume with continuous treatment may contribute to the decrease in drug half-life.[157] However, given the ability of aminoglutethimide to induce the microsome P-450-mediated metabolism of other drugs, such as dexamethasone, theophylline, and digitoxin, it would seem that induction of hepatic enzymes must be the major factor in the drug's ability to reduce its own half-life.[158]

Aminoglutethimide is metabolized by several pathways, including formation of N-acetyl, N-formyl, nitro, and hydroxylamino derivatives, and both unchanged drug and the metabolites are excreted in the urine.[159,160] The rate of metabolism to the major N-acetyl metabolite is subject to the N-acetylation polymorphism, with the half-life of the drug being 50% longer in fast acetylators.[161] The metabolites of aminoglutethimide are markedly less active than the parent drug at aromatase inhibition.[160]

Side Effects of Aminoglutethimide

Aminoglutethimide is more toxic than tamoxifen or the progestins, but it is better tolerated than estrogens or androgens. Given that the drug was originally introduced as an anticonvulsant, it is not surprising that CNS depression is the most common side effect in anticancer therapy. Many patients experience acute soporific side effects, including lethargy (40%), drowsiness, and ataxia (10%).[149] These effects

decrease in severity or disappear over the course of 6 weeks with continuation of therapy. It has been suggested that the transient nature of the CNS depression may reflect the autoinduction of metabolism and resulting tolerance based on decreased plasma levels of the drug.[149,156] Aminoglutethimide induces a maculopapular rash in 20–30% of patients, which generally appears on day 10 to 15 of drug administration and resolves spontaneously in most patients after about 5 days without withdrawal of drug.[149] Nausea and vomiting occur in about 15% of patients.

Other side effects occur infrequently. Cushingoid symptoms occur rarely with long-term administration of aminoglutethimide-plus-hydrocortisone and can be controlled by adjusting the hydrocortisone dosage.[13] Suppression of aldosterone synthesis by the adrenal cortex (see Fig. 9–10) may lead to hypotension (occasionally orthostatic). Masculinization and hirsutism have occurred in females. Rarely, patients with mild, compensated thyroid disease may become overtly hypothyroid during treatment. This reflects direct inhibition of thyroxine synthesis by the drug. Marked leukopenia and/or thrombocytopenia occur in 0.9% of patients within 3 to 7 weeks of starting therapy.[162] The bone marrow depression is reversible.[162]

Adrenocortical Suppressors

Mitotane

Mitotane is 1,1dichloro-2(o-chlorophenyl)-2-(p-chlorophenyl) ethane, best known by its trivial name, o,p'-DDD. Mitotane is used only in the palliative treatment of inoperable adrenocortical carcinoma.[163] The medical use of this compound is based on the observation that the insecticide DDD (an analog of DDT) produced necrosis and atrophy of the adrenal cortex in dogs.[164] The isomer o,p'-DDD was subsequently identified as the principal toxic agent.[165] Mitotane apparently acts directly on the adrenal glands, producing degenerative lesions of the zona reticularis and the zona fasciculata in the cortex.[166] The biochemical mechanism of its action is not known. Mitotane controls hormonal secretions in 75% of patients with adrenocortical carcinoma, but it does not have a significant effect on survival.[163]

Mitotane is administered orally, and about 40% of an oral dose is absorbed from the gastrointestinal tract (60% of the dose can be recovered unchanged in the feces), and approximately 25% of the drug absorbed each day appears in the urine as metabolites.[167,168] The major urinary form (>50%) is the metabolite 2,2-(2-chlorophenyl, 4'-chlorophenyl) acetic acid.[168,169] The drug is widely distributed in the body, but it apparently does not enter the cerebrospinal fluid.[167] Like the insecticides DDT and DDD, a significant amount of the unaltered drug is stored in fat.[168,170] On discontinuation of therapy, the drug disappears slowly from the serum over the course of several months.[170]

Some studies[171] have reported that about 75% of patients receiving mitotane have some gastrointestinal side effects, while others[163] have found a lower incidence in the range of 15%. Central nervous system side effects, which include lethargy, somnolence, ataxia, and dizziness, occur in a substantial percentage of patients.[163,171] Visual disturbances (visual blurring, diplopia, lens opacity) occur, but infrequently. In early studies, rashes (often transient) were reported in about 15% of patients.[171] Most patients have some evidence of hepatic disturbance, such as elevated serum levels of alkaline phosphatase, aspartate aminotransferase, and alanine aminotransferase.[163] Increases in serum levels of corticosteroid binding globulin, sex hormone binding globulin, and cholesterol may occur, as well as decreased levels of total and free thyroxine.[163] Male patients may develop gynecomastia.[163]

Mitotane is metabolized in the liver, and particular caution should be employed in treating patients with compromised hepatic function. Since adrenal depression is the principal action of the drug, it should be temporarily discontinued following shock or severe trauma, and because the depressed adrenal may not be able to rapidly secrete steroids, exogenous glucocorticoid should be administered. Mitotane appears to induce the hepatic metabolism of some glucocorticoids such that higher than normal amounts of steroid may be required during stress.[172] Because mitotane more or less selectively destroys the zona fasciculata and zona reticularis of the adrenal cortex and spares the zona glomerulosa, patients may have nearly normal aldosterone secretion and can withstand salt deprivation.[173] It is useful to monitor cortisol levels during treatment,[174] but conflicting data have been published regarding the usefulness of monitoring the plasma levels of mitotane itself.[167,168,175] In one study, a direct relationship was found between serum drug level and both tumor response and incidence of reversible neuromuscular toxicity,[175] whereas other studies have found no correlation of drug levels with either clinical response or side effects.[167,168] Mitotane is transferred through the placenta, and there is evidence that it is toxic to the adrenal progenitor cells of the fetus.[170]

REFERENCES

1. C. Huggins and P. J. Clark: Quantitative studies on prostate secretion. II. The effect of castration and estrogen injection on normal and on the hyperplastic prostate glands of dogs. J. Exptl. Med. 72:747 (1940).
2. C. Huggins and C. V. Hodges: Studies on prostatic cancer. I. The effect of castration, of estrogen and of androgen injection on serum phosphatases in metastatic carcinoma of the prostate. Cancer Res. 1:293 (1941).
3. C. Huggins, R. E. Stevens, and C. V. Hodges: Studies on prostatic cancer. II. The effects of castration on advanced carcinoma of the prostate gland. Arch. Surg. 43:209 (1941).
4. C. Huggins, W. W. Scott, and C. V. Hodges: Studies on prostatic cancer. III. The effects of fever, of desoxycorticosterone and of estrogen on clinical patients with metastatic carcinoma of the prostate. J. Urol. 46:997 (1941).
5. C. Huggins, M. H. Masina, L. Eichelberger, and J. D. Wharton: Quantitative studies of prostatic secretion. I. Characteristics of the normal secretion; the influence of thyroid, suprarenal, and testis extirpation and androgen substitution on the prostatic output. J. Exptl. Med. 70:543 (1939).
6. M. C. Bishop, C. Selby, and M. Taylor: Plasma hor-

mone levels in patients with prostatic carcinoma treated with diethylstilbestrol and estramustine. *Br. J. Urol.* 57:542 (1985).

7. R. Tomic: Pituitary function after orchiectomy in patients with or without earlier estrogen treatment for prostatic carcinoma. *J. Endocrinol. Invest.* 10:479 (1987).

8. C. A. Perez, W. R. Fair, and D. C. Ihde: "Carcinoma of the prostate," in *Cancer: Principles and Practice of Oncology,* ed. by V. T. DeVita, S. Hellman, and S. A. Rosenberg. Philadelphia: J.B. Lippincott Co., 1989, pp. 1023–1058.

9. G. T. Beatson: On the treatment of inoperable cases of carcinoma of the mamma: Suggestions for a new method of treatment with illustrative cases. *Lancet* 2:104,162 (1896).

10. A. Lacassagne: Apparation de cancers de la mamelle chez le souris mâle à des injections de foliculine. *Compt. Rend. Acad. Sci.* 195:630 (1932).

11. A. Haddow, J. M. Watkinson, E. Patterson, and P. C. Koller: Influence of synthetic estrogens upon advanced malignant disease. *Brit. Med. J.* 2:393 (1944).

12. I. C. Henderson, J. R. Harris, D. W. Kinne: "Cancer of the breast," in *Cancer: Principles and Practice of Oncology,* ed. by V. T. DeVita, S. Hellman, and S. A. Rosenberg. Philadelphia: J.B. Lippincott Co., 1989, pp. 1197–1268.

13. I. C. Henderson: "Endocrine therapy in metastatic breast cancer," in *Breast Diseases,* ed. by J. R. Harris, S. Hellman, I. C. Henderson, and D. W. Kinne. Philadelphia: J.B. Lippincott Co., 1987, pp. 398–428.

14. R. M. Kelley and W. H. Baker: Progestational agents in the treatment of carcinoma of the endometrium. *New Engl. J. Med.* 264:216 (1961).

15. A. T. Hertig and S. C. Sommers: Genesis of endometrial carcinoma. I. Study of prior biopsies. *Cancer* 2:946 (1949).

16. W. A. Meissner, S. C. Sommers, and G. Sherman: Endometrial hyperplasia, endometrial carcinoma, and endometriosis produced experimentally by estrogen. *Cancer* 10:500 (1957).

17. C. T. Griffiths, M. Tomic, J. M. Craig, and R. W. Kistner: Effect of progestins, estrogens, and castration on induced endometrial carcinoma in the rabbit. *Surg. Forum* 14:399 (1963).

18. B. L. G. Kneale: Adjunctive and therapeutic progestins in endometrial cancer. *Clin. Obstet. Gynecol.* 13:789 (1986).

19. K. Leung and A. Munck: Peripheral actions of glucocorticoids. *Ann. Rev. Physiol.* 37:245 (1975).

20. A. Munck and D. A. Young: "Corticosteroids and lymphoid tissue," in *Handbook of Physiology,* Section 7, *Endocrinology,* Vol. VI, *Adrenal Gland,* ed. by H. Blaschko, G. Sayers, and A. D. Smith. Washington, D.C.: American Physiological Society, 1975, pp. 231–243.

21. D. J. Ingle: Atrophy of the thymus in normal and hypophysectomized rats following administration of cortin. *Proc. Soc. Exptl. Biol. Med.* 38:443 (1938).

22. T. F. Dougherty and A. White: Functional alterations in lymphoid tissue induced by adrenocortical secretion. *Am. J. Anat.* 44:81 (1945).

23. F. R. Heilman and E. C. Kendall: The influence of 11-dehydro-17-hydroxycorticosterone (compound E) on the growth of a malignant tumor in the mouse. *Endocrinology* 34:416 (1944).

24. O. H. Pearson, L. P. Eliel, R. W. Rawson, K. Dobriner, and C. P. Rhoads: ACTH- and cortisone-induced regression of lymphoid tumors in man. A preliminary report. *Cancer* 2:943 (1949).

25. P. Fessas, M. M. Wintrobe, R. B. Thompson, and G. E. Cartwright: Treatment of acute leukemia with cortisone and corticotropin. *Arch. Int. Med.* 94:384 (1954).

26. V. T. DeVita, R. C. Young, and G. P. Canellos: Combination versus single agent chemotherapy: A review of the basis for selection of drug treatment of cancer. *Cancer* 35:98 (1975).

27. D. G. Poplack, L. E. Kun, J. R. Cassady, and P. A. Pizzo: "Leukemias and lymphomas of childhood," in *Cancer: Principles and Practice of Oncology,* ed. by V. T. DeVita, S. Hellman, and S. A. Rosenberg. Philadelphia: J.P. Lippincott Co., 1989, pp. 1671–1695.

28. S. Hellman, E. S. Jaffe, and V. T. DeVita: "Hodgkin's disease," in *Cancer: Principles and Practice of Oncology,* ed. by V. T. DeVita, S. Hellman, and S. A. Rosenberg. Philadelphia: J.B. Lippincott Co., 1989, pp. 1696–1740.

29. W. B. Pratt: Transformation of glucocorticoid and progesterone receptors to the DNA-binding state. *J. Cell. Biochem.* 35:51 (1987).

30. W. B. Pratt: Interaction of hsp90 with steroid receptors: Organizing some diverse observations and presenting the newest concepts. *Mol. Cell. Endocrinol.* 74:C69 (1990).

31. K. R. Yamamoto: Steroid receptor regulated transcription of specific genes and gene networks. *Ann. Rev. Genet.* 19:209 (1985).

32. G. M. Ringold: Steroid hormone regulation of gene expression. *Ann. Rev. Pharmacol. Toxicol.* 25:529 (1985).

33. M. Beato: Gene regulation by steroid hormones. *Cell* 56:335 (1989).

34. R. M. Evans: The steroid and thyroid hormone receptor superfamily. *Science* 240:889 (1988).

35. T. Hard, E. Kellenbach, R. Boelens, B. A. Maler, K. Dahlman, L. P. Freedman, J. Carlstedt-Duke, K. R. Yamamoto, J. A. Gustafsson, and R. Kaptein: Solution structure of the glucocorticoid receptor DNA-binding domain. *Science* 249:157 (1990).

36. L. P. Freedman, B. F. Luisi, Z. R. Korzun, R. Basavappa, P. B. Sigler, K. R. Yamamoto: The function and structure of the metal coordination sites within the glucocorticoid receptor DNA binding domain. *Nature* 334:543 (1988).

37. M. Danielsen, L. Hinck, and G. M. Ringold: Two amino acids within the knuckle of the first zinc finger specify DNA response element activation by the glucocorticoid receptor. *Cell* 57:1131 (1989).

38. W. B. Pratt, D. J. Jolly, D. V. Pratt, S. M. Hollenberg, V. Giguere, F. M. Cadepond, G. Schweizer-Groyer, M. G. Catelli, R. M. Evans, and E. E. Baulieu: A region in the steroid binding domain determines formation of the non-DNA-binding, 9 S glucocorticoid receptor complex. *J. Biol. Chem.* 263:267 (1988).

39. F. C. Dalman, L. C. Scherrer, L. P. Taylor, H. Akil, and W. B. Pratt: Localization of the 90-kDa heat shock protein-binding site within the hormone-binding domain of the glucocorticoid receptor by peptide competition. *J. Biol. Chem.* 266:3482 (1991).

40. S. M. Hollenberg, V. Giguere, P. Segui, and R. M. Evans: Colocalization of DNA-binding and transcriptional

activation functions of the human glucocorticoid receptor. *Cell.* 49:39 (1987).

41. E. R. Sanchez, S. Meshinchi, W. Tienrungroj, M. J. Schlesinger, D. O. Toft, and W. B. Pratt: Relationship of the 90-kDa murine heat shock protein to the untransformed and transformed states of the L cell glucocorticoid receptor. *J. Biol. Chem.* 262:6986 (1987).

42. S. Meshinchi, E. R. Sanchez, K. Martell, and W. B. Pratt: Elimination and reconstitution of the requirement for hormone in promoting temperature dependent transformation of cytosolic glucocorticoid receptors to the DNA-binding state. *J. Biol. Chem.* 265:4863 (1990).

43. D. Picard, S. J. Salser, and K. R. Yamamoto: A movable and regulable inactivation function within the steroid binding domain of the glucocorticoid receptor. *Cell* 54:1073 (1988).

44. M. Eilers, D. Picard, K. R. Yamamoto, and J. M. Bishop: Chimaeras of Myc oncoprotein and steroid receptors cause hormone-dependent transformation of cells. *Nature* 340:66 (1989).

45. W. B. Pratt, E. R. Sanchez, E. H. Bresnick, S. Meshinchi, L. C. Scherrer, F. C. Dalman, and M. J. Welsh: Interaction of the glucocorticoid receptor with the M_r 90,000 heat shock protein: An evolving model of ligand-mediated receptor transformation and translocation. *Cancer Res.* 49(Suppl.):2222S (1989).

46. D. C. Merkel and C. K. Osborne: "Steroid receptors in relation to response," in *Endocrine Management of Cancer: 1 Biological Bases,* ed. by B. A. Stoll. Basel: S. Karger, 1988, pp. 84–99.

47. C. K. Osborne: "Receptors," in *Breast Diseases,* ed. by J. R. Harris, S. Hellman, I. C. Henderson, and D. W. Kinne. Philadelphia: J.B. Lippincott, 1987, pp. 210–232.

48. W. B. Pratt, J. L. Kaine, and D. V. Pratt: The kinetics of glucocorticoid binding to the soluble specific binding protein of mouse fibroblasts. *J. Biol. Chem.* 250:4584 (1975).

49. J. C. Allegra, M. E. Lippman, E. B. Thompson, R. Simon, A. Barlock, L. Green, K. K. Huff, H. M. T. Do, S. C. Aitken, and R. Warren: Estrogen receptor status: An important variable in predicting response to endocrine therapy in metastatic breast cancer. *Eur. J. Cancer* 16:323 (1980).

50. I. C. Henderson: "Endocrine therapy in metastatic breast cancer," in *Breast Diseases,* ed. by J. R. Harris, S. Helleman, I. C. Henderson, and D. W. Kinne. Philadelphia: J.B. Lippincott, 1987, pp. 398–428.

51. Nolvadex Adjuvent Trial Organization: Controlled trial of tamoxifen as a single adjuvent agent in management of early breast cancer. *Lancet* 1:836 (1985).

52. M. E. Lippman, R. B. Dickson, S. Bates, C. Knabbe, K. Huff, S. Swain, M. McManaway, D. Bronzert, A. Kasid, and E. P. Gelmann: Autocrine and paracrine growth regulation of human breast cancer. *Breast Cancer Res. Treat.* 7:59 (1986).

53. G. M. Clark and W. L. McGuire: Progesterone receptors and human breast cancer. *Breast Cancer Res. Treat.* 3:157 (1983).

54. J. L. Wittliff: Steroid-hormone receptors in breast cancer. *Cancer* 53:630 (1984).

55. C. E. Ehrlich, P. C. M. Young, and R. E. Cleary: Cytoplasmic progesterone and estradiol receptors in normal, hyperplastic, and carcinomatous endometria: Therapeutic implications. *Am. J. Obstet. Gynecol.* 141:539 (1981).

56. R. C. Benson, P. A. Gorman, P. C. O'Brien, E. L. Holicky, and C. M. Veneziale: Relationship between androgen receptor binding activity in human prostate cancer and clinical response to endocrine therapy. *Cancer* 59:1599 (1987).

57. T. J. Vietti, M. P. Sullivan, D. H. Berry, T. Haddy, M. Haggard, and R. Blattner: The response of acute childhood leukemia to an initial and a second course of prednisone. *J. Pediat.* 66:18 (1965).

58. M. E. Lippman, R. H. Halterman, B. G. Leventhal, S. Perry, and E. B. Thompson: Glucocorticoid-binding proteins in human acute lymphoblastic leukemic blast cells. *J. Clin. Invest.* 52:1715 (1973).

59. C. D. Bloomfield, K. A. Smith, B. A. Peterson, L. Hildebrandt, J. Zaleskas, K. J. Gajl-Peczalska, G. Frizzera, and A. Munck: In-vitro glucocorticoid studies for predicting response to glucocorticoid therapy in adults with malignant lymphoma. *Lancet* 1:952 (1980).

60. C. H. Sibley and G. M. Tomkins: Mechanism of steroid resistance. *Cell* 2:221 (1974).

61. J. M. Harmon and E. B. Thompson: "Glucocorticoid resistance in leukemic cells," in *Resistance to Antineoplastic Drugs,* ed. by D. Kessel. Boca Raton: CRC Press, 1988, pp. 385–402.

62. K. L. Lucas, K. W. Barbour, P. R. Housley, and E. A. Thompson: Biochemical and molecular characterization of the glucocorticoid receptor of lymphosarcoma P1798 variants. *Mol. Endocrinol.* 2:291 (1988).

63. J. M. Harmon, M. S. Elsasser, L. P. Eisen, L. A. Urda, J. Ashraf, and E. B. Thompson: Glucocorticoid receptor expression in receptorless mutants isolated from the human leukemic cell line CEM-C7. *Mol. Endocrinol.* 3:734 (1989).

64. R. C. Haynes: "Adrenocorticotropic hormone: Adrenocordical steroids and their synthetic analogs: Inhibitors of the synthesis and action of adrenocortical hormones," in *The Pharmacological Basis of Therapeutics,* 8th ed., ed. by A. G. Gilman, T. W. Rall, A. S. Nies, and P. Taylor. New York: Pergamon Press, 1990, pp. 1431–1462.

65. R. P. Schleimer, H. N. Claman, and A. Oronsky (eds.): *Anti-inflammatory Steroid Action: Basic and Clinical Aspects.* San Diego: Academic Press, 1989, 564 pp.

66. A. H. Wyllie: Glucocorticoid-induced thymocyte apoptosis is associated with endogenous nuclease activation. *Nature* 284:555 (1980).

67. J. J. Cohen and R. C. Duke: Glucocorticoid activation of a calcium-dependent endonuclease in thymocyte nuclei leads to cell death. *J. Immunol.* 132:38 (1984).

68. J. J. Cohen: "Lymphocyte death induced by glucocorticoids," in *Anti-inflammatory Steroid Action: Basic and Clinical Aspects,* ed. by R. P. Schleimer, H. N. Claman, and A. Oronsky. San Diego: Academic Press, 1989, pp. 110–131.

69. W. B. Pratt: The mechanism of glucocorticoid effects in fibroblasts. *J. Invest. Derm.* 71:24 (1978).

70. M. Abramovitz, C. L. Branchaud, and B. E. P. Murphy: Cortisol-cortisone interconversion in human fetal lung: Contrasting results using explant and monolayer cultures suggest that 11β-hydroxysteroid dehydrogenase (EC 1.1.1.146) comprises two enzymes. *J. Clin. Endocrinol. Metab.* 54:563 (1982).

71. J. Q. Rose, A. M. Yurchak, and W. J. Jusko: Dose dependent pharmacokinetics of prednisone and prednisolone in man. *J. Pharmacokin. Biopharm. 9*:389 (1981).

72. S. J. Szefler: "General pharmacology of glucocorticoids," in *Anti-inflammatory Steroid Action: Basic and Clinical Aspects*, ed. by R. P. Schleimer, H. N. Claman, and A. Oronsky. San Diego: Academic Press, 1989, pp. 353–376.

73. M. L. Rocci, R. D'Ambrosio, N. F. Johnson, and W. J. Jusko: Prednisolone binding to albumin and transcortin in the presence of cortisol. *Biochem. Pharmacol. 31*:289 (1982).

74. P. J. Meffin, P. M. Brooks, and B. C. Sallustio: Alterations in prednisolone disposition as a result of time of administration, gender and dose. *Br. J. Clin. Pharmacol. 17*:395 (1984).

75. M. Bartoszek, A. M. Brenner, and S. J. Szefler: Prednisone and methylprednisolone kinetics in children receiving anticonvulsant therapy. *Clin. Pharmacol. Ther. 42*:424 (1987).

76. L. Axelrod: "Side effects of glucocorticoid therapy," in *Anti-inflammatory Steroid Action: Basic and Clinical Aspects*, ed. by R. P. Schleimer, H. N. Claman, and A. Oronsky. San Diego: Academic Press, 1989, pp. 377–408.

77. J. C. Melby: Clinical pharmacology of systemic corticosteroids. *Ann. Rev. Pharmacol. Toxicol. 17*:511 (1977).

78. *Steroid Therapy*, ed. by D. L. Azarnoff. Philadelphia: W.B. Saunders, 1975, 340 pp.

79. C. A. Mashchak, R. A. Lobo, R. Dozono-Takano, P. Eggena, R. M. Nakamura, P. F. Brenner, and D. R. Mishell: Comparison of pharmacodynamic properties of various estrogen formulations. *Am. J. Obstet. Gynecol. 144*:511 (1982).

80. F. P. Abramson and H. C. Miller: Bioavailability, distribution and pharmacokinetics of diethylstilbestrol produced from stilphostrol. *J. Urol. 128*:1336 (1982).

81. H. A. Kemp, G. F. Read, D. Riad-Fahmy, A. W. Pike, S. J. Gaskell, K. Queen, M. E. Harper, and D. Griffiths; Measurement of diethylstilbestrol in plasma from patients with cancer of the prostate. *Cancer Res. 41*:4693 (1981).

82. K. Fotherby and F. James: Metabolism of synthetic steroids. *Adv. Steroid Biochem. Pharmacol. 3*:67 (1972).

83. W. Heyns: The steroid-binding β-globulin of human plasma. *Adv. Steroid Biochem. Pharmacol. 6*:59 (1977).

84. M. Metzler: Metabolic activation of xenobiotic stilbene estrogens. *Fed. Proc. 46*:1855 (1987).

85. D. Ross, R. J. Mehlhorn, P. Moldeus, and M. T. Smith: Metabolism of diethylstilbestrol by horseradish peroxidase and prostaglandin-H synthase. *J. Biol. Chem. 260*:16210 (1985).

86. J. G. Liehr, B. B. DeGue, A. M. Ballatore, and J. Henkin: Diethylstilbestrol (DES) quinone: A reactive intermediate in DES metabolism. *Biochem. Pharmacol. 32*:3711 (1983).

87. A. L. Herbst, H. Ulfelder, and D. C. Poskanzer: Adenocarcinoma of the vagina: Association of maternal stilbestrol therapy with tumor appearance in young women. *New Engl. J. Med. 284*:878 (1971).

88. L. J. Fischer, J. L. Weissinger, D. E. Rickert, and K. L. Hintze: Studies on the biological disposition of diethylstilbestrol in rats and humans. *J. Toxicol. Environ. Health 1*:587 (1976).

89. M. Metzler and J. A. McLachlan: Oxidative metabolites of diethylstilbestrol in the fetal, neonatal and adult mouse. *Biochem. Pharmacol. 27*:1087 (1978).

90. R. Maydl, R. R. Newbold, M. Metzler, and J. A. McLachlan: Diethylstilbestrol metabolism by the fetal genital tract. *Endocrinol. 113*:146 (1983).

91. B. Epe, D. Schiffmann, and M. Metzler: Possible role of oxygen radicals in cell transformation by diethylstilbestrol and related compounds. *Carcinogenesis 7*:1329 (1986).

92. J. A. McLachlan, A. Wong, G. H. Degen, and J. C. Barrett: Morphological and neoplastic transformation of Syrian hamster embryo fibroblasts by diethylstilbestrol and its analogs. *Cancer Res. 42*:3040 (1982).

93. H. W. Rudiger, F. Haenisch, M. Metzler, F. Oesch, and H. R. Glatt: Metabolites of diethylstilbestrol induce sister chromatid exchange in human fibroblasts. *Nature 281*:392 (1979).

94. G. H. Degen and M. Metzler: Sex hormones and neoplasia: Genotoxic effects in short term assays. *Arch. Toxicol. Suppl. 10*:264 (1986).

95. K. Vallis and J. Waxman: "Tumour flare in hormonal therapy," in *Endocrine Management of Cancer: 2 Contemporary Therapy*, ed. by B. A. Stoll. Basel: Karger, 1988, pp. 144–152.

96. A. Clarysse: Hormone-induced tumor flare. *Eur. J. Cancer Clin. Oncol. 21*:545 (1985).

97. A. C. Carter, N. Sedransk, R. M. Kelley, F. J. Ansfield, R. G. Ravdin, R. W. Talley, and N. R. Potter: Diethylstilbestrol: Recommended dosages for different categories of breast cancer patients. *JAMA 237*:2079 (1977).

98. M. Bibbo, W. B. Gill, F. Azizi, R. Blough, V. Fang, R. Rosenfield, G. F. B. Schumacher, K. Sleeper, M. G. Sonek, and G. L. Wied: Follow-up study of male and female offspring of DES-exposed mothers. *J. Obst. Gynecol. 49*:1 (1977).

99. S. Shapiro, J. P. Kelley, L. Rosenberg, D. W. Kaufman, S. P. Helmrich, N. B. Rosenshein, J. L. Lewis, R. C. Knapp, P. D. Stolley, and D. Schottenfeld: Risk of localized and widespread endometrial cancer in relation to recent and discontinued use of conjugated estrogens. *New Engl. J. Med. 313*:969 (1985).

100. B. E. Henderson, R. K. Ross, M. C. Pike, and J. T. Casagrande: Endogenous hormones as a major factor in human cancer. *Cancer Res. 42*:3232 (1982).

101. J. L. Kelsey and G. S. Berkowitz: Breast cancer epidemiology. *Cancer Res. 48*:5615 (1988).

102. L. Bergkvist, H. O. Adami, I. Persson, R. Hoover, and C. Schairer: The risk of breast cancer after estrogen and estrogen-progestin replacement. *New Engl. J. Med. 321*:293 (1989).

103. Centers for Disease Control: The reduction in risk of ovarian cancer associated with oral-contraceptive use. *New Engl. J. Med. 316*:650 (1987).

104. B. J. A. Furr and V. C. Jordan: The pharmacology and clinical uses of tamoxifen. *Pharmac. Ther. 25*:127 (1984).

105. S. M. Swain and M. E. Lippman: "Endocrine therapies of cancer," in *Cancer Chemotherapy: Principles and Practice*, ed. by B. A. Chabner and J. M. Collins. New York: J.B. Lippincott, 1990, pp. 59–109.

106. K. B. Horwitz, Y. Koseki, and W. L. McGuire: Estrogen control of progesterone receptor in human breast cancer: Role of estradiol and antiestrogen. *Endocrinology* 103:1742 (1978).

107. V. C. Jordan: Metabolites of tamoxifen in animals and man: Identification, pharmacology and significance. *Breast Cancer Res. Treat.* 2:123 (1982).

108. H. K. Adam, E. J. Douglas, and K. V. Kemp: The metabolism of tamoxifen in humans. *Biochem. Pharmacol.* 27:145 (1979).

109. C. M. Sutherland, L. A. Sternson, J. H. Muchmore, J. E. Ball, and E. J. Cerise: Effect of impaired renal function on tamoxifen. *J. Surg. Oncol.* 27:222 (1984).

110. A. U. Buzdar: "Progestins in cancer treatment," in *Endocrine Management of Cancer. 2 Contemporary Therapy,* ed. by B. A. Stoll. Basel: Karger, 1988, pp. 1–15.

111. K. B. Horwitz, L. L. Wei, S. M. Sedlacek, and C. N. dArville: Progestin action and progesterone receptor structure in human breast cancer: A review. *Rec. Proc. Horm. Res.* 41:249 (1985).

112. E. Vesterinen, N. E. Backas, K. Pesonen, U. H. Stenman, and T. Laatikainen: Effect of medroxyprogesterone acetate on serum levels of LH, FSH, cortisol, and estrone in patients with endometrial carcinoma. *Arch. Gynecol.* 230:205 (1981).

113. B. I. Sikic, S. A. Scudder, S. C. Ballon, O. M. Soriero, J. E. Christman, L. Suey, M. N. Ehsan, A. E. Brandt, and T. L. Evans: High dose megestrol acetate therapy of ovarian carcinoma: A phase II study by the Northern California Oncology group. *Semin. Oncol.* 13 (Suppl. 4):26 (1986).

114. I. Hesselius and E. D. B. Johansson: Medroxyprogesterone acetate (MPA) plasma levels after oral and intramuscular administration in a long term study. *Acta Obstet. Gynecol. Scand. (Suppl. 101):*65 (1981).

115. J. Lober, H. T. Mouridsen, M. Salimtschik, and E. Johansson: Pharmacokinetics of medroxyprogesterone acetate administered by oral and intramuscular route. *Acta Obstet. Gynecol. Scand. (Suppl. 101):*71 (1981).

116. J. E. Griffin and J. D. Wilson: "The androgen resistance syndromes: 5α-reductase deficiency, testicular feminization, and related syndromes," in *The Metabolic Basis of Inherited Disease,* 6th ed., ed. by C. R. Scriver, H. L. Beaudet, W. S. Sly, and D. Valle. New York: McGraw-Hill Book Co., 1989, pp. 1919–1944.

117. K. G. Ishak: Hepatic lesions caused by anabolic and contraceptive steroids. *Semin. Liver Dis.* 2:116 (1981).

118. F. Neumann and M. Topert: Pharmacology of the antiandrogens. *J. Steroid Biochem.* 25:885 (1986).

119. G. H. Rassmussen: Chemical control of androgen action. *Ann. Rep. Med. Chem.* 21:179 (1986).

120. V. A. Knuth, R. Hano, and E. Nieshlag: Effect of flutamide or cyproterone acetate on pituitary and testicular hormones in normal men. *J. Clin. Endocrinol. Metab.* 59:963 (1984).

121. R. J. Urban, M. R. Davis, A. D. Rogol, M. L. Johnson, and J. D. Veldhuis: Acute androgen receptor blockade increases leuteinizing hormone secretory activity in men. *J. Clin. Endocrinol. Metab.* 67:1149 (1988).

122. M. Namer: Clinical applications of antiandrogens. *J. Steroid Biochem.* 31:719 (1988).

123. J. Geller, J. Albert, and A. Vik: Advantages of total androgen blockade in the treatment of advanced prostate cancer. *Semin. Oncol.* 15 (Suppl. 1):53 (1988).

124. B. Katchen and S. Buxbaum: Disposition of a new, nonsteroid, antiandrogen, α,α,α-trifluoro-2-methyl-4'-nitro-m-propionotoluidide (Flutamide), in men following a single oral 200 mg dose. *J. Clin. Endocrinol. Metab.* 41:373 (1975).

125. M. Moguilewsky, J. Fiet, C. Tournemine, and J. P. Raynaud: Pharmacology of an antiandrogen, anandron, used as an adjuvant therapy in the treatment of prostate cancer. *J. Steroid Biochem.* 24:139 (1986).

126. J. Simard, I. Luthy, J. Guay, A. Belander, and F. Labrie: Characteristics of interaction of the antiandrogen flutamide with the androgen receptor in various target tissues. *Mol. Cell. Endocrinol.* 44:261 (1986).

127. A. Belanger, M. Giasson, J. Couture, A. Dupont, L. Cusan, and F. Labrie: Plasma levels of hydroxy-flutamide in patients with prostatic cancer receiving the combined hormonal therapy: An LHRH agonist and flutamide. *Prostate* 12:79 (1988).

128. R. Neri and N. Kassem: Biological and clinical properties of antiandrogens. *Prog. Cancer Res. Ther.* 31:507 (1984).

129. P. C. Sogani, M. R. Vagaiwala, and W. F. Whitmore: Experience with flutamide in patients with advanced prostatic cancer without prior endocrine therapy. *Cancer* 54:744 (1984).

130. J. T. Grayhack, T. C. Keeler, and J. M. Kozlowski: Carcinoma of the prostate: Hormonal therapy. *Cancer* 60:589 (1987).

131. P. M. Conn, A. J. W. Hsueh, and W. F. Crowley: Gonadotropin-releasing hormone: Molecular and cell biology, physiology, and clinical applications. *Fed. Proc.* 43:2351 (1984).

132. R. J. Santen, A. Manni, and H. Harvey: Gonadotropin releasing hormone (GnRH) analogs for the treatment of breast and prostatic carcinoma. *Breast Cancer Res. Treat.* 7:129 (1986).

133. R. Linde, G. C. Doelle, N. Alexander, F. Kirchner, W. Vale, J. Rivier, and D. Rabin: Reversible inhibition of testicular steroidogenesis and spermatogenesis by a potent gonadotropin-releasing hormone agonist in normal men. *New Engl. J. Med.* 305:663 (1981).

134. C. A. Peters and P. C. Walsh: The effect of nafarelin acetate, a luteinizing-hormone-releasing hormone agonist, on benign prostatic hyperplasia. *New Engl. J. Med.* 317:599 (1987).

135. R. I. Nicholson, K. J. Walker, A. Turkes, J. Dyas, R. W. Blamey, F. C. Campbell, M. R. G. Robinson, and K. Griffiths: Therapeutic significance and the mechanism of action of the LH-RH agonist ICI118630 in breast and prostate cancer. *J. Steroid. Biochem.* 20:129 (1984).

136. Leuprolide Study Group: Leuprolide versus diethylstilbestrol for metastatic prostate cancer. *New Engl. J. Med.* 311:1281 (1984).

137. H. Parmer, L. Edwards, R. H. Phillips, L. Allen, and S. L. Lightman: Orchiectomy versus long acting D-trp-6-LHRH in advanced prostatic cancer. *Br. J. Urol.* 59:248 (1987).

138. D. J. Handelsman and R. S. Swordloff: Pharmacokinetics of gonadotropin-releasing hormone and its analogs. *Endocrine Rev.* 7:95 (1986).

139. S. R. Ahmed, J. Grant, S. M. Shalet, A. Howell, S. D. Chowdhury, T. Weatherson, N. J. Blacklock: Preliminary report on use of depot formulation of LHRH ana-

logue ICI118630 (Zoladex) in patients with prostate cancer. *Br. Med. J.* 290:185 (1985).

140. J. M. Grodin, P. K. Siiteri, and P. C. MacDonald: Source of estrogen production in postmenopausal women. *J. Clin. Endocrinol. Metab.* 36:207 (1973).

141. P. E. Lonning and S. Kvinnsland: Mechanisms of action of aminoglutethimide as endocrine therapy of breast cancer. *Drugs* 35:685 (1988).

142. D. E. Schteingart, R. Cash, and J. W. Conn: Aminoglutethimide and metastatic adrenal cancer. *JAMA* 198:1007 (1966).

143. T. Hall, J. Barlow, C. Griffiths, and Z. Saba: Treatment of metastatic breast cancer with aminoglutethimide. *Clin. Res.* 14:402 (1969).

144. R. J. Santen, S. Santner, S. Davis, J. Veldhuis, E. Samojlik, and E. Ruby: Aminoglutethimide inhibits extraglandular estrogen production in post menopausal women with breast carcinoma. *J. Clin. Endocrinol. Metab.* 47:1257 (1978).

145. J. Kitawaki, T. Yamamoto, M. Urabe, T. Tamura, S. Inoue, H. Honjo, and H. Okada: Selective aromatase inhibition by pyridoglutethimide, an analogue of aminoglutethimide. *Acta Endocrinologica* 122:592 (1990).

146. R. J. Santen, E. Samojlik, and S. A. Wells: Resistance of the ovary to blockade of aromatization with aminoglutethimide. *J. Clin. Endocrinol. Metab.* 51:473 (1980).

147. P. E. Lonning, D. C. Johannessen, and T. Thorsen: Alterations in the production rate and the metabolism of oestrone and oestrone sulfate in breast cancer patients treated with aminoglutethimide. *Br. J. Cancer* 60:107 (1989).

148. R. J. Santen: Suppression of estrogens with aminoglutethimide and hydrocortisone (medical adrenalectomy) as treatment of advanced breast carcinoma: A review. *Breast Canc. Res. Treat.* 1:183 (1981).

149. R. J. Santen, T. J. Worgul, A. Lipton, H. Harvey, A. Boucher, E. Samojlik, and S. A. Wells: Aminoglutethimide as treatment of postmenopausal women with advanced breast carcinoma. *Ann. Int. Med.* 96:94 (1982).

150. T. Nemoto, D. Rosner, J. K. Patel, and T. L. Dao: Aminoglutethimide in patients with metastatic breast cancer. *Cancer* 63:1673 (1989).

151. F. R. Ahmann, E. D. Crawford, W. Kreis, Y. Levasseur, and the Aminoglutethimide Study Group: Adrenal steroid levels in castrated men with prostatic carcinoma treated with aminoglutethimide plus hydrocortisone. *Cancer Res.* 47:4736 (1987).

152. A. Y. C. Chang, J. M. Bennett, K. J. Pandya, R. Asbury, and C. McCune: A study of aminoglutethimide and hydrocortisone in patients with advanced and refractory prostate carcinoma. *Am. J. Clin. Oncol.* 12:358 (1989).

153. P. N. Plowman, L. A. Perry, and T. Chard: Androgen suppression by hydrocortisone without aminoglutethimide in orchiectomised men with prostatic cancer. *Br. J. Urol.* 59:255 (1987).

154. A. S. Bhatnagar, C. Nadjafi, and R. Steiner: "Aromatase inhibitors in cancer treatment," in *Endocrine Management of Cancer. 2. Contemporary Therapy,* ed. by B. A. Stoll. Basel: Karger, 1988, pp. 30–42.

155. T. A. Thompson, J. D. Vermeulen, W. E. Wagner, and A. R. Le Sher: Aminoglutethimide bioavailability, pharmacokinetics, and binding to blood constituents. *J. Pharmaceut. Sci.* 70:1041 (1981).

156. F. T. Murray, S. Santner, E. Samojlik, and R. J. Santen: Serum aminoglutethimide levels: studies of serum half-life, clearance, and patient compliance. *J. Clin. Pharmacol.* 19:704 (1979).

157. P. E. Lonning, J. S. Schanche, S. Kvinnsland, and P. M. Ueland: Single-dose and steady state pharmacokinetics of aminoglutethimide. *Clin. Pharmacokin.* 10:353 (1985).

158. H. K. Adam: "Pharmacokinetics of agents in relation to response," in *Endocrine Management of Cancer. 1. Biological Bases,* ed. by B. A. Stoll. Basel: Karger, 1988, pp. 112–124.

159. M. H. Baker, A. B. Foster, S. J. Harland, and M. Jarman: Metabolism of aminoglutethimide in humans: Formation of N-formylaminoglutethimide and nitroglutethimide. *Br. J. Pharmacol.* 74:243P (1981).

160. A. B. Foster, L. J. Griggs, I. Howe, M. Jarman, C. S. Leung, D. Manson, and M. G. Rowlands: Metabolism of aminoglutethimide in humans. Identification of four new urinary metabolites. *Drug. Metab. Disp.* 12:511 (1984).

161. A. M. Adam, H. J. Rogers, S. A. Amiel, and R. D. Rubens: The effect of acetylator phenotype on the disposition of aminoglutethimide. *Br. J. Pharmac.* 18:495 (1984).

162. A. A. Messeih, A. Lipton, R. J. Santen, H. A. Harvey, A. E. Boucher, R. Murray, J. Ragaz, A. U. Buzdar, G. A. Nagel, and I. C. Henderson: Aminoglutethimide-induced hematologic toxicity: Worldwide experience. *Cancer Treat. Rep.* 69:1003 (1985).

163. J. P. Luton, S. Cerdas, L. Billaud, G. Thomas, B. Guilhaume, X. Bertagna, M. H. Laudat, A. Louvel, Y. Chapius, P. Blondeau, A. Bonnin, and H. Bricaire: Clinical features of adrenocortical carcinoma, prognostic factors, and the effect of mitotane therapy. *New Engl. J. Med.* 322:1195 (1990).

164. A. A. Nelson and G. Woodard: Severe adrenal cortical atrophy (cytotoxic) and hepatic damage produced in dogs by feeding 2,2-*bis*(parachlorophenyl)-1,1-dichloroethane (DDD or TDE). *Arch. Pathol.* 48:387 (1949).

165. C. Cueto and J. H. Brown: Biological studies on an adrenocorticolytic agent and the isolation of the active components. *Endocrinology* 62:334 (1958).

166. O. Vilar and W. W. Tullner: Effects of o,p'-DDD on histology and 17-hydroxycorticosteroid output of the dog adrenal cortex. *Endocrinology* 65:80 (1959).

167. R. H. Moy: Studies of the pharmacology of o,p'-DDD in man. *J. Lab. Clin. Med.* 58:297 (1961).

168. Y. Touitou, A. Bogdan, J. C. LeGrand, and P. Desgrez: Metabolism de 1'o,p'-DDD (mitotane) chez l'homme et l'animal. *Annal. Endocrinol.* (Paris) 38:13 (1977).

169. M. Inouye, T. Mio, and K. Sumino: Metabolism of o,p'-DDD in humans: A novel metabolic pathway forming methylthio-containing metabolites. *Japanese J. Med.* 28:41 (1989).

170. S. Leiba, R. Weinstein, B. Shindel, M. Lapidot, E. Stern, H. Levavi, Y. Rusecki, and A. Abramovici: The protracted effect of o,p'-DDD in Cushing's disease and its impact on adrenal morphogenesis of young human embryo. *Annal. Endocrinol.* (Paris) 50:49 (1989).

171. J. A. Lubitz, L. Freeman, and R. Okun: Mitotane use in inoperable adrenal cortical carcinoma. *J. Am. Med. Assoc.* 223:1109 (1973).

172. R. V. Hague, W. May, and D. R. Cullen: Hepatic microsomal enzyme induction and adrenal crisis due to o,p'

-DDD therapy for metastatic adrenocortical carcinoma. *Clin. Endocrinol. 31*:51 (1989).

173. T. E. Temple, D. J. Jones, G. W. Liddle, and R. N. Dexter: Treatment of Cushing's disease: Correction of hypercorticolism by o,p'-DDD without induction of aldosterone deficiency. *New Engl. J. Med. 281*:801 (1969).

174. D. N. Orth and G. W. Liddle: Results of treatment in 108 patients with Cushing's syndrome. *New Engl. J. Med. 285*:244 (1971).

175. H. Van Slooten, A. J. Moolenaar, A. P. Van Seters, and D. Smeenk: The treatment of adrenocortical carcinoma with o,p'-DDD: Prognostic simplications of serum monitoring. *Eur. J. Clin. Oncol. 20*:47 (1984).

Clinical Cancer Chemotherapy

Choice of Drugs for Cancer Chemotherapy

The Clinical Situation

Choosing anticancer drugs for clinical use is more difficult than preclinical animal studies would suggest. Cancer appearing spontaneously in the human population is intrinsically much more heterogeneous than cancer transplanted in rodent models. Progress in chemotherapy is limited by this heterogeneity and by the fact that the population cannot be divided into homogeneous subgroups. Ideally, each treatment subgroup should include all patients likely to respond and should exclude all patients unlikely to respond to specific drug regimens. Although it is expected that better understanding of the molecular biology of cancer will improve treatments for genetically defined lesions, such an approach is not yet possible. Recent studies suggest that there may not be a correlation between the histopathologic type of tumor and a defined genetic lesion responsible for that cancer in all patients.[1] At present, the choice of agents for use in clinical cancer chemotherapy requires a knowledge of the clinical situation that the physician encounters in the individual patient. Decision making is guided by a synthesis of information concerning the relevant characteristics of both the tumor and the patient.[2-5]

Choice of the appropriate therapeutic agent or agents is based upon prior clinical experience as defined both by accepted clinical trials and by the accumulated medical knowledge of the treating physician. In order to successfully apply this clinical knowledge, the physician must make an accurate assessment of the state of the tumor and the state of the patient. This assessment is used to match the given patient with the best fit in a historically defined and relevant subgroup.

The Tumor

Meaningful categorization of tumors requires the definition of tumor type, which usually means knowing the site in the body where the cancer originated as well as the cell type—e.g., breast adenocarcinoma, colorectal adenocarcinoma, squamous cell carcinoma of the skin. Additional information as to the degree of differentiation is often useful. Neoplasms that display the least retention of normal differentiated histologic characteristics, that is, poorly differentiated cancers—usually grow faster, metastasize more readily, are more lethal, and may be more responsive to drug therapy in the short run than the more slowly growing, well-differentiated cancers. Stage of the tumor is another major consideration in categorization. When localized, each type of primary (site) tumor has accepted staging criteria taking size of tumor, depth of invasion, local lymph node involvement, and sometimes degree of differentiation into account.[6] When a tumor has spread to multiple sites within the body, knowledge of these sites and of the amount of tumor (burden) in each site helps in selecting the treatment and in estimating the outcome with given treatment programs.

The Patient

Antitumor drugs can be extremely toxic agents (Table 10–1). Hence, the condition of the host (patient) is the other half of the equation. Patient factors are not always independent of the tumor. Such factors, however, have a profound influence on the ability of the patient to tolerate drug therapy of sufficient dose intensity to cause tumor regression. The patient must obviously survive the treatment if it is to be effective. Antineoplastic drug tolerance is determined primarily by the metabolic capacity of the liver and kidneys and by the host's ability to produce blood cells under stress (the bone marrow reserve). In some instances, the ability of the rapidly proliferating cells of the gastrointestinal tract to withstand and recover from a drug-induced cytotoxic insult may be dose-limiting.

The state of the host's ability to metabolize and eliminate the drug is an especially important consideration when administering the widely used and extremely valuable agents cisplatin and doxorubicin. Cisplatin is excreted by the kidneys and can cause renal failure. Knowledge of baseline renal function and vigorous attention to hydration are necessary to prevent renal damage. Renal functional impairment, should it occur during cisplatin treatment, can limit future drug use even in patients where it is efficacious. Doxorubicin is metabolized by the liver, and administration to jaundiced patients can cause severe toxicity.

Patients with a diminished bone-marrow capacity to produce blood cells may suffer overwhelming toxicity (infection due to lack of white blood cells and bleeding due to lack of platelets) after standard dosages of myelosuppressive drugs. Such patients may even show some blood count depression when treated with agents that are usually not myelosuppressive.

Organ functions (including bone marrow reserve) may be influenced by age, other illnesses, prior injury, prior chemotherapy, prior radiotherapy, or tumor infiltration. When combined with knowledge of a patient's organ function, an understanding of the routes of metabolism and elimination and the anticipated toxicities of agents (Table 10–1) can guide the selection of a tolerable regimen for that patient. For example, patients with a decreased bone-marrow reserve are best treated with nonmyelosuppressive regimens when possible, or with agents, such as antimetabolites, that do not produce additional permanent marrow damage.

Scales for assessing performance status are also useful in assessing suitability of a particular treatment. Patients who are asymptomatic, fully active, have good appetites, and have not lost weight do better with any given drug regimen than patients who have unremitting pain, are bedridden, have no appetite, and have lost 10–15% of their body mass. Apart from cancers of the reproductive organs, gender is usually not a relevant factor in categorizing patients for drug treatment.

Satisfactory categorization of the patient using the characteristics described above enables the physician to define the possible and probable clinical course on a historical basis. One should know the natural history untreated, the natural history with standard drug treatments, and, to the extent possible, the natural history with research treatments as presented in recent clinical trials. Such information is important in evaluating risk versus benefit in the individual patient. For example, if a patient is expected to have a relatively long natural history without significant symptoms, use of a drug program with severe or potentially lethal toxicity might be unwise unless it offered curative potential. On the other hand, even early on, when the natural history without treatment or with standard treatment is poor (short survival, severe symptoms), aggressive drug therapy in a research setting becomes one option to be balanced against the equally reasonable option of no drug treatment with only palliative care.

Figure 10–1 schematically depicts the considerations in question using the concept of "life force." In this analogy, vigor and organ performance usually produce a maximum life force in the individual during their teen years. Death is represented by a life force of zero. The loss of life force per unit time is greater with an aggressive cancer than an indolent cancer (Fig. 10–1A). Figure 10–1B shows that treatment usually causes an immediate loss (cost) in

Table 10–1   Potential for Moderate to Severe Organ System Toxicities of Anticancer Drugs

Bone Marrow (Depressed Blood Counts)	Gastrointestinal Tract (Irritation, Ulceration, Diarrhea)	Oral Mucosa (Irritation, Ulceration)	Heart (Heart Failure)	Lung (Pneumonitis, Fibrosis)	Renal (Various Degrees of Failure)	Liver (Enzyme Elevations, Jaundice, Cirrhosis)	Nervous System		Skin (Dermatitis)
							Central (Depression)	Peripheral (Paresthesias, Functional Loss)	
All agents *except:* Hormones Asparaginase Bleomycin Cisplatin Floxuridine Streptozotocin Vincristine	Fluorouracil Floxuridine Methotrexate Mercaptopurine Cytarabine	Fluorouracil Methotrexate Cytarabine Dactinomycin Daunorubicin Doxorubicin Idarubicin Bleomycin Procarbazine Hydroxyurea	Daunorubicin Doxorubicin	Bleomycin Busulfan Methotrexate	Cisplatin Streptozocin Methotrexate Mitomycin	Methotrexate Mercaptopurine Thioguanine Cytarabine	Mitotane Procarbazine	Cisplatin Vincristine Vinblastine	Bleomycin Methotrexate Fluorouracil Dactinomycin Doxorubicin

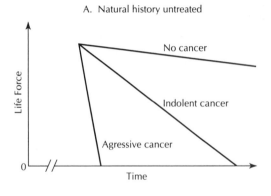

A. Natural history untreated

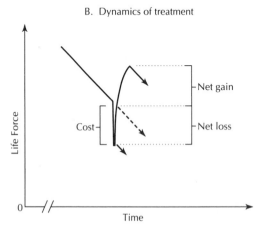

B. Dynamics of treatment

Figure 10–1 Influence on host function (life force) over time of the nature of cancer, treatment cost, and therapeutic outcome.

life force. Various treatments cost relatively more or less. If the loss exceeds what the patient possesses, death from toxicity ensues. This means that waiting too long in the course of a cancer may preclude use of certain treatments that cost too much in terms of life force. When benefit is achieved by treatment, the patient is able to recover after paying the cost and there may be actual net gain, as depicted in Figure 10–1B. Treatments that shift the curve upward until it overlaps that seen with "no cancer" in Figure 10–1A have achieved, in effect, a cure of the cancer.

Determination of Therapeutic Goals

CURE. The choice of drugs for treatment must be guided by the therapeutic objectives that could reasonably apply in a given case. The most valued objective is *cure*. The ability of chemotherapy regimens to effect a cure is improving with time (Table 10–2). Unfortunately, this objective does not apply for patients who are afflicted with such common diseases as non-small-cell lung cancer and pancreatic cancer. Cure is fully satisfactory only if it is associated with resumption of a functional, relatively asymptomatic life. Quality-of-life issues pertain when there are many years to live after achievement of cure.[7,8] Thus, even after cure is achieved in a given tumor type, considerable effort is directed toward finding improved regimens of diminished toxicity.[9]

PROLONGATION OF LIFE. Prolongation of life is a reasonable goal when cure is not possible. This endpoint is much less distinct than cure and assumes accurate knowledge as to survival without drug treatment. Prolongation of life is an endpoint best identified in randomized studies in which one or more treatment groups demonstrate statistically improved survival.[10] Median duration of survival is a parameter often used to compare treatments. It should be noted that, in addition to this parameter, the shape of the survival curve for the entire population is important as well. Early toxic deaths and/or the generation of a small subset of patients with marked prolongation of survival may have little or no effect on the median duration of survival yet be important in judging the value of the treatment. With prolongation of life, quality of life may become an issue, especially if treatment induces chronic or protracted toxicity.[11]

PALLIATION OF SYMPTOMS AND QUALITY OF LIFE. Palliation of symptoms is another valuable therapeutic objective.[12] Inasmuch as symptoms are a subjective measure of disease state, symptomatic improvement may not necessarily correlate with an objective therapeutic effect on the tumor. Aggressive efforts directed to symptom control may lead to a diminution of symptoms even while the cancer is growing. For example, narcotic administration may alleviate pain due to progressive cancer. Alternatively, the generation of toxicity may lead to worsening of symptoms despite regression of the tumor.

Table 10–2   Tumor Types Where Chemotherapy Can Effect a Cure

Chemotherapy-Induced Cures Possible (Standard Therapy)	Adjuvant or Neoadjuvant Chemotherapy–Induced Cures Probable
Gestational choriocarcinoma	Breast cancer
Testicular cancer	Colorectal cancer
Ovarian cancer	Head and neck cancer
Small cell lung cancer	Osteogenic sarcoma
Burkitt's lymphoma	Soft tissue sarcoma
Hodgkin's disease	Anal carcinoma
Diffuse large cell lymphoma	
Lymphoblastic lymphoma	
Acute myelogenous leukemia	
Ewing's sarcoma	
Neuroblastoma	
Wilm's tumor	
Embryonal rhabdomyosarcoma	
Childhood acute lymphocytic leukemia	

Another aspect of response highlighted in recent years is quality of life. Various schemes for evaluating changes in the function and symptomatology of patients with treatment have been developed.[13,14] Quality of life tends to be a more subjective measure of response than measurable tumor regression and is, by itself, an ill-defined endpoint for defining improved drug therapy. Whereas objective measurements of tumor regression allow translation of knowledge from cells to animals to humans, quality of life is uniquely human. Fortunately, there is evidence that treatments of improved efficacy can generate improved quality of life over time.[7]

RELIEF OF FEAR AND ANXIETY. A more subjective aim than symptom palliation is relief of fear and anxiety effected by "doing something." Many patients want something done to try to stop their cancer from growing and are not satisfied with symptomatic relief alone. When there is little recognized effective therapy, this creates a problem. One approach has been to enter such patients into Phase I research studies of new drugs aimed at defining dose-dependent toxicities. When such studies are not available or when the patient is not a candidate for such studies due to inadequate organ function or inadequate survival to allow for drug evaluation, the problem remains. In such a situation, the use of standard drugs in relatively nontoxic dose schedules provides some chance of antitumor effect while generating subjective benefits. In addition, this alternative maintains the therapeutic relationship between physician and the individual patient. Inasmuch as the dose-response relationship for antitumor effect may be shallow in any given patient, perhaps little is lost by this approach. While this approach may be appropriate in individual circumstances, its widespread use must be tempered with the realization that dose-response effects may be operative when considering populations of patients having common diseases such as breast cancer, colorectal cancer, ovarian cancer, and lymphomas.[15]

OBJECTIVE, MEASURABLE TUMOR RESPONSE. The most common aim that guides the choice of drugs is a response that is defined by an objective, measurable decrease in tumor mass (a regression). In the treatment of solid tumors, relatively standard definitions apply for complete response, partial response, stable disease, and progressive disease. Complete response is the disappearance of all evidence of tumor. Partial response is a 50% reduction in the sum of the products of the largest diameters of all measurable lesions by their perpendiculars without appearance of any new lesions. Progressive disease is an increase by greater than 25% in the sum of the products of the appropriate diameters of measurable lesions and/or the appearance of new lesions. Stable disease is the category used when lesions persist, but fall neither into the partial response nor progressive disease category. It is important to remember that a complete disappearance of tumor may be brought about by only a relatively small (one- or two-log) reduction in tumor cell number when there are a large number (nine or more logs) of cells that need to be killed for cure to be achieved. Another consideration is that the tumor mass itself may contain varying amounts of connective tissue and inflammatory cells. It is possible that a tumor mass or nodule can change in cellularity yet not change in size with treatment. Biopsy of representative tumor masses is a necessity in situations where more benign cells or fibrous tissue may replace tumor cells killed by drugs or where benign nodules may coexist with cancer nodules. One noteworthy example of this phenomenon is in testicular cancer, where nodules remaining after chemotherapy may be either benign or malignant.[16]

NEED TO RESEARCH BETTER THERAPY. Depending on the setting, a major determinant in the choice of drugs can be the need to do research. The drug therapy of many cancers is unsatisfactory, and research offers the only chance for improvement. Research studies range from dose-tolerance studies of new drugs in Phase I clinical trial to comparisons between defined treatments in Phase III trial. When standard therapy has been exhausted or is ineffective in a given patient or group of patients, a clinical trial of a new drug regimen is a reasonable option. Other considerations may enter into whether a given patient will be entered into a drug trial. Availability of pertinent studies may be limited to particular academic institutions or clinical investigators. Some patients may not wish to take the risks involved in research studies. Primary-care physicians may be more or less supportive of experimental studies. For whatever the reasons, it is clear that only a minority of eligible patients end up being treated in investigational studies.

DELIVERY OF THERAPY THAT IS COST EFFECTIVE. It is likely that the choice of drugs will become increasingly constrained by cost/benefit considerations.[17-19] Costs involve monetary expenditures as well as toxic effects. When two drug regimens produce the same objective tumor response yet one is slightly more expensive than the other, it is problematic as to which should be used. It only complicates matters if the more expensive regimen is marginally less toxic and better tolerated.

Financial constraints generated at the federal level, effected as well through insurance companies and health-maintenance organizations, already influence both doctor and patient. One example of this sort of situation occurs with the use of autologous bone-marrow transplants in support of high-dose chemotherapy for women with breast cancer. The argument rages as to whether this is experimental or the best conventional, aggressive treatment.[20] Such therapy greatly increases toxicity and cost (> $100,000/patient), yet may cure only a minority of patients.[21-23] From the patient's point of view, it is her only chance of cure. Yet, from a societal perspective, what fraction of patients needs to be cured to justify such a large outlay of money? Are future advances being delayed or are other patients receiving less effective care because of such large expenditures per patient?

Another example of financial constraints is seen when third-party carriers do not pay for treatment with "experimental" regimens. This is an important constraint, since many regimens are identified as being effective by the clinical oncologist some time (up to years) before regulatory bodies/agencies certify their effectiveness. It is likely that physicians and patients will become more public in advocating particular drug regimens, as such activity may be the only way to gain the support necessary to have third-party payers cover the costs of such treatments.

Choice of Drug Therapy for a Given Patient

The choice of drug or a drug regimen for a given patient is influenced most directly by the likelihood of efficacy in that patient. The probability of response (or activity) of a given drug regimen in a population of patients having relevant characteristics is defined in clinical studies. Phase II studies determine whether a drug has antitumor activity and estimate the response rate in a defined patient population.

Large-scale Phase III studies in defined patient populations compare two or more drug regimens in terms of response rate and, ideally, survival and quality of life. As noted earlier, a major role for the clinical oncologist is to categorize a given patient into the most appropriate group so that prior clinical studies are relevant in guiding the choice of a treatment regimen. The goodness of fit of a particular patient with a particular historical group has a direct bearing on predictability of treatment outcome for that patient. It should be noted that even the best of drug regimens will not produce a beneficial response in all patients.

Types of Treatment Involving Chemotherapy

Combination Chemotherapy

Anticancer drugs are rarely used individually. Generally, combinations of agents are used based upon a rationale developed in preclinical cell culture or animal studies or earlier clinical studies.[24-27] Preclinical studies in animal models first demonstrated the improved efficacy of drug combinations in producing cures as compared to single agents. In the clinic, combination chemotherapy regimens generally lead to higher response rates and account for the ability to cure patients in most diseases where cure is possible (Table 10-2). Several generally accepted guidelines are utilized in selecting drugs for use in combination chemotherapy. These are:

1. To utilize drugs that have been shown to possess antitumor activity when used alone.
2. To utilize drugs that have nonoverlapping toxicities and/or produce relevant toxicities at different times after treatment.
3. To utilize drugs that have different mechanisms or targets of action and/or do not display cross-resistance.

As will be discussed below, there have been recent permutations of these guidelines both in terms of dose intensity of each drug used in a combination and in the use of combinations of myelosuppressive drugs with autologous bone marrow transplantation. Specific applications of drug regimens in clinical cancer treatment will be discussed in the next chapter.

There are several specific areas of chemotherapy that take into account the definite, yet limited, ability of drugs to kill tumor cells with sufficient selectivity to allow host benefit. Studies with transplantable animal tumors have shown that drug regimens capable of eradicating a smaller number of tumor cells will fail if the tumor-cell burden is too large. Both adjuvant chemotherapy and combined modality therapy represent an attempt to initiate drug treatment at a time when the tumor cell burden is low.

Adjuvant Chemotherapy

Adjuvant chemotherapy is the application of drug treatment to a patient population in which a portion of the patients will harbor small numbers of occult metastatic cells despite eradication of a primary tumor with either surgery, radiotherapy, or a combination of surgery and radiotherapy. For example, women with stage II breast cancer who have had successful eradication of the tumor in the breast (with surgery ± irradiation) have about a 40% chance of dying of residual, occult metastatic disease.[28] Adjuvant chemotherapy administered to such women appears to decrease the probability of dying to about half of that, or 20%. Recently, studies have shown that adjuvant chemotherapy in colorectal cancer appears to decrease mortality by about one-third.[29-30] The objective of adjuvant chemotherapy is cure. The surrogate parameter for cure is length of disease-free survival. It should be noted that even without chemotherapy, some patients will be cured and some will not. Hence, those patients rendered free of cancer by eradication of the primary tumor and those patients who still die despite adjuvant chemotherapy all receive no benefit from the adjuvant treatment. Risk/benefit considerations are especially important, as toxicity from chemotherapy could lead to the death of a patient already cured by eradication of the primary tumor. Although a statistical benefit can be seen in a treated population of patients, it is currently impossible to say whether a given patient is cured because of eradication of the primary tumor by surgery and/or radiotherapy alone, or because adjuvant chemotherapy has been administered.

Combined Modality Therapy

Adjuvant chemotherapy is but one of several variations of combined modality therapy, that is, treatment in which chemotherapeutic agents are used in conjunction with surgery and/or radiotherapy. Surgery and conventional external beam radiotherapy are applicable only to localized, bulk tumor masses. Conventional chemotherapy is a systemic modality, most effective against small amounts of tumor irrespective of localization within the body. Thus, it makes sense to combine focal treatment (surgery, radiotherapy) of large primary tumor masses with systemic treatment of smaller, often microscopic, metastatic cancer deposits.

PRIMARY OR NEOADJUVANT CHEMOTHERAPY. One useful variant of such combined modality therapy is "primary" or "neoadjuvant" chemotherapy.[31,32] Ordinary adjuvant chemotherapy is applied after the tumor is eradicated at its site of origin either by surgical excision and/or by radiotherapy. Neoadjuvant or primary chemotherapy is given to shrink the tumor in its site of origin prior to surgery or irradiation of the focal tumor. Advantages of neoadjuvant chemotherapy include being able to determine whether the chemotherapy regimen is effective against a given tumor, to shrink bulk tumor to facilitate focal treatment of bulk tumor with surgery or radiotherapy, and to treat for microscopic systemic disease immediately. Neoadjuvant therapy has been most notably applied in head and neck cancer and esophageal cancer.[32,33] Reduction in the size of the local tumor with chemotherapy may allow less locally destructive focal treatments. With equivalent chance for achieving cure, patients with laryngeal cancer who receive initial chemotherapy followed by radiotherapy may have voice preservation by being spared surgery to remove their voice box.[34,35]

RADIOSENSITIZATION. In addition to having antitumor effect on their own, several commonly used anticancer drugs interact with radiotherapy to produce radiosensitization. Such radiosensitization can create added toxicity such as can be seen with the use of adriamycin with or after irradiation of the heart or gastro-intestinal tract.[36,37] Fluorouracil (FU) has radiosensitizing properties *in vitro* that have been borne out clinically in the treatment of localized head and neck, esophageal, gastric, pancreatic, and rectal cancers.[38] Cisplatin, an agent demonstrating radiosensitizing abilities in cell culture systems, has been combined with FU in head and neck and esophageal cancer, in particular.[38-40]

Principles and Concepts Applicable to the Clinical Use of Anticancer Drugs

In general, all agents used in the clinical treatment of cancer possess a substantial preclinical rationale as defined elsewhere in this book. Such a rationale includes a reasonably defined mechanism of action, as well as evidence that the agent either kills cells or stops cell growth in culture and does so selectively (affecting cancers more than normal tissues) in animal models. Preclinical investigation over the past fifty years has defined a set of principles subsequently found to be useful in the clinical (human) situation (Table 10–3).

Large Tumors Are Less Effectively Treated Than Small Tumors

As was first demonstrated in preclinical models, tumor burden is a major factor in determining probable clinical outcome in a given patient. The principle of proportional cell kill (Chapter 3) states that the proportion of tumor cells killed is a constant percentage of the total number of cells present. To the degree that this principle pertains, it means that the probability of killing the last tumor cell and generating a cure is greater with smaller tumor burdens. Furthermore, the probability of resistance to a given regimen increases with increasing tumor burden. Finally, the growth fraction of small tumors is higher than for large tumors and, since growing cells are more likely to be killed than resting cells, smaller tumors should be more sensitive to treatment. The increased likelihood of success with a smaller tumor burden has been the basis for the major success of chemotherapy in the adjuvant therapy of breast and colon cancer. This concept also contributes to the rationale for combined modality therapy

Table 10–3   Principles and Concepts Developed in Preclinical Cell Culture and Animal Tumor Models Found to Be Useful in Human Therapy

Principle/Concept	Provides Rationale (In Part) For
1. Proportional cell kill (a set fraction of cells will be killed with any given drug treatment)	Adjuvant therapy (treatment when tumor burden is lowest), combined modality therapy (debulking, decreasing number of tumor cells with another modality)
2. Dose-response effects (tumor cell kill increases with dosage increase)	Dose-intensification (see 4 below) Regional chemotherapy
3. Resistance a. is acquired with treatment b. varies with individual drugs/regimens	Intense initial therapy Use of non-cross-resistant drugs and drug combinations

4. Toxicity is reproducible and understandable Cyclic treatment allows differential recovery of normal over tumor tissue Permanent damage can be done to normal tissue acutely or cumulatively	Cyclic therapy
	Safe drug usage
	Supportive care
	  Cytokines
	  Bone marrow transplantation
	  Antibiotics
	  Blood products
	  Close monitoring, dosage adjustment, selection of drugs that will be tolerated

5. Drug combination therapy is better than single agent therapy (see 3 and 4 above).	Combination chemotherapy
6. Drug combinations may show antagonistic, additive, or synergistic actions	Use of combinations that are at least additive in preclinical studies
7. Drug actions may be schedule dependent	Testing a variety of schedules

in which surgery or radiotherapy is used to debulk and reduce the tumor burden prior to or in combination with chemotherapy to treat small amounts of residual systemic disease.

Dose-Response Effects Apply

Dose-response considerations defined in animal tumor models appear to have clinical relevance. The probability of tumor regression increases with increasing dose of drug administered. Unfortunately, with even more certainty, toxicity increases as well, giving rise to attempts to diminish toxicity selectively for an improved therapeutic index. Methods for dose escalation with diminished toxicity developed in animal models and extended into the clinic include dose-schedule manipulation, use of bone-marrow colony stimulating factors or cytokines, and bone marrow transplantation.[23,41,42]

Retrospective analyses of clinical data suggest that it is not simply dose that counts, but rather the amount of drug delivered per unit time—i.e., dose intensity (mg/m^2/week). There is an excellent correlation between increasing dose intensity (on a wide variety of schedules) and response rate in breast cancer, small-cell lung cancer, colorectal cancer, and ovarian cancer.[15] There is a positive correlation as well between dose intensity and median survival time in breast cancer and ovarian cancer and relapse-free survival in adjuvant breast cancer regimens. The relevance of dose intensity to antitumor effect appears to hold for many antitumor drugs, and tumor types and can be extended to combination drug regimens.[15]

Regional infusion of an appropriate drug is a special application of dose-response effects.[43] Higher regional drug levels may increase the cytotoxicity for regionally confined tumors. When regional drug extraction provides for a lower systemic drug level, systemic toxicity may be decreased as well. A common regional drug infusion is the hepatic arterial infusion of 5-fluoro-2'-deoxyuridine. Such an infusion increases the drug exposure of liver metastases from colorectal cancer by over 100-fold and doubles the response rate.[44]

One important application of regional drug administration is direct injection into the cerebrospinal fluid (CSF) to treat tumor cells growing in the fluid and upon adjacent meningeal surfaces. Restricted access to many common anticancer drugs limits the effectiveness of intravenous administration in the treatment of tumors within the CSF. For example, successful therapy in childhood acute lymphocytic leukemia usually requires the direct injection of methotrexate into the CSF space. Meningeal spread of lung and breast cancer is similarly treated.

Resistance Is Relevant

High levels of intrinsic resistance to chemotherapeutic agents account for low initial response rates in some tumor types (e.g. non-small cell lung cancer). Relapse in other, initially responsive tumor types (e.g., breast cancer) is due to acquired resistance. Therapeutic improvements in the clinic brought about by the use of combination chemotherapy and the timely application of non-cross-resistant drug regimens were first defined in preclinical animal models. Dose intensification, made possible by improved supportive care (antibiotics, blood products, cytokines, and bone-marrow transplant), is another means of overcoming low levels of drug resistance.

Toxicities Must Be Reproducible and Manageable

Drugs used in the clinical treatment of cancer must have predictable and reproducible side effects or toxicities (Table 10–1). If a drug is to be safe to use, a consistent pattern of dose-related toxicity should be found both in a given patient and in a given patient population. Prior to clinical testing for efficacy, all anticancer drugs are evaluated for toxicities in small (rodents) and large (dogs, monkeys) animal models. Animal toxicity studies allow a first approximation of the dose likely to be tolerated in humans.[45] Phase I dose escalation studies are conducted in patients to determine the maximum tolerated dose. Phase I clinical studies additionally define the types of toxicities, the

schedule for toxicity development and reversal, and the relative severity of organ toxicities a given drug can generate as the dose is escalated to tolerance.

Combination Chemotherapy Is Generally Most Effective

As discussed earlier, the use of multiple drugs in combination chemotherapy is standard in the clinic. Individually active agents are first identified in the tumor type in question. The predictable nature of the individual drug-induced toxicities (Table 10–1) guides the use of active drugs in combinations that have nonoverlapping toxicities. Alternatively, drugs that produce dose-limiting myelosuppression can be combined when bone-marrow transplantation is used to prevent lethal depression of bone-marrow function.[21-23]

As predicted from preclinical studies, drug combinations generally produce higher response rates in treated populations than those produced by single agents alone. It is likely, however, that for a given patient, some of the drugs in a combination are not effective and their use dilutes the possible dose intensity of the effective agents. Attempts to overcome this problem and to develop individual regimens based on *in vitro* culturing of tumors from individual patients have not yet been successful enough to warrant widespread application in the clinic.[46]

Summary

Preclinical investigations and subsequent clinical trials have defined useful therapeutic principles and continue to generate a variety of options for treating patients. For an individual patient, it can be seen that the choice of drugs should be a decision taking into account pertinent host factors and tumor factors matched to a historical experience that defines potential outcomes. Each decision represents, in large part, the outcome of a synthesis of the physician's own knowledge and experience with the patient's personality, needs, and risk-taking ability. Recently, considerations of the quality of life with and without treatment have become more prominent. Choice of drugs in the future is likely to be more constrained than in past years by economic considerations. The value (in dollars to be paid by society) placed on a day, a month, or a year or more of additional life is a question being debated more intensely as treatments become more expensive.

REFERENCES

1. P. C. Nowell: Commentary: How many human cancer genes? *J. Natl. Cancer Inst. 83*:1061 (1991).

2. M. N. Levine, G. P. Browman, M. Gent, R. Roberts, and M. Goodyear: Review: When is a prognostic factor useful?: A guide for the perplexed. *J. Clin. Oncol. 9*:348 (1991).

3. C. K. Osborne: "Prognostic factors in breast cancer," in *Principles & Practice of Oncology Updates,* Vol. 4, ed. by (V. T. DeVita, Jr., S. Hellman, and S. A. Rosenberg, J. B. Lippincott, Philadelphia: 1990, pp. 1–11.

4. U. Sagman, E. Maki, W. K. Evans, D. Warr, F. A. Sheperd, J. P. Sculier, R. Haddad, D. Payne, J. F. Pringle, J. L. Yeoh, A. Ciampi, G. DeBoer, S. McKinney, R. Ginsberg, and R. Feld: Small-cell carcinoma of the lung: Derivation of a prognostic staging system. *J. Clin. Oncol 9*:1639 (1991).

5. R. T. Skeel: "Systemic assessment of the patient with cancer," *Handbook of Cancer Chemotherapy,* 3rd ed., ed. by R. T. Skeel. Boston: Little, Brown and Company Inc., 1991, pp. 55–70.

6. International Union Against Cancer: *TNM-Atlas Illustrated Guide to the Classification of Malignant Tumours,* ed. by B. Spiessl, O. Scheibe, and G. Wagner, Heidelberg: Springer-Verlag, 1989, 350 pp.

7. R. D. Gelber, A. Goldhirsch, and F. Cavalli: Quality-of-life-adjusted evaluation of adjuvant therapies for operable breast cancer. *Ann. Intern. Med. 114*:621 (1991).

8. L. Schwab: ABMT trials evaluate quality of life. *J. Natl. Cancer Inst. 83*:1136 (1991).

9. R. L. Schilsky and C. Erlichman: "Infertility and carcinogenesis: Late complications of chemotherapy," in *Cancer Chemotherapy Principles & Practice,* ed. by B. A. Chabner and J. M. Collins. Philadelphia: J. B. Lippincott Company, 1980, pp. 32–58.

10. S. Kaasa, E. Lund, E. Thorud, R. Hatlevoll, and H. Host: Symptomatic treatment versus combination chemotherapy for patients with extensive non-small cell lung cancer. *Cancer 67*:2443 (1991).

11. P. A. Singer, E. S. Tasch, C. Stocking, S. Rubin, M. Siegler, and R. Weichselbaum: Sex or survival: Trade-offs between quality and quantity of life. *J. Clin. Oncol. 9*:328 (1991).

12. B. R. Cassileth, E. J. Lusk, D. Guerry, A. D. Blake, W. P. Walsh, L. Kascius, and D. J. Schultz: Special Article: Survival and quality of life among patients receiving unproven as compared with conventional cancer therapy. *New Engl. J. Med. 324*:1180 (1991).

13. N. K. Aaronson, B. E. Meyerowitz, M. Bard, J. R. Bloom, F. L. Fawzy, M. Feldstein, D. Fink, J. C. Holland, J. E. Johnson, J. T. Lowman, B. Patterson, and J. E. Ware, Jr.: Quality of life research in oncology. *Cancer 67*:839 (1991).

14. I. R. Gough and L. I. Dalgleish: What value is given to quality of life assessment by health professionals considering response to palliative chemotherapy for advanced cancer? *Cancer 68*:220 (1991).

15. W. M. Hryniuk: "The importance of dose intensity in the outcome of chemotherapy," in *Important Advances in Oncology 1988,* ed. by V. T. DeVita Jr., S. Hellman, and S. A. Rosenberg. Philadelphia: J. B. Lippincott Company, 1988, pp. 121–141.

16. S. D. Williams, R. Birch, L. H. Einhorn, L. Irwin, F. A. Greco, and P. J. Loehrer: Treatment of disseminated germ-cell tumors with cisplatin, bleomycin, and either vinblastine or etoposide. *New Engl. J. Med. 316*:1435 (1987).

17. W. H. Ettinger, Jr.: Forces of change in the health care system. *Cancer 67*:1728 (1991).

18. B. E. Hillner, and T. J. Smith: Special Article: Efficacy and cost effectiveness of adjuvant chemotherapy in women with node-negative breast cancer. *New Engl. J. Med. 324*:160 (1991).

19. J. W. Yarbro: Changing cancer care in the 1990s and the cost. *Cancer 67*:1718 (1991).

20. I. C. Henderson: Editorials: Window of opportunity. *J. Natl. Cancer Inst. 83*:894 (1991).

21. S. J. Forman, G. M. Schmidt, A. P. Nademanee, M. D. Amylon, N. J. Chao, J. L. Fahey, P. N. Konrad, K. A. Margolin, J. C. Niland, M. R. O'Donnell, P. M. Parker, E. P. Smith, D. S. Snyder, G. Somio, A. S. Stein, and K. G. Blume: Allogeneic bone marrow transplantation as therapy for primary induction failure for patients with acute leukemia. *J. Clin. Oncol. 9*:1570 (1991).

22. M. J. Kennedy, R. A. Beveridge, S. D. Rowley, G. B. Gordon, M. D. Abeloff, and N. E. Davidson: Articles: High-dose chemotherapy with reinfusion of purged autologous bone marrow following dose-intense induction as initial therapy for metastatic breast cancer. *J. Natl. Cancer Inst. 83*:920 (1991).

23. W. P. Peters: "High-dose chemotherapy and autologous bone marrow support for breast cancer," in *Important Advances in Oncology 1991,* ed. by (V. T. DeVita Jr., S. Hellman, and S. A. Rosenberg. Philadelphia: J. B. Lippincott Company, 1991, pp. 135–150.

24. B. A. Chabner: Editorial: In defense of cell-line screening. *J. Natl. Cancer Inst. 82*:1083 (1990).

25. B. A. Chabner: "Clinical strategies for cancer treatment: The role of drugs," in *Cancer Chemotherapy, Principles & Practice,* ed. by B. A. Chabner and J. M. Collins. Philadelphia: J. B. Lippincott Company, 1990, pp. 1–15.

26. R. K. Johnson: Editorial: Screening methods in antineoplastic drug discovery. *J. Natl. Cancer Inst. 82*:1082 (1990).

27. B. I. Sikic: Editorial: Anticancer drug discovery. *J. Natl. Cancer Inst. 83*:738 (1991).

28. G. Bonadonna: Karnofsky Memorial Lecture: Conceptual and practical advances in the management of breast cancer. *J. Clin. Oncol. 7*:1380 (1989).

29. J. S. Macdonald and S. F. Schnall: "The role of 5-FU plus levamisole in the therapy of colon cancer," in *Principles & Practice of Oncology Updates,* Vol. 5, ed. by V. T. DeVita Jr., S. Hellman, and S. A. Rosenberg. Philadelphia: J. B. Lippincott Company, 1991, pp. 1–9.

30. C. G. Moertel, T. R. Fleming, J. S. Macdonald, D. G. Haller, J. A. Laurie, P. J. Goodman, J. S. Ungerleider, W. A. Emerson, D. C. Tormey, J. H. Glick, M. H. Veeder, and

J. A. Mailliard: Levamisole and fluorouracil for adjuvant therapy of resected colon carcinoma. *New Engl. J. Med.* 322:352 (1990).

31. E. Frei III: What's in a name—Neoadjuvant. *J. Natl. Cancer Inst.* 80:1088 (1989).

32. F. M. Muggia and I. Gill: "Primary chemotherapy," in *Principles & Practice of Oncology Updates,* Vol. 4, ed. by V. T. DeVita Jr., S. Hellman, and S. A. Rosenberg. Philadelphia: J. B. Lippincott Company, 1990, pp. 1–12.

33. D. Kelsen: "Chemotherapy for local-regional and advanced esophageal cancer," Vol. 2, in *Principles & Practice of Oncology Updates,* ed. by V. T. DeVita Jr., S. Hellman, and S. A. Rosenberg. Philadelphia: J. B. Lippincott Company, 1988, pp. 1–12.

34. D. G. Pfister, E. Strong, L. Harrison, I. E. Haines, D. A. Pfister, R. Sessions, R. Spiro, J. Shah, F. Gerold, T. McLure, B. Vikram, D. Fass, J. Armstrong, and G. L. Bosl: Larynx preservation with combined chemotherapy and radiation therapy in advanced but resectable head and neck cancer. *J. Clin. Oncol.* 9:850 (1991).

35. The Department of Veterans Affairs Laryngeal Cancer Study Group: Induction chemotherapy plus radiation compared with surgery plus radiation in patients with advanced laryngeal cancer. *New Engl. J. Med.* 324:1685 (1991).

36. R. A. Minow, R. S. Benjamin, and J. A. Gottlieb: Adriamycin (NSC 123127) cardiomyopathy—an overview with determination of risk factors. *Cancer Chemother. Rep.* 6:195 (1975).

37. T. L. Phillips, M. D. Wharam, and L. W. Margolis: Modification of radiation injury to normal tissues by chemotherapeutic agents. *Cancer* 35:1678 (1975).

38. J. E. Byfield: "Combined modality infusional chemotherapy with radiation," in *Cancer Chemotherapy by Infusion* ed. by J. J. Lokich. 1990, Chicago: Precept Press, pp. 521–551.

39. E. B. Douple and R. C. Richmond: "A review of interactions between platinum coordination complexes and ionizing radiation: Implications for cancer therapy," in *Cisplatin Current Status and New Developments,* ed. by A. W. Prestayko, S. T. Crooke, and S. K. Carter. 1980, New York: Academic Press, pp. 125–147.

40. P. F. Engstron, L. R. Coia, and E. M. Soffen: "Esophageal and anal carcinoma," in *Cancer Chemotherapy by Infusion,* ed. by J. J. Lokich. 1990, pp. 313–322 (1990).

41. M. H. Bronchud, A. Howell, D. Crowther, P. Hopwood, L. Souza, and T. M. Dexter: The use of granulocyte colony-stimulating factor to increase the intensity of treatment with doxorubicin in patients with advanced breast and ovarian cancer. *Br. J. Cancer* 60:121 (1989).

42. J. Crawford, H. Ozer, R. Stoller, D. Johnson, et al.: Reduction by granulocyte colony-stimulating factor of fever and neutropenia induced by chemotherapy in patients with small-cell lung cancer. *New Engl. J. Med.* 325:164 (1991).

43. W. D. Ensminger and J. W. Gyves: Regional cancer chemotherapy. *Cancer Treat. Rep.* 68:101 (1984).

44. N. Kemeny, J. Daly, B. Reichman, N. Geller, J. Botet, and P. Oderman: Intrahepatic or systemic infusion of fluorodeoxyuridine in patients with liver metastases from colorectal carcinoma. *Ann. Intern. Med.* 107:459 (1987).

45. J. M. Collins, C. K. Grieshaber, and B. A. Chabner: Review: Pharmacologically guided phase I clinical trials based upon preclinical drug development. *J. Natl. Cancer Inst.* 82:1321 (1990).

46. D. D. Von Hoff, R. Kronmal, S. E. Salmon, J. Turner, J. B. Green, J. S. Bonorris, E. L. Moorhead, H. E. Hynes, R. E. Pugh, R. J. Belt, and D. S. Alberts: A Southwest Oncology Group Study on the use of a human tumor cloning assay for predicting response in patients with ovarian cancer. *Cancer* 67:20 (1991).

CHAPTER ELEVEN

Cancer Treatment

Introduction

The major types of cancer treatment are surgery, radiotherapy, and chemotherapy. Successful treatment involves the integration of these methods to take advantage of the strengths of each one. Surgery and radiotherapy are local treatments that either remove or sterilize defined tumor masses. When a tumor is locally confined, surgery and/or radiotherapy often proves curative. Even when the cancer is not totally confined to one body region, direct eradication of large, focal tumor masses may help by lowering the overall tumor-cell number or burden. Chemotherapy, as commonly practiced, is a systemic therapy delivered most often intravenously. Thus, chemotherapy can kill tumor cells located throughout the body. Its success is inversely related to the tumor-cell burden, and this provides the rationale for adjuvant chemotherapy after eradication of bulk tumor masses with surgery or radiotherapy.

Much has been written about the success of chemotherapy in pediatric cancers and in hematological malignancies (lymphomas and leukemias). The most frequent use of cancer chemotherapy by far, however, is in the treatment of the common malignant solid tumors in adults. In this chapter, therefore, we have chosen to examine the role of chemotherapy in the treatment of four important solid tumors affecting the adult population (Table 11-1). Breast cancer, colon cancer, and lung cancer are the most prevalent malignancies of adult

life. Testicular cancer, due to its responsiveness to chemotherapy, has a relevance far greater than its prevalence would dictate. Taken together, these four tumors span the spectrum of chemotherapeutic responsiveness from testicular cancer, which is usually cured by chemotherapy, to non-small-cell lung (NSCL) cancer, which rarely responds to any meaningful degree (Table 11-2). Treatments for these cancers are prototypic for many other solid malignancies and illustrative of the application of most of the principles described in the preceding chapter.

In the discussion below, little emphasis has been placed on the details of specific drug regimens, as these are more subject to change with time and are more thoroughly described in current medical oncology texts and journals.

Testicular Cancer

With 6,300 cases per year, testicular cancer accounts for only 1% of all new male cancer cases in the United States. Nonetheless, it has become a noteworthy cancer to medical oncologists because of the high rate of cure achievable with chemotherapy in widespread disease. The relative 5-year survival for testicular cancer in white males improved from 63% in 1960-63 to 93% in 1981-87 due to the impact of curative chemotherapy on metastatic disease (Table 11-3). Survival rates of 80% to 90% are now possible even in those patient subgroups where death was uniform before 1960. The success of chemotherapy in testicular cancer rep-

247

Table 11-1 Estimated New Cases and Deaths in 1992 in U.S. From Testicular, Breast, Colorectal, and Lung Cancer (From Boving et al.[1])

Cancer	New Cases	Deaths
Testicular	6,300	350
Breast (female)	180,000	46,000
Colorectal		
Colon	111,000	51,000
Rectal	45,000	7,300
Lung	168,000	146,000

resents a driving force in attempts to replicate such results in the more common and much more refractory cancers of the breast, colon, and lung (Table 11–3).

Curative chemotherapy in testicular cancer is based on the use of combinations of individually active drugs. In the 1960s, combination chemotherapy regimens based on actinomycin D were found to generate a 50% objective response rate in disseminated testicular cancer.[2] Subsequently, mithramycin and vinblastine used as single agents were found to have the same level of efficacy.[3,4] Complete responses (CRs) were generated in 10% to 20% of patients, and about half the patients achieving CRs were cured. Those patients who relapsed after a chemotherapy-induced CR usually did so within 12 months of initiation of chemotherapy. The lack of late relapses (beyond two years) meant that the tumor cell population was uniformly highly prolific and drug sensitive. Such rapid proliferation was consistent with a heightened sensitivity to chemotherapeutic agents. The ability to determine success or failure in 1–2 years instead of 5 or more years, as was necessary with breast cancer, for example, meant that new regimens could be evaluated for efficacy and that progress could be defined in relatively short time periods.

Improvement in the therapy of testicular cancer has depended on the introduction of new, effective agents over time. During the 1970s, bleomycin was found to have definite activity in testicular cancer.[5] Its lack of myelosuppression allowed it to be combined successfully with vinblastine, a myelosuppressive drug. A series of trials demonstrated that there was clinical synergism with the vinblastine-bleo-

mycin (VB) combination and that high complete response rates (57%) and survival rates (45%) were possible.[6] VB represented a major advance in the treatment of disseminated testicular cancer. The discovery that cisplatin, another nonmyelosuppressive agent, had activity in testicular cancer represented another major advance.[7] Cisplatin (P) provided an additional active agent with nonoverlapping toxicities that could be combined with vinblastine-bleomycin ($\pm$ other agents) to form new, PVB-based regimens for evaluation.

In an initial study of a PVB regimen conducted by Einhorn, all patients responded, there being a 70% complete response rate and a 30% partial response rate.[8] About one-third of patients with a partial response were rendered free of evidence of disease by surgical resection of all residual localized disease remaining after chemotherapy. The 5-year survival rate of patients treated in the study was 64%, and 57% survived beyond 10 years and were considered cured. Although initial studies utilized maintenance therapy after induction of a response with PVB, a subsequent randomized study failed to demonstrate any benefit from maintenance therapy after four courses of PVB.[9]

Surgical resection of residual "masses" in patients who achieved partial responses became standard treatment. Early on, it was recognized that surgical resection after cytoreductive chemotherapy could render many patients disease-free. Tumor nodules remaining after three or four cycles of chemotherapy were found at the time of resection to be necrotic debris, teratoma, or viable testicular cancer.[10] Although teratoma is histologically benign, if left in place it may grow, obstruct, or invade local structures and become unresectable. In addition, residual teratoma might undergo malignant transformation and thus must be resected. The finding of viable testicular cancer upon resection of residual disease proved to be indicative for the presence of additional, as yet unrecognized, microscopic cancer in other metastatic sites. Hence, further courses of platinum-based chemotherapy (generally including one agent not utilized in initial treatment) were administered as an effective salvage regimen to this group of patients.[11]

Despite the initial successes of the PVB-based

Table 11–2 *Parameters of Chemotherapy Effect in Selected Solid Tumors*

Tumor Type	Drug Efficacy			Sites of Failure		Curative Potential With Chemotherapy	
	Single-Agent Activity	Number of Active Agents	Combinations Activity	Locoregional	Systemic	As Adjuvant	With Metastases
Testicular	Good	Many	Excellent	Common	Common		High
Breast	Fair	Many	Good	Occasional	Common	Good	Low—with bone marrow transplant
Colon	Fair	1–2	Fair	Occasional	Common	Fair	None
Non-small-cell lung	Poor-Fair	Few	Poor-Fair	Occasional	Common	None	None

Table 11–3   Trends in 5-Year Survival Rates in U.S. (From Boving et al.[1])

| Site | Percent Five-Year Survival For Diagnosis In | | | | | |
| | 1960–63 | | 1974–76 | | 1981–87 | |
	White	Black	White	Black	White	Black
Testicular	63		79	77	93	94
Breast (female)	63	46	75	63	78	63
Colon	43	34	50	46	58	47
Rectal	38	27	49	41	55	44
Lung	8	5	12	11	13	11

drug regimens, a number of problems remained to be addressed. Not all patients were cured. Hence, attention turned to the definition of those prognostic factors that made for a favorable response (cure) and of those factors that were associated with death from cancer. Table 11–4 outlines the University of Indiana group's classification system in which patients with minimal and moderate disease are likely to have a favorable outcome and patients with advanced disease are likely to have a poor outcome.[12] A favorable outcome is defined as achievement of a complete response with chemotherapy or of a disease-free state by complete resection of residual teratoma after achievement of a partial response with chemotherapy. Whereas 99% of patients with minimal disease and 90% with moderate disease have a favorable response to PVB, only 58% of patients with advanced disease have such a response.[12] The values of the three known tumor markers (lactate dehydrogenase, alpha fetoprotein, and human chorionic gonadotropin) have been shown to provide further prognostic information within the advanced group of patients. In advanced disease (Table 11–4), the response rate is 73% when only one marker is elevated, but falls to 45% when all three markers are elevated.[12]

The definition of two prognostic groups (favorable and unfavorable) has allowed investigators to focus on different challenges in the treatment of each group. For the favorable group, the challenge has been to decrease toxicity while retaining the high response and cure rate. For the unfavorable group, the challenge

has been to develop improved regimens for refractory disease.

Several initial measures were taken to reduce toxicity. One approach to reducing toxicity involved reduction by 25% of the vinblastine dose in PVB regimen.[13] With such dosage reduction, hematological toxicity decreased without a reduction in therapeutic efficacy, as shown by a randomized study.[8] Furthermore, additional courses of PVB beyond four did not improve the overall response rate or the therapeutic benefit in any given patient. Hence, prolonged, intensive PVB treatment that would generate greater toxicity without therapeutic gain was omitted in subsequent patients. In early studies, maintenance therapy with vinblastine was given for a total of two years of treatment. As noted above, additional investigations aimed at reducing toxicity subsequently demonstrated that continued maintenance therapy after four courses of PVB (given over three months) did not improve the response rate and survival.[9]

The recognition that etoposide (VP-16) is an active agent in testis cancer represented an advance relevant to both the prognostically favorable and prognostically unfavorable patient groups.[14] This drug (the semisynthetic podophyllotoxin derivative) has now replaced vinblastine in the PVB regimen largely because it causes much less neuromuscular toxicity. Reduction of neuromuscular toxicity is especially important in the prognostically favorable patient population. For patients in the unfavorable group, the response rate for etoposide is higher than that for vinblastine.[15]

Additional improvements of the treatment of patients in the prognostically unfavorable group include the recognition that another new agent, ifosfamide, has significant activity even after patients have received heavy pretreatment with other agents.[16] Most recently, massive doses of carboplatin and etoposide have been administered with autologous bone-marrow support to achieve long-term disease-free survival in patients whose tumor had been highly refractory to prior chemotherapy including the best cisplatin-based and ifosfamide-based salvage regimens.[17]

Clearly, the successes in the treatment of testicular cancer are gratifying to all chemotherapists. Patients are cured using a well-defined and soundly based therapeutic approach. But several unique aspects of the disease and the patient population must be considered when comparing progress in testicular cancer to that in the other, more common tumor types discussed below. Disease-specific aspects include a highly and uniformly prolific cancer sensitive to multiple drugs, most of which can be effectively combined. Testicular cancer patients do not often develop significant liver, bone marrow, and brain metastases. Tumor largely confined to lymph nodes does not compromise vital organ function, thus allowing for better tolerance of chemotherapy. In addition, the patient population is a major factor in determining tolerance to aggressive and toxic chemotherapy regimens. In one study of the long-term effects of chemotherapy in testicular cancer, for example, the mean age was 29.5 years (range 19–53 years) and none of the patients had preexisting renal or pulmonary disease.[18] Such patients can tolerate more chemotherapy-related physiological stress than patients in the 60–70 year-old age group, which is the patient population most affected by the major cancers of adult life.

Breast Cancer

In the United States, breast cancer accounts for 32% of new cases of cancer in women and 19% of female cancer deaths.[1] In 1992, there will be an estimated 180,000 newly diagnosed cases of breast cancer and 46,000 deaths from breast cancer in American women (Table 11-1). It is currently the second leading cause of death from cancer in women and the leading cause of death in women aged 35–54. Nearly

Table 11-4   Indiana Classification of Extent of Disease

Minimal—favorable outcome

1. Elevated HCG and/or αFP-only
2. Cervical nodes ($\pm$ nonpalpable, retroperitoneal nodes)
3. Unresectable, but nonpalpable, retroperitoneal disease
4. Minimal pulmonary metastases—less than five per lung field and the largest <2 cm ($\pm$ nonpalpable abdominal disease)

Moderate—favorable outcome

5. Palpable abdominal mass as only anatomical disease
6. Moderate pulmonary metastases—five to ten pulmonary metastases per lung field and the largest <3 cm or a mediastinal mass $<50\%$ of the intrathoracic diameter or a solitary pulmonary metastasis any size >2 cm ($\pm$ nonpalpable abdominal disease)

Advanced—poor outcome

7. Advanced pulmonary metastases—mediastinal mass $>50\%$ of the intrathoracic diameter or greater than ten pulmonary metastases per lung field or multiple pulmonary metastases >3 cm ($\pm$ nonpalpable abdominal disease)
8. Palpable abdominal mass plus pulmonary metastases
   8.1 Minimal pulmonary
   8.2 Moderate pulmonary
   8.3 Advanced pulmonary
9. Hepatic, osseous, or CNS metastases

all women who develop breast cancer now receive some form of drug therapy. Due to the size of the population afflicted with the disease, even small percentage improvements in outcome such as those generated by adjuvant therapy positively affect thousands of patients. Accordingly, clinical research efforts have been commensurate with the scope of the problem. Due to its high visibility, breast cancer may well be the most important disease in defining the public's perception of cancer and in providing impetus to the science and practice of medical oncology.

Death from breast cancer occurs from metastases to lung, liver, bone marrow, brain, and other sites. Drug therapy for breast cancer is given either to cause regression of demonstrable metastatic disease or to prevent the growth of possible occult metastatic disease after eradication of the primary cancer (i.e., adjuvant therapy).

METASTATIC, ADVANCED DISEASE. When breast cancer has spread from the breast (and local lymph nodes) to other parts of the body, it has been considered an incurable disease.[19] Due to considerable heterogeneity in survival, no major impact of drug therapy in prolonging life has been convincingly demonstrated through randomized trials.[20] Yet in clinical practice almost all patients with metastatic disease will receive drug therapy and many patients appear to benefit from it. The major therapeutic goals of metastatic disease treatment are palliation of symptoms with an improved quality of life and an objective, measurable tumor response. Although palliation of symptoms may be the treatment objective for the individual patient, most studies of the efficacy of various treatments have focused on objective, measurable tumor responses within defined groups of patients. Methods for assessing changes in the quality of life are being increasingly incorporated into current studies, however.

Drug therapy for breast cancer involves two categories of pharmaceuticals, hormonal agents and cytotoxic, chemotherapeutic agents. The hormonal agents such as tamoxifen, progestins, aminoglutethimide, and estrogens are all equivalent in terms of response rate and survival benefit.[19] Tamoxifen produces the

least toxicity and is the best tolerated agent and therefore the treatment of first choice. In metastatic breast cancer, hormonal agents produce a 50–60% response rate in patients whose tumors are estrogen receptor positive (ER+).[21] In patients with estrogen receptor negative tumors, the response rate is significantly lower, at 6–9%. Hormonal agents tend to be more effective against metastatic disease in bone, lung, and skin and less effective against liver and brain metastases. Occasionally, complete responses in patients having only bone, lung, or skin metastases may last for many years. Patients with primary tumors displaying higher estrogen-receptor levels not only respond more readily to hormonal agents when metastatic disease develops, but also tend to have a longer disease-free interval before it develops.[22]

Many chemotherapeutic agents can produce measurable regressions in breast cancer. Due to higher response rates with combinations of drugs, such regimens are standard. Multiple trials of various combinations of chemotherapeutic drugs have not defined any single markedly superior regimen.[23] The most frequent combinations have included various permutations of cyclophosphamide (C), adriamycin (A), fluorouracil (F), and methotrexate (e.g., FAC or CAF, CMF, FA, AC). Although overall response rates (percent partial plus percent complete responses) as high as 80% have been reported in several small series of patients, a recent review of 45 trials indicates that the complete response rate is around 8% and the overall response rate 39% for conventional chemotherapy.[23] This statistical assessment gave a median duration of response of 9.6 months, a median survival of 16.6 months, and a two-year survival rate of 39%.

The question of dose-response in breast cancer chemotherapy has generated much controversy in recent years.[24] Retrospective analyses have combined multiple series of patients and examined the response rate versus average relative dose intensity of either CMF or CAF. Such analyses have been interpreted as demonstrating a significant increase in response rate with dose intensity in patients with advanced breast cancer.[25] Although only a few studies have been conducted, one randomized trial of low-dose CMF versus a two-fold higher dose of CMF found a significant difference in response

Table 11-5 *Five-Year Breast Cancer Survival Rates by Tumor Size and Lymph Node (LN) Status.* (Adapted from Carter et al.[29])

Size	LN Status	Relative Survival (%)
<2.0	Negative nodes	96.3
	1–3 Pos. nodes	87.4
	4+ Pos. nodes	66.0
2–5 cm	Negative nodes	89.4
	1–3 Pos. nodes	79.9
	4+ Pos. nodes	58.7
>5.0 cm	Negative nodes	82.2
	1–3 Pos. nodes	73.0
	4+ Pos. nodes	45.5

rate (11% versus 30%) and in toxicity.[26] Patients receiving the high-dose CMF had more vomiting, myelosuppression, conjunctivitis, and alopecia. Survival was 15.6 months in the high-dose group versus 12.8 months in the low-dose group, which was not a statistically significant difference. Quality-of-life scales confirmed greater immediate toxicity with the high-dose treatment, but a trend to improvement in general health and several disease-related indices in these patients. Thus, despite the general feeling that there should be a dose-response effect in breast cancer chemotherapy, the magnitude and value of that effect in light of the increasing toxicity has not been clarified. It is clear that normal tissue toxicity can be described by a reproducible dose-response curve. What is not settled, however, is whether the dose-response curve for antitumor effect is such that the clinically achievable increase in dose intensity will be meaningful. As noted below, the value of the dose-response effect is most controversial as it applies to high-dose chemotherapy with autologous bone-marrow-transplant support (HDC with ABMT).

Multiple studies of HDC with ABMT have established that such aggressive treatment leads to a higher response rate in breast cancer than seen with conventional dosages of similar drugs.[27] A recent review of most of the relevant literature indicated that the complete response rate and overall response rate are 36% and 70%, respectively, for HDC with ABMT ver-

sus 8% and 39% for conventional dosage chemotherapy.[23] This same review concluded, however, that the data did not indicate any improvement in survival for HDC with ABMT over conventional treatment. To that end, several trials randomizing patients between HDC with ABMT and conventional therapy have been initiated in metastatic disease. In addition, HDC with ABMT is being tested as an adjuvant therapy in very high-risk patients, such as those with large primary tumors and involvement of multiple axillary lymph nodes (Tables 11-5, 11-6).

There appears to be no benefit for women who have only partial responses to HDC with ABMT. This is understandable, since even a complete response may represent only a 2- to 3-log reduction in tumor-cell number in a situation where 9 to 11 logs of cell kill would be necessary for cure. It is for this reason that some investigators are restricting HDC with ABMT in advanced disease to those patients who respond first to several courses of conventional chemotherapy.[27] On the other hand, there may be some durability of improvement in a small portion of the patients with complete responses to HDC and ABMT.[27] Although not proven, the potential that 10% or so of patients might achieve long-term survival with HDC and ABMT exists. This hope and the high response rate have driven women to seek this as yet ill-defined chance for cure. On the other hand, the constraints of cost ($100,000/patient), toxicity (10% treatment-related

Table 11-6 *Breast Cancer Recurrence Rate As Related to Number of Involved Axillary Lymph Nodes.* (Adapted from Nemoto et al.[30])

Number Positive Nodes	Percent Without Recurrence
0	81
1	77
2	60
3	57
4	56
5	46
6–10	37
11–15	28
>21	18

deaths), and lack of defined benefit in controlled studies have provoked opposition to this approach as standard therapy.[23]

EARLY (RESECTABLE) PRIMARY DISEASE. Progress in the clinical treatment of breast cancer has been greatest in early-stage disease—that is, in women who appear to have cancer confined to the primary site. Breast conservation with lumpectomy followed by local radiotherapy is equally effective in terms of survival as the more mutilating technique of surgical mastectomy.[28] Even early on, it was realized that as many as 50% of women with no clinical evidence of disease at the time of radical mastectomy would ultimately die of metastatic breast cancer. The last two decades of breast cancer research have focused on this problem. One aim has been to define prognostic factors that correlate with the probability of development of manifest clinical disease and death in women who appear free of such disease at the time of eradication of the primary tumor within the breast (Tables 11–5, 11–6). A second aim has been to develop adjuvant drug treatments in an attempt to prevent relapse of disease in metastatic sites after eradication of the primary tumor in the breast.

The two major prognostic factors used to characterize patients in adjuvant drug studies have been the size of the primary tumor and the number of axillary lymph nodes involved. Five-year survival after eradication of the primary tumor declines with increasing size of the primary tumor and number of involved lymph nodes (Table 11–5). Recurrence at five years is directly correlated to the number of axillary lymph nodes infiltrated by the cancer (Table 11–6).

In recent years, it has been recognized that certain subgroups of lymph node-negative patients do poorly and may be appropriate candidates for adjuvant therapy.[31–33] Among prognostic factors of importance are the level of estrogen receptor and the presence of progesterone receptors, both of which correlate with survival.[31] In addition, increased proliferative activity as measured by the S-phase fraction (determined by flow cytometry) appears to predict an increased risk of recurrence.[31,32] Ploidy, presence of the HER-2 oncogene, and high ca-

thepsin levels also appear to correlate with survival, but these measures are still under investigation and not in routine clinical use.[31] The definition of prognostic factors is of critical importance to adjuvant breast cancer therapy. Identification of patients who have a good prognosis spares them the cost and toxicity of adjuvant therapy. For those with a prognosis that indicates the need for further therapy, the intensity of the treatment applied can be proportional to the risk of tumor recurrence and death.

The Early Breast Cancer Trialists' Collaborative Group has recently analyzed and published data on 75,000 women (about 90% of those ever randomized) entered into adjuvant breast cancer trials.[34,35] Highly significant reductions in the annual rates both of recurrence and of death from breast cancer were found in treated patients compared to untreated control patients. Combination chemotherapy produced a 28% reduction in recurrence and a 16% reduction in mortality. Long-term chemotherapy (e.g., 12 months) was shown to be no better than short-term treatment (e.g., 6 months). Survival (not adjusted for other causes of death) at ten years for node-negative patients was 67.2% for the treated and 63.3% for the untreated control groups. For node-positive patients, survival at ten years was 46.6% for the treated and 39.8% for the untreated, control groups. Tamoxifen treatment reduced annual rates of recurrence and of death from breast cancer by 25% and 17%, respectively. Survival (not adjusted for other causes of death) in node-negative patients was 74.5% for those who received chemotherapy and 71.0% for untreated control patients. For node-positive patients, survival at ten years was 50.4% for those who received chemotherapy and 42.2% for untreated control patients. Long-term (two years or more) treatment with tamoxifen was found to be significantly more effective than shorter tamoxifen regimens.

Data presented at an NIH Consensus Development Conference on Adjuvant Chemotherapy and Endocrine Therapy for Breast Cancer in 1985 led the panel of experts to recommend chemotherapy for premenopausal women with positive lymph nodes as standard care, regardless of hormonal status.[36] For postmenopausal women with positive nodes and positive hormonal receptor levels, tamoxifen was recommended as the treatment of choice. A National Cancer Institute Clinical Alert of May 18, 1988, and the NIH Consensus Development Conference Statement for a second consensus conference held June 18–21, 1990, declared that the rate of local and distant relapse following local therapy for node-negative breast cancer was decreased by both combination chemotherapy and by tamoxifen.[37,38] Both NIH consensus conferences encouraged continued enrollment of patients in clinical trials but maintained that treatment was appropriate for most patients whether in a trial or not.

Hence, most of the 180,000 patients in the U.S. newly diagnosed with breast cancer are likely to receive drug therapy either as treatment for metastatic disease or as adjuvant therapy in early stages to prevent the development of metastatic disease and death. In actuality, the pharmaceutical attack has gone even further. Based on the low toxicity of tamoxifen and its ability to retard breast cancer in the remaining breast of patients on adjuvant therapy, a chemoprevention trial is being conducted to determine whether chronic administration will prevent the development of breast cancer in women at high risk.[39]

Colorectal Cancer

In the United States, colorectal cancer is the third leading cause of cancer death in men and in women, and second only to lung cancer as a cause of death in men and women combined.[1] There were about 156,000 new cases of colorectal cancer diagnosed in the United States and 58,000 deaths from this cancer in 1992 (Table 11–1). Deaths from colorectal cancer occur most frequently after age 55. Although it is generally thought that chemotherapy is less effective in the treatment of colorectal cancer than in the treatment of breast cancer, recent developments are such that most patients will receive chemotherapy either for metastatic disease or as adjuvant therapy. As with breast cancer, the size of the population afflicted with colorectal cancer is so large that even a small (percentage) improvement in survival with adjuvant therapy can benefit thousands of patients.

METASTATIC DISEASE. Fluorouracil (FU) has been singularly the mainstay of chemotherapy for colorectal cancer for over 30 years. The lack of other active agents has generated a variety of permutations in drug scheduling, ranging from a standard bolus administration through protracted outpatient infusions of 30 days or longer. In one major study, for example, prolonged continuous infusions of FU were found to yield a higher response rate (30%) when compared to an equitoxic bolus regimen (7%), although survival was not affected.[40] Further efforts to boost the activity of FU had their genesis in preclinical studies of biochemical modulation with other antimetabolites, such as methotrexate, or with metabolites such as leucovorin (formyltetrahydrofolic acid). In the most successful of these efforts, the addition of leucovorin (LV) to FU markedly increased the response rate from the low levels seen with FU alone (Table 11–7). Although in most studies the increased response rate had little impact on survival[44] (Table 11–7), one well-designed study demonstrated a statistically significant increase in median survival from 7.7 months for FU alone to 12 months for FU plus LV.[45] Based on these results, the use of regimens with FU plus LV has become standard therapy for metastatic colorectal cancer. Nonetheless, a 30–40% response rate and a 12-month median survival must be seen as providing only limited benefit for patients with a disease in which continued research is essential.

Certain patients with metastatic colorectal

Table 11–7 *Comparison of Fluorouracil (FU) Alone Versus FU Plus Leucovorin (LV) Against Colorectal Cancer*

	Response Rate (%)		Survival (Median) (Weeks)	
Reference	FU	FU + LV	FU	FU + LV
41	12	30	46	55
42	13	44	55	62
43	7	33	41	54

Table 11–8   Response Rates for Hepatic Arterial Versus Intravenous
Chemotherapy for Hepatic Metastases Fom Colorectal Cancer
(Comparative studies)

Reference	Hepatic Arterial		Intravenous	
	Drug	Response (%)	Drug	Response (%)
47	FUDR	50	FUDR	20
48	FUDR	42	FUDR	10
49	FUDR	62	FUDR	17
50	FUDR	48	FU	21

cancer seem to be curable. Those with three or fewer metastatic tumor nodules in the liver as the sole site of metastatic colorectal cancer appear to be cured 25–30% of the time by resection of the nodules.[46] This surgical experience and the frequent occurrence of hepatic metastases has made hepatic arterial chemotherapy the most prominent form of regional chemotherapy. Due to improved selectivity in regional delivery, 5-fluoro-2'-deoxyuridine (FUDR) is often used instead of FU for hepatic arterial chemotherapy. A number of studies have demonstrated that hepatic arterial FUDR generates a significantly higher response rate than intravenous therapy (Table 11–8). Very little FUDR reaches the systemic circulation due to high hepatic extraction.[51] Unfortunately, other metastases in extrahepatic sites frequently develop. It is perhaps for this reason that the survival benefit for hepatic arterial FUDR is ill-defined and controversial.[52,53]

ADJUVANT CHEMOTHERAPY. Colorectal cancer can be divided into two anatomically distinct types, nonrectal colon cancer and rectal cancer. Due to the frequent inability to achieve adequate surgical margins within the pelvis, rectal cancer recurs locally much more frequently than does colon cancer.

The prognosis for patients having tumor involvement of lymph nodes immediately adjacent to the primary tumor in the colon can be fairly poor, depending on a variety of factors (Table 11–9). The recent demonstration that FU plus levamisole could improve the chances of survival for such patients with nonrectal colon cancer has been heralded as a therapeutic advance (Table 11–10). In the largest study to date, FU with levamisole reduced the overall

death rate by 33% in patients with involved lymph nodes, while levamisole alone had no effect.[54] Based on that study, adjuvant therapy with FU and levamisole has become the standard regimen for colon cancer whenever there is local nodal involvement. A large nationwide study is currently underway to determine whether the addition of LV will be of further benefit in adjuvant therapy.

The propensity for rectal carcinoma to recur in the pelvis close to the site of resection of the primary tumor has led investigators to examine the effect of radiotherapy of that area. In some studies, chemotherapy has been added for its potential adjuvant effect against occult systemic disease. Several large series have demonstrated that combining chemotherapy with radiotherapy facilitates the control of local disease and improves disease-free survival and overall survival rates (Table 11–11). Locoregional control with chemotherapy added to radiotherapy has been better than that achieved with radiotherapy alone. Perhaps improved locoregional control is due to the radiosensitizing as well as the chemotherapeutic effect of FU. Although combined therapy (with pelvic radiotherapy and an FU regimen) is now standard therapy, investigations are underway to determine whether leucovorin and levamisole may further increase the modest effect found to date.

Lung Cancer

Lung cancer is the leading cause of death from cancer in the United States (Table 11–1). Despite more than two decades of effort to reduce mortality, the five-year survival rate is only 11–13%. In terms of treatment, lung cancer is di-

Table 11-9   Significant Prognostic Variables in Colon Cancer When Regional Lymph Nodes Are Involved (Dukes' C Stage). (Adapted from Moertel et al.[54])

Variable	Recurrence At 3½ Years (%)	Surviving By 3½ Years (%)
Depth of invasion into:		
Submucosa or muscular layer	76	84
Serosa	49	56
Stuck onto adjacent organ		
Yes	46	45
No	54	63
Invasion of adjacent organ		
Yes	43	29
No	54	61
Obstruction		
Yes	46	47
No	55	63
Regional peritoneal implants		
Yes	38	42
No	54	61
No. of nodes involved		
1-4	61	70
>4	33	34
Histologic differentiation		
Well	56	57
Moderately well	55	64
Poor	40	42

Table 11-10   Adjuvant FU Plus Levamisole in Colon Cancer

Reference	Treatment	Survival	
		% Disease-Free at (Years)	% Alive at (Years)
55	None		56 (5)
	Drugs		68 (5)
56	None	50 (5)	58 (5)
	Drugs	60 (5)	64 (5)
54	None	47 (3)	55 (3)
	Drugs	63 (3)	71 (3)

Table 11–11   Effect of Adjuvant Chemotherapy and Radiotherapy in Rectal Cancer

Reference	Treatment	Local Failure (%)	Distant Metastases (%)	Survival Disease-Free	Survival Overall (%)	Follow-Up (Months)
57,58	None	24	34	48	28	72
	ChemoRx	27	27	54	43	72
	RadioRx	20	30	52	43	72
	Both	11	26	67	57	72
59	None	25	26	37	48	64
	ChemoRx	21	24	46	58	64
	RadioRx	16	31	39	50	64
60	RadioRx	25	46	38	38	84
	Both	14	29	58	53	84

vided into two categories, small-cell lung cancer (SCLC) and non-small-cell lung cancer (NSCLC). Small-cell lung cancer differs from NSCLC in that it is usually widely metastatic at the time of diagnosis, grows more rapidly, and responds better to a wide variety of chemotherapeutic agents. NSCLC grows more slowly, is less likely to be overtly metastatic at the time of diagnosis, and does not respond as well to chemotherapy. NSCLC lumps together epidermoid carcinoma, adenocarcinoma, and large-cell carcinoma of the lung. NSCLS accounts for about 80% of all lung cancer and lung cancer deaths.[61] The use of chemotherapy for NSCLC will be discussed below as an example of chemotherapy for a "nonresponsive" tumor type. In metastatic NSCLC, in particular, there is considerable controversy as to whether chemotherapy is worthwhile.[62] As discussed in the previous chapter, a variety of reasons for treatment other than cure come into play in NSCLC.

ADVANCED METASTATIC DISEASE. Drug combinations containing cisplatin or the more recently introduced platinum analog, carboplatin, are most commonly used in the treatment of metastatic or advanced, inoperable NSCLC. Table 11–12 presents representative results for therapy achieved in one large group trial.[63] Response rates are low and median survival is short. A number of randomized trials have compared cisplatin-based combinations to best supportive care (Table 11–13). The results of these studies demonstrate an improved survival

for chemotherapy treatment over best supportive care, but the magnitude of this effect is small and perhaps clinically insignificant.[62] Toxicity in those regimens showing improved duration of survival is generally severe, and patients do not generally experience any improvement in their performance status.[64,67] Knowledgeable chemotherapists in this area have suggested that chemotherapy should be limited to the use of moderately intense regimens and restricted to patients who are in good physical condition.[64] Continued therapy should be given only if there is evidence of tumor regression after several courses. Furthermore, it is clear that patients who have significant symptoms and weight loss due to tumor do not benefit from chemotherapy in NSCLC. Regionally confined, but inoperable, NSCLC is usually treated with radiotherapy. The addition of cisplatin-based chemotherapy to radiotherapy appears to improve median survival and increase the proportion of patients alive at three years from 11% to 23%.[68]

ADJUVANT THERAPY. Only one published trial used cisplatin-based chemotherapy adjuvantly after surgical resection in NSCLC.[69] This trial by the Lung Cancer Study Group randomized patients to a postoperative cytoxan/adriamycin/cisplatin (CAP) regimen versus immunotherapy. Median time to death was delayed by seven months (from 17 months to 24 months) in the CAP-treated group. The investigators questioned whether the benefit of a seven-month increase in disease-free survival out-

Table 11–12 *Trial Comparing Carboplatin to Multidrug Cisplatin-Based Combinations.* (Adapted from Bonomi et al.[63])

Treatment	No. of Patients	Response Rate (%)	Median Survival (Weeks)	% Severe Toxicity
MVP	176	20	23	26
VP	175	13	25	36
MVP/CAMP	172	13	25	26
Carboplatin	88	9	32	4

MVP = mitomycin + vinblastine + cisplatin; VP = vinblastine + cisplatin; CAMP = cyclophosphamide + doxorubicin + methotrexate + procarbazine

weighed the discomforts of chemotherapy and represented any improvement in the quality of life for patients. They concluded that any improvement in the surgical adjuvant therapy for lung cancer would require a more effective systemic regimen.

Summary

This chapter has summarized the role of chemotherapy in four important types of cancer. Three of them taken together, breast cancer, colorectal cancer, and NSCLC, account for over 50% of annual cancer deaths in the United States. The fourth, testicular cancer, afflicts far fewer people, yet is significant as the prime example of chemotherapeutic success in a metastatic solid tumor. Clinical treatment for these tumor types illustrates the application and usefulness of principles and concepts derived from preclinical model systems (Table 10–3).

The various treatment regimens described in this chapter fulfill the spectrum of therapeutic goals defined in the previous chapter. Cure is the intent for metastatic testicular cancer. Cure or at least prolongation of survival time is the therapeutic goal in adjuvant breast cancer and colon cancer treatment. Palliation of symptoms and an improved quality of life are major objectives in the treatment of metastatic breast cancer. In metastatic colorectal cancer and NSCLC, major reasons for treatment are to obtain even the small improvement in survival possible for some patients and to conduct research to improve therapy. There is a tendency for patients and their physicians to be activists

Table 11–13 *Randomized Trials Comparing Cisplatin-Based Combinations to Best Supportive Care (BSC) in Advanced NSCLC*

Reference	Treatment	No. of Patients	Response (%)	Median Survival (Weeks)	Survival Difference
64	VP	44	25	33	P = 0.01
	BSC	50		17	
64	CAP	43	13	25	P = 0.05
	BSC	50		17	
65	VP	24	42	28	P < 0.001
	BSC	22		10	
66	VP	44	11	22	NS (P = 0.5)
	BSC	43		16.5	

VP = vinca alkaloid + cisplatin; CAP = cyclophosphamide + doxorubicin + cisplatin; CEP/MEC = cyclophosphamide + epirubicin + cisplatin alternating with methotrexate + etoposide + lomustine and to believe that "active intervention" (i.e., using chemotherapy) is better than supportive care alone. At this juncture, the chemotherapeutic regimens being used appear to be achieving these therapeutic aims, although often for too short a time or for too few of the patients. Nonetheless, it is a reasonable expectation that the conceptual framework and research approach that have developed over time will continue to guide future efforts.

REFERENCES

1. C. C. Boring, T. S. Squires, and T. Tong: Cancer statistics, 1992. *CA—A Cancer Journal For Clinicians* 42:19 (1992).

2. M. C. Li, W. F. Whitmore, R. Golby, and H. Grabstad: Effects of combined drug therapy on metastatic cancer of the testis. *J. Am. Med. Assoc.* 174:145 (1960).

3. B. J. Kennedy: Mithramycin therapy in advanced testicular neoplasms. *Cancer* 26:755 (1970).

4. M. L. Samuels and C. D. Howe: Vinblastine in the management of testicular cancer. *Cancer* 25:1009 (1970).

5. R. H. Blum, S. Carter, and K. A. Agre: A clinical review of bleomycin: A new antineoplastic agent. *Cancer* 31:903 (1973).

6. M. L. Samuels, V. J. Lanzotti, L. E. Boyle, P. Y. Holoye, and D. E. Johnson: "An update of the Velban-bleomycin program in testicular neoplasia with a note on cis-dichlorodiammineplatinum," in *Cancer of the Genitourinary Tract*, ed. by D. E. Johnson and M. Samuels. New York: Raven Press, 1979, pp. 159–172.

7. D. J. Higby, H. J. Wallace, D. J. Albert, and J. F. Holland: Diaminodichloroplatinum: A phase I study showing responses in testicular and other solid tumors. *Cancer* 33:1219 (1974).

8. L. H. Einhorn and J. Donohue: Cis-diamminedichloroplatinum, vinblastine and bleomycin combination chemotherapy in disseminated testicular cancer. *Ann. Intern. Med.* 87:293 (1977).

9. L. H. Einhorn, S. D. Williams, M. Troner, R. Birch, and F. A. Greco: The role of maintenance therapy in disseminated testicular cancer. *New Engl. J. Med.* 305:727 (1981).

10. L. H. Einhorn, S. D. Williams, I. Mandelbaum, and J. P. Donohue: Surgical resection in disseminated testicular cancer following chemotherapeutic cytoreduction. *Cancer* 48:904 (1981).

11. D. F. Bajorin, H. Herr, R. J. Motzer, and G. J. Bosl: *Semin. Oncol.* 19:148 (1992).

12. R. Birch, S. Williams, A. Cone, L. Einhorn, P. Roark, S. Turner, and F. A. Greco: Prognostic factors for favorable outcome in disseminated germ cell tumors. *J. Clin. Oncol.* 4:400 (1986).

13. L. H. Einhorn and S. D. Williams: Chemotherapy of disseminated testicular cancer: A random prospective study. *Cancer* 46:1339 (1980).

14. S. D. Williams, L. H. Einhorn, F. A. Greco, R. Old-

ham, and R. Fletcher: VP-16-213 salvage therapy for refractory germinal neoplasms. *Cancer* 46:2154 (1980).

15. G. C. Garrow and D. H. Johnson: Treatment of "good risk" metastatic testicular cancer. *Semin. Oncol.* 19:159 (1992).

16. P. J. Loehrer, R. Lauer, B. J. Roth, S. D. Williams, L. A. Kalasinski, and L. H. Einhorn: Salvage therapy in recurrent germ cell cancer: Ifosfamide and cisplatin plus either vinblastine or etoposide. *Ann. Int. Med.* 109:540 (1988).

17. C. R. Nichols, J. Andersen, H. M. Lazarus, H. Fisher, J. Greer, E. A. Stadtmauer, P. J. Loehrer, and D. L. Trump: High-dose carboplatin and etoposide with autologous bone marrow transplantation in refractory germ cell cancer: An Eastern Cooperative Oncology Group Protocol. *J. Clin. Oncol.* 10:558 (1992).

18. S. Osanto, A. Bukman, F. Van Hoek, P. J. Sterk, J. A. P. M. De Laat, and J. Hermans: Long-term effects of chemotherapy in patients with testicular cancer. *J. Clin. Oncol.* 10:574 (1992).

19. I. C. Henderson, J. R. Harris, D. W. Kinne, and S. Hellman: "Cancer of the breast," in *Cancer Principles & Practice of Oncology*, ed. by V. T. DeVita, Jr., S. Hellman, and S. A. Rosenberg. Philadelphia: J.B. Lippincott, 1989, pp. 1197–1268.

20. G. P. Canellos: "Treatment of metastases; selection of therapy," in *Breast Diseases*, ed. by J. R. Harris, S. Hellman, I. C. Henderson, and D. W. Kinne. Philadelphia: J.B. Lippincott, 1987, pp. 385–391.

21. I. C. Henderson: "Treatment of metastases; endocrine therapy in metastatic breast cancer," in *Breast Diseases*, ed. by J. R. Harris, S. Hellman, I. C. Henderson, and D. W. Kinne. Philadelphia: J.B. Lippincott, 1987, pp. 398–399.

22. G. M. Clark, W. L. McGuire, C. A. Hubay, O. H. Pearson, and J. S. Marshall: Progesterone receptors as a prognostic factor in stage II breast cancer. *New Engl. J. Med.* 309:1343 (1983).

23. D. M. Eddy: High-dose chemotherapy with autologous bone marrow transplantation for the treatment of metastatic bone cancer. *J. Clin. Oncol.* 10:657 (1992).

24. I. C. Henderson, D. F. Hayes, and R. Gelman: Dose-response in the treatment of breast cancer: A critical review. *J. Clin. Oncol.* 6:1501 (1988).

25. W. M. Hryniuk: "The importance of dose intensity in the outcome of chemotherapy," in *Important Advances in Oncology 1988*, ed. by V. T. DeVita, Jr., S. Hellman, and S. A. Rosenberg. Philadelphia: J.B. Lippincott Company, 1988, pp. 121–141.

26. I. F. Tannock, N. F. Boyd, G. DeBoer, C. Erlichman, S. Fine, G. Larocque, C. Mayers, D. Perrault, and H. Sutherland: A randomized trila of two dose levels of cyclophosphamide, methotrexate, and fluorouracil chemotherapy for patients with metastatic breast cancer. *J. Clin. Oncol.* 6:1377 (1988).

27. K. Antman, L. Ayash, A. Elias, C. Wheeler, M. Hunt, J. P. Eder, B. A. Teicher, J. Critchlow, J. Bibbo, L. E. Schnipper, and E. Frei III: A phase II study of high-dose cyclophosphamide, thiotepa, and carboplatin with autologous marrow support in women with measurable advanced breast cancer responding to standard-dose therapy. *J. Clin. Oncol.* 10:102 (1992).

28. B. Fisher, M. Bauer, R. Margolese, R. Poisson, Y.

Pilch, C. Redmond, E. Fisher, N. Wolmark, M. Deutsch, E. Montague, E. Saffer, L. Wickerham, H. Lerner, A. Glass, H. Shabata, P. Deckers, A. Ketcham, R. Oishi, and I. Russell: Five-year results of a randomized clinical trial comparing total mastectomy and segmental mastectomy with or without radiation in the treatment of breast cancer. *New Engl. J. Med. 312*:665 (1985).

29. C. L. Carter, C. Allen, and D. E. Henson: Relation of tumor size, lymph node status, and survival in 24,740 breast cancer cases. *Cancer 63*:181 (1989).

30. T. Nemoto, J. Vana, R. N. Bedwani, H. W. Baker, F. H. McGregor, and G. P. Murphy: Management and survival of female breast cancer: Results of a national survey by the American College of Surgeons. *Cancer 45*:2917 (1980).

31. W. L. McGuire, A. K. Tandon, C. Allred, G. C. Chamness, and G. M. Clark: Commentaries: How to use prognostic factors in axillary node-negative breast cancer patients. *J. Natl. Cancer Inst. 82*:1006 (1990).

32. H. Sigurdsson, B. Baldetorp, A. Borg, M. Dalberg, M. Ferno, D. Killander, and H. Olsson: Indicators of prognosis in node-negative breast cancer. *New Engl. J. Med. 322*:1045 (1990).

33. D. Rosner and W. W. Lane: Should all patients with node-negative breast cancer receive adjuvant therapy? *Cancer 68*:1482 (1991).

34. Early Breast Cancer Trialists' Collaborative Group: Systemic treatment of early breast cancer by hormonal, cytotoxic, or immune therapy. 133 randomised trials involving 31,000 recurrences and 24,000 deaths among 75,000 women. *Lancet 339*:1 (1992).

35. Early Breast Cancer Trialists' Collaborative Group: Systemic treatment of early breast cancer by hormonal, cytotoxic, or immune therapy. 133 randomised trials involving 31,000 recurrences and 24,000 deaths among 75,000 women. *Lancet 339*:71 (1992).

36. M. E. Lippman (ed.): *Proceedings of the NIH Consensus Development Conference on Adjuvant Chemotherapy and Endocrine Therapy for Breast Cancer.*

37. *Clinic Alert from the National Cancer Institute,* May 18, 1988.

38. Treatment of Early Stage Breast Cancer, June 18–21, 1990. *National Institutes of Health Consensus Development Conference Statement.*

39. *National Surgical Adjuvant Breast and Bowel Project Protocol PI:* "A Clinical Trial to Determine the Worth of Tamoxifen for Preventing Breast Cancer." Activated 4/29/92.

40. J. J. Lokich, J. D., Ahlgren, J. L. Gullo, J. A. Phillips, and J. G. Fryer: A prospective randomized comparison of continuous infusion fluorouracil with a conventional bolus schedule in metastatic colorectal carcinoma: A Mid-Atlantic Oncology Program Study. *J. Clin. Oncol. 7*:425 (1989).

41. N. Petrelli, H. O. Douglass, Jr., L. Herrera, D. Russell, D. M. Stablein, M. D. Green, F. M. Muggia, A. Megibow, E. S. Greenwald, R. M. Bukowski, J. Harris, B. Levin, E. Gaynor, A. Loutfi, M. H. Kalser, J. S. Barkin, P. Benedetoo, P. V. Woolley, R. Nauta, D. W. Weaver, and L. P. Leichman for the Gastrointestinal Tumor Study Group. *J. Clin. Oncol. 7*:1419 (1989).

42. J. H. Doroshow, P. Multhauf, L. Leong, K. Margolin, T. Litchfield, S. Akman, B. Carr, M. Bertrand, D. Goldberg, D. Blayney, O. Odujinrin, R. DeLap, J. Shuster, and E. Newman: Prospective randomized comparison of fluorouracil versus fluorouracil and high-dose continuous infusion leucovorin calcium for the treatment of advanced measurable colorectal cancer in patients previously unexposed to chemotherapy. *J. Clin. Oncol. 8*:491 (1990).

43. C. Erlichman, S. Fine, A. Wong, and T. Elhakim: A randomized trial of fluorouracil and folinic acid in patients with metastatic colorectal carcinoma. *J. Clin. Oncol. 6*:469 (1988).

44. F. H. Valone, M. A. Friedman, P. S. Wittlinger, T. Drakes, P. D. Eisenberg, M. Malec, J. F. Hannigan, and B. W. Brown, Jr.: Treatment of patients with advanced colorectal carcinomas with fluorouracil alone, high-dose leucovorin plus fluorouracil, or sequential methotrexate, fluorouracil, and leucovorin: A Randomized Trial of the Northern California Oncology Group. *J. Clin. Oncol. 7*:1427 (1989).

45. M. A. Poon, M. J. O'Connell, C. G. Moertel, H. S. Wieand, S. A. Cullinan, L. K. Everson, J. E. Krook, J. A. Mailliard, J. A. Laurie, L. K. Tschetter, and M. Wiesenfeld: Biochemical modulation of fluorouracil: Evidence of significant improvement of survival and quality of life in patients with advanced colorectal carcinoma. *J. Clin. Oncol. 7*:1407 (1989).

46. P. H. Sugarbaker and N. Kemeny: "Treatment of metastatic cancer to liver," in *Cancer Principles & Practice of Oncology,* ed. by V. T. DeVita, Jr., S. Hellman, and S. A. Rosenberg. Philadelphia: J.B. Lippincott Company, 1989, pp. 2275–2298.

47. Y. Z. Patt, A. W. Boddie, Jr., and C. Charnsangaavej: Hepatic arterial infusion with floxuridine and cisplatin: Overriding importance of antitumor effect versus degree of tumor burden as determinants of survival among patients with colorectal cancer. *J. Clin. Oncol 4*:1356 (1986).

48. A. M. Cohen, N. Schaeffer, and J. Higgins: Treatment of metastatic colorectal cancer with hepatic artery combination chemotherapy. *Cancer 57*:1115 (1986).

49. N. Kemeny, J. Daly, and Reichman: Intrahepatic or systemic infusion of fluorodeoxyuridine in patients with liver metastases from colorectal carcinoma. *Ann. Int. Med. 107*:459 (1987).

50. D. C. Hohn, R. J. Stagg, and M. A. Friedman: A randomized trial of continuous intravenous versus hepatic intraarterial floxuridine in patients with colorectal cancer metastatic to the liver: The Northern California Oncology Group Trial. *J. Clin. Oncol. 7*:1646 (1989).

51. W. Ensminger, A. Rosowski, V. Raso, D. C. Levin, M. Glode, S. Come, G. Steele, and E. Frei III: A clinical-pharmacological evaluation of hepatic arterial infusions of 5-fluoro-2'-deoxyuridine and 5-fluorouracil. *Cancer Res. 38*:3784 (1978).

52. N. E. Kemeny: "Is hepatic infusion of chemotherapy effective treatment for liver metastases? Yes!" in *Important Advances in Oncology 1992,* ed. by V. T. DeVita, Jr., S. Hellman, and S. A. Rosenberg. Philadelphia: J.B. Lippincott Company, 1992, pp. 207–227.

53. M. J. O'Connell: "Is hepatic infusion of chemotherapy effective treatment for liver metastases? No!" in *Important Advances in Oncology 1992,* ed. by V. T. DeVita, Jr., S. Hellman, and S. A. Rosenberg. New York: J.B. Lippincott Company, 1992, pp. 229–234.

54. C. G. Moertel, T. R. Fleming, J. S. Macdonald, D. G. Haller, J. A. Laurie, P. J. Goodman, J. S. Ungerleider, W.

A. Emerson, D. C. Tormey, J. H. Glick, M. H. Veeder, and J. A. Mailliard: Levamisole and fluorouracil for adjuvant therapy of resected colon carcinoma. *New Engl. J. Med.* 322:352 (1990).

55. R. Windle, P. R. F. Bell, and D. Shaw: Five year results of a randomized trial of adjuvant 5-fluorouracil and levamisole in colorectal cancer. *Br. J. Surg.* 74:569 (1987).

56. J. A. Laurie, C. G. Moertel, T. R. Fleming, H. S. Wieand, J. E. Leigh, J. Rubin, G. W. McCormack, J. B. Gerstner, J. E. Krook, J. Malliard, D. I. Twito, R. F. Morton, L. K. Tschetter, and J. F. Barlow for the North Central Cancer Treatment Group and the Mayo Clinic: Surgical adjuvant therapy of large-bowel carcinoma: An evaluation of levamisole and the combination of levamisole and fluorouracil. *J. Clin. Oncol.* 7:1447 (1989).

57. Gastrointestinal Tumor Study Group: Prolongation of the disease-free interval in surgically treated rectal carcinoma. *New Engl. J. Med.* 312:1465 (1985).

58. Gastrointestinal Tumor Study Group: Survival after postoperative combination treatment of rectal cancer. *New Engl. J. Med.* 315:1294 (1986).

59. B. Fisher, N. Wolmark, H. C. Redmond, D. L. Wickerham E. R. Fischer, J. Jones, A. Glass, H. Lerner and W. Lawrence Rockette: Postoperative adjuvant therapy or radiation therapy for rectal cancer: Results from NSABP protocol R-01. *J. Natl. Cancer Inst.* 80:21 (1988).

60. J. E. Krook, C. G. Moertel, L. L. Gunderson, H. S. Wieand, R. T. Collins, R. W. Beart, T. P. Kubista, M. A. Poon, W. C. Meyers, M. H. Veeder, T. E. Witzig, S. Cha, and S. C. Vidyarthi: Effective surgical adjuvant therapy for high-risk rectal carcinoma. *New Engl. J. Med.* 324:709 (1991).

61. J. D. Minna, J. Pass, E. Glatstein, D. C. Ihde: "Cancer of the lung," in *Cancer Principles & Practice of Oncology*, ed. by V. T. DeVita, Jr., S. Hellman, and S. A. Rosenberg. Philadelphia: J.B. Lippincott, 1989, pp. 591–705.

62. J. C. Ruckdeschel: Editorial: Is chemotherapy for metastatic non small-cell lung cancer "Worth It"? *J. Clin. Oncol.* 8:1293 (1990).

63. P. D. Bonomi, D. M. Findelstein, J. C. Ruckdeschel, R. H. Blum, M. D. Green, B. Mason, R. Hahn, D. C. Tormey, J. Harris, R. Comis, and J. Glick: Combination chemotherapy versus single agents followed by combination chemotherapy in state IV non-small-cell lung cancer: A Study of the Eastern Cooperative Oncology Group. *J. Clin. Oncol.* 7:1602 (1989).

64. E. Rapp, A. Pater, Y. Cormier, N. Murray, W. K. Evans, D. I. Hodson, D. A. Clark, R. Feld, A. M. Arnold, J. I. Ayoub, K. S. Wilson, J. Latreille, R. F. Wierzbicki, and D. P. Hill: Chemotherapy can prolong survival in patients with advanced non-small-cell lung cancer: Report of a Canadian multicenter randomized trial. *J. Clin. Oncol.* 6:633 (1988).

65. E. Quoix, A. Dietemann, and J. Charbonneau: Is cisplatin-based chemotherapy useful in disseminated non-small lung cancer (NSCLC)? Report of a French multicenter randomized trial. *Cancer Bull.* 78:341 (1991).

66. S. Kaasa, E. Lund, E. Thorud, R. Hatlevoll, and H. Host: Symptomatic treatment versus combination chemotherapy for patients with extensive non-small cell lung cancer. *Cancer* 67:2433 (1991).

67. J. C. Ruckdeschel, D. M. Findelstein, D. S. Ettinger, R. H. Creech, B. A. Mason, R. A. Joss, and S. Vogl: A randomized trial of the four most active regimens for metastatic non-small-cell lung cancer. *J. Clin. Oncol.* 4:14 (1986).

68. R. O. Dillman, S. L. Seagren, K. J. Propert, J. Guerra, W. L. Eaton, M. C. Perry, R. W. Carey, E. F. Frei, Jr., and M. R. Green: A randomized trial of induction chemotherapy plus high-dose radiation versus radiation alone in stage III non-small-cell lung cancer. *New Engl. J. Med.* 323:940 (1990).

69. E. C. Holmes and M. Gail for the Lung Cancer Study Group: Surgical adjuvant therapy for stage II and stage III adenocarcinoma and large-cell undifferentiated carcinoma. *J. Clin. Oncol.* 4:710 (1986).

New Directions in Cancer Chemotherapy

CHAPTER TWELVE

Anticancer Drug Development

Screening Methods in Antineoplastic Drug Discovery

As we have seen, cancer chemotherapy alone is often not very effective in producing long-range survival or cures of the most common solid tumors—e.g., carcinomas of lung, colon-rectum, and advanced breast. One reason for this may be the prolonged mass doubling time and low growth fraction of these tumors. By contrast, most of the animal tumors that were used in the past as primary screens to test the antitumor effectiveness of new drugs have a very short mass doubling time (Table 12–1). Thus, a certain bias favoring the selection of agents presumed to be effective against tumors of high growth fraction—e.g. leukemias and lymphomas—was introduced into the screening for new anticancer agents. Nonetheless, almost all currently used antitumor drugs were shown to have antitumor activity in one or more animal models before clinical efficacy was demonstrated. A few agents are clinically effective and yet without effect in the most commonly used *in vivo* animal screens—i.e., the L1210, P388, B16, and Lewis lung tumors. Examples of such drugs are busulfan and hexamethylmelamine (shown to be effective in the Walker 256 carcinosarcoma and Dunning leukemia of rats), L-asparaginase (effective against tumors lacking L-asparagine synthetase), o', p' DDD (introduced because of its selective adrenal cortical toxicity in animals), and hormones (introduced because of the known hormonal dependence of certain tumors). There are also a number of drugs that were selected for preclinical or clinical testing based on their activity in experimental animal systems but that have not become clinically useful agents.[2] Some of these were dropped because of their severe or unpredictable toxicity, others because of their lack of any therapeutic advantage.

Potential new anticancer agents come from a number of sources (Table 12–2).[3] Some are synthetic analogs of known effective agents, some are "natural products" isolated from microorganisms or plants, and some represent attempts at "rational" drug design based on potential inhibitors of enzymes or other components that appear essential for tumor cell growth. The number of potential new agents screened annually by the National Cancer Institute of the United States has varied over the years. In 1973, the peak year for new drug screening, 51,334 compounds were submitted to the Drug Development Program of NCI, but that same year only 13 IND (Investigation of New Drug) applications were filed for clinical testing.[4] In order to develop screens that would have a better chance of detecting agents with activity against solid tumors and to limit the input to the screening program, the NCI Division of Cancer Treatment began placing greater emphasis on the testing of new synthetic compounds and natural products against a panel of cultured human cancer cell lines and against human tumor xenografts in immunologically incompetent (athymic) mice (see below).

After antitumor activity has been deter-

Table 12–1 *Doubling Times of Several Mouse Tumors That Have Been Used to Determine the Antitumor Effects of Drugs.* (Adapted from Zubrod[1])

Tumor	Doubling Time (Days)
L1210	0.5
S180	0.6
CA755	0.5
P388	0.6
B16 Melanoma	2.0
Lewis lung	2.3
AKR Leukemia	5.0

mined and sufficient information gathered on the formulation, toxicology, and dosage scheduling in animal systems, a drug may be submitted for Phase I clinical trials. The primary purpose of the Phase I trial is to determine toxicity and maximum tolerated dose (MTD) in patients with cancer. If no untoward effects that would severely limit or preclude further use are evident, Phase II trials are then initiated. The purpose of Phase II studies is to identify the presence or absence of significant antitumor effects and to determine the antitumor spectrum of action. The response of individual patients' cancers to the drug and the number of patients who achieve complete or partial remission are noted. A positive response is usually defined as

greater than 50% reduction of measurable tumor mass lasting longer than one month. Complete remission means disappearance of observable tumor and return to a normal Karnofsky performance status (see Chapter 3). If Phase II studies indicate a reasonable response rate or novel antitumor spectrum, Phase III trials, which are designed to compare a given drug with other drugs or treatment modalities, may be undertaken. If a drug shows definite activity against a certain tumor type, it may be added to a proven drug combination or adjuvant therapeutic regimen. From this whole process, only a few drugs eventually are accepted into clinical practice.

In 1984, the Division of Cancer Treatment of the National Cancer Institute undertook an extensive review of its 30-year-old screening program for new anticancer drugs.[5] At its peak in the mid to late 1970s, the NCI screening program tested up to 40,000 compounds per year, mostly in the L1210 and P388 murine leukemia models. The results from this program were relatively modest. The most important drugs that came out of it were the nitrosoureas, hydroxyurea, mitoxantrone, and deoxycoformycin.

The cost of this drug discovery program, including the screening operation and preclinical development, was $29 million in 1984. On the average, only three to five new chemical agents reached clinical trial annually as a result of this

Table 12–2 *Pathways to the Discovery of Current Anticancer Drugs.* (From Sikic[3])

Targeted Synthesis	Screening of Natural Products	Screening of Chemicals	Analogue Synthesis	Serendipity and Rational Application
Antimetabolites:	Dactinomycin	Busulfan	Cyclophosphamide	Mechlorethamine
Methotrexate	Vincristine	Dacarbazine	Chlorambucil	Asparaginase
Thioguanine	Vinblastine	Procarbazine	Melphalan	Mitotane
Mercaptopurine	Plicamycin	Hydroxyurea	Ifosfamide	Cisplatin
Fluorouracil	Daunorubicin	Thiotepa	Etoposide	Levamisole
Cytarabine	Doxorubicin	Carmustine	Teniposide	Interferons
PALA	Mitomycin C	Lomustine	Carboplatin	
Hormones:	Bleomycin	Mitoxantrone		
Steroids	Streptozocin	Altretamine		
Tamoxifen	Taxol	Pentostatin		
Flutamide				
Leuprolide				
Octreotide				

large screening program. Obviously, there had to be a better way to develop anticancer drugs.

In January 1985, the Board of Scientific Counselors of the Division of Cancer Treatment approved a pilot effort to examine the use of a rapid *in vitro* screening procedure utilizing a panel of cultured human cancer cell lines.[5] The purpose of this study was to determine whether such an approach could predict more rapidly and reliably the activity of new compounds and whether it would predict activity against some human solid tumors that the mouse leukemia models might miss. In addition, the NCI placed more emphasis on the screening of natural products from unique sources such as soil fungi, tropical plants, and marine animals, since recent history had suggested that the success rate for finding cytotoxic substances from these sources was much higher than that from randomly selected synthetic chemicals.

Although the new NCI screening effort is still undergoing evolution, it can apparently predict antitumor activity, because when drugs known to be clinically effective were tested retrospectively in the human cell culture screen they showed activity.[6] Agents with significant activity in the *in vitro* growth-inhibition screening system are then evaluated in athymic mice bearing human tumor xenografts of the cell lines found to be sensitive *in vitro*.

The current testing procedure is designed to examine the *in vitro* cytotoxicity of potential anticancer agents against 60 human tumor cell lines organized into subpanels representing leukemia, melanoma, and cancers of the lung, colon, kidney, ovary, and central nervous system.[7] The goal of this screen is to provide initial evaluation of 10,000 compounds annually for activity against a diverse group of cancers. Subsequently, compounds showing activity are tested against xenografts of these cell lines, as noted above.

The *in vitro* screening procedure has utilized two measures of cell viability after exposure of cultured cells to drugs. One is the staining of cells with 3-(4,5-dimethylthiazole-2-yl)-2,5-diphenyltetrazolium bromide (MTT). This assay is based on the metabolic reduction of MTT to formazan, a colored substance that can be detected at a wavelength of 550 nm in a spectrophotometer. The amount of reduction is pro-

portional to the metabolic "intactness" of a cell—i.e., its viability. An advantage of this assay is that it can be run in microtiter dishes on hundreds of cell samples at one time so that various drug concentrations can be used to get an idea of the dose-response relationships for each drug tested. The other assay, which has some advantages over the MTT test, is the staining of cells with a protein-binding dye, sulforhodamine (SRB), that can also be measured colorimetrically. The SRB assay measures whole-culture protein content, and since dead cells either lyse or are lost during the procedure, the amount of SRB binding is proportional to the number of live cells left in a culture after drug exposure.[8] The cost of this screening procedure is $200 to $300 per compound, and it could be used to screen about 20,000 compounds annually in the NCI testing facility.[7]

However, there are, several pitfalls in the use of these *in vitro* screening methods to predict clinical activity of new anticancer drugs.[9] A number of drugs may require metabolic activation to be effective. A classic example of this is cyclophosphamide (Chapter 6). This difficulty can be circumvented if liver microsomal preparations are added to the *in vitro* cell culture medium or if cells that express various cytochrome P-450 mixed-function oxidases, such as hepatoma cell lines, are added to the panel of cell lines tested.

A second pitfall is that the role of pharmacokinetics and biodistribution in determining drug effects cannot be evaluated *in vitro*. Many host factors, such as the route of drug administration, extent of drug metabolism, rate of clearance, and tissue distribution will determine whether or not a drug works *in vivo*. Moreover, the geometry of solid tumor growth *in vivo* is very different from that of cells growing in suspension or in monolayer cultures. Some drugs may not be able to penetrate well into the core of solid tumors because of their chemical characteristics (e.g., lipid solubility, ionic charge, hydrophilic properties, molecular size). Also, because the cells in the central part of solid tumors are more distant from the blood supply and may be more hypoxic, have a lower pH in the microenvironment, which is more hypertonic, and have different cell-cycle kinetics than tumor cells nearer to the blood supply, a drug that looks active against a monolayer of cultured tumor cells may or may not have equivalent activity in vivo.[9]

Various means to circumvent the in vitro/in vivo problem have been envisioned. As noted above, a secondary screen for antitumor activity using human tumor xenografts in athymic mice is used to gauge in vivo activity. The implantation of human tumor cells into the subrenal capsule of mice has also been used as an in vivo screen for antitumor activity.[10] More recently, an assay based on the encapsulation of human tumor cells in 1 mm-diameter microcapsules surrounded by a semipermeable membrane has been used as a short-term in vivo evaluation of the effects of anticancer drugs versus human tumors.[11] The microcapsules containing human cancer cells are injected intraperitioneally into athymic or C57BL/6 mice, and drugs are administered intravenously. The microcapsules are removed at various intervals during treatment and the number of viable tumor cells compared between drug-treated and control animals. Advantages of the microencapsulation assay are that activity can be assessed against tumors that have a three-dimensional geometry more closely resembling tumors growing in vivo and that various pharmacokinetic and biodistribution factors can be evaluated.

Ideally, future anticancer drug discovery will be based on more rational and mechanism-based approaches. As more is learned about the biology of cancer cells—e.g., the role of oncogenes, tumor suppressor genes, tumor growth factors, hormone-drug-receptor interactions, signal transduction mechanisms, and positive and negative regulators of cell proliferation and differentiation—the more likely it is that rational drug design will be possible (see Chapter 14).

One way to test the effects of compounds developed by mechanism-based design is to use transgenic models of tumor development. A wide variety of cancer-prone strains of mice have been created by the introduction of putative cancer-related genes (Table 12–3).[12] Such models may be more likely to mimic the so-called spontaneously arising cancers in humans. They will also provide a way to test the role of various mutated or activated oncogenes and mutated or inactivated tumor suppressor

genes in tumor development in various target organs. When "metastasis genes" are isolated and characterized, they too may be introduced into such transgenic models to determine what genes play a role in the aggressiveness of various tumor types. In addition, drug resistance genes such as the mdr gene (see Chapter 4) can be introduced to see what effect they have on the drug responsiveness of tumors that develop in various tissue types. Finally, the ability to develop tumors in vivo in selected animal tissues will allow the testing of various drugs and drug combinations against specific tumors in an in vivo setting in which the crucial pharmacokinetic and biodistribution parameters can be evaluated.

Indicators of Patient Response to Therapy

Chemosensitivity Testing

A clinical oncologist's dream would be fulfilled if he or she could obtain a culture of a patient's tumor before treatment and test it against a battery of drugs to see which one the tumor would respond to. Indeed, such testing has been going on since the late 1950s[13]; from its outset, however, in vitro sensitivity testing of human tumors was fraught with the difficulties of obtaining enough viable cells from a given tumor, getting them to grow in culture, and finding a practical concentration of cytotoxic drugs that can be achieved in vivo. In 1978, Salmon and his colleagues[14] developed a soft agar cloning assay that made growth of freshly obtained tumor cells more feasible. Since that time, numerous modifications of this assay have been made (reviewed in ref. 15). A review of studies carried out with 2,300 patients at various institutions indicated that 69% of those whose cancer cells were sensitive in vitro responded to the in vitro–selected therapy (true positives), whereas 91% of those whose cells did not respond in vitro did not have a clinical response (true negatives). In a clinical trial in which patients were randomized into a "drug choice by clinician" or a "drug choice by cloning assay," 21% of patients had a partial response to a single agent selected by cloning assay, but only 3% had a positive response to a drug chosen by a clinician without using cloning data.[16] Although a significant differ-

Table 12–3 Transgenic Models of Tumor Development. Only the tissue or cell type of the predominant tumor type provoked by the transgene is indicated. (From Adams and Cory[12])

Tissue or Cell Type	Gene	Regulator	Tissue or Cell Type	Gene	Regulator
Hematopoietic			Mammary	myc	MMTV WAP
B (or T) lymphoid	myc	Eμ		c-H-ras	WAP
	N-myc	Eμ		v-H-ras	MMTV
	SV40 Tag	Eμ		N-ras	MMTV
	bcl-2	Eμ		erbB2	MMTV
	erbB2 (neu)	Eμ		ret	MMTV
	v-abl	Eμ		wnt-1 (int-1)	MMTV
	bcr-v-abl	Eμ or MPSV		int-2	MMTV
	bcr-abl	MT-1		TGF-α	MMTV
T lymphoid	myc	Thy-1	Hepatic	SV40 Tag	MT-1 urinary protein antitrypsin albumin
	L-myc	Eμ			
	SV40 Tag	lck		HBV antigen	Albumin
	N-ras	Eμ		myc	Albumin, antitrypsin
	pim-1	Eμ or H-2K		TGF-α	MT-1
	lck	lck		c-H-ras	Albumin
Erythroid	FSFV gp55	β-actin or FSFV		HBx	HBx
Neuronal				Growth hormone	MT-1
Retinal	SV40 Tag	PNMT	Pancreatic		
Hypothalamic	SV40 Tag	GnRH	Islet	SV40 Tag	Insulin
Retinoblast	SV40 Tag	LHβ	Acinar	SV40 Tag	Glucagon
Adrenal	JCV early	JCV		SV40 Tag	Elastase
Perineuronal	HTLV-1tat	HTLV-1		c-H-ras	Elastase
Skin and soft tissue			Other tissues	myc	Elastase
Dermal	BPV	BPV	Kidney	BKV early	BKV
	v-jun	H-2K	Heart	SV40 Tag	ANF, protamine
Epidermal	c-H-ras	Keratin	Lung	v-H-ras	MMTV
	v-H-ras	Zeta-globin		c-H-ras	Eμ
	TGF-α	Keratin	Stomach	Ad12 early	MMTV
Adipose	SV40 Tag	α-Amylase	Bone	SV40 Tag	Amylase, protamine
Melanocytic	SV40 Tag	Tyrosinase	Cartilage	c-fos	H-2K
Mesenchymal	HTLV-1 tat	HTLV-1	Lens	SV40 Tag	αA-crystallin
	SV40 Tag	Renin	Pituitary	SV40 Tag	Vasopressin
Vascular			Diverse types	SV40 Tag	MMTV, H2-K
Choroid plexus	SV40 T	SV40		myc	MMTV
	LPV early	LPV		p53	p53
Endothelial	HIV tat	HIV		Py mTag	Eμ
	Py mTag	Polyoma		v-fps	Globin

Abbreviations are as follows: SV40 Tag, either the large T antigen gene or the complete SV40 early region; FSFV gp55, the spleen focus-forming virus Env protein, which binds to the erythropoietin receptor; LPV, lymphotropic papovavirus; HTLV-1 *tat*, the trans-activator gene of human T-cell leukemia virus-1; JCV and BKV, human papovaviruses; HIV, human immunodeficiency virus; Py mTag, the middle T antigen gene from polyoma virus; and Ad12, the early region (*E1A* and *E1B* genes) of adenovirus type 12. Regulators include the long terminal repeat from myeloproliferative sarcoma virus (MPSV), Friend spleen focus-forming virus (FSFV), or MMTV; and enhancers and promoters from the genes for immunoglobulin heavy chains (Eμ), metallothionein-1 (MT-1), phenylethanolamine N-methyltransferase (PNMT), gonadotropin-releasing hormone (GnRH), leuteinizing hormone β subunit (LHβ), the H-2K antigen of the major histocompatibility locus, whey acidic protein (WAP), and atrial natriuretic factor (ANF).

ence in response rate was observed, no difference in survival was seen in the two arms of the study, and this 133-patient study took 4½ years to complete. In another clinical trial in patients with small-cell carcinoma of the lung, cell lines were able to be grown from only 28 out of 80 patients and chemosensitivity data were obtained in 26 patients (33% of total).[17] Four of 16 patients (25%) who received secondary therapy based on *in vitro* sensitivity testing had a complete response, compared with 3 of 43 (7%) who received an empirically chosen drug regimen.

Such results show both the promise and the pitfalls of *in vitro* chemosensitivity testing. The latter include: 1) low patient accrual to such trials, 2) the difficulty of obtaining viable cultures of cancer cells, and 3) the difficulty of translating effective cytotoxic concentrations *in vitro* to pharmacologically realistic and effective doses *in vivo*. Despite these difficulties, improved knowledge of the growth factors and other conditions required for the growth of specific tumor cell types *in vitro*, as well as improved microsurgical techniques to obtain cells, may make more patients' tumors available for chemosensitivity testing. Moreover, the use of such assays could significantly improve the

testing of new drugs.[18] What better way to find out if a potential new therapeutic agent works than to test it against real cancer cells from real patients?

Tumor Markers

Three of the most important questions facing any cancer therapist are: 1) How can I diagnose a cancer earlier in order to maximize the patient's chance for survival? 2) How can I determine whether the patient's disease is responding to treatment? 3) How long should I treat the patient in the face of clinically apparent remission? These questions are central to any good program of cancer management, but they are very difficult to answer. Definite progress has been made in the earlier diagnosis of malignant disease, exemplified by advances in exfoliative cytology (e.g., the Papanicolaou test for cervical cancer), radiographic detection techniques (e.g., CT, MRI, PET), and endoscopic examination. The limits of the sensitivity of these methods at their best, however, probably still precludes the detection of cancers at less than the 10^9 cell stage (Fig. 12–1).[19] More-sensitive tests would be beneficial.

The question of response to therapy is less

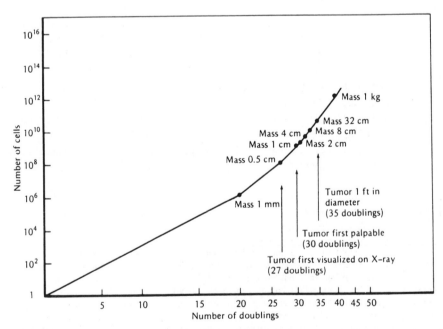

Figure 12–1 Theoretical growth curve relating number of tumor doublings to number of tumor cells present and levels of clinical awareness of tumor. (From DeVita *et al.*[19])

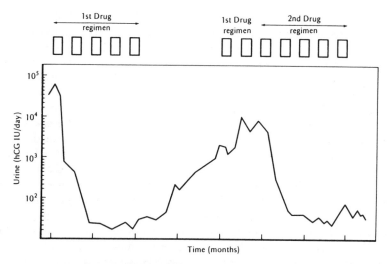

Figure 12-2 Human chorionic gonadotropin (hCG) excretion in a patient with gestational choriocarcinoma whose tumor was not eliminated by initial therapy. The tumor then showed resistance to the drugs that induced the first remission, but it responded to other drugs. The hCG levels are expressed as International Units excreted in the urine per day. (From Bagshawe[20])

difficult to answer when a cancer is clinically detectable. Obviously, a shrinkage in tumor mass or a decrease in the number of leukemia cells in the blood and marrow, coupled with the improvement of a patient's performance status, are indicators of a positive response. But even when there is no clinical evidence of tumor, the patient may still be harboring a significant number of malignant cells. How, then, does one know how long to treat the patient? Ideally, what is needed is some sensitive indicator or "biological marker," the level of which would correspond to the tumor load in the patient. The need for biological markers of malignant neoplastic disease has become increasingly apparent in recent years. At least for the immediate future, improvement in cancer therapy will continue to depend on early diagnosis and better use of currently available treatment modalities. Both early diagnosis and improved use of therapeutic modalities will be greatly facilitated by the identification of tumor markers that 1) are tumor-type specific, 2) are readily detectable in body fluids and tissue extracts, 3) appear early in the course of disease before it is clinically detectable, 4) are indicative of the overall tumor cell burden in the body, 5) correlate with the degree of success of anticancer therapy, 6) indicate the presence of micrometastases, and 7) predict the return of disease after apparently successful treatment.

The "ideal" biological tumor marker has not been found for any neoplasm. Human chorionic gonadotropin (hCG) comes closest to the ideal among the currently available markers. Elevated levels of hCG are indicative of the presence of choriocarcinoma, and a decrease in hCG correlates well with successful therapy (Fig. 12-2). The level of hCG production has been determined by both *in vitro* and *in vivo* measures to be about 10^{-5} International Units per cell per day.[20] In addition, the decrease in urinary hCG levels following successful chemotherapy correlates with the killing of choriocarcinoma cells. Thus, by determining the slope of the hCG decrement with time, one can extrapolate to theoretical zero tumor burden, which is the sine qua non of successful therapy. The validity of extrapolating the data in this manner depends on certain assumptions: (1) that the patient's tumor continues to be eliminated at a constant rate throughout treatment, (2) that the production of hCG per cell stays relatively constant during the response to therapy, (3) that the plasma half-life of hCG doesn't change significantly during treatment. These assumptions are probably not quantitatively precise, but from a practical point of view it has been observed that if patients are treated until the projected "zero tumor burden" is achieved, a high percentage of them will be cured. However, any decrease in the rate of response after hCG levels drop below detectable amounts would increase the treatment time to achieve total elimination of the tumor. For this reason, additional clinical information must be taken into account as part of the decision to terminate therapy. For example, if there were a long latent period between the suspected onset of tumor and the initiation of treatment, if there were large metastases, or if metastatic spread to the central nervous system had occurred, treatment should be continued for up to five months after "zero tumor burden" is reached.[20] The fortunate fact in the case of choriocarcinoma is that recurrence is usually detectable by elevation of hCG levels well before any other clinical evidence of disease is present. Clearly, the ability to follow the therapeutic response of other cancers in a similar manner would be a tremendous boon to cancer chemotherapy.

The report of Abelev[21] that alpha fetoprotein reappears in the serum of adults with hepatomas or teratocarcinomas, and the demonstration by Gold and his colleagues[22] of the presence of carcinoembryonic antigen (CEA) in human colon cancer, have been a stimulus to the search for embryonic gene products that are expressed by cancer cells and that may be utilized as indicators of malignant disease. Unfortunately, CEA and other fetal antigens of this type are also associated with a number of nonmalignant disease states.[23] A number of other fetal antigens, placental hormones, enzymes, and biochemical products of cell metabolism have been found to be associated with human malignant disease (Table 12–4).[24] Many of these markers lack specificity in that they may reflect tissue damage resulting from any of a number of mechanisms or they may indicate states of hypermetabolism and increased cell turnover that occur in a number of nonmalignant proliferative disorders. Nevertheless, in cases where a certain marker is elevated, even if it is not specific to that tumor type, it may still be very useful in following the course of a patient's disease and response to therapy.

Research aimed at discovering biological markers specific to the malignant process and, it is hoped, also to the tissue of origin is continuing. In order for a marker to have a significant impact in cancer diagnosis, it should be possible to detect the marker in body fluids when a tumor is smaller than one cubic centimeter (10^9 cells) in size. This will require very sensitive assays, probably severalfold more sensitive than currently available radioimmunoassays.

Unfortunately, since specific, sensitive markers are not yet available for most neoplastic diseases, less direct approaches must still be taken to answer the question of treatment duration. One approach is based on the cytokinetics of the tumor involved (if it is known or if reasonable assumptions can be made), and another depends on the observed relationship between treatment duration and the duration of complete remission following treatment. Both are somewhat empirical and are based on certain assumptions for which experimental animal data are available but that may be unsupported by hard clinical evidence. One of the more successful examples of the cytokinetic approach is in the treatment of Hodgkin's disease with the MOPP regimen (mustargen, vincristine [Oncovin®], prednisone, and procarbazine). With this regimen the median time to nearly complete remission (about a 90% reduction in tumor mass) is one and a half months.[25] If one assumes that it takes the presence of 10^{12} cells for a lymphoma to be clinically detectable and that a 90% reduction of tumor mass occurs after 1.5 months of treatment,[25] it would take 19.5 months of treatment to induce a "cellular cure." Assuming a 1-log kill per 1.5 months and no significant tumor regrowth during treatment, 1.5 months after the initiation of treatment there would be 10^{11} cells, at 3.0 months there would be 10^{10} cells, at 4.5 months 10^9 cells, etc. By 19.5 months there would be 0 cells left in 90% of the patients. Interestingly, it has been found that 24 months of treatment with MOPP produces a significantly greater duration of remission than six months of treatment.[25] To achieve complete cure for leukemias and lymphomas (except Burkitt's lymphoma), it appears that a minimum of two years of treatment is warranted, and for acute leukemia of childhood three years of treatment may be required.[26] For testicular cancer, the disease-free survival plateau is reached at about one year after induction of complete remission.[27]

Drug-Delivery Systems

The goal of selective chemotherapy aimed at killing cancer cells with minimal cytotoxicity to normal cells would be greatly advanced if

Table 12–4 *Selected Antigenic Moieties of Diagnostic Value in Practical Immunohistochemistry.* (From Pfeifer and Wick[24])

Antigen	Predominant Distribution	Diagnostic Use
Cytokeratin	Epithelial cells	Distinction between lymphoma or melanoma and carcinoma
Epithelial membrane antigen	Epithelial cells	Distinction between melanoma and carcinoma
Leukocyte common antigen	Leukocytes	Distinction between lymphoma, carcinoma, and melanoma
Desmin	Myogenous cells	Identification of myogenic sarcomas
Muscle-specific actin	Myogenous cells	Identification of myogenic sarcomas
Thyroglobulin	Thyroid follicular cells	Identification of certain thyroid carcinomas
Prostate-specific antigen	Prostatic epithelium	Identification of metastatic prostatic carcinomas
Calcitonin	Parafollicular thyroid epithelium	Distinction of medullary thyroid carcinoma from other thyroid tumors
Carcinoembryonic antigen	Endodermally derived epithelium	Identification of certain carcinomas; distinction of mesothelioma and adenocarcinoma
Placental alkaline phosphatase	Placental tissue and germ cell tumors	Screening identification of possible germ cell and trophoblastic tumors
Alpha-fetoprotein	Neoplastic hepatic tissue and selected germ cell tumors	Identification of possible hepatocellular carcinoma, embryonal carcinoma, and endodermal sinus tumor
Beta-human chorionic gonadotropin	Placental tissue; trophoblastic and germ cell tumors	Identification of possible trophoblastic and germ cell tumors
CA 125	Mullerian epithelium	Identification of possible female genital tract carcinomas
CA 19-9	Alimentary tract epithelium	Identification of gastrointestinal and pancreatic carcinomas
Gross cystic disease fluid protein-15	Pathologic mammary epithelium	Identification of metastatic breast carcinomas
HMB-45	Melanocytic cells	Identification of melanomas
Chromogranin-A	Neuroendocrine cells	Identification of neuroendocrine carcinomas
Synaptophysin	Neuroendocrine cells	Identification of neuroendocrine carcinomas and neuroectodermal tumors

anticancer drugs could be targeted specifically to tumor tissue. Several kinds of approaches have been tried. These include encapsulation of drugs into liposomes or microspheres, targeting tumor tissue with monoclonal antibodies to tumor-associated antigens, and implantable drug-delivery devices such as pumps and injection ports. Some of these are briefly discussed here (and are reviewed in refs. 28–32).

Liposomes

Liposomes are unilamellar or multilamellar vesiclelike structures that can be formulated with varying amounts and types of lipids. They can also be formulated so that their size and *in vivo* distribution can be varied to favor their disposition in liver, spleen, or lung.[28]

Attempts have been made to use liposomes for the selective delivery of anticancer drugs (e.g., doxorubicin and bleomycin), antifungal agents (e.g., amphotericin B), biological response modifiers, and enzymes.[28]

A number of different formulations of doxorubicin have been tested in clinical trials. Several studies have shown that its myelosuppressive and cardiotoxic effects can be moderated by drug administration in liposomes and that the size and lipid composition of the liposomes can determine the toxic and antitumor effects.[31,32] The reduction in cardiotoxicity has been correlated with lower cardiac distribution of liposome-encapsulated drug, which in turn is determined by the lipid composition of the liposome carrier. Doxorubicin incorporated in small (0.1 μm) lipid vesicles has greater antitumor activity than drug in large vesicles (1.0 μm), and in addition, drug contained in small vesicles usually has less myelosuppressive activity in mice.[31]

A very successful clinical use of liposomal drug delivery is the administration of liposome-encapsulated amphotericin B for fungal infections associated with a depressed immune state in patients with hematologic malignancies. Since such fungal infections frequently involve the reticuloendothelial system (RES), liposome-targeted drug delivery is ideal because liposomes are avidly taken up by cells of the RES. This approach has a high therapeutic efficacy with much reduced drug toxicity, compared to free amphotericin B.[28]

The ardent RES uptake of liposomes, though, is sometimes a bane rather than a blessing. For example, some anticancer drugs are hepatotoxic, and high uptake of drug-bearing liposomes by RES cells of the liver could increase this toxic effect. Another problem with liposomes as they are frequently formulated is that they are unstable and have to be prepared fresh before injection. Moreover, they may break and release free drug in the bloodstream before they reach the target organ.

One way to improve tissue targeting and get around nonspecific uptake of liposomes by RES cells is to embed in the surface of the liposomes antibodies that recognize cell surface antigens on tumor cells. Such an approach has been tried by Rahman et al.,[33] who embedded antilaminin receptor antibody into liposomes encapsulated with doxorubicin. The rationale for this is that cancer cells with high metastatic potential often have an increased number of laminin receptors on their surface. Rahman and his colleagues showed that cultured human breast carcinoma cells bound more antibody-coupled liposomes and were more growth inhibited than normal breast epithelial cells, which had a lower content of laminin receptors than did the carcinoma cells. Moreover, antibody-coupled liposomes encapsulating doxorubicin were more cytotoxic to tumor cells than unencapsulated doxorubicin or drug-containing liposomes without antilaminin receptor antibody.

Another potential use of liposomes is to activate tumor-cell-killing macrophages *in vivo*. It has been shown, for instance, that tumoricidal macrophages can be activated in mice with a renal adenocarcinoma by intravenous injection of liposomes bearing a macrophage activator that is a synthetic lipoprotein analog of the outer cell wall from a gram-negative bac-

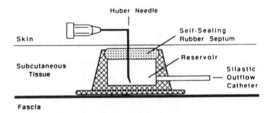

Figure 12–3 Cross-sectional schematic illustrating the basic design of injection and/or infusion ports. (From Ensminger and Wollner[37])

Table 12–5   Investigational New Anticancer Agents in Early Clinical Trials (1992–93)

Cytotoxic Agents	Biological Response Modifiers
Phase I	**Phase I**
BSO	Auto. tumor vaccine/BCG (Tice)/IL-2
Chloroquinoxaline sulfonamide	CSF-M (Cetus)
Hepsulfam	IFN-Beta (Mochida)
Ipomeanol	IL-1 Beta (Syntex)
Liposome-encapsulated doxorubicin	IL-1 Alpha (Dainippon)
Mafosfamide	IL-2 (Cetus)/BCG (Tice)/TCV
Ormaplatin (Tetraplatin)	IL-2 (Cetus)/IL-4 (Sterling)
Pentosan	IL-2 (HLR)/IL-4 (Sterling)
Porfiromycin	IL-2/A-LAK (Cetus)
Pyrazine Diazohydroxide	IL-2/AEL (HLR)
Pyrazoloacridine	IL-2/MDELAK (Cetus)
Terephthalamidine	IL-2 (PEG)
Teroxirone	IL-3
Topotecan (Hycamptamine)	IL-4
Uridine	MoAb: Lym-1
Phase II	MoAb: 14G2A
Acivicin	MoAb: Melanoma (9.2.27)
Aclacinomycin	MoAb: R24 with GM-CSF/Yeast
Amonafide	MoAb: D612
Bisantrene	MoAb: L6
Caracemide	MoAb: BL3-GD
Deazauridine	MoAb: HeFi-1
Deoxyspergualin	MoAb: Bombesin (2Al1)
DFMO	MoAb: CC-49 (Dow)
Didemnin B	MoAb: IMMU-4
Dichloromethotrexate	MoAb: T-cell (3A1, 95-5-49, 95-6-22)
Dihydro-5-azacytidine	MoAb: Colorectal (LiCo 16.88, 28A32)
Echinomycin	MoAb: Chimeric B72.3
Fazarabine	MoAb: B72.3 Chimeric gamma-1
Hexamethylene bisacetamide	MoAb: RG83852 Anti-EGFR (Rorer)
Homoharringtonine	MoAb: 225 (Anti-EGFR IgG1)
Menogaril	N-2 transduced TIL
Merbarone	TIL transduced with TNF gene
Methyl G	Tumor primed anti-CD3 activated
MMPR	lymphocytes
N-Methylformamide	**Phase II**
Pibenzimol	Asparaginase-PEG
Piroxantrone	Cis-Retinoic Acid
Spirogermanium	CSF-GM (Schering)
Spiromustine	CSF-GM (Hoechst)
Suramin	IFN: Rec Beta (Berlex)
Thiadiazole	IFN: Rec Gamma (Biogen)
Thioguanine (IV)	IFN: Rec Gamma (Schering)
Tiazofurin	IL-2/TIL (Cetus, Bioreactor Expanded)
TMCA	IL-2/TIL (Cetus)
	(continued)

Table 12–5   Investigational New Anticancer Agents in Early Clinical Trials (continued)

Cytotoxic Agents	Biological Response Modifiers
Triciribine phosphate	IL-2/TIL (HLR)
Trimetrexate	MoAb: 111InT101
	MoAb: B72.3
	MoAb: R24
	MoAb: Colorectal (17-1A)
	Poly ICLC
	TNF (Genentech)

terium.[34] Injection of these liposomes significantly reduced the number of lung metastases in nephrectomized mice, and this effect depended on dose and frequency of administration.

Microspheres

Another possible way to deliver more drug to tumors and prolong the exposure time of cancer cells in a tumor is to trap drug in the capillary bed supplying the tumor. If the blood supply to a tumor can be determined and can be reached by catheter, a technique called regional perfusion can be applied. To gain improved regional drug delivery, tiny (15–80 μm) starch microspheres have been infused into the arterial blood supply of a tumor. The microspheres briefly interrupt the blood supply, and since they degrade rapidly (within 10 to 30 minutes), they do not permanently shut off the vascular flow to a tissue. Thus, if an anticancer drug is administered along with, or shortly following, the creation of this artificial "embolism," a larger dose of drug can theoretically be delivered to a tumor while decreasing the amount of drug that circulates to the rest of the body. This technique has been tried with some success in the treatment of patients with hepatic metastases by the delivery of BCNU, 5-fluorouracil, FUDR, mitomycin C, or doxorubicin.[28,35,36] Because the blood supply of hepatic tumors is usually via the hepatic artery, while most of the blood supply to the normal liver parenchyma is via the portal vein, this type of therapy is ideally suited to cancer in the liver. Similar approaches to "arterial chemoembolization" have been attempted with ethylcellulose microcapsules, albumin microspheres, and polymethacrylate nanoparticles (reviewed in ref. 28).

Antibody-based Delivery Systems

The use of antibodies to tumor-associated antigens as a way to target drugs and toxic substances to tumors is not a new idea. Indeed, this approach has been thought of as the ideal way to develop a "magic bullet" for treating cancer. With the development of monoclonal antibodies (Moabs) to tumor-associated antigens, this approach has become more realistic because now much more specificity can be obtained in the recognition of tumor cells. This will be discussed in more detail in Chapter 13. Suffice it to say here that numerous experimental animal studies have been carried out with monoclonal antibody-drug, -toxin, and -radionuclide complexes and it has been shown that such complexes can bind to tumor cells with some specificity as well as increase biodistribution to tumor tissue when compared to free drug. Problems with this therapeutic method include nonspecific binding to normal tissues, host antibody formation against the injected monoclonal antibodies (which have usually been of murine origin), and heterogeneity of the targeted tumor with respect to cell surface antigens in the tumor cell population. Nevertheless, a number of clinical trials are underway with Moab conjugates, most often of the radionuclide-Moab type, with some indication of success (see Chapter 13).

Implantable Drug Delivery Devices

For certain cancers, such as those in the liver where a catheter can be inserted into blood ves-

Table 12–6 *New Therapeutic Agents.* (From *The Cancer Letter*)[38]

Cancer Type	Drug Name	Sponsor	FDA Official Designation	Development Status
Adrenal	Gossypol	Marcus Reidenberg, M.D. New York Hospital-Cornell Medical Center (New York, NY)	Treatment of cancer of the adrenal cortex	Phase II
Bladder	INTRON® A, interferon alfa-2b (recombinant)	Schering-Plough (Madison, NJ)	Treatment of carcinoma *in situ* of the urinary bladder	Application submitted
	Photofrin® (profimer sodium)	QLT Phototherapeutics (Pearl River, NY)	Photodynamic therapy in patients with transitional cell carcinoma *in situ* of urinary bladder	Phase III
Brain	Adenosine (MEDR-340)	Medco Research (Los Angeles, CA)	Treatment of brain tumors in conjunction with BCNU	Phase II
	INTRON® A, interferon alfa-2b (recombinant)	Schering-Plough (Madison, NJ)	Treatment of primary malignant brain tumors	Phase II
	serratia marcescens extract (polyribosomes)	Cell Technology (Boulder, CO)	Treatment of primary brain malignancies	Phase II
Cervical	INTRON®, interferon alfa-2b (recombinant)	Schering-Plough (Madison, NJ)	Treatment of invasive carcinoma of the cervix	Phase III
	Mitolactol®, Elobromal dibromodulcitol	Amswiss Scientific (New York, NY)	Treatment of recurrent invasive metastatic squamous carcinoma of the cervix	Phase II/III
Colorectal	5-fluorouracil (5-FU)	Hoffmann-La Roche (Nutley, NJ)	For use in combination with Roferon®-A for the treatment of advanced colorectal carcinoma	Phase III
	Adrucul (fluorouracil)	Lederle (Wayne, NJ)	Combination with leucovorin for therapy of metastatic adenocarcinoma of the colon and rectum	Application submitted
	d,l-Leucovorin calcium	Lederle (Wayne, NJ)	For use in combination with 5-FU for the treatment of metastatic adenocarcinoma of the colon and rectum	Application submitted

Continued

277

Table 12-6 New Therapeutic Agents. (continued)

Cancer Type	Drug Name	Sponsor	FDA Official Designation	Development Status
	Immther (disaccharide tripeptide glycerol dipalmitoyl)	Immuno Therapeutics (Moorhead, MN)	Treatment of pulmonary and hepatic metastases in patients with colorectal adenocarcinoma	Phase II/III
	Isovorin (l-leucovorin calcium)	Lederie (Wayne, NJ)	For use in combination with 5-FU for the treatment of metastatic adenocarcinoma of the colon and rectum	Phase III
	Roferon®-A, interferon-alfa-2a (recombinant)	Hoffmann-La Roche (Nutley, NJ)	For use in combination with 5-FU for the treatment of advanced colorectal carcinoma	Phase III
	Trimetrexate glucuronate	Warner-Lambert (Morris Plains, NJ)	Treatment of metastatic colorectal adenocarcinoma	Phase II
	XomaZyme®-791 (anti-TAP-72 immunotoxin)	Xoma (Berkeley, CA)	Treatment of metastatic colorectal adenocarcinoma	Phase I
Esophageal	5-fluorouracil (5-FU)	Hoffmann-La Roche (Nutley, NJ)	For use in combination with Roferon®-A for the treatment of esophageal carcinoma	Phase III
	Photofrin® (porfimer sodium)	QLT Phototherapeutics (Pearl River, NY)	Photodynamic therapy in patients with primary or recurrent obstructing (either partially or completely) esophageal carcinoma	Phase III
	Roferon®-A, interferon-alfa-2a (recombinant)	Hoffmann-La Roche (Nutley, NJ)	For use in combination with 5-FU for the treatment of esophageal carcinoma	Phase III
Germ cell	Iodine-131 murine MAb to human alpha-fetoprotein	Immunomedics (Warren, NJ)	Treatment of alpha-fetoprotein producing germ cell tumors	Phase I
	Iodine-131 murine MAb to human chorionic gonadotropin (hCG)	Immunomedics (Warren, NJ)	Detection of hCG-producing tumors, such as germ cell and trophoblastic cell tumors	Phase I
Head and neck	Trimetrexate glucuronate	Warner-Lambert (Morris Plains, NJ)	Treatment of metastatic carcinoma of the head and neck (i.e., buccal cavity, pharynx and larynx)	Phase II

Category	Agent	Company	Indication	Status
Hepatic	Iodine-131 murine MAb to human alpha-fetoprotein	Immunomedics (Warren, NJ)	Treatment of hepatocellular carcinoma and hepatoblastoma	Phase I
	Technetium Tc-99m murine MAb to human AFP	Immunomedics (Warren, NJ)	Detection of hepatocellular carcinoma and hepatoblastoma	Phase I
Leukemia	2'-Chloro-2'-deoxyadenosine	St. Jude Children's Hospital (Memphis, TN)	Treatment of acute myeloid leukemia	Phase I/II
	2-Chlorodeoxy-adenosine	Ortho Biotech (Raritan, NJ)	Treatment of chronic lymphocytic leukemia	Phase II
	2-Chlorodeoxy-adenosine	Ortho Biotech (Raritan, NJ)	Treatment of hairy cell leukemia	Phase II
	5-AZA-2'-deoxycytidine	Pharmachemie (Oradell, NJ)	Treatment of acute leukemia	Phase I
	All-trans retinoic acid	Hoffmann-La Roche (Nutley, NJ)	Treatment of acute promyelocytic leukemia	Phase II/III
	Anagrelide	Bristol-Myers Squibb (New York, NY)	Treatment of thrombocytosis in chronic myelogenous leukemia (CML)	Phase III
	Anti-my9-blocked ricin	Immunogen (Cambridge, MA)	Treatment of myeloid leukemia, including AML and blast crisis of CML	Phase I
	Erwinase® (erwinia L-asparaginase)	Porton International (Washington, DC)	Treatment of acute lymphocytic leukemia (ALL)	Application submitted
	Fludara® (fludarabine monophosphate)	Berlex (Wayne, NJ)	Treatment of chronic lymphocytic leukemia (CLL)	Phase II
	INTRON® A, interferon alfa-2b (recombinant)	Schering-Plough (Madison, NJ)	Treatment of chronic myelogenous leukemia (CML)	Phase III
	Leucomax® (granulocyte/macrophage-colony stimulating factor)	Schering-Plough (Madison, NJ)	Treatment of chronic lymphocytic leukemia to increase granulocyte count	In clinical trials
	Monoclonal antibodies (PM-81 and AML-2.23)	Medarex (West Lebanon, NH)	Treatment of patients with acute myelogenous leukemia undergoing bone marrow transplantation	Phase I

Continued

Table 12-6 *New Therapeutic Agents* (continued)

Cancer Type	Drug Name	Sponsor	FDA Official Designation	Development Status
	Oncolysin B (anti-b4-blocked ricin)	Immunogen (Cambridge, MA)	Treatment of B-cell leukemia and B-cell lymphoma	Phase II
	PEG-L-asparaginase	Enzon (S. Plainfield, NJ)	Treatment of acute lymphocytic leukemia	Application submitted
	Pentostatin	Warner-Lambert (Morris Plains, NJ)	Treatment of hairy cell leukemia	Application submitted
	Roferon®-A, interferon alfa-2a (recombinant)	Hoffmann-La Roche (Nutley, NJ)	Treatment of chronic myelogenous leukemia (CML)	Phase III
	VeeM-26, teniposide (VM-26)	Bristol-Myers Squibb (New York, NY)	Treatment of refractory childhood acute lymphocyte leukemia (ALL)	Application submitted
Lung	Trimetrexate glucuronate	Warner-Lambert (Morris Plains, NJ)	Treatment of advanced nonsmall cell carcinoma of the lung	Phase II
Lymphoma	Fludara® (fludarabine phosphate)	Berlex (Wayne, NJ)	Treatment and management of non-Hodgkin's lymphoma (NHL)	Phase III
	Iodine-1-131 lym-1 monoclonal antibody	Lederie (Wayne, NJ)	Treatment of B-cell lymphoma	Phase I
	Methotrexate with laurocapram	Whitby Research (Richmond, VA)	Topical treatment of mycosis fungoides	Phase II
	Oncolysin B (anti-b4-blocked ricin)	Immunogen (Cambridge, MA)	(See Leukemia)	
	Specifid® murine monoclonal antibodies to human B-cell lymphomas (anti-idiotypes)	IDEC Pharmaceuticals (Mountain View, CA)	Treatment of B-cell lymphoma	Phase III
	Sterecyt® (prednimustine)	Kabi-Pharmacia (Piscataway, NJ)	Treatment of malignant non-Hodgkin's lymphomas	Phase III
Melanoma	Ethyol® (amifostine)	U.S. Bioscience (W. Conshohocken, PA)	Use as a chemoprotective agent for cisplatin in the treatment of metastatic melanoma	Phase III

	Interleukin-2	Hoffmann-La Roche (Nutley, NJ)	Treatment of metastatic malignant melanoma	Phase III
	Melacine® (melanoma vaccine)	Ribi ImmunoChem (Hamilton, MT)	Treatment of stage III-IV melanoma	Phase II
	OncoTrac® Melanoma (technetium Tc-99m antimelanoma murine MAb)	NeoRX (Seattle, WA)	For use in detecting by imaging metastases of malignant melanoma	Application submitted
	Roferon®-A, interferon-alfa-2a (recombinant) with interleukin-2	Hoffmann-La Roche (Nutley, NJ)	Treatment of metastatic malignant melanoma	Phase III
	XomaScan-Mel (indium IN 111 antimelanoma antibody XMMME-0001-DTPA)	Xoma (Berkeley, CA)	Diagnostic use in imaging systemic and nodal melanoma metastases	Phase III
	XomaZyme®-Mel XMMME-001-RTA	Xoma (Berkeley, CA)	Treatment of stage III melanoma not amenable to surgical resection	Phase II
Ovarian	Decapeptyl® Injection (triptorelin pamoate)	Organon (West Orange, NJ)	For use in the palliative treatment of advanced ovarian carcinoma of epithelial origin	Phase II
	Ethyol® (amifostine)	U.S. Bioscience (W. Conshohocken, PA)	Use as a chemoprotective agent for cisplatin in the treatment of advanced ovarian carcinoma	Phase III
	Ethyol® (amifostine)	U.S. Bioscience (W. Conshohocken, PA)	Use as a chemoprotective agent for cyclophosphamide in the treatment of advanced ovarian carcinoma	Phase III
	INTRON® A, interferon alfa-2b (recombinant)	Schering-Plough (Madison, NJ)	Treatment of ovarian carcinoma	Phase III
	OncoRad OV103 (yttrium labeled MAb)	CYTOGEN (Princeton, NJ)	Treatment of ovarian cancer	Phase II

Continued

Table 12–6 *New Therapeutic Agents* (continued)

Cancer Type	Drug Name	Sponsor	FDA Official Designation	Development Status
	OncoScint OV103 (indium IN 111 murine MAb B72.3)	CYTOGEN (Princeton, NJ)	Detection of ovarian cancer	Application submitted
	Taxol (BMY-45622)	Bristol-Myers Squibb (New York, NY)	Treatment of ovarian cancer	Phase II/III
Pancreatic	Panorex® (monoclonal antibody 17-1A)	Centocor (Malvern, PA)	Treatment of pancreatic cancer	Phase II
	Trimetrexate glucuronate	Warner-Lambert (Morris Plains, NJ)	Treatment of pancreatic adenocarcinoma	Phase II
Renal	interleukin-2	Hoffmann-La Roche (Nutley, NJ)	Treatment of metastatic renal cell carcinoma	Phase III
	INTRON® A, interferon alfa-2b (recombinant)	Schering-Plough (Madison, NJ)	Treatment of metastatic renal cell carcinoma	Phase III
	Proleukin-PEG®, interleukin-2 (recombinant)	Cetus (Emeryville, CA)	Treatment of metastatic renal cell carcinoma	Application submitted
	Roferon®-A, interferon alfa-2a (recombinant)	Hoffmann-La Roche (Nutley, NJ)	Treatment of metastatic renal cell carcinoma	Phase III
	Roferon®-A, interferon alfa-2a (recombinant) with interleukin-2	Hoffmann-La Roche (Nutley, NJ)	Treatment of metastatic renal cell carcinoma	Phase III

sels that perfuse the tumor bed, it is feasible to place indwelling catheters hooked to a subcutaneously implanted infusion port or implantable pump to provide an access route to deliver drug in a continuous or carefully programmed manner. In colorectal cancer, carcinoid tumors, or hepatocellular cancers, where control of the tumor within the liver has a good possibility of improving survival and quality of life, it is often worth the expense and effort to utilize such implantable devices.[37]

The objective of such devices is to achieve continual access to the arterial blood supply restricted to the liver and the tumor within the liver. The correct placement of a catheter and access of the infused material is monitored by angiography using a radioactive tracer like technetium-99m aggregated with albumin (TcMAA) followed by γ-camera scanning. The TcMAA scan can also rule out drug flow to undesired areas, such as the stomach and duodenum.

Hepatic arterial infusion of FUDR via implanted pumps has produced some striking results in the treatment of liver metastasis[37] and has led to the development of implantable injection ports (Fig. 12–3). These subcutaneously implanted ports provide continual access for infusion of drugs and circumvent the problems of multiple venipunctures and the resulting vessel sclerosis or thrombosis that goes with it. These ports have been utilized in well over 200 patient-years with relatively few untoward effects and with excellent patient acceptance. Side effects include occlusion of the catheter (4–21%, depending on the study), thrombosis (4–16%), extravasation (3–9%), and local infection (2–6%) (reviewed in ref. 37). Thus, implantable injection ports can be a good solution for patients requiring chemotherapy involving repeated drug injections, protracted infusions, or multiple blood sampling.[37]

Some Newer Drugs in the Pipeline

Table 12–5 lists new investigational anticancer agents in clinical trials in the early 1990s provided by the Cancer Therapy Evaluation Program of the Division of Cancer Treatment of NCI. It includes both drugs and biological substances and the phase of clinical trial in which

they were being tested. Table 12–6 is a similar list of new agents by disease category. It is obvious from a perusal of Table 12–6[38] that not all the agents in clinical trials are new. Some of them are being used in different settings or in different combinations than before. For example, 5-fluorouracil is in a clinical trial with interferon-α2a for advanced colorectal carcinoma, and this combination has shown some promising results.

How many of these new agents will become accepted for general clinical use in cancer treatment isn't clear at this point, but the diversity of types of agents indicates some of the new thrusts in cancer research. For example, the introduction of cytokines such as IL-1, -2, -3, and -4, colony-stimulating factors such as GM-CSF, retinoic acid analogs, tumor-infiltrating lymphocytes (TIL), a host of monoclonal antibody preparations, as well as a number of new chemical entities, reflects these new directions.

REFERENCES

1. C. G. Zubrod: Chemical control of cancer. *Proc. Natl. Acad. Sci. USA* 69:1042 (1972).

2. R. K. Johnson and A. Goldin: The clinical impact of screening and other experimental tumor studies. *Cancer Treatment Rev.* 2:1 (1975).

3. B. I. Sikic: Anticancer drug discovery. *J. Natl. Cancer Inst.* 83:738 (1991).

4. S. A. Schepartz: "Report of the Associate Director, Drug Research and Development," in the *1976 Report of the Division of Cancer Treatment, NCI* (V. T. DeVita, Director), Vol. 1, p. 13, June 1976.

5. B. A. Chabner: In defense of cell-line screening. *J. Natl. Cancer Inst.* 82:1083 (1990).

6. M. C. Alley, D. A. Scudiero, A. Monks, M. L. Hursey, M. J. Czerwinski, D. L. Fine, B. J. Abbott, J. G. Mayo, R. H. Shoemaker, and M. R. Boyd: Feasibility of drug screening with panels of human tumor cell lines using a microculture tetrazolium assay. *Cancer Res.* 48:589 (1988).

7. A. Monks, D. Scudiero, P. Skehan, R. Shoemaker, K. Paull, D. Vistica, C. Hose, J. Langley, P. Cronise, A. Vaigro-Wolff, M. Gray-Goodrich, H. Campbell, J. Mayo, and M. Boyd: Feasibility of a high-flux anticancer drug screen using a diverse panel of cultured human tumor cell lines: *J. Natl. Cancer Inst.* 83:757 (1991).

8. L. V. Rubinstein, R. H. Shoemaker, K. D. Paull, R. M. Simon, S. Tosini, P. Skehan, D. A. Scudiero, A. Monks, and M. R. Boyd: Comparison of in vitro anticancer-drug-screening data generated with a tetrazolium assay versus a protein assay against a diverse panel of human tumor cell lines. *J. Natl. Cancer Inst.* 82:1113 (1990).

9. R. M. Phillips, M. C. Bibby, and J. A. Double: A critical appraisal of the predictive value of in vitro chemosensitivity assays. *J. Natl. Cancer Inst.* 82:1457 (1990).

10. J. A. Bennett, V. A. Pilon, and R. T. MacDowell: Evaluation of growth and histology of human tumor xenografts implanted under the renal capsule of immunocompetent and immunodeficient mice. *Cancer Res.* 45:4963 (1985).

11. E. Gorelik, A. Ovejera, R. Shoemaker, A. Jarvis, M. Alley, R. Duff, J. Mayo, R. Herberman, and M. Boyd: Microencapsulated tumor assay: New short-term assay for in vivo evaluation of the effects of anticancer drugs on human tumor cell lines. *Cancer Res.* 47:5739 (1987).

12. J. M. Adams and S. Cory: Transgenic models of tumor development. *Science* 254:1161 (1991).

13. J. C. Wright, J. P. Cobb, S. L. Gumport, F. M. Golomb, and D. Safadi: Investigation of the relation between clinical and tissue culture response to chemotherapeutic agents of human cancer. *New Engl. J. Med.* 257:1207 (1957).

14. S. E. Salmon, A. W. Hamburger, B. Soehnlen, B. G. M. Durie, D. S. Alberts, and T. E. Moon: Quantitations of differential sensitivity of human-tumor stem cells to anticancer drugs. *New Engl. J. Med.* 298:1321 (1978).

15. D. Von Hoff: He's not going to talk about in vitro predictive assays again, is he? *J. Natl. Cancer Inst.* 82:96 (1990).

16. D. Von Hoff, J. F. Sandbach, G. M. Clark, J. N. Turner, B. F. Forseth, M. J. Piccart, N. Colombo, and F. M. Muggia: Selection of cancer chemotherapy for a patient by an in vitro assay versus a clinician. *J. Natl. Cancer Inst.* 82:110 (1990).

17. A. F. Gazdar, S. M. Steinberg, E. K. Russell, R. Ilona Linnoila, H. K. Oie, B. C. Ghosh, J. D. Cotelingam, B. E. Johnson, J. D. Minna, and D. C. Ihde: Correlation of in vitro drug-sensitivity testing results with response to chemotherapy and survival in extensive-stage small cell lung cancer: A prospective clinical trial. *J. Natl. Cancer Inst.* 82:117 (1990).

18. S. E. Salmon: Chemosensitivity testing: Another chapter. *J. Natl. Cancer Inst.* 82:82 (1990).

19. V. T. DeVita, Jr., R. C. Young, and G. P. Canellos: Combination versus single agent chemotherapy: A review of the basis for selection of drug treatment of cancer. *Cancer* 35:98 (1975).

20. K. D. Bagshawe: Recent observations related to the chemotherapy and immunology of gestational choriocarcinoma. *Adv. Cancer Res.* 18:231 (1973).

21. G. I. Abelev: Alpha-fetoprotein in oncogenesis and its association with malignant tumors. *Adv. Cancer Res.* 14:295 (1971).

22. P. Gold and S. O. Freedman: Demonstration of tumor-specific antigens in human colonic carcinomata by immunological tolerance and absorption techniques. *J. Exptl. Med.* 121:439 (1965).

23. N. Zamcheck and G. Pusztaszeri: CEA, AFP, and other potential tumor markers. *CA—A Cancer Journal for Clinicians* 25:204 (1975).

24. J. D. Pfeifer and M. R. Wick: "The pathological evaluation of neoplastic diseases," in *American Cancer Society Textbook of Clinical Oncology,* ed. by A. I. Holleb, D. J. Fink, and G. P. Murphy. Atlanta: The American Cancer Society, Inc., 1991, pp. 7–24.

25. E. Frei III: "Effect of dose and schedule on response," in *Cancer Medicine,* ed. by J. F. Holland and E. Frei III. Philadelphia: Lea and Febiger, 1973, p. 717.

26. R. J. A. Aur, J. V. Simone, H. O. Husto, and M. S. Vevzosa: A comparative study of central nervous system irradiation and intensive chemotherapy early in remission in childhood acute lymphocytic leukemia. *Cancer* 29:381 (1972).

27. L. H. Einhorn: Testicular cancer as a model for a curable neoplasm. *Cancer Res.* 41:3275 (1981).

28. P. K. Gupta: Drug targeting in cancer chemotherapy: A clinical perspective. *J. Pharm. Sci.* 79:949 (1990).

29. R. Langer: New methods of drug delivery. *Science* 249:1527 (1990).

30. D. H. Robinson and J. W. Mauger: Drug delivery systems. *Am. J. Hosp. Pharm.* 48 *(Suppl. 1):*14 (1991).

31. M. B. Bally, R. Nayar, D. Masin, P. R. Cullis, and L. D. Mayer: Studies on the myelosuppressive activity of doxorubicin entrapped in liposomes. *Cancer Chemother. Pharmacol.* 27:13 (1990).

32. A. Gabizon, A. Dagan, D. Goren, Y. Barenholz, and Z. Fuks: Liposomes as in vivo carriers of adriamycin: Reduced cardiac uptake and preserved antitumor activity in mice. *Cancer Res.* 42:4734 (1982).

33. A. Rahman, M. Panneerselvam, R. Guirguis, V. Castronovo, M. E. Sobel, K. Abraham, P. E. Daddona, L. A. Liotta: Anti-laminin receptor antibody targeting of liposomes with encapsulated doxorubicin to human breast cancer cells in vitro. *J. Natl. Cancer Inst.* 81:1794 (1989).

34. C. P. N. Dinney, C. D. Bucana, Y. Utsugi, I. J. Fidler, A. C. von Eschenbach, and J. J. Killion: Therapy of spontaneous lung metastasis of murine renal adenocarcinoma by systemic administration of liposomes containing the macrophage activator CGP 31362. *Cancer Res.* 51:3741 (1991).

35. W. D. Ensminger, J. W. Gyves, P. Stetson, S. Walker-Andrews: Phase I study of hepatic arterial degradable starch microspheres and mitomycin. *Cancer Res.* 45:4464 (1985).

36. J. W. Gyves, W. D. Ensminger, D. Van Harken, J. Niederhuber, P. Stetson, and S. Walker. Improved regional selectivity of hepatic arterial mitomycin by starch microspheres. *Clin. Pharmacol. Ther.* 34:259 (1983).

37. W. D. Ensminger and I. S. Wollner: Implantable drug delivery devices (pumps, ports) in cancer therapy. *Rational Drug Therapy* 22:1 (1988).

38. "Cancer Economics," supplement in *The Cancer Letter,* Vol. 17, ed. by K. Boyd Goldberg, March 1991, pp. 6–8.

CHAPTER THIRTEEN

Biological Treatments of Cancer

In recent years, biological approaches to treating cancer have received a lot of attention, both in the research laboratory and in the clinic. Although many of these have shown great promise in the laboratory for selected types of cancer, they have not yet provided the quantum leap in cancer treatment that was hoped for. Nevertheless, new biological agents and new combinations of agents continue to be discovered and to show activity against cancer in both experimental animal and clinical studies. Thus, it is important to place these agents in their proper context in the armamentarium against cancer and to be aware that this is an area where future breakthroughs will probably occur.

In this chapter we will focus on immune system modulators such as extracts from microorganisms, polypeptides, polyribonucleotides, cytokines, and tumor necrosis factors. We will also discuss adoptive immunotherapy, monoclonal antibodies (Mabs) and Mab-toxins or—radionuclide conjugates, tumor vaccines, and genetic therapy.

Modulators of the immune system include both naturally occurring materials isolated from microorganisms, synthetic or semisynthetic polypeptides, synthetic compounds, and cytokines produced by cells of the immune system in the body that are involved in the cascade of events leading to an immune response against cancer cells. This group of agents is often included under the heading "biological response modifiers" or biomodulators. A partial list of these is shown in Table 13–1.[1]

Microorganisms

BCG, a member of the *Mycobacterium* family, or extracts thereof (e.g., BCG-Mer), has been tried therapeutically in a number of ways. These include adjuvant therapy for metastatic disease, intralesional injection for cutaneous melanoma, topical instillation for urinary bladder cancer, and in combination with tumor cell vaccines or with chemotherapy (reviewed in ref. 1). Other than intralesional use for cutaneous melanoma and instillation therapy for bladder cancer, BCG has not shown a great deal of activity and its current use is limited.

Among other microorganisms tested, *C. parvum* has probably received the most clinical testing, and it has shown some activity intraperitoneally in refractory ovarian cancer. It is thought that these bacterial preparations act primarily to augment the activity of cytotoxic lymphocytes, macrophages, and natural killer (NK) cells. There is evidence that bacterial extracts can induce the production of cytokines such as interleukin-1 (IL-1) and tumor necrosis factor (TNF) (discussed below). This is most likely the mechanism of action of products such as lipopolysaccharide (LPS) and other polysaccharides.[1,2]

Polypeptides

Polypeptides useful as immune system modulators are most often synthetic peptides modeled after naturally occurring ones—e.g.,

Table 13–1   Examples of Biological Response Modifiers. (Adapted from Talmadge and Clark[1])

Microorganisms: whole, extracts, and cell-wall
skeletons
Bacillus Calmette-Guérin (BCG)
Methanol extractable residue (MER from BCG)
Corynebacterium parvum (*C. parvum* or, more
correctly, *Propionibacterium acnes*)
Brucella abortus
Bru-Pel (*Brucella abortus* extract)
Pseudomonas aeruginosa (Pseudogen)
Bordetella pertussis
Norcardia rubra (also cell-wall extract (N-CWS)
Picibanil (OK-432, *Streptococcus pyogenes*)
Klebsiella spp.
Micrococcus spp.
Lactobacillus casei (LC 9018)

Chemically identified compounds from natural
sources
Peptidoglycan (gram-negative bacteria)
WSA (disaccharide bound to a peptidoglycan,
Micrococcus smegmatis)
Lipopolysaccharide (LPS, from *Escherichia, coli,
Salmonella typhimurium)*
Monophosphoryl lipid A (detoxified LPS)
Biostim (glycoprotein, *Klebsiella pneumoniae*)

Polysaccharides
Krestin (PSK)
Glucan (β1-3 polyglucose, *Saccharomyces cerevisiae*)
Lentinan (B1-3 polyglucose, *Lentinus edodes*)
Pustulon
Levan
Mannozym

Polypeptides
Bestatin *(Streptomyces olivoreticuli)*
Tuftsin (part of Fc portion of leukokinin)
Muramyldipeptide (MDP, BCG, also a large
number of analogs)
Muramyltripeptide (MTP-PE, a lipophilic analog of
MDP, also a large number of similar analogs)
FK-565
Complement C5a analogs

Synthetic compounds
Levamisole
Isoprinosine
Pyrimidinols (ABPP)
Anthraquinone (Tilorone)
Azimexone BM 12.531
Cimexone
Alkyl-lysophospholipids (a large
number of analogs)
Sodium diethylthiocarbamate
Thiabendazole
Methylfurylbutyrolactones (Nafocare B)

Polyribonucleotides
Poly IC
Poly ICLC
Poly AU
Ampligen

Vaccines/inducers of specific immune
response
Viral oncolysates
Chemically modified tumor vaccines
Hapten-modified tumor vaccines
Normal tumor vaccine with or without
adjuvant
Xenogenized tumor cell vaccine
Immune RNA
Transfer factor

---

bestatin, tuftsin, muramyldipeptide, and complement component C5a analogs.

Bestatin, originally isolated from a *Streptomyces* species, has been used in clinical trials in Japan and Europe.[1] It has been shown to activate NK cells and macrophages and to be of

some benefit as an adjuvant to chemotherapy in acute myelogenous leukemia. Tuftsin is a tetrapeptide that acts as an activator of macrophages and may have some clinical use as an adjuvant to chemotherapy. It stimulates tumor cell killing by macrophages and cytotoxic T cells. FK-565 is a synthetic acyltripeptide analog of an immunoactive peptide isolated from a *Streptomyces* species and has been shown to inhibit metastasis in a murine model.[3] It also apparently acts by activating macrophages. Analogs of complement component C5a have been synthesized and tested for their ability to stimulate macrophages to produce IL-1 and IL-6, which in turn stimulate other cells in the immune cascade.[4]

The above are just some examples of synthetic peptide analogs that have immune modulatory activity. A growing number of these are being synthesized and tested for activity. Theoretically at least, such peptides could be designed so that they would resist degradation by proteases, have high affinity for cytokine receptors, be orally absorbable, and have pharmacokinetics and biodistribution properties that would make them ideal therapeutic agents to augment a patient's immune system. This would circumvent many of the problems of treating patients with the naturally occurring immunomodulatory polypeptides, many of which are more difficult to use because of their pharmacologic properties (e.g., poor oral absorption, rapid destruction by proteases in the body) or their propensity to induce antipolypeptide antibodies and thus limit their continued use in a given patient.

Other Synthetic Compounds

Examples of other synthetic compounds with immunomodulatory activity are listed in Table 13–1. Of these, levamisole has been shown to have the most clinical utility so far. In patients with stage B2 or C colon cancer, levamisole plus 5-fluorouracil, as adjuvants to surgical resection, have been shown to provide a longer survival than has surgery alone.[5] Alkyl-lysophospholipids can induce interferon production by cells, but they have significant systemic toxicity in animals. Azimexone and cimexone are inducers of colony stimulating factors (CSFs, discussed below) and foster bone marrow stem cell regeneration. The pyrimedinedione compound 2-amino-5-bromo-6-phenyl-4(3H)-pyrimidinedione (ABPP) is an interferon inducer that has shown some immune system stimulating activity in tumor-bearing animals.

Other than levamisole, these synthetic compounds have not demonstrated great clinical utility. However, they may well represent only the first generation of such drugs that could act similarly to endogenous activators of the immune system and that would be easier from a pharmacologic standpoint to administer to patients.

Polyribonucleotides

These agents were developed for clinical use because of their ability to induce interferon production *in vivo*. They are synthetic double-stranded polymers of nucleic acid bases. In addition to inducing interferon, these agents appear to have other immune system and tumoricidal effects. Poly IC, poly ICLC, poly AU, and ampligen have also been tested clinically (reviewed in ref. 1). Poly IC is a poor inducer of interferon in humans, probably because it is rapidly degraded by serum ribonucleases. Poly IC complexed with poly-L-lysine (poly ICLC) is less sensitive to ribonucleases and is a potent inducer of interferon production in mice. In Phase I clinical trials of poly ICLC, some responses were observed in patients with leukemia, myeloma, and renal cell carcinoma. Phase II clinical trials of ICLC are in progress. Overall response rates to all these interferon inducers have been low, and it is likely their usefulness will be limited to augmentation of other treatment modalities.

Cytokines

The term "cytokines," used in its broadest sense, defines a large group of secreted polypeptides, released by living cells that act nonenzymatically in picomolar to nanomolar concentrations to regulate cellular functions.[6] These cellular functions include regulation of immune cell activity (interferons and interleukins), hematopoiesis (colony stimulating factors, or CSFs), and regulation of proliferation and differentiation of a wide variety of cell types (peptide growth factors such as EGF, FGF, TGFα, and TGFβ, etc.). Here we will discuss the cytokines that affect the immune system and hematopoiesis. The other peptide growth factors are discussed in Chapter 14.

Interferons

As mentioned in Chapter 1, interferon was discovered in 1957 by two virologists, A. Isaacs and J. Lindenmann, who were looking for a substance that blocks viral infection of cells.[7] Their research was prompted by the clinical observation that patients seldom come down with two virally induced diseases at the same time. They showed that the medium removed from influenza virus-infected chicken cells grown in culture, when added to other cultures of chicken cells, prevented infection of the second cultures by a different virus. They named this interfering substance interferon. Since that time, numerous studies aimed at isolating and characterizing interferon have been carried out.

Human interferons are classified into three general groups: IFN-α, -β, and -γ.[8] IFN-α is produced by leukocytes and lymphoblastoid cells stimulated by viruses or by microbial cell components. The α interferons are members of a multigene family; they are acid stable (M_r = 16–25 kDa) polypeptides. IFN-β is a 20-kDa glycoprotein produced by fibroblasts in culture after exposure to various microorganisms, microbial components, or high-molecular-weight polyanions (e.g., poly IC). Two IFN-β genes have been identified. IFN-γ, so-called immune interferon, is produced by T lymphocytes in response to antigenic or mitogenic stimulation. There are at least two species of IFN-γ, a 20 kDa and a 25 kDa glycoprotein, and they are acid-labile. The antiviral action of the interferons appears to involve interference with viral nucleic acid and protein synthesis via an increased rate of viral RNA degradation and decreased rate of peptide chain initiation.

The antitumor effects of interferons appear to result from a stimulation of natural killer (NK) cells and macrophages, and from a direct cytotoxic effect on tumor cells. The evidence that multiple actions are involved comes from studies in tumor-bearing animals before and after depletion of NK cells. For example, in a study of the growth of tumors produced by Moloney sarcoma virus–transformed cells in mice, it was found that a mixture of IFN-α and -β markedly stimulated NK-cell activity at the site of the tumor and inhibited tumor growth; however, when NK cells were depleted by *in vivo* treatment with an antibody to NK cells, tumor growth was still inhibited.[9] When the tumor load was very high, however, NK-cell depletion did reduce the antitumor effect of IFN, suggesting that IFN has dual actions: direct inhibition of tumor cell multiplication and stimulation of NK-cell activity, the latter of which plays a more apparent role in IFN action when the tumor burden is high.

IFN-γ, isolated initially from activated T lymphocytes and later produced by recombinant DNA techniques, is a potent activator of tumoricidal macrophages.[10] It also has marked macrophage migration inhibitory factor (MIF) activity. Thus, IFN-γ may be responsible for the immunomodulating activities previously ascribed to the lymphokines macrophage-activating factor (MAF) and MIF. One of the mechanisms by which IFN-γ also increases the cellular killing effect of macrophages mediated by IgG antibodies involves induction of F_c receptors on the macrophage surface.[11]

The antitumor immune modulating effect of IFN *in vivo* and the relatively low host toxicity of IFN led to a number of clinical trials. The greatest therapeutic usefulness of IFN has been in the treatment of a relatively rare form of leukemia, called "hairy cell" leukemia because of the spiked appearance of the cell surface. Most of the earlier clinical trials used IFN-α purified from human leukocytes and later obtained by recombinant DNA techniques. Currently, various recombinant forms of IFN-α, -β, and -γ are in clinical trials for various malignancies and for AIDS-related Kaposi's sarcoma.

An intriguing approach to the activation of tumoricidal macrophages involves the use of liposomes to deliver macrophage-activating factors directly to these phagocytic cells.[12] Liposomes, containing phosphatidylcholine and phosphatidylserine, are selectively taken up by phagocytic cells, including reticuloendothelial cells in the liver, spleen, lymph nodes, and bone marrow, as well as by circulating monocytes. Incorporation of agents that activate macrophages, such as crude macrophage-activating factor (MAF), IFN-γ, and the low molecular weight (M_r = 459) synthetic compound muramyl dipeptide (N-acetylmuramyl-L-alanyl-Disoglutamine; MDP) into liposomes provides a delivery system for these factors to macrophages. Once the carrier liposomes are engulfed, the macrophages become tumoricidal against target cells *in vivo*. The macrophages thus activated recognize and lyse neoplastic cells *in vitro* by a mechanism that requires cell-to-cell contact but apparently is independent of MHC antigens.[12] Intravenous administration of liposomes containing MAF plus MDP to nude mice, who were previously injected with B16 melanoma cells and who had spontaneous metastases in the lungs and lymph nodes by the time of liposome treatment, produced 9/18 250-day survivors, compared to 2/18 250-day survivors in the liposome-only control group.[12] These data indicate that activation of macrophages *in vivo* is possible and hold out the possibility that metastatic tumor sites can also be recognized and destroyed by such activated macrophages.

Interleukins

The interleukins belong to a family of polypeptide growth and differentiation factors called "lymphokines." These are factors, produced by lymphocytes or macrophages, that stimulate the proliferation, differentiation, and function of T lymphocytes, B lymphocytes, and certain other cells involved in the immune response. Initially discovered as soluble factors present in the growth medium of cultured lymphocytes, several such activities have been now identified (reviewed in ref. 13). These activities were usually defined by their role in simulating an *in vitro* immune reaction—i.e., promoting the activation and/or proliferation of immune system cells. Accordingly, the following kinds of activities were identified: T-cell mitogenesis factor (TMF), or T-cell-stimulating factor (TSF), which fostered T-cell proliferation in response to added plant lectins; killer/helper factors (KHFs), which stimulated *in vitro* generation of antigen-specific cytolytic T cells; B-cell helper factors, which could replace T cells in fostering differentiation of B cells into antibody-producing cells; and T-cell growth factor (TCGF), which was produced by mitogen-stimulated lymphocytes and promoted proliferation of antigen-activated T cells. By the use of cloned lymphocyte populations, more exten-

sive purification of lymphokine-containing media, and specific monoclonal antibodies, it was possible to catalogue these factors more definitively. It became clear that several of the previously described activities could be attributed to two distinct polypeptides. The renaming of these factors was adopted at the Second International Lymphokine Workshop held in Ermattingen, Switzerland, in 1979. One of these is interleukin-1 (IL-1) and the other interleukin-2 (IL-2). The term "interleukin" was chosen because it indicates the basic property of these secreted mediators—i.e., to serve as intercellular signals between leukocytes. Several additional interleukins have now been identified and their cellular source and functions characterized (Table 13–2).[14]

IL-1 is produced by activated macrophages and acts as a cofactor along with other mitogens in proliferation of T cells and promotes production of IL-2 by T cells; it also fosters B-cell proliferation and antibody production by B cells. Fully processed IL-1 is a 17,500-Da polypeptide originally isolated from both murine and human monocyte/macrophage cells.

Cloning of the IL-1 genetic sequences indicated that there are at least two genes, termed IL-1α and IL-1β, with only about 25% sequence homology.[13,15] IL-1 has a broad spectrum of activities, including maturation of hematopoietic stem-cell precursors, induction of synthesis of other interleukin receptors on T lymphocytes, and maturation of T lymphocytes. IL-1 also has proinflammatory effects by stimulating arachidonic acid metabolism, prostaglandin production, and secretion of proteases and collagenases by cells involved in the inflammatory response. It also acts as a pyrogen by raising body temperature. Thus, the IL-1 polypeptide family has broad target cell specificity.

Interleukin-2 (IL-2) was originally discovered in the growth medium of mitogen-stimulated murine and human peripheral blood lymphocytes (reviewed in ref. 13) and shown to foster T-cell proliferation and maintenance in culture; hence it was originally called T-cell growth factor. Human IL-2 is a 17,200 Da glycoprotein with a slightly basic isoelectric point. Although initially thought to be only a mitogen for T cells, IL-2 is now known to foster growth and differentiation of B lymphocytes,

Table 13–2 Characteristics of Some Human Interleukins and Hematopoietic Growth Factors. (Modified from Laver and Moore[14])

Factor	Molecular Weight	Cellular Source	Hematopoietic Activities
IL-1 alpha	17,500	Macrophages, epithelial cells	Affects early hematopoietic progenitors, making them more sensitive to "later" acting factors (hematopoietin 1 activity); induces CSF production by accessory cells; causes multiple effects on lymphoid and other nonhematopoietic cells
IL-1 beta	17,500	Endothelial cells, fibroblasts, other cell types	
IL-2	17,200	Activated T cells	Is a cofactor for growth and differentiation of T and B cells; augments lymphocyte-activated killer activity; induces production of other lymphokines
IL-3	25,000	Activated T cells	Stimulates early growth of granulocyte, monocyte, erythroid, and megakaryocyte progenitor cells; supports mast cell growth; induces acute nonlymphocytic leukemia blasts to proliferate
IL-4	20,000	T cells	Promotes secretion of IgG; induces B-cell growth; synergizes with other growth factors to promote colony growth; enhances growth of mast cell lines
IL-5	18,000	Activated T cells	Induces proliferation and differentiation of eosinophil progenitors
IL-6	21,000	Fibroblasts, macrophages, some T-cell and tumor cell lines	Induces differentiation of B cells; enhances Ig secretion by B cells; synergizes with other growth factors to promote colony growth

	Molecular weight	Source cells	Function
IL-7	17,500	Marrow stromal cells	Supports growth of pre-B cells
IL-8	10,000	Activated T cells and monocytes; endothelial cells	Activates neutrophils; attenuates inflammatory events at blood-vessel endothelium
HILDA	38,000	T-cell clones	Supports growth of Da-2 murine cell line; has chemotactic and activating properties on eosinophils; affects early hematopoietic progenitors by synergizing with other growth factors; suppresses M1 murine myeloid leukemia cell line
M-CSF	45,000	Monocytes, fibroblasts, endothelial cells	Stimulates growth of monocyte colonies; supports survival of monocytes *in vitro*; activates mature monocytes; enhances ADCC against tumor cell lines
G-CSF	19,600	Monocytes, fibroblasts, endothelial cells	Stimulates growth of granulocyte colonies and activates mature granulocytes; induces *in vitro* differentiation of leukemia cell lines; stimulates proliferation of leukemic progenitors; increases ADCC of neutrophils
GM-CSF	22,000	Monocytes, fibroblasts, endothelial cells, T cells	Stimulates growth of granulocytic, monocytic, and early erythroid progenitors and to a lesser extent also megakaryocytic progenitors; activates mature granulocytes and monocytes; enhances ADCC; may stimulate leukemic progenitors' proliferation
Erythropoietin	34,000	Renal and hepatic cells	Stimulates proliferation of committed erythroid progenitors; induces hemoglobin formation

induce the production of other lymphokines, and stimulate the activity of peripheral lymphokine-activated killer (LAK) cells (see below). High-affinity receptors for IL-2 have been identified on activated T cells, and the signal transduction mechanism of these receptors appears to involve activation of a *src* proteinlike tyrosine protein kinase.

Interleukin-3 is a 25,000 Da glycoprotein produced by activated T cells and has broad activity in stimulating the proliferation of hematopoietic stem cells. It can stimulate the colony growth of progenitor cells in the granulocyte, monocyte, erthryoid, and megakaryocyte series as well as the proliferation of mast cells and enhanced phagocytosis by macrophages.[13,14] Like IL-2, target cells for IL-3 express high-affinity receptors coupled to a *src*-like tyrosine kinase activity.

Interleukin-4 was discovered in 1983 when it was observed that a murine thymoma cell line (EL4) produced a factor that stimulated the growth in culture of B lymphocytes activated with antiimmunoglobulin antibodies (reviewed in ref. 16). This B-cell growth factor, derived from T cells, turned out to be a 20,000-Da glycoprotein now called interleukin-4. IL-4 also enhances expression of class II major histocompatibility antigens and stimulates immunoglobulin synthesis. It enhances proliferation of mast cells and acts synergistically with other cytokines to promote granulocyte and erythroid progenitor cell colony growth. IL-4 also appears to have a negative regulatory effect on production of IL-1, tumor necrosis factor, and prostaglandin E_2 by macrophages, suggesting an antiinflammatory action.[13]

An activity secreted by mitogen-stimulated murine T lymphocytes and found to promote B-lymphocyte and eosinophil proliferation and differentiation was found to be a distinct factor and was termed interleukin-5. Human recombinant IL-5 has predominantly the eosinophil-stimulating activity.

As is true for a number of the other interleukins, IL-6 has broad target-cell specificity. IL-6 is a glycoprotein of about 21,000 Da, but demonstrates significant microheterogeneity due to differential glycosylation. It is produced by a wide variety of cells, including fibroblasts, monocytes/macrophages, T and B lymphocytes, endothelial cells, keratinocytes, and a number of tumor cell types.[13,17] Inducers of IL-6 production by normal cells include IL-1, tumor necrosis factor-α, PDGF, virus infection, double-stranded RNA, and cAMP.[13] IL-6 and IL-1 are synergistic in the induction of T-cell proliferation, and this action appears to be at least in part due to up-regulation of IL-2 receptors on T cells. B-cell differentiation is also enhanced by IL-6. IL-3 and IL-6 act synergistically to support proliferation of pluripotent hematopoietic progenitor cells.[18] IL-6, like IL-1, plays a role in inflammatory responses. These interleukins have a synergistic effect on the induction of acute phase protein production by hepatocytes, and both act as pyrogens to increase body temperature. Human tumor cells, particularly myeloma cells, produce and respond to IL-6, suggesting an autocrine growth factor–type stimulatory effect in multiple myeloma.

IL-7 has been identified as a B-cell growth-promoting factor produced by bone-marrow stromal cells.[19] Its effect seems to be primarily on B-lymphocyte progenitor cells rather than mature B cells.

IL-8 is produced by activated T cells and endothelial cells.[20] It activates neutrophils and, in addition, may play a role in dampening inflammatory damage to blood vessels by inhibiting adhesion of neutrophils to endothelial cells.

Additional interleukins continue to be discovered and characterized. As of this writing, interleukins up to IL-13 have been characterized. For example, IL-12 is a recently described cytokine that stimulates IFN-α production, induces T_{helper} cell differentiation, and thus plays a role in initiating cell-mediated immunity.[21,22] IL-12's action in stimulating NK cells to produce IFN-α is inhibited by IL-10.[22] IL-13 is a 10,000 Da protein produced by activated T_{helper} cells that elicits differentiation of human monocytes and proliferation and differentiation of human cells.[23]

Potential Clinical Usefulness of Interleukins

IL-1, -2, -3, and -4 have been introduced into clinical trial for a variety of malignant diseases. IL-1α and -1β have been employed to reverse bone marrow suppression due to chemotherapy or radiotherapy and to augment immunotherapy. IL-2 has been used in adoptive immunotherapy to stimulate clonal expansion of lymphokine-activated killer (LAK) cells and tumor-infiltrative lymphocytes (TIL) (see below). IL-3 has been utilized to stimulate bone marrow recovery in bone marrow or peripheral stem cell transplantation. IL-4 has been introduced as an immune system stimulator in various cancer treatment regimens.

Adoptive Immunotherapy

Adoptive immunotherapy is "a treatment approach in which cells with antitumor reactivity are administered to a tumor-bearing host and mediate either directly or indirectly the regression of established tumor."[24] Several types of approaches have been tried. One idea is to take tumor cells from a patient (removed by biopsy or surgery), inactivate the cells by X-irradiation, and then use these cells plus bacterial-derived adjuvants such as BCG or *C. parvum* to attempt to induce an immune response in the patient to his own tumor cells.[25] Another idea is to take the patient's own lymphocytes and activate them *in vitro* with appropriate activating factors and then inject them back into the patient. The latter approach has been taken by Rosenberg and his colleagues,[24] who have obtained, by leukapheresis, large quantities of patients' leukocytes, from which lymphocytes are separated. The lymphocytes are then incubated with recombinant interleukin-2, which stimulates a population of lymphocytes that when activated can lyse fresh, noncultured, natural killer cell–resistant tumor cells but not normal cells.[26] These cells have been termed lymphokine-activated killer (LAK) cells. In earlier animal studies, Rosenberg *et al.* have demonstrated that the adoptive transfer of LAK cells, incubated in culture with IL-2 followed by additional treatment *in vivo* with IL-2, induced the regression of pulmonary and hepatic metastases from a wide variety of murine tumors, including melanomas, sarcomas, a colon adenocarcinoma, and a urinary bladder carcinoma (reviewed in ref. 24). In these model systems, the *in vivo* administration of both IL-2-activated LAK cells plus subsequent IL-2 was required for tumor regression. Expansion of the LAK cell population *in vivo* has been shown to occur after injection of more IL-2.

This rationale was then utilized in clinical trials. *In vitro* IL-2-activated LAK cells have been infused intravenously followed by IV infusion of IL-2 every 8 hours for several days, depending on patient tolerance. With the high doses of IL-2 used in the earlier studies, patients experienced pulmonary edema with dyspnea and several pulmonary complications. Other side effects include malaise, fever, chills, nausea, vomiting, diarrhea, erythema, pruritus, and fluid retention.[24] These toxic effects are reversible when IL-2 treatment is stopped. Autologous LAK cell infusion by itself has minimal toxicity. Partial or complete responses have been seen in 13% to 57% of patients with advanced cancer, depending on the tumor type.[27] At least partial responses were seen in patients with renal cell cancer, melanoma, non-Hodgkin's lymphoma, and colorectal cancer. However, a recent prospective randomized trial of high dose IL-2 plus LAK cells produced complete remissions only in 3/27 melanoma patients and 7/46 renal cell cancer patients.[28] Though it remains to be seen whether this or other forms of adoptive immunotherapy can cure patients with advanced disease, this approach shows promise of becoming an important addition to the armamentarium of the clinical oncologist.

Although lymphocytes circulating in the peripheral blood of cancer patients can in certain cases be activated to become cytotoxic tumor-killer cells, these cells are apparently a relatively small percentage of circulating lymphocytes, and it requires high doses of IL-2 *in vivo* to keep these cells active. As noted above, these high doses of IL-2 have significant host toxicity.

Techniques have now been developed to isolate T lymphocytes directly from a patient's tumor, and these tumor-infiltrative lymphocytes (TIL) can also be clonally expanded in culture by adding IL-2. TIL cells bear a cell-surface marker called CD8 (and are thus CD8+). They can kill the hosts' tumor cells in culture in a major histocompatibility complex (MHC) class I–restricted manner and are 50 to 100 times more potent than LAK cells in reducing lung metastases in mouse model systems.[27] In order for TIL cells to be effective *in vivo*, IL-2 must also be injected, but it requires lower doses of IL-2 than for LAK-cell therapy. However, adjuvant treatment with cyclophosphamide or irradiation is required for TIL therapy to work. The reason for this isn't clear, but it may be that inhibition of T suppressor cells and/or the reduction of total tumor burden (with subsequent improved access of TIL to tumor tissue) are necessary for this approach to be effective.

Clinical trials have been initiated with TIL + IL-2 with or without cyclophosphamide. Results are better in regimens with cyclophosphamide, and overall about 38% of patients with melanoma have had at least a partial response.[27]

Studies with [111]Indium-labeled TIL have shown that up to 0.015% of injected TIL localize in each gram of tumor tissue. This localization effect has suggested another approach—i.e., using these cells to deliver cytotoxic products directly to tumors. This is discussed below under "Gene Therapy."

Colony Stimulating Growth Factors

The colony stimulating factors are a subset of regulatory polypeptides of the cytokine family that are involved in the proliferation and differentiation of granulocytes and monocyte/macrophages. They were originally called colony stimulating factors because they were discovered as a result of their ability to allow colonies of hematopoietic cells to grow in semisolid culture medium. The term "CSF" has stuck, and subsets of CSFs, based on their ability to stimulate particular pathways of hematopoietic cell differentiation, have been identified. These are granulocyte-macrophage stimulating (GM-CSF), granulocyte stimulating (G-CSF), monocyte/macrophage stimulating (M-CSF), and multicell type stimulating (multi-CSF or interleukin-3). Some of the other interleukins discussed above also foster early

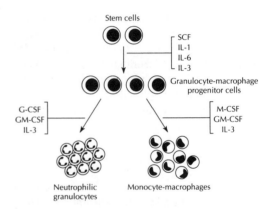

Figure 13–1   The four CSFs stimulate a population of committed granulocyte-macrophage progenitor cells to generate populations of maturing granulocytes or monocyte-macrophages. Several growth factors can influence the formation of progenitor cells by some cells in the more ancestral hematopoietic stem-cell compartment. (From Metcalf.[29])

progenitor-cell proliferation, as does a polypeptide called stem cell factor (SCF). (Figure 13–1).[29]

The CSFs are glycoproteins with 15,000–21,000 Da polypeptide chains and variable amounts of carbohydrate (Table 13–3). They consist of a single polypeptide chain, except M-CSF, which is a homodimer. They are produced by multiple cell types, including fibroblasts, placenta, endothelial cells, lymphocytes, and bone marrow stromal cells. Blood levels of CSFs are normally low, but their production can be rapidly elevated in response to infection. *In vitro*, some cell-type specificity can be demonstrated: GM-CSF and IL-3 stimulate formation of granulocyte and macrophage colonies; G-CSF favors granulocyte colony formation; and M-CSF fosters macrophage colony growth. In addition to stimulating progenitor cell pro-

Table 13–3   The Human CSFs. (From Metcalf[29])

Acronym	Polypeptide Chain (kD)	Native Glycosylated (kD)	Chromosomal Location
GM-CSF	14.7	18–30	5q23–31
G-CSF	18.6	20	17q11.2–21
M-CSF	21, 18	45–90	1p13–21
IL-3	15.4	15–30	5q23–31

liferation and cellular commitment to a particular differentiation pathway, the CSFs also are necessary to maintain functional activity of mature cells—e.g., chemotaxis, phagocytosis, and production and release of cytotoxic factors.[29]

Interestingly, receptors for multiple CSFs are present on many hematopoietic progenitor-cell types. There is a sort of redundancy in the signaling process for hematopoietic cell proliferation, as if nature has built in multiple mechanisms to protect the host from invading organisms and other stresses. For example, granulocyte-macrophage progenitor cells and their maturing progeny express membrane receptors for GM-, G-, M-, and multi-CSF. In addition, CSF-occupied receptors can initiate multiple functions in responding cells, implying that broad signaling cascades are initiated by receptor occupancy. As one might expect from these observations, there are numerous potential interactions among CSFs. For instance, combinations of two CSFs can produce additive or synergistic responses. Because CSF receptor levels are low (a few hundred per cell),[29] occupancy of more than one type of CSF receptor may be required for an optimal proliferative response. Alternatively, progenitor cells may have multiple receptor types so that they are able to respond either to their normal, most appropriate ligand, and secondarily to another, less optimal ligand that may be turned on by a different stress and/or a different CSF-producing cell type, so that the host can respond to any of a number of emergencies.

Other ligand-receptor interactions have also been observed. Binding of GM-CSF to its receptor down-regulates expression of G-CSF receptors. GM-CSF and IL-3 compete for binding to the same receptor. Macrophages are induced by IL-3 and M-CSF to produce G-CSF and also by GM-CSF to produce M-CSF. Obviously, there is a great deal of cross-talk between cells in the hematopoietic system, and it must require some finely tuned regulation, the mechanisms for which are only vaguely understood.

In spite of all the redundancies in the system, it is clear that in populations of bipotential progenitor cells, G-CSF fosters development of the cells in the granulocyte lineage and M-CSF fosters development of cells in the monocyte/macrophage lineage. This is borne out *in vivo* in that injection of G-CSF into mice induces a greater increase in peripheral blood granulocytes than other blood cells, whereas GM-CSF induces a rise in both macrophages and granulocytes (reviewed in ref. 29). IL-3 administration elicits a rise in granulocytes, macrophages, eosinophils, and megakaryocytes, as might be expected from its broad target-cell specificity.

Clinically, the CSFs have been used in treatment of AIDS, aplastic anemia, congenital or cyclic neutropenia, and in cancer. The latter use has been to restore bone marrow function after chemotherapy, often accompanied by bone marrow transplantation. Both G-CSF and GM-CSF have been shown to replenish peripheral blood neutrophils after high-dose chemotherapy followed by autologous bone-marrow transplantation.[30,31] Positive benefits include decreasing the frequency of infections and shortening the stay in the hospital.

An intriguing sidelight of CSF therapy was the observation of a dramatic rise in the number of progenitor cells in the peripheral blood.[32] Usually, these cells are largely restricted to the bone marrow. This raises the possibility of harvesting stem cells from the peripheral blood rather than the marrow. Advantages of this are the ability to recover many more stem cells and decreased trauma to the patient. A number of cytokines are currently being evaluated to attain maximal mobilization of stem cells into the peripheral blood. Clinical trails are being done to evaluate the use of peripheral stem cells rather than bone marrow cells, and the results are encouraging.

Tumor Necrosis Factor

In the late 1800s it was observed that a few cancer patients had regression of their tumors after a full-blown systemic bacterial infection. This led a handful of investigators, including William Coley in the United States, to attempt to treat cancers by infecting patients with certain bacteria (reviewed in ref. 33). The infectious process proved difficult to control, although a few positive responses were noted. There was sufficient encouragement, however, from this approach to prompt Coley in 1893 to try a mixture of killed bacteria (*Streptococcus pyogenes* and *Serratia merescens*). When he injected his "Coley's toxins" directly into tumors he got, in a few cases, some remarkable remissions of the tumor. This approach was taken by a number of investigators and continued on an experimental basis for a number of years. In fact, Coley's toxins were considered to be the only systemic therapy for cancer until the 1930s. With the advent of radiotherapy, chemotherapy, and improved cancer surgery, this treatment was abandoned and forgotten until the early 1980s.

It has been known for a long time that filtrates of certain bacteria such as the mycobacterium BCG and the corynebacterium C. parvum can induce a hemorrhagic necrosis of tumors when injected into tumor-bearing mice. Later work showed that an extract of gram-negative bacteria, known as endotoxin or bacterial pyrogen, could induce similar effects. Endotoxin was subsequently identified as a lipopolysaccharide (LPS). Because LPS is quite toxic, it never found its way into clinical use, but BCG and C. parvum have received extensive clinical trials and were not found to be very effective. The effectiveness of BCG and LPS against certain murine tumors in vivo, however, stimulated continued interest in finding the mechanism of this effect. The evidence pointed to the fact that these agents acted by modulating the host's immune response, probably by stimulating macrophages.

Attempts to define the antitumor mechanism of BCG and LPS led Old and his colleagues to test the serum of mice injected with BCG or LPS or both for antitumor activity. The serum of BCG-infected, LPS-injected mice produced hemorrhagic necrosis of mouse sarcomas in vivo. This effect required both BCG and LPS. Moreover, serum from BCG- and LPS-treated mice was also cytotoxic for a line of transformed mouse fibroblasts (L cells) in culture, but BCG and LPS added directly to the cultures were not, indicating that these agents were eliciting the release of some cytotoxic factor into the serum. It was also found that the in vivo necrotizing factor and the factor cytotoxic to cultured cells were one and the same. The factor was named tumor necrosis factor (TNF).[34]

TNF has also been shown to be identical to a cachexia-inducing factor called "cachectin."[35] This factor, also produced by macrophages, suppresses lipogenic enzymes such as

glycero-3-phosphate dehydrogenase. It has been postulated that the cachexia associated with cancer may involve endogenous release of TNF. In addition to macrophages and certain lymphoid cell lines, there is evidence that TNF can also be produced by NK cells and enodthelial cells. What role release from these latter cell types might play in vivo isn't yet clear. A variety of agents can modulate cellular release of TNF. TNF expression by producer cells is increased by IFN-γ and indomethacin and decreased by glucocorticoids and PGE$_2$.

The normal biological function of TNF also is a little vague. Since bacterial and parasitic infections stimulate TNF release by immune system cells, it is thought that the normal function of TNF is to help fight off these infectious processes. The role of TNF in increasing phagocytotic activity of PMNs, fat mobilization from adipocytes, and fever induction are most likely involved in TNF's infection fighting action.

It is likely that TNF is one of a family of tumor cell cytotoxic factors produced in the body. Another biological factor with TNF activity is lymphotoxin (LT), which is produced by mitogen-stimulated T lymphocytes and is thought to play a role in T-cell-mediated tumor cell killing.[33] It is now known that the genes for TNF and lymphotoxin are related but not identical. There is about 30% sequence homology at the amino acid level. These gene products have been termed TNF-α (has cachectin activity) and TNF-β (has lymphotoxin activity). TNF-α is produced primarily by monocyte/macrophage cells, although it is also produced by T and B lymphocytes, LAK cells, NK cells, neutrophils, astrocytes, endothelial cells, smooth muscle cells, and a variety of tumor cell lines, whereas TNF-β is produced almost exclusively by lymphoid cells (reviewed in ref. 36). TNF-α and -β are considered members of the "inflammatory cytokines" and are released at sites of inflammation. They also act as immunostimulants and mediators of host resistance to infectious agents and malignant cells. Overproduction of TNF-α during infection can lead to the septic shock syndrome.

The TNF-α and TNF-β genes are single-copy genes and closely linked within the MHC locus on chromosome 6 in humans. TNF-α is a trimer made up of 17,000 Da polypeptide chains. Native TNF-β is also a trimer; it consists of 25,000 Da subunits, each with one N-linked carbohydrate chain. TNF receptors of 55 kDa and 75 kDa have been identified, and most cell types examined have both types. Each receptor type binds TNF-α and -β with similar high affinity, and they appear to transduce signals via G-protein-mediated activation of protein kinases. The TNFs have a large number of biological activities and can induce a large number of genes in multiple target cells. These genes include transcription factors, cytokines, growth factors, adhesion molecules, inflammatory mediators, and acute-phase proteins.[36]

The tumor cell killing effect of TNF may be both direct and indirect. There is evidence that cells that bind TNF can be killed by induction of a cytolytic cascade of events, including generation of oxygen radicals, DNA fragmentation, and apoptosis.[37] Why TNF tends to kill tumor cells preferentially over normal cells isn't clear, but it may be related to a higher number of TNF receptors on tumor cells, more active internalization of TNF into tumor cells, ability of tumor cell lysosomes to more effectively process TNF into a cytotoxic form, or lack of some protective factor in tumor cells. There is evidence that TNF has to be internalized and processed in lysosomes to be cytotoxic, since resistant cells do not degrade TNF as avidly as sensitive cells and inhibitors of lysosomal enzymes reduce TNF cytotoxicity.[37] Indirect killing could occur by TNF-induced activation of macrophages and cytotoxic T cells at the site of the tumor.

The clinical usefulness of TNF has been relatively limited.[38] However, some responses have been observed, and in a study of patients with metastatic renal cell carcinoma who responded to IL-2 therapy, the serum levels of TNF correlated with response: 48 hours after IL-2 infusion, both TNF serum levels and biological activity were higher in the responders than in the nonresponders.[39]

Although TNF-α has some promising antitumor effects, the systemic toxicity observed after intravenous infusion limits its utility. Therefore, efforts have been made to deliver TNF more directly to tumors. One such approach is to encapsulate TNF in liposomes. Liposome-encapsulated recombinant human TNF-α has been reported to retain full immunostimulatory effects but have much-reduced toxic effects compared to free TNF-α when injected IV into normal rats.[40] Moreover, a new gene therapy approach incorporates the TNF-α gene into TIL cells in order to deliver TNF-producing cells directly to the tumor site (see "Gene Therapy" below).

Gene Therapy

The recently developed ability to clone specific human genes suggests another way to treat cancer. If the malignant phenotype results from the expression of certain "cancer genes," or the lack of expression of certain tumor suppressor genes, as the diminished tumorigenicity of hybrid cells derived from the fusion of normal and malignant cells suggests, then alteration of a cell's "gene dosage" for specific genes could significantly affect the outcome of a malignant growth. For example, if a tumor suppressor gene or a gene for the expression of a key differentiation factor could be delivered to leukemic cells in the bone marrow, the malignant process could be stopped or reversed. If the DNA coding for a particular gene were incorporated into the cell's genetic apparatus, a permanent reprogramming of the cell, which would be passed on to progeny cells, might be achieved. This could conceivably be done with bone marrow cells removed from a patient through the use of an appropriate physical means of DNA transfer or by a viral vector. This might also be achieved *in vivo* by injection of a viral vector targeted to the desired cell type.

Gene transfer has been successfully carried out *in vitro* and *in vivo* (reviewed in ref. 41) by physical/chemical means and by viral vectors. "Naked" functional DNA can be transferred into mammalian cells by: (1) coprecipitation of DNA with calcium phosphate and calcium phosphate–mediated cellular uptake, (2) use of polycation-or lipid-DNA complexes, (3) encapsulation of DNA into liposomes or erythrocyte ghosts, (4) microinjection of DNA into cells directly or via high-velocity tungsten "microprojectiles," and (5) exposure of cells to rapid pulses of high-voltage current (electrocorporation).

All of these methods have worked *in vitro*. A

general characteristic of these methods is the integration into the genome of multiple tandem repeats. These integrated sequences, however, may be unstable, and the overall efficiency of these physical/chemical transfection methods is reported to be only about 1% of treated cells.[41]

The use of viral vectors for transferring genes into cells is more efficient than physical/chemical means, and potentially, by the use of viruses with the right tissue tropism, every cell in a targeted tissue could be infected, delivering thereby the gene of interest. A wide variety of transducing viral vectors have been employed, including DNA viruses such as SV40, polyoma, and adenoviruses as well as retroviruses. The idea here is to insert the gene of interest into a virus that is nonpathogenic or genetically manipulated to be nonpathogenic and that efficiently infects host cells. The virus must also be able to stably integrate its genome bearing the desired gene into the host's genome. Another desirable characteristic, though it is not so easy to achieve, is that the integrated gene sequences be under the control of tissue specific promoters.

The transfer of functional genes into mammalian cells has been carried out *in vitro* and *in vivo*. For example, partial correction of a murine hereditary growth disorder has been achieved by germ-line incorporation of a growth-promoting gene.[42] Murine renal cell carcinoma cells transfected with a bovine papilloma virus expression vector bearing a murine interleukin-4 (IL-4) gene, and then injected into mice, secreted IL-4 *in vivo*.[43] This led to the infiltration of $CD8^+$ cytotoxic lymphocytes and activated macrophages into the tumor site and subsequent tumor rejection. *In vivo,* direct transfer of the normal human cystic fibrosis transmembrane conductance regulator (CFTR) gene into airway epithelial cells of the rat has been achieved.[44] This was done by intratracheal instillation of a replication-deficient recombinant adenovirus vector containing normal human CFTR cDNA. Two days after intratracheal introduction of the adenovirus vector, *in situ* analysis demonstrated CFTR gene expression in lung epithelium, and the CFTR gene continued to be expressed for up to 6 weeks after treatment. The CFTR protein was also detected in lung epithelial cells. These experiments illustrate the feasibility of gene therapy

in vivo and hold out the exciting possibility of correcting human genetic defects.

The effectiveness of gene therapy in humans is being examined. Several clinical trials are underway, including therapy for adenosine deaminase deficiency in which the adenosine deaminase (ADA) gene, transfected into the patient's own lymphocytes and then reinjected, can be expressed in patients with ADA deficiency and relieves symptoms related to that disease (reviewed in ref. 45). The TNF gene has been successfully transfected into human TIL cells *in vitro,* and clinical trials are underway to see whether these TNF-expressing cells will provide a local cell killing effect in patients' tumors.[27] Additional cytokine genes are also being considered for insertion into human TIL, including the genes for γ-interferon (IFN-γ), IL-2, IL-6, and T-cell receptors.[27] Clinical trials, based on the delivery system for CFTR used in rodents, were begun in 1993.

Antisense Oligonucleotide Therapy

Another potential approach to regulating gene expression in cancer cells is by introducing an antisense piece of DNA or RNA into such cells. The molecular trick here can be achieved either by DNA transfer of a coding sequence that has the reverse (complementary) sequence of the normal gene and that has a promoter on the "wrong end"—i.e., such that an RNA transcription product will be complementary to the normal mRNA transcript and be able to hybridize with it, or by introducing a smaller piece of DNA (an oligodeoxynucleotide) that can do the same thing. It has been shown that antisense transcripts form RNA–RNA duplexes with the normal transcript[46] and that insertion of "flipped gene" constructions of the thymidine kinase (TK) gene can inhibit expression of TK four- to fivefold in intact mouse L cells.[47] Such an approach might be used to inhibit the expression of cancer-associated genes if an antisense gene or oligodeoxynucleotide could be directed to cancer cells.

This approach will be discussed in more detail in Chapter 14. Suffice it to say here that this idea works *in vitro* with cultured human cancer cells. There are a number of examples. Retrovirus-mediated gene transfer has been used to introduce antisense RNA complementary to human creatine kinase mRNA into human histiocytic lymphoma cells, and this blocked translation of creatine kinase in these cells.[48] Antisense oligodeoxynucleotides specific for the BCL-2 gene in B-cell lymphomas has been shown to induce cell death of human pre-B-cell acute lymphocytic leukemia cells.[49] Antisense oligodeoxynucleotides to the N-*myc* gene have been shown to block N-*myc* expression and inhibit proliferation of human neuroblastoma cells.[50] Transfection of a recombinant plasmid containing a genomic segment of the K-*ras* protooncogene in the antisense orientation by electrocorporation into a human lung cancer cell line inhibited expression of K-*ras* and proliferation of the cells.[51]

Such a therapeutic approach remains to be proven in patients, but if *in vivo* stability and tissue specific targeting problems can be solved, such therapy would be very attractive because it could produce tumor-specific cell killing with minimal toxicity to the patient.

Monoclonal Antibodies

A remarkable advance in the preparation of antibodies that recognize specific antigenic determinants has been provided by the work of Köhler and Milstein.[52] They showed that fusion of an antigenically stimulated lymphocyte with a malignant myeloma cell, whose whole protein-synthetic machinery is geared to make immunoglobulins, results in the formation of a hybrid cell (hybridoma) that produces large amounts of antibody against the antigenic determinant originally recognized by the stimulated lymphocyte. In an immunized animal, different clones of lymphocytes that recognize different antigenic determinants on the injected antigen are produced. The fusion of a population of antibody-producing lymphocytes obtained from the spleen of an immunized animal with myeloma cells will result in clones of hybridomas, each producing antibodies highly specific for a given antigenic determinant recognized by the injected animal as foreign. These highly specific antibodies arising from discrete hybridoma clones are called monoclonal antibodies.

The hybridoma clones are obtained by fusing cells in the presence of Sendai virus or polyethylene glycol to make cell membranes soft and sticky, such that two cells in contact will fuse to form a heterokaryon containing nuclei from both cell types. With continued passage in culture, the nuclei ultimately fuse to form a true hybrid cell. The myeloma cell line that is usually used in these fusions is one that has been selected by development of resistance to 8-azaguanine for a deficiency in an enzyme involved in nucleic acid synthesis, hypoxanthine-guanine phosphoribosyl transferase (HGPRT). The cultures are then grown in a medium in which only hybrid cells will survive. The fused cells are then cloned to select for hybridomas making specific antibodies. Once it is determined which clones make antibody, these clones can be grown in large cultures or injected back into the peritoneal cavity of animals who become living incubators for the proliferation of antibody-producing cells. Incredible amounts of specific, high-titer antibody can be obtained from the ascites fluid of a relatively few animals. Thus, one can obtain a panel of highly specific antibodies directed at different antigenic determinants of a single antigen in a relatively inexpensive manner. Another advantage of this technique is that it is not necessary to have pure antigen to obtain specific antibodies. Specific antibodies have been obtained, for example, by the injection of whole tumor cells or cell homogenates into mice, followed by hybridoma formation and cloning. In this way, specific antibodies directed against animal and human cancer cells have been obtained.

The potential use of monoclonal antibodies that recognize tumor-associated antigenic determinants is far-reaching. Monoclonal antibodies directed against tumor cell surface components can inhibit tumor cell proliferation in culture and in whole animals.[53,54] Administration of monoclonal antibodies directly to patients has been tried, with limited success so far. Monoclonal antibodies by themselves will most likely be of therapeutic benefit in clearing circulating tumor cells from the blood, in diminishing the amount of circulating tumor antigen, which could have a blocking effect on subsequent immunotherapy, and in clearing the bone marrow of tumor cells so that it can be used for autologous transplantation in patients after they have been treated with bone marrow suppressive therapy.[55-57] In the latter case, samples of the patient's marrow are removed, treated with antibody directed against the type of tumor antigen present on the surface of their cells (determined by "typing" of the patient's tumor cells with a panel of monoclonal antibodies prepared against the particular type of tumor that they have), and stored frozen until after the patient is treated. Then the patient's own bone marrow is injected in order to restore normal bone marrow function.

Monoclonal antibodies can also be complexed with antitumor drugs, toxins, or radionuclides. The rationale of this approach is to target toxic substances directly to the tumor cells and spare normal cells. This approach has been tried experimentally with some success. For example, conjugates of antitumor antibody and the anticancer drug daunomycin have been shown to inhibit the growth of lung carcinomas and hepatomas in animals with more efficacy than the drug or the antibody alone or than an unconjugated mixture of drug and antibody.[58,59]

Doxorubicin conjugated with a monoclonal antibody directed to a human melanoma-associated proteoglycan has been shown to suppress growth of human melanomas growing in nude mice.[60] Coupling of bacterial toxins such as diphtheria toxin or plant toxins such as abrin and ricin, all of which are potent inhibitors of protein synthesis and extremely toxic for mammalian cells, has also been tried as an approach to more selective tumor cell killing. For example, conjugates of ricin A chain to monoclonal antibodies against T-cell leukemias or Burkitt's lymphoma cells are specifically toxic for the malignant cells bearing the tumor-associated antigen [61-63] and can be shown to selectively kill tumor cells mixed with normal bone marrow.[63] Such toxin-monoclonal antibody conjugates may be useful in clearing tumor cells from the bone marrow prior to autologous marrow transplantation as indicated above. Whether such drug-antibody or toxin-antibody conjugates will provide an advantage for systemic cancer therapy, however, remains an open question.

A number of clinical trials with Mab-toxin conjugates have been initiated (reviewed in ref. 64). Although some responses have been observed, a number of problems with this approach have emerged. Some of these problems are common to all monoclonal antibody therapy. The problems include: (1) the difficulty of Mabs' being able to penetrate into solid tumor masses in such a way as to deliver pharmacologically effective concentrations of drug or toxin, (2) the heterogeneity of tumors such that in any given tumor cell population only a minority of cells may have the targeted tumor antigen, (3) formation of anti-IgG antibodies by the patient, (4) the possible toxicity of antigen-antibody complexes (e.g., renal failure), and (5) the blocking effect of high circulating tumor antigen, which could neutralize the antibody conjugate. A higher rate of success will likely be achieved by the use of monoclonal antibody-radionuclide complexes, because sufficient radioactivity may be able to be delivered to the area of the tumor regardless of the facts that the complex doesn't penetrate all the way into the interior of the tumor and that there is heterogeneity with respect to display of surface antigen. Moreover, such monoclonal antibody-radionuclide conjugates can be used to localize tumors diagnostically. Iodine-125, iodine-131, and technetium-99m have been coupled to monoclonal antibodies and been used successfully to radiolocalize human tumor xenografts growing in nude mice.[65-68] The feasibility of this approach has been shown in patients by the successful localization of colon carcinoma with ^{131}I-labeled monoclonal antibodies to colon cancer antigens[69] and of hepatocellular carcinoma with ^{131}I-labeled antiferritin.[70] Thus, this approach using radiolabeled antibodies holds diagnostic as well as therapeutic potential for the treatment of cancer.

An advantage of radiolabeled monoclonal antibody conjugates for diagnosis and therapy is that regardless of tumor cell antigenic heterogeneity, as long as a significant number of the cells in the tumor bear the antigens recognized by the antibody, the Mab should be taken up by the tumor. The localized radioisotope should then be effective. For diagnostic purposes, localized radioisotope of appropriate energy can be detected by external radioimaging devices. For a therapeutic goal, the radiolabeled Mabs can kill cells that are millimeters away and thus be effective even against antigen-negative cells close to the antigen-expressing cells.

For a radiolabeled monoclonal antibody conjugate to be effective, it must possess the following characteristics: (1) the radionuclide must be tightly linked to the antibody so that significant amounts of free radioactivity aren't released from the antibody; (2) the chelating agent and the coupling reaction cannot compromise antibody specificity or negatively affect the pharmacokinetics and biodistribution of the Mab; and (3) the Mab conjugate should not cross-react with normal tissues. Several β-emitters have been used for Mab conjugates, including ^{131}I, ^{90}Y, ^{186}Re, and ^{67}Cu.[71]

Future directions in isotopic labeled monoclonal antibody research will focus on the development of better localizing Mabs, the use of α-emitters that have higher energy and better localized cell-killing effects, and the development of genetically engineered or human Mabs that are less likely to generate an anti-antibody immune response than the currently used murine antibodies. In addition, other cell targets will be used to direct Mabs to tumors. These include tumor cell surface mucins, for which there is evidence for some tumor type specificity,[72] and cell surface cytokine receptors such as the inducible α chain of the interleukin-2 receptor (IL-2Rα) expressed on the surface of abnormal T lymphocytes.[71] The latter target has been utilized in a clinical study of patients with adult T-cell leukemia. An Mab targeted to the IL-2Rα receptor has been shown to induce remission in about one-third of patients without significant toxicity.[71] This selectivity is presumably due to the fact that resting T cells do not express IL-2Rα, whereas abnormal T cells do. Similar approaches can be visualized for the development of antireceptor Mabs targeted to receptors for tumor-derived paracrine or autocrine growth factors.

To circumvent the problems with murine Mabs, genetically engineered antibodies combining mouse variable or hypervariable regions (the specific antigen-binding region) with human constant and variable framework regions have been produced. This is done by transfecting hybrid mouse-human immunoglobulin genes into lymphoid cells that can express a chimeric protein from such genes. In this way, human-mouse Mabs to human colorectal, mammary, pancreatic, and B- and T-cell lymphomas have been made (reviewed in ref. 71). Although such "humanized" Mabs appear to be less immunogenic, the presence of human

allotypes on the hybrid immunoglobulin may still provide a "foreign" determinant. Early clinical trials suggest, nevertheless, that the hybrid Mabs are less immunogenic and have a longer plasma half-life.

An ultimate goal is the development of totally human Mabs against cancer cells. A number of approaches have been tried. Human B-cell lymphoid cell lines immortalized by Epstein-Barr virus have been employed as the antibody-producing cell type, but these cells produce low amounts of the expected IgM-type antibodies. Human antibodies produced in severe combined immunodeficient (SCID) mice by reconstituting their bone marrow and lymphoid tissue with human counterpart cells has been attempted and may work, but clinical trials have not yet been done with such Mabs to prove this.

Another approach bypasses hybridoma technology altogether. In this procedure, immunoglobulin variable-region genes from human B cells are cloned by the polymerase chain-reaction technique and then expressed in *E. coli* and screened for ability to bind antigen. By this technique, large libraries of immunoglobulin genes can be generated and screened for antigen-binding specificity. Another advantage of this system is that such clones of Ig genes can be genetically manipulated to generate immunoglobulins of desired antigen specificity.

Modification of Tumor-cell Antigenicity

Since many tumors are apparently not immunogenic enough to stimulate an effective immune response against them, increasing their antigenicity could be a way to induce a more effective host immune response. For example, one way might be to remove tumor cells from a patient, modify them with chemicals or viruses to make them more immunogenic, and then inject them back into the patient after sterilizing them by X-irradiation or cytotoxic drugs.

Tumor cell immunogenicity could also be increased by modulating expression of MHC gene products on tumor cells. Since class I MHC antigens are necessary for the presentation and recognition of tumor cell neoantigens by cytolytic T lymphocytes, their masking or absence on tumor cell surfaces may be key to their ability to escape an immune response of the host. One way to alter this is to introduce—by DNA-mediated gene transfer, for example—the genes for the missing MHC class I molecules. This has been done in adenovirus 12–transformed cells that lack expression of an H-2 class I gene product and that produce lethal tumors in syngeneic mice.[73] The induced expression of a single type of class I gene was sufficient to block the *in vivo* tumorigenicity of these cells. Thus, an approach to cancer therapy may be to increase or modulate expression of class I genes in tumor cells. IFN-γ can increase expression of class I antigens in certain cells.[73] Other such modulators may also be found.

Another method to boost a patient's response to a tumor is to transfect cytokine genes into surgically removed tumor cells followed by reimplantation or to deliver such genes by tumor-targeted gene therapy *in vivo* so that their recognition by immune cells is increased. Insertion of genes for IL-4, IL-2, TNF, IFN-γ, and GM-CSF into tumor cells has been attempted (reviewed in ref. 27).

Tumor Vaccines

For those cancers that are initiated or promoted by infectious viruses, it is conceivable that a vaccine derived from inactivated viruses or a preparation of viral antigens would prevent the onset of the disease. For example, there is a strong correlation between hepatitis B virus (HBV) infection and hepatocellular carcinomas. In a number of countries where hepatitis B infection is widespread, there is a high incidence of liver cancer. In China and twenty other countries where infection is endemic and liver cancer rates are high, an active immunization program against HBV is underway. Although HBV vaccination is not expected to eliminate liver cancer entirely because some liver tumors are HBV-negative, it is predicted that the rate of liver cancer in endemic areas might be reduced by as much as 80%. However, this might take twenty to thirty years to be evident, since the infant population receiving immunization now wouldn't be expected to develop liver carcinomas until age 20 to 40.

Other cancers with a likely viral etiology include adult T-cell leukemia associated with HTLV-1 infection endemic in certain parts of Japan and the Caribbean, cervical carcinoma associated with human papilloma virus (HPV), and certain B-cell lymphomas (e.g., Burkitt's) and nasopharyngeal carcinoma associated with Epstein-Barr virus (EBV). Effective vaccines have not yet been developed or clinically tested for these latter viruses, however, and it remains to be seen if these diseases could be prevented by such an approach.

Vaccination of patients who already have cancer is entirely another matter, and will likely be much more difficult to accomplish successfully. As noted above, several attempts have been made to elicit tumor immunity by inoculation of sterilized tumor cells or tumor associated antigen-containing cell lysates, sometimes with adjuvants such as BCG, or by injection of antiidiotypic antibodies directed against tumor associated antigens (reviewed in refs. 74 and 75). Such approaches have in certain instances shown some promising results, but overall these therapies have met with limited success.

Another idea is to construct recombinant viruses that express tumor associated antigens so that infected tumor cells will display the target antigen together with host MHC antigens and immunogenic viral proteins (via the normal cellular mechanism for antigen processing). This has achieved some success in experimental animal studies. For instance, vaccinia virus recombinants expressing a breast cancer-associated mucin called H23 epithelial tumor antigen (ETA) have been utilized to inoculate Fisher rats that were subsequently challenged with *ras*-transformed tumorigenic cells bearing H23 ETA.[75] Vaccination of rats with the recombinant virus expressing H23 ETA prior to challenge with the tumorigenic cells prevented tumor development in 82% of animals, whereas all animals inoculated with tumorigenic cells without prior vaccination developed tumors. These and other data encourage the idea that if an appropriate immune stimulus can be provided to an immunocompetent patient, at least a partial rejection reaction may be mounted in that patient. It is important to point out that this is unlikely to be effective in patients with a large tumor burden or in immunocompromised patients. Nevertheless, as an adjuvant to other treatment modalities such as surgery, radiation, or chemotherapy, immunotherapy may provide the extra needed "punch" to completely eliminate the residual tumor or silent metastases present in a patient, leading to more cures than are currently achievable by standard therapy.

REFERENCES

1. J. E. Talmadge and J. Clark: "Biological response modifiers: Preclinical and clinical results," in *Cancer Chemotherapy and Biological Response Modifiers,* Annual 9, ed. by H. M. Pinedo, D. L. Longo, and B. A. Chabner. Amsterdam: Elsevier 1987, pp. 454–472.

2. R. Engelhardt, A. Mackensen, and C. Galanos: Phase I trial of intravenously administered endotoxin (*Salmonella abortus equi*) in cancer patients. *Cancer Res.* 51:2524 (1991).

3. N. Inamura, K. Nakahara, T. Kino, T. Gotoh, I. Kawamura, H. Aoki, H. Imanaka, and S. Sone: Activation of tumoricidal properties in macrophages and inhibition of experimentally-induced murine metastases by a new synthetic acyltripeptide, FK-565. *J. Biol. Response Modif.* 4:408 (1985).

4. E. L. Morgan, S. D. Sanderson, W. Scholz, D. J. Noonan, W. O. Weigle, and T. E. Hugli: Identification and characterization of the effector region within human C5a responsible for stimulation of interleukin-6 synthesis. *J. Immunol.* 148:3937 (1992).

5. C. G. Moertel T. R. Fleming, J. S. MacDonald, D. G. Haller, J. A. Laurie, P. J. Goodman, J. S. Ungerleider, W. A. Emerson, D. C. Tormey, J. H. Glick, M. H. Veeder, and J. A. Mailliard: Levamisole and fluorouracil for adjuvant therapy of resected colon carcinoma. *New Engl. J. Med.* 322:352 (1990).

6. C. Nathan and M. Sporn: Cytokines in context. *J. Cell Biol.* 113:981 (1991).

7. A. Isaacs and J. Lindenmann: Virus interference. I. The interferon. *Proc. Roy. Soc. Ser. B* 147:258 (1957).

8. K. C. Zoon and R. Wetzel: "Comparative structures of mammalian interferons," in *Interferons and Their Applications,* ed. by P. E. Came and W. A. Carter. New York: Springer-Verlag, 1984.

9. K. L. Fresa and D. M. Murasko: Role of natural killer cells in the mechanism of the antitumor effect of interferon on Moloney sarcoma virus-transformed cells. *Cancer Res.* 46:81 (1986).

10. L. Varesio, E. Blasi, G. B. Thurman, J. E., Talmadge, R. H. Wiltrout, and R. B. Herberman: Potent activation of mouse macrophage by recombinant interferon-γ. *Cancer Res.* 44:4465 (1984).

11. Y. Akiyama, M. D. Lubeck, Z. Steplewski, and H. Koprowski: Induction of mouse IgG2a- and IgG3-dependent cellular cytotoxicity in human monocytic cells (U937) by immune interferon. *Cancer Res.* 44:5127 (1984).

12. I. J. Fidler: Macrophages and metastasis—A biological approach to cancer therapy. *Cancer Res.* 45:4714 (1985).

13. S. B. Mizel: The interleukins. *FASEB J.* 3:2379 (1989).

14. J. Laver and M. A. S. Moore: Clinical use of recombinant human hematopoietic growth factors. *J. Natl. Cancer Inst.* 81:1370 (1989).

15. C. A. Dinarello: Biology of interleukin 1. *FASEB J.* 2:108 (1988).

16. W. E. Paul and J. Ohara: B-cell stimulatory factor—1/interleukin 4. *Annu. Rev. Immunol.* 5:429 (1987).

17. S. Akira, T. Hirano, T. Taga, and T. Kishimoto: Biology of multifunctional cytokines: IL 6 and related molecules (IL 1 and TNF) *FASEB J.* 4:2860 (1990).

18. K. Ikebuchi, G. G. Wong, S. C. Clark, J. N. Ihle, Y. Hirai, and M. Ogawa: Interleukin 6 enhancement of interleukin 3-dependent proliferation of multipotential hemopoietic progenitors. *Proc. Natl. Acad. Sci. USA* 84:9035 (1987).

19. A. E. Namen, S. J. Lupton, K. Hjerrild, J. Wignall, A. Schmierer, B. Mosley, C. J. March, D. Urdal, S. Gillis, D. Cosman, and R. G. Goodwin: Stimulation of B-cell progenitors by cloned murine interleukin-7. *Nature* 333:571 (1988).

20. M. A. Gimbrone, Jr., M. S. Obin, A. F. Brock, E. A. Luis, P. E. Hass, C. A. Hebert, Y. K. Yip, D. W. Leung, D. G. Lowe, W. J. Kohr, W. C. Darbonne, K. B. Bechtol, and J. B. Baker: Endothelial interleukin-8: A novel inhibitor of leukocyte-endothelial interactions. *Science* 246:1601 (1989).

21. P. Scott: IL-12: Initiation cytokine for cell-mediated immunity. *Science* 260:496 (1993).

22. C. S. Tripp, S. F. Wolf, and E. R. Unanue: Interleukin 12 and tumor necrosis factor α are costimulators of interferon γ production by natural killer cells in severe combined immunodeficiency mice with listeriosis, and interleukin 10 is a physiologic antagonist. *Proc. Natl. Acad. Sci. USA* 90:3725 (1993).

23. A. N. J. McKenzie, J. A. Culpepper, R. De Waal Malefyt, F. Briére, J. Punnonen, G. Aversa, A. Sato, W. Dang, B. G. Cocks, S. Menon, J. E. De Vries, J. Banchereau, and G. Zurawski: Interleukin 13, a T-cell-derived cytokine that regulates human monocyte and B-cell function. *Proc. Natl. Acad. Sci. USA* 90:3735 (1993).

24. S. A. Rosenberg, M. T. Lotze, L. M. Muul, S. Leitman, A. E. Chang, S. E. Ettinghausen, Y. L. Matory, J. M. Skibber, E. Shiloni, J. T. Vetto, C. A. Seipp, C. Simpson, and C. M. Reichert: Observations on the systemic administration of autologous lymphokine-activated killer cells and recombinant interleukin-2 to patients with metastatic cancer. *New Engl. J. Med.* 313:1485 (1985).

25. M. G. Hanna, J. S. Brandhorst, and L. C. Peters: Active specific immunotherapy of residual micrometastases: An evaluation of sources, doses, and ratios of BCG with tumor cells. *Cancer Immunol. Immunother.* 7:165 (1979).

26. J. J. Mule, S. Shu, S. L. Schwarz, and S. A. Rosenberg: Adoptive immunotherapy of established pulmonary metastases with LAK cells and recombinant interleukin-2. *Science* 225:1487 (1984).

27. S. A. Rosenberg: Immunotherapy and gene therapy of cancer. *Cancer Res. (Suppl.)* 51:5074s (1991).

28. S. A. Rosenberg, M. T. Lotze, J. C. Yang, S. L. Topalian, A. E. Chang, D. J. Schwartzentruber, P. Aebersold, S. Leitman, W. M. Linehan, C. A. Seipp, D. E. White, and S. M. Steinberg: Prospective randomized trial of high-dose

interleukin-2 alone or in conjunction with lymphokine-activated killer cells for the treatment of patients with advanced cancer. *J. Natl. Cancer Inst.* 85:622 (1993).

29. D. Metcalf: Control of granulocytes and macrophages: Molecular, cellular, and clinical aspects. *Science* 254:529 (1991).

30. W. P. Hammond IV, T. H. Price, L. M. Souza, and D. C. Dale: Treatment of cyclic neutropenia with granulocyte colony-stimulating factor. *New Engl. J. Med.* 320:1306 (1989).

31. J. Vose, P. Bierman, A. Kessinger, P. Coccia, J. Anderson, F. Oldham, C. Epstein, J. Armitage: The use of recombinant human granulocyte-macrophage colony stimulating factor for the treatment of delayed engraftment following high dose therapy and autologous hematopoietic stem cell transplantation for lymphoid malignancies. *Bone Marrow Transp.* 7:139 (1991).

32. U. Duhrsen, J.-L. Vileval, J. Boyd, G. Kannourakis, G. Morstyn, and D. Metcalf: Effects of recombinant human granulocyte colony-stimulating factor on hematopoietic progenitor cells in cancer patients. *Blood* 72:2074 (1988).

33. L. J. Old: Tumor necrosis factor (TNF). *Science* 230:630 (1985).

34. E. A. Carswell, L. J. Old, R. L. Kassel, S. Green, N. Fiore, and B. Williamson: An endotoxin-induced serum factor that causes necrosis of tumors. *Proc. Natl. Acad. Sci. USA* 72:3666 (1975).

35. B. Beutler and A. Cerami: Cachectin and tumor necrosis factor as two sides of the same biological coin. *Nature* 320:584 (1986).

36. J. Vilcek and T. H. Lee: Tumor necrosis factor: New insights into the molecular mechanism of its multiple actions. *J. Biol. Chem.* 266:7313 (1991).

37. J. W. Larrick and S. C. Wright: Cytotoxic mechanism of tumor necrosis factor-α. *FASEB J.* 4:3215 (1990).

38. J. K. McIntosh, J. J. Mule, W. D. Travis, and S. A. Rosenberg: Studies of effects of recombinant human tumor necrosis factor on autochthonous tumor and transplanted normal tissue in mice. *Cancer Res.* 50:2463 (1990).

39. J-Y. Blay, M. C. Favrot, S. Negrier, V. Combaret, S. Chouaib, A. Mercatello, P. Kaemmerlen, C. R. Franks, and T. Philip: Correlation between clinical response to interleukin 2 therapy and sustained production of tumor necrosis factor. *Cancer Res.* 50:2371 (1990).

40. R. J. Debs, H. J. Fuchs, R. Philip, E. N. Brunette, N. Duzgunes, J. E. Shellito, D. Liggitt, and J. R. Patton: Immunomodulatory and toxic effects of free and liposome-encapsulated tumor necrosis factor α in rats. *Cancer Res.* 50:375 (1990).

41. T. Friedmann: Progress toward human gene therapy. *Science* 244:1275 (1989).

42. R. E. Hammer, R. D. Palmiter, and R. L. Brinster: Partial correction of murine hereditary growth disorder by germ-line incorporation of a new gene. *Nature* 311:65 (1984).

43. P. T. Golumbek, A. J. Lazenby, H. I. Levitsky, L. M. Jaffee, H. Karasuyama, M. Baker, and D. M. Pardoll: Treatment of established renal cancer by tumor cells engineered to secrete interleukin-4. *Science* 254:713 (1991).

44. M. A. Rosenfeld, K. Yoshimura, B. C. Trapnell, K. Yoneyama, E. R. Rosenthal, W. Dalemans, M. Fukayama, J. Bargon, L. E. Stier, L. Stratford-Perricaudet, M. Perricau-

det, W. B. Guggino, A. Pavirani, J-P. Lecocq, and R. G. Crystal: In vivo transfer of the human cystic fibrosis transmembrane conductance regulator gene to the airway epithelium. *Cell* 68:143 (1992).

45. L. Thompson: At age 2, gene therapy enters a growth phase. *Science* 258:744 (1992).

46. J. Tomizawa, T. Itoh, G. Selzer, and T. Som: Inhibition of ColE1 primer formation by a plasmid-specified small RNA. *Proc. Natl. Acad. Sci. USA* 78:1421 (1981).

47. J. G. Izant and H. Weintraub: Inhibition of thymidine kinase gene expression by antisense RNA: A molecular approach to genetic analysis. *Cell* 36:1007 (1984).

48. J. L. C. Ch'ng, R. C. Mulligan, P. Schimmel, and E. W. Holmes: Antisense RNA complementary to 3' coding and noncoding sequences of creatine kinase is a potent inhibitor of translation in vivo. *Proc. Natl. Acad. Sci. USA* 86:10006 (1989).

49. J. C. Reed, C. Stein, C. Subasinghe, S. Haldar, C. M. Croce, S. Yum, and J. Cohen: Antisense-mediated inhibition of BCL2 protooncogene expression and leukemic cell growth and survival: Comparisons of phosphodiester and phosphorothioate oligodeoxynucleotides. *Cancer Res.* 50:6565 (1990).

50. A. Rosolen, L. Whitesell, N. Ikegaki, R. H. Kennett, and L. M. Neckers: Antisense inhibition of single copy N-myc expression results in decreased cell growth without reduction of c-myc protein in a neuroepithelioma cell line. *Cancer Res.* 50:6316 (1990).

51. T. Mukhopadhyay, M. Tainsky, A. C. Cavender, and J. A. Roth: Specific inhibition of K-ras expression and tumorigenicity of lung cancer cells by antisense RNA. *Cancer Res.* 51:1744 (1991).

52. G. Köhler and C. Milstein: Continuous cultures of fused cells secreting antibody of predefined specificity. *Nature* 256:495 (1975).

53. H. P. Vollmers, B. A. Imhof, I. Wieland, A. Hiesel, and W. Birchmeier: Monoclonal antibodies. NORM-1 and NORM-2 induce more normal behavior of tumor cells in vitro and reduce tumor growth in vivo. *Cell* 40:547 (1985).

54. H. Masui, T. Kawamoto, J. D. Sato, B. Wolf, G. Sato, and J. Mendelsohn: Growth inhibition of human tumor cells in athymic mice by anti-epidermal growth factor receptor monoclonal antibodies. *Cancer Res.* 44:1002 (1984).

55. L. M. Nadler, P. Stashenko, R. Hardy, W. D. Kaplan, L. N. Button, D. W. Kufe, K. N. Antman, and S. F. Schlossman: Serotherapy of a patient with a monoclonal antibody directed against a human lymphoma-associated antigen. *Cancer Res.* 40:3147 (1980).

56. R. C. Bast Jr., P. DeFabritiis, J. Lipton, R. Gelber, C. Mauer, L. Nadler, S. Sallan, and J. Ritz: Elimination of malignant clonogenic cells from human bone marrow using multiple monoclonal antibodies and complement. *Cancer Res.* 45:499 (1985).

57. J. J. Vredenburgh, Jr., and E. D. Ball: Elimination of small cell carcinoma of the lung from human bone marrow by monoclonal antibodies and immunomagnetic beads. *Cancer Res.* 50:7216 (1990).

58. E. Hurwitz, B. Schechter, R. Arnon, and M. Sela: Binding of anti-tumor immunoglobulins and their daunomycin conjugates to the tumor and its metastasis. In vitro and in vivo studies with Lewis lung carcinoma. *Int. J. Cancer* 24:461 (1979).

59. Y. Tsukada, W. K.-D. Bischof, N. Hirai, H. Hirai, E.

Hurwitz, and M. Sela: Effect of a conjugate of daunomycin and antibodies to rat α-fetoprotein on the growth of α-fetoprotein-producing tumor cells. *Proc. Natl. Acad. Sci. USA* 79:621 (1982).

60. H. M. Yang and R. A. Reisfeld: Doxorubicin conjugated with a monoclonal antibody directed to a human melanoma-associated proteoglycan suppresses the growth of established tumor xenografts in nude mice. *Proc. Natl. Acad. Sci. USA* 85:1189 (1988).

61. V. Raso, J. Ritz, M. Basala, and S. F. Schlossman: Monoclonal antibody-ricin A chain conjugate selectively cytotoxic for cells bearing the common acute lymphoblastic leukemia antigen. *Cancer Res.* 42:457 (1982).

62. B. K. Seon: Specific killing of human T-leukemia cells by immunotoxins prepared with ricin A chain and monoclonal anti-human T-cell leukemia antibodies. *Cancer Res.* 44:259 (1984).

63. M. Bregni, P. DeFabritiis, V. Raso, J. Greenberger, J. Lipton, L. Nadler, L. Rothstein, J. Ritz, and R. C. Bast, Jr.: Elimination of clonogenic tumor cells from human bone marrow using a combination of monoclonal antibody: Ricin A chain conjugates. *Cancer Res.* 46:1208 (1986).

64. I. Pastan and D. FitzGerald: Recombinant toxins for cancer treatment. *Science* 254:1173 (1991).

65. T. Nakamura, H. Sakahara, S. Hosoi, T. Yamamuro, S. Higashi, H. Mikawa, K. Endo, and S. Toyama: In vivo radiolocalization of antiosteogenic sarcoma monoclonal antibodies in osteogenic sarcoma xenografts. *Cancer Res.* 44:2078 (1984).

66. D. Colcher, A. M. Kennan, S. M. Larson, and J. Schlom: Prolonged binding of a radiolabeled monoclonal antibody (B72.3) used for the in situ radioimmunodetection of human colon carcinoma xenografts. *Cancer Res.* 44:5744 (1984).

67. S. A. Shah, B. M. Gallagher, and H. Sands: Radioimmunodetection of small human tumor xenografts in spleen of athymic mice by monoclonal antibodies. *Cancer Res.* 45:5824 (1985).

68. D. R. Elmaleh, P. C. Zamecnik, F. P. Castronovo, Jr., H. W. Strauss, and E. Rapaport: ^{99m}Tc-labeled nucleotides as tumor-seeking radiodiagnostic agents. *Proc. Natl. Acad. Sci. USA* 81:918 (1984).

69. J.-P. Mach, J.-F. Chatal, J.-D. Lumbroso, F. Buchegger, M. Forni, J. Ritschard, C. Berche, J.-Y. Douillard, S. Carrel, M. Herlyn, Z. Steplewski, and H. Koprowski: Tumor localization in patients by radiolabeled monoclonal antibodies against colon carcinoma. *Cancer Res.* 43:5593 (1983).

70. P. K. Leichner, J. L. Klein, S. S. Siegelman, D. S. Ettinger, and S. E. Order: Dosimetry of ^{131}I-labeled antiferritin in hepatoma: Specific activities in the tumor and liver. *Cancer Treat. Rep.* 67:647 (1983).

71. T. A. Waldmann: Monoclonal antibodies in diagnosis and therapy. *Science* 252:1657 (1991).

72. R. S. Metzgar, M. A. Hollingsworth, and B. Kaufman: "Pancreatic Mucins," in *The Pancreas*, Vol. 2, ed. by V. L. Go, E. Dimagno, J. Gardner, I. Lebenthal, H. Reber, and G. Scheele. New York: Raven Press, 1993, pp. 351–367.

73. K. Tanaka, K. J Isselbacher, G. Khoury, and G. Jay: Reversal of oncogenesis by the expression of a major histocompatability complex class I gene. *Science* 228:26 (1985).

74. F. K. Stevenson: Tumor vaccines. *FASEB J.* 5:2250 (1991).

75. M. Hareuveni, C. Gautier, M-P. Kieny, K. Wreschner, P. Chambon, and R. Lathe: Vaccination against tumor cells expressing breast cancer epithelial tumor antigen. *Proc. Natl. Acad. Sci. USA* 87:9498 (1990).

CHAPTER FOURTEEN

Potential Targets for New Anticancer Drugs

Advancing knowledge of the cellular and molecular biology of processes that regulate cell proliferation, cell differentiation, and cellular responses to external signals has provided a number of potential targets for new approaches to treating cancer.

We now know a lot more than we did even a few years ago about what regulates gene transcription and translation, what factors control cell proliferation and differentiation, how a cell interacts with external signals such as hormones and growth factors, and what mechanisms transduce these signals into stimulatory or inhibitory cellular responses. In addition, we know quite a bit more about the alterations of gene expression that occur in cancer cells and about how cancer cells can grow in an unregulated fashion, resist the action of drugs, and metastasize.

This new knowledge has provided a wealth of information about the biochemistry and biology of the cancer cell and about how a cancer cell differs from the normal cells in tissues in which cancer arises. It is these differences that must be exploited in the development of the next generation of anticancer agents. The dictum in the development of these new agents is: Kill cancer cells, but do as little damage as possible to normal cells. This is usually difficult to do, but it is the standard by which new therapies must be measured.

In this chapter we explore a number of potential targets for new drug development. Where possible, we mention some potential agents that can attack these targets in cancer cells. However, in many instances, effective inhibitors may not be available or may not be practical for systemic use in humans. These targets, then, await some innovative schemes for drug development.

DNA Replication and Repair

DNA Polymerase

Research on bacterial DNA replication in the 1970s indicated that there were at least two DNA polymerases, pol I and pol III, involved in the process. Although research on eukaryotic DNA polymerases lagged behind that in *E. coli*, it soon became clear that multiple polymerases were also involved in DNA replication in higher cells. Several eukaryotic DNA polymerases have now been identified,[1] and they are listed in Table 14–1. Pol α is a key component of the DNA replicative complex and is ubiquitous among eukaryotic cells. Pols α, δ, and ϵ show increased activity in proliferating cells.[2] Pol δ activity depends on the presence of a cofactor called proliferating cell nuclear antigen (PCNA). Pol β is primarily a repair enzyme; its activity doesn't vary with the cell cycle, but it is induced by DNA-damaging agents. Pol γ is the mitochondrial DNA replicative enzyme.

Although the power of reverse genetic analysis in yeast has established the uniqueness of several DNA polymerases, the precise function

Table 14–1 Eukaryotic DNA Polymerases. (From Linn[1])

	α	β	γ	δ	ε
Subunits (kd)[a]					
Catalytic	165	40	125	125	255 (145)
Associated	70, 58, 48	None	35	48	55 (HeLa) 80, 34, 30, 29 (yeast)
Yeast catalytic subunit gene[b]	POL1 = CDC17		MIP1	POL3 = CDC2	POL2
Observed in Drosophila	+	+	+	–	–
Processivity	Moderate	Low	High	PCNA-dependent[c]	Very high
Associated 3'→5' exonuclease	–[d]	–[e]	+	+	+
Polarity of stimulatory ATPase/helicase[f]	3'→5'	–	–	5'→3'	3'→5'
Miscellaneous	58- and 48-kd subunits catalyze primase		Mitochondrial	α Family	α Family

[a]Apparent subunit sizes vary to ±10% owing to variations among species as well as differing techniques. Glycosylation and phosphorylation of pol α also change its apparent molecular weight. Active proteolytic fragments of the catalytic subunits of pols α, ε, and γ are also observed.

[b]Pol β has not been observed in yeast. However, a gene, REV3, containing motifs of the α family encodes a 173-kd polypeptide that appears to be nonessential but required for induced mutagenesis. It would presumably have a role in DNA repair. Other yeast genes include RP11 and RP12, the large and small primase subunits, respectively; DPB2, the 80-kd subunit of pol ε; POL30, PCNA.

[c]Pol δ is very processive in the presence of PCNA; it is nonprocessive in its absence.

[d]Drosophila pol α has a cryptic exonuclease that is exposed upon removal of the 70-kd subunit. A multimeric complex of HeLa pol α has been reported to contain 3'→5' and 5'→3' exonuclease activities, and a 3'→5' exonuclease activity (with properties not resembling those of an editor) has been reported for a preparation of the yeast catalytic subunit.

[e]Pol β complexes to DNAase V; the complex can nick translate as well as remove damaged 3' termini.

[f]Polarity is with respect to the strand bound by the helicase.

of each polymerase has not in every case been determined. Indeed, the various polymerases appear to function somewhat differently in different cell types or even at different parts of the genome in the same cell type.[1] The latter may reflect the complexity of the eukaryotic chromosome and its replication process. What is intriguing, though, is that if different regions of the chromosome utilize different combinations of DNA polymerases, as has been suggested,[1] or if areas of chromosomes bearing genetic insertions, deletions, or amplifications use different combinations of polymerases, it may be possible to inhibit, somewhat selectively, the replication of specific genomic regions that are involved in the proliferation and uncontrolled growth of cancer cells.

Suramin may be an example of such an inhibitor. Although by no means a new drug (it has been used for many ears in the treatment of trypanosomal infections), it has shown activity against some acute leukemias, several carcinomas, and adrenocortical tumors.[3] Suramin is a 1,400-dalton, sulfated polycyclic compound, based on the chemical structure of dyes such as trypan red, which was shown in the 1920s to have trypanocidal activity. It has been shown to inhibit DNA polymerase pol α activity *in vitro* and DNA synthesis in HeLa cells as well as SV40 viral DNA replication in SV40 transformed cells.[4] Suramin may, therefore, serve as a prototype drug for the development of future agents that can inhibit the function of replicative DNA polymerases. The drug has shown some activity in clinical trials.[5]

Topoisomerases

DNA topoisomerases are nuclear enzymes that affect the structure of DNA by breaking-rejoining actions. Topoisomerase I acts on single-stranded DNA, and topoisomerase II produces double-stranded DNA breakage-rejoining. These enzymes are important in DNA replication, recombination, and repair and in chromosomal condensation.[6]

Recently, topo-II activity has been found to be decreased or altered in cells resistant to a variety of drugs, including acridines, etoposide, teniposide, doxorubicin, daunorubicin, and mitoxantrone.[7,8] All of these drugs are thought to exert their cytotoxic action by forming a stable ternary DNA–topo II–drug complex, which maintains a cleaved state of DNA and interferes with DNA replication, repair, and transcription. In a study by Eder et al.,[9] it was found that an inhibitor of topo II, novobiocin, potentiated the antitumor effects of cyclophosphamide, BCNU, and cisplatin in tumor-bearing mice without markedly affecting the bone marrow toxicity of these drugs. These data suggest that an enhanced selective toxicity may be achieved by combinations of DNA-damaging drugs with topo-II inhibitors that have a greater effect on tumor DNA replication and/or repair than on those processes in normal cells. In addition, one could conceive of strategies to design analogs of drugs that form DNA–topo II complexes in resistant cells with altered topo II. Such a strategy has been employed by Finlay *et al.*,[10] who found that chemical modifications of the drug amsacrine restored drug sensitivity in cells made resistant to the parent amsacrine compound, which is a known topo-II inhibitor.

DNA Repair

A number of chemically active anticancer drugs act by damaging DNA (Chapter 6). Cancer cells, particularly resting G_0 cells, may escape lethality by repairing their DNA prior to cell division. Moreover, cancer cells can become resistant to DNA-damaging drugs by having increased repair enzyme activity. Thus, if one could design relatively nontoxic inhibitors of DNA repair processes that have some selectivity for cancer cells over normal cells, by virtue of selective uptake, activation, or affinity for repair enzymes in cancer cells, conceivably one could have a synergistic and selective cell-killing effect between such an inhibitor and a DNA-damaging drug. One approach to this is the use of inhibitors of the enzyme O^6 alkylguanine-DNA alkyl transferase, an enzyme that removes alkyl groups from DNA damaged by various DNA-alkylating agents including those used as anticancer drugs. O^6-benzylguanine is such an inhibitor, and it has been found to increase the antitumor effect of the drug BCNU when given in combination to male mice bearing human tumor xenografts.[11]

Other inhibitors of DNA repair, including methylxanthines such as caffeine; nicotinamide analogs such as 3-aminobenzamide; and β-lapachone, a naturally occurring tricyclic o-naphthoquinone, have been shown to potentiate the cytotoxic effects of alkylating agents in cultured human cancer cells.[12] β-lapachone was also shown to enhance the cytotoxic effects of DNA-damaging agents that induce DNA-strand breaks, such as neocarzinostatin or X rays, in a cultured radioresistant human malignant melanoma derived from a patient with a resistant tumor. This action of β-lapachone is apparently due to an effect on the DNA-unwinding activity of topoisomerase I and occurred at a concentration (4 μM) that did not affect undamaged DNA in normal human fibroblasts, suggesting a specific drug effect on DNA repair.[13]

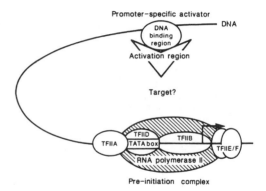

Figure 14–1 A possible mechanism for transcription stimulation by promoter-specific activators. The activator enhances a step following assembly of the general factors into a preinitiation complex. The promoter-specific activator is shown bound to its site on the DNA loop and brings the promoter region into proximity with the preinitiation complex. The site of transcription initiation is indicated by the dark arrow. (From Lillie and Green.[15])

Gene Transcription and Translation

Transcription Factors

Regulation of gene expression in eukaryotic cells involves both *cis* elements (DNA sequences that act as regulators—e.g., promoters or enhancers—of genes upstream or downstream from them) and *trans*-acting factors (usually polypeptides that bind to regulatory sequences of DNA and modulate the transcription of genes into RNA). Regulatory processes of gene expression utilize a large array of *cis* DNA elements and protein *trans*-activators, which receive cues or signals from exogenous stimulatory or inhibitory agents (ligands) such as hormones and growth factors. These ligand–transcription factor complexes then direct spatial rearrangements of DNA that modulate the start of transcription of a protein-encoding gene.[14]

There are two kinds of transcription factors: general and promoter DNA-sequence specific. The general factors are called TFIIA, TFIIB, TFIID, TFIIE, and TFIIF. These form a transcription initiation complex with RNA polymerase II and DNA (Fig. 14–1).[15] Promoter-specific *trans*-activators include the AP-1 and ATF families of proteins that bind to specific DNA sequences. For example, the AP-1 activator

protein binds to a phorbol-ester-responsive *cis*-element called TRE (for TPA-responsive element), whose consensus sequence is TGACTCA. The ATF-binding site contains the base sequence TGACGTCA, which is the consensus sequence of the cyclic AMP responsive element (CRE). It is now known that there are subfamilies of each of these *trans*-acting factors. The AP-1/TRE site is recognized by a group of proteins encoded by the c-*fos* and c-*jun* gene families, which are protooncogenes and have cell-transforming variants known as v-*fos* and v-*jun*. The proteins coded for by these genes are induced by mitogenic, differentiation-inducing, and neuronal-specific stimulatory agents.[16] The ATF/CRE *cis*-acting sequence is recognized by a family of proteins known as CRE-binding proteins (CREB), which respond to cellular signals generated by cAMP, calcium, and virally induced factors.[16]

Numerous other transcriptional regulatory factors (both positive and negative) have been discovered and continue to be discovered. They share a number of common features: they assume a conformational structure that allows them, frequently after interaction with a ligand and/or dimerization with another protein, to bind in a sequence-specific way to DNA. What makes transcriptional regulatory proteins attractive targets for chemotherapeutic intervention is the fact that they play such a key role in the whole phenotypic program of a cell. By controlling either the expression or the function of these factors, one could alter the entire program of a cell's existence: its response to exogenous signals such as growth factors, its rate of cell division, its ability to express genes controlling cell motility and invasiveness, and its ability to differentiate. Even though many of these transcriptional regulatory factors are phylogenetically very old (similar proteins are found in bacteria, yeast, and fruit flies), there is evidence for developmental and cell-type specificity in their expression, posttranslational modifications, and function.[17] For example, the Fos protein can be posttranslationally modified to produce isomeric forms separable by electrophoresis. Depolarizing agents and calcium-channel agonists induce the c-fos gene in PC12 pheochromocytoma cells, but the Fos protein is differently modified after induction by depolarization or calcium channel agonists than the Fos protein that accumulates after treatment of PC12 cells with nerve growth factor.[18] Variable posttranslational modifications of Fos could lead to different interactions with its dimerizing partner protein Jun, leading in turn to differential effects on gene transcription.[17] There may also be developmentally regulated differences in the expression, posttranslational modification, and function of transcriptional factors that could distinguish less-well-differentiated cells, including cancer cells, from more-well-differentiated normal cells.

Now, how could one get at modifying the activity of transcriptional regulatory factors in cancer cells? At least two ways come to mind. One is by using specific ligands or combinations of ligands to differentially modify trans-acting factors in different cells—e.g., the differentiating effects of various ligands on PC12 cells noted above. Another is to specifically shut off the expression of transcriptional activators in cancer cells—for example, by using a delivery system (e.g., a specific monoclonal antibody or viral vector) to deliver an inhibitory factor or gene to a cancer cell. A variation on the latter theme would be to employ antisense oligonucleotides to shut off the expression of transcriptional activators (see section below). Both anti-Fos antibodies and antisense oligonucleotides to the fos gene have been shown to inhibit cell proliferation enhanced by mitogens in 3T3 cells.[19,20] Another example is the shutting off of the myc gene in human promyelocytic leukemia (HL-60) cells, which decreases cell proliferation and favors cell differentiation.[21,22]

Antisense Oligonucleotides

During the process of gene transcription, an mRNA coding for a protein is made from a DNA gene sequence that produces a complementary base pair in the mRNA. For example:

$$DNA{:}3'{-}A{-}T{-}G{-}C{-}5'$$
$$RNA{:}5'{-}U{-}A{-}C{-}G{-}3'$$

The mRNA is made in a 5'-to-3' direction. If a transcribable DNA sequence has the reverse orientation of complementary bases—e.g., 5'-T-A-C-G-3'—it will transcribe an "antisense" mRNA with the following orientation: 5'-C-G-U-A-3'. This mRNA can then hybridize with the normal mRNA as follows:

$$5'{-}U{-}A{-}C{-}G{-}3' \text{ (normal)}$$
$$3'{-}A{-}U{-}G{-}C{-}5' \text{ (antisense)}$$

This double-stranded RNA is a substrate for ribonucleases (i.e., RNase H) in cells and is degraded before it can be translated into protein. Hence, the product of the targeted gene is not formed. Since each protein-coding gene in the cell has a specific base sequence that makes it unique, one can, theoretically at least, specifically shut off only one gene in a cell—a highly desirable outcome if that happens to be a cancer-related gene.

Although there is some evidence to suggest that mechanisms by which antisense oligonucleotides work is more complicated than this, the strategy nevertheless works. One of the first demonstrations of this in mammalian cells was the use of an antisense gene to thymidine kinase (TK) transfected into mouse L cells,[23] which inhibited the expression of the TK protein four- to fivefold.

It is now known that the whole antisense base sequence is not required in order to destroy the function of an mRNA. Small stretches of oligodeoxynucleotides—e.g., 15 to

18 deoxynucleotides long ("15-mer," "18-mer," etc.)—can eliminate the function of an mRNA. Favorite "targets" used to design an antisense base sequence are the initiation codon and those codons immediately downstream.[24] Several examples of the use of antisense gene therapy are now extant. For example, Szczylik et al.[25] have shown that a synthetic 18-mer oligodeoxynucleotide complementary to the bcr-abl gene mRNA inhibited the proliferation of cultured blast cells from patients with chronic myelocytic leukemia (CML), whereas colony formation of normal granulocyte-macrophage precursor cells was not affected. The bcr-abl gene results from the chromosome 9 to 22 translocation known as the Philadelphia chromosome in CML.

Watson et al.[26] have reported that exposure of MCF-7 human breast carcinoma cells to an antisense oligodeoxynucleotide to the c-myc cellular oncogene inhibited by 75% estrogen-stimulated cell proliferation. These data support the hypothesis that c-myc expression is an important component of estrogen's stimulatory effect on breast cancer cells.

Melani et al.[27] have described an inhibitory effect of an antisense oligodeoxynucleotide to the c-myb protooncogene in human colon carcinoma cells that express c-myb, and the observed level of inhibition of cell proliferation was directly related to the level of c-myb expression by the colon cancer cells.

Cell Cycle Factors

Cyclins and cdc Kinases

Cyclins are a family of proteins, originally discovered in sea urchins and clams, that are synthesized and degraded at various times during the cell cycle. They have subsequently been shown to act by complexing with and activating a 34,000 dalton cell division control protein called cdc2 or $p34^{cdc2}$, which has protein kinase activity (reviewed in refs. 28–30). There are three families of cyclins: G_1, A type, and B type. The genes for many of these have been cloned from various organisms, from clams to man, and they have sequence homology in a region called the "cyclin box."

G_1 cyclins complex with cdc2 kinase, and the formation of this complex appears to be required for cells to cross a critical point in the G_1 phase of the cell cycle, known as START or "the restriction point," prior to their entry into S phase. The activated cyclin/cdc2 complex appears to phosphorylate a number of proteins critical for entry into S phase, and the cyclin is then degraded.

A-type cyclins complex with cdc2 in S phase, and there is evidence to suggest that the cyclin A/cdc complex phosphorylates components of the DNA replication machinery to promote DNA synthesis.

B-type cyclins associate with cdc2 during S phase and stimulate progression through mitosis. Cyclin B degradation then occurs, a required step in the cell's exit from mitosis. Both A-type and B-type cyclins are degraded by an ubiquitin-mediated pathway, the A type during metaphase and the B type at the end of metaphase.

The kinase activity of cdc2 is regulated not only by its association with cyclins but also by its phosphorylation state because, although the cyclin B/cdc 2 complex forms as soon as cyclin B is synthesized in late S phase, the complex is inactive until cdc2 is dephosphorylated by a phosphatase called cdc25 at a specific tyrosine in the molecule. At the end of G_2 phase, cdc2 is inactivated by dephosphorylation at a threonine residue, via a specific phosphatase. Taken together, the evidence indicates that the cyclin B/cdc2 complex is the major mitotic kinase whose activity is regulated by specific phosphorylation/dephosphorylation steps and that the proteins phosphorylated by this complex are key to the mitotic process.

There are several implications of the formation and function of cyclin/cdc2 complexes for cancer. For example, some cyclins appear to be induced by growth factors and overexpression of cyclins and/or their decreased degradation might continue to drive cells through the cell cycle. Moreover, the accumulation of persistently activated cyclin/cdc2 complexes could allow cells to continue cycling even when exogenous growth factors are subsequently absent or lowered in concentration.

There is also evidence that alteration of cyclins is involved in cell transformation events produced by transforming viruses. A fragment of the hepatitis B viral genome has been found integrated into a regulatory site of the cyclin A gene in human hepatocarcinoma cells, and this integration appears to activate the cyclin A gene. The cyclin A protein complexes with the adenovirus-transforming protein E1a in adenovirus-transformed cells. The *mos* oncogene appears to act by stabilizing cyclins and may thus prevent cells from entering the resting phase of the cell cycle, G_0.

Certain oncogene proteins, such as c-Src and c-Abl, are substrates for cyclin B/cdc2 kinase activity, and this may be involved in the regulation of the activity of these oncoproteins. The products of the tumor suppressor genes RB and p53 form complexes with, and appear to be phosphorylated by, cyclin A/cdc2, and the phosphorylation of RB keeps it in its inactive state, thus allowing cell proliferation to proceed. Aberrant expression of cyclin/cdc kinase activity could keep RB in its inactive, phosphorylated state. Finally, the aneuploid chromosomal state of many cancer cells implies a loss of finely tuned cell cycle events such that some chromosomal replication can go on without mitosis, or duplication of some chromosomes and not others can occur prior to cell mitosis. This, in turn, implies a loss or abnormality in the carefully regulated and timed events of cyclin synthesis, complex formation with cdc2, and/or cyclin degradation.

How would one attack this problem therapeutically? Clearly, there are several possible points of potential attack. One could think of antisense oligonucleotides to shut off cyclin or cdc2 kinase gene expression, but that would require selective cell targeting of the antisense agents in order to protect normal cycling cells, such as those of the bone marrow or GI mucosa. One could think of specific cdc2 kinase inhibitors or activators of proteases that would degrade cyclins, but again that would most likely require cell-specific drug delivery. If tumor cell-specific alterations in any of these proteins can be found, the job of the "cancer chemist" will be made easier. It is clear that cycling cells go through a number of "checkpoint" controls as they traverse the cell cycle, and our emerging understanding of the regulatory events at these checkpoints should provide future targets for therapeutic intervention.[31]

Growth Factors

Growth factors are small polypeptides, often in the 6,000–25,000-molecular weight range, that stimulate proliferation and influence differentiation of normal cells. They may also be overexpressed or inappropriately expressed in cancer cells. Malignant cells may have unregulated expression of growth factors, their receptors, or components of their signal transduction mechanisms.

Growth factors that stimulate cell division are of two types: factors such as PDGF, EGF, and FGF that provide "competence" for transversing the G_1 phase of the cell cycle, and factors such as IGF-1 that stimulate "progression" into S phase and beyond. There is also a critical time in G_1 when both types of factors are required (the "restriction point" noted above). After this time, only the presence of the "progression" factor is required. The products of several oncogenes mimic growth factors or their receptors (see below) and can substitute for competence factors. For some cell types, the absence of growth factors at critical times causes the cells to undergo programmed cell death (apoptosis).

Many of the receptors for growth factors possess tyrosine kinase activity (Fig. 14–2).[32] They have extracellular ligand-binding domains and intracellular tyrosine kinase domains, which when activated can phosphorylate proteins involved in cell proliferation and/or differentiation events.

A variety of human tumor cells have been shown to produce their own growth factors (reviewed in ref. 32). Growth factor stimulation of cells can be endocrine (one cell type produces the factor that circulates and affects a distant target cell), paracrine (producing and responding cell are localized in the same tissue), or autocrine (producing cell also has receptors to respond to the growth factor). Various tumors are known to have one or more of these mechanisms of response to growth factors.

One can think, then, of several possible mechanisms by which to attack cancer cells in their growth factor-responding Achilles' heel. One could design antagonists that bind to the receptor, for example, but do not produce a response. Since more cancer cells than normal cells in a given tissue usually are cycling at any

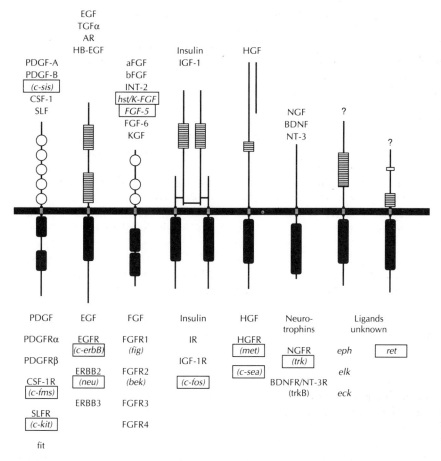

Figure 14-2 Transmembrane tyrosine kinases. Structural features of various receptor tyrosine kinase receptors are shown. Each receptor family is designated by a prototype ligand. Growth factors known to bind to receptors of a given family are listed above, and receptors that constitute each family are listed below. Boxes denote those growth factors or receptors whose genes were initially identified as activated oncogenes. The *c-onc* designation is used to specify cellular homologs of retroviral oncogenes. Open circles illustrate immunoglobulin-like repeats. Dashed boxes indicate cysteine-rich domains. Dark boxes indicate conserved tyrosine kinase domains. (From Aaronson.[32])

point in time, the cancer cells would presumably be more susceptible to apoptosis by growth factor deprivation. Another method would be to design monoclonal antibodies to a growth factor receptor that is crucial for cancer cells to proliferate. This could lead to down-regulation of the receptor and loss of responsiveness to the factor. If the monoclonal antibody were bound to a radioactive atom such as ^{131}I, a local cell killing of receptor-bearing cells could also be achieved. Since cancer cells may have an up-regulated or higher receptor content than nearby normal cells, some selectivity might be achieved. One could also think about ways to

attack the signal transduction mechanisms by which the growth factor–receptor complexes trigger intracellular events.

Signal-Transduction Mechanisms

In general, there are four types of signal transduction mechanisms for growth-modulating substances: (1) receptors coupled to tyrosine kinase activity, (2) receptors coupled to guanine nucleotide-binding proteins, which in turn may activate or inhibit adenylate cyclase, activate phosphoinositide hydrolysis leading to protein kinase C activation and intracellular Ca^{++} release, or modulate cell membrane ion channels, and (3) intracellular receptors such as those for steroid hormones, thyroid hormone, and retinoic acid, all of which have DNA-binding domains as well as ligand-binding domains and can interact directly with DNA to modulate gene transcription. All of these receptor-mediated signal transduction mechanisms are potential sites for chemotherapeutic attack, depending on which ones are up-regulated or deregulated in cancer cells—for example, by oncogene activation or overexpression, or by tumor suppressor gene inactivation.

Protein Kinases

The tyrosine kinase-coupled receptors mentioned above are one potential target. Activation of these receptors can lead to phosphorylation of a number of key substrates (Fig. 14–3). Many growth factor receptors mediate their cellular effects by intrinsic tyrosine kinase activity, which in turn may phosphorylate other substrates involved in mitogenesis. A number of transforming oncogene products have growth factor or growth factor receptorlike activities that work via a tyrosine kinase-activat-

ing mechanism (see below). For example, the v-src gene product is itself a cell membrane-associated tyrosine kinase. The v-sis oncogene product is virtually homologous to the B chain of platelet-derived growth factor (PDGF). The v-erb product is a truncated form of the epidermal growth factor (EGF) receptor. The fms gene product is analogous to the receptor for colony stimulating factor CSF-1. The met and tck protooncogene products turn out to be receptors for hepatocyte growth factor (HGF) and nerve growth factor (NGF), respectively.

Some of the key substrates for receptor tyrosine kinase coupled activity (Fig. 14–3) include: (1) phospholipase C (PLCγ), which in turn activates phosphatidyl inositol hydrolysis, releasing the second messengers diacylglycerol (DAG) and inositol trisphosphate (InsP$_3$), which activate protein kinase C (PKC) and mobilize intracellular calcium release (a number of tumor promoters also activate PKC), (2) the GTPase activating protein GAP that modulates ras protooncogene protein function, (3) Src-like tyrosine kinases, (4) PI-3 kinase that associates with and may modulate the transforming activity of polyoma middle T antigen and the v-src and v-abl gene products, (5) the raf protooncogene product that is itself a serine/threonine protein kinase.

Thus, activation of protein kinases is a key

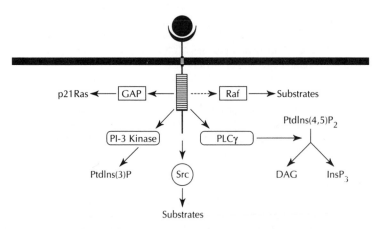

Figure 14–3 Substrates of receptor tyrosine kinases. A prototype receptor tyrosine kinase and known intracellular substrates are shown. The substrate specificity of different receptors is described in the text. The dashed line leading to Raf indicates that its activation may be by mechanisms other than direct tyrosine phosphorylation in response to some growth factor receptors. (From Aaronson[32])

Abbreviations: Ptdins(4,5)P$_2$, phosphatidylinositol 4,5-bisphosphate; PLC$_\gamma$, phospholipase C$_\gamma$; Ptdins(3)P, phosphatidylinositol 3-phosphate; DAG, diacylglycerol; InsP3, inositol trisphosphate.

mechanism in regulating signals for cell proliferation. The substrates of these kinases include
transcription regulatory factors such as those
linked to mitogenic signaling pathways—e.g.,
proteins encoded by the *jun, fos, myc, myb, rel,*
and *ets* protooncogenes.

The central role of tyrosine phosphorylation
in cell proliferative signaling mechanisms provides another target for chemotherapy. Tyrosine analogs that block tyrosine phosphorylation by acting selectively on tyrosine kinases
may provide such agents. For example, if one
could selectively block the tyrosine-phosphor-
ylating activity of an overexpressed or inappropriately activated *src, fms,* or *erb* B oncogene,
one might be able to shut off a proliferative signal in certain kinds of cancer cells. Similarly, if
one could design a peptide that would mimic
an overexpressed protein kinase substrate such
as Src or Raf, one might be able to specifically
block their activation. Tyrphostins might be
examples of such agents. They are a group of
natural tyrosine analogs that block phosphorylation of tyrosine residues. They have
been shown to block proliferation of cultured
cells.[33]

Other protein kinases may also be targets for
chemotherapeutic intervention. In recent
years, protein kinases have been discovered at
a rapid pace. The catalytic domains of these enzymes share a significant amount of sequence
homology, yet the cellular localization, substrate specificity, and ligands that activate
them may vary among cell types. While there
may not be "1,001 kinases" in mammalian
cells, the number discovered is well over 100
and may well go a lot higher (Table 14–2).[34] In
view of the importance of phosphorylation-de-
phosphorylation reactions in cellular regulatory mechanisms, this provides a rich pool of
targets indeed.

demonstrated that phosphatases play a role in
the activity of various receptors and in the
function of certain cell cycle regulating genes
(reviewed in refs. 35 and 36). For example, expression of a truncated, abnormal protein tyrosine phosphatase in baby hamster kidney
(BHK) cells produces multinucleated cells, possibly by dephosphorylating p34^{cdc2}.[36] Activation
of p34^{cdc2} requires dephosphorylation of a tyrosine residue, and this activation drives the
cell from G_2 into M phase. The truncated phosphatase apparently interferes with the normal
synchrony between nuclear formation and cell
division.

Protein tyrosine phosphatases (PTPase), it is
now known, are a diverse family of enzymes
that exist in cell membranes. Some of them are
associated with receptors that have tyrosine kinase activity. Phosphatases are also in other intracellular locations. The aberrant phosphorylation state of tyrosine in certain key proteins,
such as c-Src or c-Raf, that can lead to cellular
transformation could theoretically come about
due to deregulation of a protein kinase or
under expression of a protein phosphatase. For
example, cells treated with vanadate, a PTPase
inhibitor, had increased protein phosphotyrosine levels and a transformed phenotype.[37] Further evidence that PTPases are involved in cancer is the observation that receptor-linked
PTPase γ (one of the PTPase isozymes) is located on chromosome 3, which is deleted in
renal cell and lung carcinomas, suggesting that
the PTPase γ gene may act as a tumor suppressor gene. Thus, one could predict that a
high level of expression of specific PTPases may
be able to reverse the malignant phenotype, and one can think of strategies, then, to
transfect these genes into tumor cells or
deliver inducers of the enzymes to tumor
cells.

Protein Phosphatases

Let us not forget the catalysts for the other half
of this reaction—the phosphatases. Although it
has been known for a long time that protein
phosphatases play a regulatory role in certain
cellular metabolic functions—e.g., in the acti-
vation-inactivation steps for glycogen synthase
and phosphorylase—it has only recently been

G protein–linked Receptors

As noted above, guanine nucleotide-binding
protein-coupled receptors are a diverse set of li-
gand-activated receptors that regulate adenylate cyclase, ion channels, certain protein
kinases, and other signal transduction mechanisms. They all share a common general structure (Fig. 14–4),[38] with an external ligand-bind-

Table 14-2 *Examples of Mammalian Protein Kinases.* (From Hunter[34])

Protein-Serine/Threonine Kinases (50)	Protein-Tyrosine Kinases (29)
Cyclic nucleotide-regulated	*src* gene family
cAMP-dependent protein kinases (C_α, C_β)	pp60[c-src] (fibroblast, neuronal forms)
cGMP-dependent protein kinase	pp62[c-yes], pp56[lck]
Calmodulin-regulated	*fgr, hck, fyn, lyn* proteins
Phosphorylase kinase (distinct liver and muscle forms?)	*abl* gene family
Myosin light chain kinases (skeletal, smooth muscle)	p150[c-abl] (Type I and Ty$_{1\text{-}2}$ II N-terminus)
Type II-calmodulin dependent protein kinase	*arg* protein
(brain α, β, β' subunits; liver α, α' subunits; muscle β, β' subunits)	*fps* gene family
Calmodulin-dependent protein kinases I and III	p98[c-fps]
Diacylglycerol-regulated	NCP94
Protein kinase Cs (α, β and β', γ, δ [RP14])	*c-fps*-related proteins (TKR11 and TKR16)
Others	Growth factor receptors
Casein kinases I and II	EGF receptor family
Nuclear protein kinases N1 and N2	EGF receptor (*c-erbB* protein)
Protease-activated kinases I and II	*neu* protein (*erbB2* protein)
Glycogen synthase kinases 3 and 4	Insulin receptor family
Heme-regulated protein kinase	Insulin receptor
Double-stranded RNA regulated protein kinase	IGF-1 receptor
Double-stranded DNA regulated protein kinase	*c-ros, met, trk* proteins
S6 kinase	PDGF receptor family
β-adrenergic receptor kinase	PDGF receptor
Rhodopsin kinase	CSF-1 receptor (*c-fms* protein)
Histone H1 kinase	*c-kit* protein
Hydroxymethylglutaryl-CoA reductase kinase	*c-sea, ret* proteins
Pyruvate dehydrogenase kinase	Others
Branched chain ketoacid dehydrogenase kinase	p75 (liver)
Polypeptide-dependent protein kinase	p120 (brain)
Polyamine-stimulated protein kinase	
c-mos, c-raf, A-raf, pks, pim-1 proteins	
CDC-R (PSK-J3), CDC2Hs, PSK H1, PSK-C3	

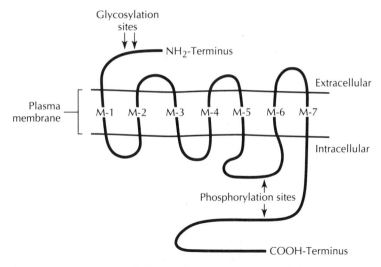

Figure 14–4 Schematic representation of the membrane organization of plasma membrane receptors (such as adrenergic receptors, muscarinic acetylcholine receptors, substance K receptors, or opsins; see text) that are linked to G proteins. An extracellular amino terminal region with sites of glycosylation on asparagine residues is followed by seven membrane-spanning domains (M1 to M7) interspersed with three intracellular and three extracellular loops and then an intracellular carboxy terminus. The consensus sequences expected at sites for phosphorylation are found in the third intracellular loop and carboxy terminal regions. (From Taylor and Insel[38])

ing domain, membrane-spanning domains, and an intracellular domain that interacts with various G-protein complexes and contains sites for phosphorylation. The ligands that interact with such receptors include α and β adrenergic agonists and antagonists, angiotensin, serotonin, bombesin, bradykinin, acetylcholine (muscarinic type), vasopressin, and vasoactive intestinal polypeptide (VIP).

Several lines of evidence implicate G protein–coupled receptors in malignant transformation.[32] Overexpression of acetylcholine or serotonin receptors in NIH 3T3 cells causes ligand-dependent transformation. Bombesin-like peptides are secreted by some small-cell lung carcinoma cells and stimulate their growth, and antibodies to bombesin inhibit tumor cell proliferation. Some pituitary, adrenal cortical, and ovarian tumors have point mutations in G proteins coupled to adenylate cyclase that could lead to constitutive overproduction of cAMP.

The $\alpha_{1\beta}$-adrenergic receptor is a member of the G protein–coupled receptor superfamily and activates PI hydrolysis, a signaling pathway that is activated by a number of growth factors and that plays a crucial role in mitogenesis. Mutation of three amino acid residues in the 3rd intracellular loop (see Fig. 14–4) increases the binding affinity of norepinephrine and its ability to stimulate PI hydrolysis by two to three orders of magnitude.[39] Moreover, this activating mutation renders the receptor constitutively active, stimulating PI turnover even in the absence of ligand. When the wild-type gene for the $\alpha_{1\beta}$ receptor is transfected into rat or NIH 3T3 fibroblasts, the cells express high levels of this receptor, become transformed in response to norepinephrine, and form tumors when injected into nude mice. When the mutated gene is transfected into fibroblasts, the cells spontaneously form transformed foci in the absence of ligand and have an enhanced ability to form tumors in nude mice. Thus, the $\alpha_{1\beta}$-adrenergic receptor gene acts like a protooncogene and when activated or overexpressed is a transforming oncogene. These data suggest that other G protein–coupled receptors of this type can act as oncogenes in certain cell types. This further suggests a host of strategies for chemotherapeutic interdiction of this system—for example, the design of specific antagonists of the G protein–coupled receptors that may be activated or overexpressed in tumor cells.

There is also evidence that alteration of G protein subunits themselves can cause alterations in fibroblast growth characteristics. For example, transfection and overexpression of a mutated G protein α_{i2} subunit gene, a gene shown to be involved in proliferation of fibroblasts and differentiation of myeloid cells, in fibroblasts produces increased cell proliferation and anchorage-independent growth, indicating a role for this G protein subunit in regulation of fibroblast cell proliferation and in transformation events.[40]

In view of the apparent central role of protein kinase C (PKC) in cell proliferation and the observations that overexpression of two isoforms of PKC, PKCβ and PKCγ, in rodent cells correlates with their tumorigenicity in nude mice and that expression of mutant forms of PKCα increases metastatic potential of tumor cells, it seems logical that inhibitors of overexpressed or mutant forms of PKC may have some therapeutic value. Some known PKC inhibitors have been examined for their effects on tumor cell growth *in vitro* and *in vivo*. Two such inhibitors, (4E)-N,N,-dimethyl-D-*erthryo*-sphingenine (DMS) and (4E)-N,N,N,-trimethyl-D-*erythro*-sphingenine (TMS), have been shown to inhibit the growth of human gastric cancer cells in culture and in nude mice.[41]

Oncogenes

Oncogenes and their normal cellular counterparts, the protooncogenes, can be classified by their function into several different categories, as reviewed by Hunter (Table 14–3).[42] A number of these genes encode growth factors—e.g., *sis* (PDGF B-chain), *int*-2, and *hst* (FGF-like factor). These oncogene growth factors can stimulate tumor cell proliferation by paracrine or autocrine mechanisms, but by themselves may not be sufficient to sustain the transformed phenotype.

A second type of oncogene codes for altered growth factor receptors, many of which, as noted above, have associated tyrosine kinase activity. These include the *src* family of oncogenes, *erb* B (EGF receptor), and *fms* (CSF-1 receptor). For some of these receptorlike, tyrosine kinase-associated membrane proteins the actual ligand is not known (e.g., *trk*, *met*, and *ros*). A third receptor class, without associated tyrosine kinase activity, is the *mas* gene product (angiotensin receptor) and the $\alpha_{1\beta}$ adrenergic receptor.

A fourth class of oncogene products are membrane-associated, guanine nucleotide-binding proteins, such as the Ras family of proteins. These proteins bind GTP, have associated GTPases, and act as signal transducers for cell surface growth factor receptors. The transforming *ras* oncogenes have been mutated in such a way to render them constitutively active by maintaining them in a GTP binding state, most likely because of a defect in the associated GTPase activity.

A fifth category are the cytoplasmic oncoproteins with serine/threonine protein kinase activity. These include the products of the *raf*, *pim*-1, *mos*, and *cot* genes. A prototype of this class is the c-Raf protein, which is activated by a variety of tyrosine kinase-associated receptors (see above). There is some evidence that c-Raf can translocate to the nucleus and may act as a "shuttle" to convey membrane-activated cytoplasmic signals to the nucleus.[42] The oncogenic form of Raf has lost part of its regulatory amino terminal sequence and appears to be constitutively active. c-Crk is also a cytoplasmic protein, and it appears to act by stabilizing tyrosine kinases associated with the Src family of oncoproteins.

A seventh, large class of oncogenes are those that code for nuclear transcription factors, such as *myc*, *myb*, *fos*, *jun*, *erb* A, and *rel*. For a number of these, the oncogenic alteration that makes them transforming oncoproteins is a mutation that leads to loss of negative regulatory elements (e.g., for *jun*, *fos*, and *myb*), and in other cases (e.g., *erb*-A and *rel*), the activating mutations cause the loss of their active domains, producing a mutant protein that prevents the activity of the normal gene product—a so-called dominant negative mutation. It is interesting that mutations of the tumor suppressor gene p53, in sort of a "reverse twist," produce a dominant negative effect by

Table 14-3 *Functions of Cell-Derived Oncogene Products.* The table is somewhat selective and obviously incomplete. These oncogenes were originally detected as retroviral oncogenes or tumor oncogenes. Others were identified at the boundaries of chromosomal translocations and at sites of retroviral insertions in tumors, or were found as amplified genes in tumors and shown to have transforming activity. (From Hunter[42])

Class 1—Growth Factors	
sis	PDGF B-chain growth factor
int-2	FGF-related growth factor
hst (KS3)	FGF-related growth factor
FGF-5	FGF-related growth factor
int-1	Growth factor?
Class 2—Receptor and Nonreceptor Protein-Tyrosine Kinases	
src	Membrane-associated nonreceptor protein-tyrosine kinase
yes	Membrane-associated nonreceptor protein-tyrosine kinase
fgr	Membrane-associated nonreceptor protein-tyrosine kinase
lck	Membrane-associated nonreceptor protein-tyrosine kinase
fps/fes	Nonreceptor protein-tyrosine kinase
abl/bcr-abl	Nonreceptor protein-tyrosine kinase
ros	Membrane associated receptor-like protein-tyrosine kinase
erbB	Truncated EGF receptor protein-tyrosine kinase
neu	Receptor-like protein-tyrosine kinase
fms	Mutant CSF-1 receptor protein-tyrosine kinase
met	Soluble truncated receptor-like protein-tyrosine kinase
trk	Soluble truncated receptor-like protein-tyrosine kinase
kit (W locus)	Truncated stem cell receptor protein-tyrosine kinase
sea	Membrane-associated truncated receptor-like protein-tyrosine kinase
ret	Truncated receptor-like protein-tyrosine kinase
Class 3—Receptors Lacking Protein Kinase Activity	
mas	Angiotensin receptor
α1B	Adrenergic R
Class 4—Membrane-Associated G Proteins	
H-ras	Membrane-associated GTP-binding/GTPase
K-ras	Membrane-associated GTP binding/GTPase
N-ras	Membrane-associated GTP-binding/GTPase
gsp	Mutant activated form of $G_s \alpha$
gip	Mutant activated form of $G_i \alpha$
Class 5—Cytoplasmic Protein-Serine Kinases	
raf/mil	Cytoplasmic protein-serine kinase
pim-1	Cytoplasmic protein-serine kinase
mos	Cytoplasmic protein-serine kinase (cytostatic factor)
cot	Cytoplasmic protein-serine kinase?
Class 6—Cytoplasmic Regulators	
crk	SH-2,-3 protein that binds to (and regulates?) phosphotyrosine-containing proteins
Class 7—Nuclear Transcription Factors	
myc	Sequence-specific DNA-binding protein
N-*myc*	Sequence-specific DNA-binding protein?

Continued

Table 14–3   Functions of Cell-Derived Oncogene Products. (continued)

L-*myc*	Sequence-specific DNA-binding protein?
myb	Sequence-specific DNA-binding protein
lyl-1	Sequence-specific DNA-binding protein?
p53	Mutant form may sequester wild-type p53 growth suppressor
fos	Combines with c-*jun* product to form AP-1 transcription factor
jun	Sequence-specific DNA-binding protein: part of *AP-1*
erbA	Dominant negative mutant thyroxine (T$_3$) receptor
rel	Dominant negative mutant NF-κB-related protein
vav	Transcription factor?
ets	Sequence-specific DNA-binding protein
ski	Transcription factor?
evi-1	Transcription factor?
gli-1	Transcription factor?
maf	Transcription factor?
pbx	Chimeric E2A-homeobox transcription factor
Hox2.4	Transcription factor?
	Unclassified
abl	Cytoplasmic truncated cytoskeletal protein?
bcl-2	Plasma membrane signal transducer?

producing a protein that in this case prevents the action of a tumor suppressor function (see below).

It has been noted that the detection of activated or mutated oncogenes in human cancers could have diagnostic and therapeutic implications, a sort of "oncogenes at the bedside" approach[43] (Table 14–4). For example, the detection of the *bcr/abl* gene in leukemic cells could confirm the diagnosis of chronic myelogenous leukemia. The levels of the *neu* oncogene product can be used to determine the prognosis in breast cancer. Loss or damage to the RB or p53 genes can be used to determine susceptibility to certain cancers, and so on.

What could one do to alter oncogene expression and could that favorably affect the outcome of cancer therapy? As Bishop[43] concludes, it seems unlikely that in the near future we will be able to replace or repair mutated or activated oncogenes or tumor suppressor genes in all cancer cells in a given tumor, particularly a solid tumor such as those of the lung, breast, colon, etc. However, it may be more feasible to achieve this in leukemias and lymphomas, where it is easier to expose the cells to injected monoclonal antibodies, viral vectors carrying corrected tumor suppressor genes, or antisense

oligonucleotides designed to shut off activated or mutated oncogenes. There is evidence that transfection of the RB or p53 tumor suppressor genes into transformed cells can reverse the malignant phenotype of these cells (reviewed in ref. 43).

It may be more feasible, at least for the near future, to think in terms of producing peptides or other ligands that overcome the activity of oncogene protein products themselves. As more is learned about the structure and function of these oncoproteins, this approach is becoming more and more realistic. A good example is the Ras oncoprotein. A number of the protein–protein interactions required for Ras activity and the posttranslational modification of Ras that must occur for it to be functional are now known (reviewed in ref. 44). The mitogenic activity of Ras is modulated by its interaction with the GTPase-activating protein (GAP), which down-regulates Ras activity by hydrolyzing GTP to GDP. It is the GTP-bound state of Ras that is required for its signal-transducing functions. The mutated Ras oncoprotein appears to be deficient in its ability to associate with GAP and be down-regulated by hydrolysis of GTP to GDP. Thus, the design of modified peptides with GTPase activity and higher affinity for mutated Ras than for normal Ras might be a possibility.

A more feasible approach, though, may be to think in terms of altering the posttranslational modifications of Ras that are necessary for its activity. For example, for Ras to be active it must become associated with cell membranes, and this requires that it be isoprenylated on its carboxy terminal end. This step is catalyzed by an enzyme called farnesyl-protein transferase (FPT), which recognizes a specific amino acid sequence at the C-terminus of Ras. Inhibitors of the synthesis of the isoprenoid substrate for this enzyme are known (e.g., lovastatin and compactin), and they have been shown to inhibit cell proliferation of Ras-transformed cells.[44] However, since isoprenoid biosynthesis is critical for several other important processes, including cholesterol and heme production, these compounds could also be quite toxic to normal cells at the concentrations needed to inhibit tumor cell proliferation. A better approach would be to design inhibitors of the farnesyl-protein transferase-mediated isoprenylation of the mutated Ras oncoprotein, if that could be done selectively or with minimal effects on other crucial normal cellular components. The essential interactions between Ras and farnesyl-protein transferase appear to involve a tetrapeptide (CAAX) sequence in Ras. Adding or deleting an amino acid from this sequence inhibits the ability of Ras to act as a substrate for FPT, and perhaps even more interesting is the fact that octa- or even tetrapeptides can effectively compete with Ras as substrates for FPT. An octapeptide mimicking the C-terminus of Ras has been shown to block Ras function when the octapeptide was microinjected into Xenopus oocytes (data reviewed in ref. 44). Again, for this to be an effective cancer chemotherapeutic approach, such peptide inhibitors would either have to block selectively the isoprenylation of mutated Ras or be selectively delivered to cancer cells.

Tumor Suppressor Genes

Knowledge of the existence of tumor suppressor genes came from somatic cell hybridization

Table 14–4 *Oncogenes at the Bedside.* (Modified from Bishop[43])

Tumor	Locus	Applicable Feature	Application[a]
Acute lymphocytic leukemia	*BCR/ABL*	Distinctive translocation	Distinguish from chronic myelogenous leukemia
Adenocarcinoma of lung	K-*RAS*	Point mutations	Prognosis
Chronic myelogenous leukemia	*BCR/ABL*	Translocation breakpoint detectable	Diagnosis in absence of Philadelphia chromosome
Carcinoma of breast	*ERBB-1*	Overexpression	Prognosis
	NEU	Amplification	Prognosis
	11q13	Amplification	Prognosis
	11p	Deletion	Prognosis
	MYC	Amplification	Prognosis
Myelodysplasia	N-*RAS*/K-*RAS*	Point mutations	Prognosis
Neuroblastoma	N-*MYC*	Amplification	Prognosis and selection of therapy
Retinoblastoma	*RB1*	Loss or damage	Detection of predisposition
P53		Loss or damage	Detection of predisposition

[a]The list offers representative examples of varying certainty and prospect.

experiments in which tumor cells were fused with normal cells and their malignant phenotype examined.[45,46] The resulting cell hybrids were usually, though not always, nontumorigenic, and this loss of tumorigenicity was found to be associated with the presence of certain chromosomes. If these chromosomes were lost during subsequent passage of the cultured hybrid cells, they reverted to a malignant phenotype. These results suggested the presence of a tumor suppressor function coded for by genes on the lost chromosomes. This evidence was greatly strengthened by experiments utilizing the transfer of the missing putative suppressor chromosome into malignant cells and showing that the phenotype reverted to normal.[47]

Evidence supporting the two-hit hypothesis of Knudson[48] also strengthened the argument for the loss of some genetic function being important in carcinogenesis. The two-hit theory states that at least two genetic mutations are necessary for a cell to become malignant. In the case of hereditary cancers, such as the hereditary form of retinoblastoma, one mutation would be present in the germ line and a second one would occur sometime after conception. The identification of the retinoblastoma (RB) gene and the demonstration that both alleles are lost or inactivated in retinoblastoma definitively showed that tumor suppressor genes exist.

It is now known that a number of other gene deletions or allelic inactivations occur in a wide variety of human cancers, and a number of additional putative tumor-suppressor genes have been localized to specific chromosomes (Table 14–5).[49]

The p53 tumor suppressor gene was discovered by a totally different route (reviewed in ref. 49). The p53 protein was initially found in SV40 virus-transformed cells in association with the SV40 large T antigen, which is critical for cell transformation by SV40. It was also found that cotransfection of rodent cells with ras and p53 genes produced cell transformation. Thus, p53 originally was thought to be an oncoprotein or at least a cofactor to an oncoprotein. It was later found that the p53 protein that had transforming capability was in fact a mutated form of the protein and that the wild-type protein had a tumor suppressor function in that it inhibited cell transformation and cell

proliferation. It has also been found that there are germline mutations of the p53 gene in Li-Fraumeni syndrome, a genetically inherited trait that makes individuals susceptible to certain cancers such as rhabdomyosarcomas, leukemias, melanomas, and carcinomas of the brain, breast, lung, larynx, colon, and adrenal cortex at an early age.[50] Somatic mutations in the p53 gene have now been implicated in a wide variety of human cancers, including leukemias, lymphomas, sarcomas, and carcinomas of the lung, breast, colon, esophagus, liver, bladder, ovary, and brain.[51]

The ubiquitous nature of alterations of p53 in human cancer indicates that p53 has a central role in transformation of cells to a malignant phenotype. The function of p53 isn't exactly clear, but like the RB protein, it appears to play a central role in cell cycle events: it appears to be a substrate for cyclin/cdc2 kinase; it has a DNA-binding domain that implies a transcriptional regulatory function; and it is bound up by certain transforming oncoproteins, such as SV40 large T, adenovirus E1B, and papilloma virus E6. Interestingly, the p53 protein is also found intracellularly in complexes with the heat shock cognate protein hsc 70, a "chaperonin" (see below) that may be involved in the assembly of p53 subunits, which is a necessary event for p53 to function normally. Mutant p53 appears to bind normal (wild-type) p53 into a tight complex with hsc 70, preventing the normal assembly and release of functional p53 oligomers. This may explain how one mutated allele of the p53 gene can function in a "dominant negative" way to inhibit the function of the normal protein.

One might ask how the activation of oncogenes and the inactivation of tumor suppressor genes act in concert to bring about cancer. One interesting model of how this occurs has been proposed by Vogelstein and his colleagues[52] (Fig. 14–5). In this model, the loss of certain tumor suppressor genes and the activation of oncogenes occur at various steps in the progression from normal colonic epithelium to metastatic carcinoma. For example, the activation of the K-ras gene by mutation occurs at the transition from early to intermediate adenoma, and the loss of the p53 gene occurs during the progression from late adenoma to carcinoma.[53]

Table 14–5   Examples of Suppressor Genes in Human Tumors. (From Weinberg[49])

Detected by Cell Hybridization or Chromosome Transfer

Chromosomal Location	Tumor Type
1p	Neuroblastoma
3p	Renal cancer
6	Endometrial cancer
9	Endometrial cancer
11	Neuroblastoma; cervical cancer; Wilm's tumor

Detected Through Loss of Heterozygosity or Direct Molecular Probing

Chromosomal Location	Tumor Type
1p	Melanoma; MEN type 2; neuroblastoma; medullary thyroid ca; pheochromocytoma; ductal cell cancer
1q	Breast cancer
3p	SCLC; adenocarcinoma of lung; cervical cancer; von Hippel-Lindau disease, renal cell cancer
5q	Familial adenomatous polyposis; colorectal cancer
9q	Bladder cancer
10q	Astrocytoma; MEN type 2
11p	Wilm's tumor; rhabdomyosarcoma; breast cancer; hepatoblastoma; transitional cell bladder cancer, lung cancer
11q	MEN type 1
13q	Retinoblastoma; osteosarcoma; SCLC; ductal breast cancer; stomach cancer; bladder cancer; colon cancer
17p	SCLC; colorectal cancer; breast cancer, osteosarcoma; astrocytoma, squamous-cell lung cancer
17q	NF type 1
18q	Colorectal cancer
22q	NF type 2; meningioma; acoustic neuroma; pheochromocytoma

MEN, multiple endocrine neoplasia; SCLC, small-cell lung carcinoma; NF, neuroribromatosis.

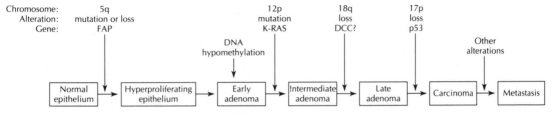

Figure 14–5   A model for colorectal tumorigenesis. Tumorigenesis proceeds through a series of genetic alterations involving tumor suppressor genes (particularly those on chromosomes 5, 17, and 18) and oncogenes *(ras)*.Although these alterations occur during characteristic phases of tumor development, the total accumulation of alterations, rather than their order with respect to one another, seems most important for determining tumor behavior. (From Vogelstein et al.[52])

A therapeutic approach designed to replace defective tumor suppressor genes or inhibit the expression of oncogenes by antisense oligonucleotides might be thought of; however, this approach is subject to many of the caveats already discussed, including the difficulties in targeting them to tumor cells and in getting penetration into solid tumors, as well as possible degradation of the nucleic acid material in the bloodstream and in cells by nucleases before they reach the target gene. Nevertheless, in certain situations this may work. For example, it has been shown by Bayever et al.[54] that an antisense phosphorothioate oligodeoxynucleotide to p53 is cytotoxic to human acute myelogenous leukemia (AML) cells in culture but not to normal bone marrow cells. Pharmacokinetic data on similar phosphorothioate antisense compounds indicate that they achieve inhibitory concentrations in the blood of rodents and have plasma half-lives that are sufficiently long to make systemic therapy for leukemia, lymphoma, and possibly other tumors feasible.[55] It isn't entirely clear how the antisense oligo to p53 works against AML cells, but it may be inhibiting the function of an overexpressed or mutated p53 gene.

Cell Surface and Extracellular Matrix

Cell Surface Carbohydrates

Malignant transformation of mammalian cells is accompanied by multiple changes in the cell surface or plasma membrane of cells.[56] These alterations are morphological, functional, and immunological in nature. For instance, changes in membrane fluidity, cell surface ionic charge, lectin-binding affinity, cell permeability and transport mechanisms, intercellular communication, cell surface-associated enzymes and receptors, turnover and shedding of cell surface components, activity of cell surface associated proteases, cellular adhesion to extracellular matrix, and reactivity with antibodies have all been observed in one or more types of malignantly transformed cells.

While the biochemical basis for all these changes is often not clear several generalizations can be made. One fact that is clear is that there are compositional changes in cell surface glycoproteins, glycolipids, and mucins that occur, and many of these may help explain the differences between cancer and normal cells noted above. It is becoming increasingly clear that many changes occurring on the cell surface of cancer cells are related to changes in cell surface carbohydrates. One of the commonly observed alterations in cell surface carbohydrates is a shift to higher molecular weight glycans caused by one or more of the following: increased branching on the trimannosyl core of asparagine-linked oligosaccharides, increased polylactosaminoglycan chain formation, and increased sialylation (reviewed in ref. 57). These changes in carbohydrates have also been associated with reduced cellular adhesion to the extracellular matrix and with increased invasiveness and metastatic potential of tumor cells.

Recently, the enzymatic basis for some of these changes has been found. There are several glycosyltransferase activities in mammalian cells that are responsible for the synthesis and processing of oligosaccharides on cell surface glycoproteins and glycolipids. One important family of these are the N-acetyl-glucosaminyl transferases. Six of these have been identified: GlcNAc transferases I through VI. The activities of certain of these are altered during transformation of cells by oncogenic viruses or in cancer tissues. Examples include an increase in GlcNAc transferase V in BHK cells transformed with polyoma viruses or Rous sarcoma virus, increases in GlcNAc transferase III in hepatomas, and increases of both GlcNAc III and V in ras-transformed NIH 3T3 cells (data reviewed in ref. 57). In addition, alterations in the levels of oligosaccharide-elongating enzymes have been found in virally transformed cells. These changes in enzyme activities appear to explain the increased branching of N-linked oligosaccharides, the elongated polylactosaminoglycan chains, and the increased sialylation of carbohydrates often observed in cancer cells. This in turn explains, at least in part, the altered antigenicity of tumor cells and the fact that many monoclonal antibodies made against animal and human tumor cells recognize a carbohydrate-determined epitope. As yet, many of the genes for these carbohydrate synthesis and processing enzymes have not been cloned and their regulatory mechanisms are yet to be clarified. Nor have specific inhibitors been found. Yet these enzymes clearly represent a future target for the development of anticancer drugs.

Extracellular Matrix

The extracellular matrix (ECM) is the complex structure of carbohydrate- and protein-containing components that make up the basement membranes underlying epithelial tissues and that surround structural tissues such as bone and muscle. The ECM forms sheetlike structures that appear early in the differentiation steps of development and that serve as a support and a barrier for cell layers (reviewed in ref. 58). It is now apparent that the basement membranes of epithelial tissues, first seen in the light microscope years ago, serve a complicated role in cell–cell adhesion and in the regulation of cell proliferation and differentiation. The ECM that makes up basement membranes is a target for the lytic enzymes secreted by metastatic cancer cells (see below). The biochemical components of the ECM of epithelial tissues include laminin, type-IV collagen, heparan sulfate proteoglycan, entactin, and fibronectin, as well as other components that contribute to the ECM of specific tissues—e.g., osteonectin in bone.

ECM components are produced early in the development of multicellular organisms by cells in tissues undergoing differentiation. It is now known that the ECM is not an inert structural element in tissues but that it provides important signals that regulate gene expression, cell proliferation, and cell differentiation. Cells' interactions with the ECM are mediated by cell surface receptors that link the ECM to the internal cellular skeletal network via a transmembrane component of the receptors. One of the important ECM components in this transmembrane signaling process is laminin, which is a large (450,000 molecular weight) glycoprotein, cruciate in structure, and with multiple binding domains for cell surface receptors and other components of the ECM (reviewed in ref. 59). Several types of laminin-binding proteins have been identified on cell surface membranes. Those include a high affinity 67 kDA receptor, galactoside-binding lectins, galactosyltransferase, sulfatides, and integrins, a family of cell surface receptors that bind various ECM components, including fibronectin, vitronectin, thrombospondin, collagen, and von Willebrand factor, as well as laminin.

The interactions of tumor cells with the ECM are important in determining the invasiveness and metastatic potential of cancer cells, and the ability of cancer cells to attach to laminin correlates with their metastatic potential (reviewed in ref. 60). The 67 kDa high affinity laminin receptor has been particularly associated with a cancer cell's metastatic capability, in that highly metastatic cells express higher levels of laminin receptors on their surface than do less metastatic or benign tumor cells of the same tissue type. A number of examples can be cited: the number of laminin receptors on breast carcinoma cells correlates with the extent of lymph node metastases in patients; the number of 67 kDa laminin receptors also correlates with the degree of invasiveness and metastasis of colon carcinoma cells in patients with that disease.[60]

Thus, for cancer cells to be invasive and metastatic they apparently need to attach to the ECM, locally degrade it to slip into the bloodstream or lymphatic channels and circulate to distant organs, attach to endothelium, invade again, and set up housekeeping in the new target organ. (This process will be described in greater detail in the next section.) Attachment of cells via laminin receptors is thus important for at least two of the steps involved in metastasis: initial attachment to the ECM and attachment to the endothelium in target organs.

Other attachment factors, however, are also important in the metastatic process. One of these attachment factors is a type of cell–cell adhesion molecule (CAM) called E-cadherin. It acts as a calcium-dependent adhesion factor for cell–cell interactions of epithelial cells and plays a key role in the normal development of epithelial tissues (reviewed in ref. 61). Loss or aberrant expression of E-cadherin has been implicated in the invasive and metastatic potential of tumor cells. Invasive, ras-transformed Madin-Darby canine kidney (MDCK) cells lacked E-cadherin expression, but if the E-cadherin cDNA was transfected into these cells, they lost their invasiveness.[61] Similarly, noninvasive clones of ras-transformed MDCK cells were rendered invasive by transfection of a plasmid-encoding E-cadherin-specific antisense RNA. Moreover, human cancer cell lines from bladder, breast, lung, and pancreas carcinomas were found to be noninvasive by an *in vitro* assay if they expressed E-cadherin and invasive if they did not.[62] The former could be rendered invasive if treated with monoclonal antibodies to E-cadherin, and the latter could be made noninvasive by transfection with E-cadherin cDNA.

Taken together, these data indicate the importance of cell adhesion to the ECM and of cell–cell adhesion molecules (CAMs) in the expression of the metastatic phenotype. Strategies, then, to increase the expression of normal CAMs in tumor tissue might be thought of as ways to modulate this phenotype.

Tumor Metastasis

For the most part, the reason that cancer is a fatal disease is that cancer cells can invade through tissues and metastasize to distant organs in the body. Not all the cells in a tumor mass have equal metastatic potential, but those that do represent a significant population of the cells in a malignant tumor that has reached a progressive stage.[63,64] Those cells have some special attributes that render them invasive and metastatic, and if one could design therapeutic modalities to block these special functions one might be able to inhibit the invasive and metastatic process.

Invasion and metastasis are facilitated by attachment factors that tumor cells use to attach to the ECM and endothelium of blood vessels as noted above, by lytic enzymes such as proteases, collagenases, and glycosidases that allow tumor cells to penetrate through tissue barriers, by an increased motility, and possibly by tissue chemoattractants that may play a role in the selective "homing" of tumor cells to certain organs.[63] Any or all of the steps in the metastatic process are potential sites for chemotherapeutic intervention—i.e., tumor cell attachment, ECM degradation, tumor cell locomotion, circulation in lymphatic channels or blood vessels, attachment to endothelium in selective tissues, reinvasion, and growth at a new organ site.

Proteases and Collagenases

The invasive and metastatic potential of tumor cells has been correlated in a number of studies with the activity of various protease activities, including serine proteases such as plasmin (activated by plasminogen activator), thiol proteases such as the cathepsins, and metalloproteases such as type-IV collagenase. These proteolytic activities don't go unabated in tissues, even tumor tissues, because there are a number of tissue protease inhibitors that keep them in check under normal conditions. Proteases, after all, are needed for a number of natural processes such as normal tissue repair, tissue remodeling during development, and implantation of the blastocyst and growth of the placenta during normal pregnancy. In these instances, as opposed to highly malignant tumors, the proteases and antiproteases are kept in a tightly regulated balance, the mechanisms for which aren't entirely clear but probably involve the local release of growth factors, feedback from the ECM, etc. For example, metalloproteases are induced by interleukin-1, EGF, and PDGF,[65] whereas TGF-β has been shown to induce the production of plasminogen activator inhibitor type 1 and to decrease the degradation of the ECM by human fibrosarcoma cells in culture.[66] Thus, normally there is a stringently regulated process that controls the release of proteases and their inactivation once they have done their job. Tumor cells of the metastatic variety have lost or don't respond to this control mechanism.

Another point that is clear is that individual proteases don't act alone in the metastatic process but act as part of a cascade of lytic activity. For instance, plasminogen activator activates plasmin, which in turn can activate type IV collagenase. Of the plasminogen activators, the urokinase type (u-PA) has been most closely linked to the metastatic phenotype.[63] Several studies also support an important role for type-IV collagenase in tumor metastasis.[63] Moreover, benign proliferative lesions of the breast, benign polyps of the colon, as well as normal colon and gastric mucosa have low levels of a 72 kDa form of type-IV collagenase, but their invasive counterparts express this enzyme. Also, type-IV collagenolytic activity can be inhibited by retinoic acid, and this correlates with loss of the invasive phenotype in cultured human melanoma cells.[67]

Another important concept for understanding the biology of tumor metastasis is the interaction of cancer cells with the surrounding stroma in which they grow. Cross talk among the cancer cells, the ECM, and the supporting stroma occurs. As an epithelial tumor grows and breeches the ECM, the tumor cells come into contact with the fibroblasts and other mesenchymal cells in the supporting stroma. Via production and secretion of various growth factors and cytokines and interaction among tumor cells, stromal cells, and ECM components, the process of invasion and metastasis goes on. This is also, apparently, part of the process by which tumors become vascularized. They secrete factors called tumor angiogenesis factors that induce the growth of vascular endothelial channels through the stroma and ECM to reach the tumor, and that appears to be the time in the life cycle of a malignant neoplasm when it undergoes a spurt of growth and becomes more aggressive.[68]

Interestingly, Chambon and his colleagues[69] have isolated a gene of the ECM-degrading metalloprotease family that they've called stromolysin-3, which is expressed in stromal cells of invasive breast carcinomas but not in less advanced *in situ* breast carcinomas. Furthermore, the fact that the gene is expressed at high levels in the stromal cells of invasive breast carcinomas, but not in carcinoma cells themselves, suggests that release of a factor from the carcinoma cells induces the expression of the stromolysin-3 gene and that this event is related to tumor progression. Thus, the products of the stromolysin gene family are an important potential target for breast cancer therapy.

An important family of metalloprotease inhibitors found in tissues are the tissue inhibitors of metalloprotease (TIMPs). Two of these have been identified: TIMP-1 and TIMP-2. In some animal models, administration of TIMP-1 inhibits metastasis, and transfection of antisense TIMP-1 RNA induces oncogenicity in murine 3T3 cells (reviewed in ref. 63). Addition of TIMP-2 to the cell culture medium has been shown to block the invasiveness of human fibrosarcoma cells in an *in vitro* assay.[70] These

and other data, taken together, suggest a therapeutic approach to block tumor cell metastasis by administration of metalloprotease inhibitors or inducers of inhibitor activity. However, it must be kept in mind that metalloproteases are important for normal functions such as wound healing, so any therapeutic approach using protease inhibitors would most likely have to be directed to the tumor itself.

The cathepsins are a family of cysteine proteases that also appear to be involved in the metastatic process. Cathepsin B activity is elevated in a variety of human and animal tumors and is found at higher levels in metastatic as opposed to nonmetastatic B16 melanoma cells.[71] Cathepsin L is expressed at higher levels in a wide variety of human cancers than in their normal counterpart tissues.[72] These enzymes are also capable of degrading components of the ECM, and, potentially at least, could be a target for therapy. Other proteases and protease inhibitors have been found in tumor tissue, including tumor-associated trypsinogen-2 (TAT-2) and a corresponding inhibitor (TATI).[73] Undoubtedly, more tumor-associated proteases and tissue protease inhibitors will be found in the future, and this whole area is a fertile ground for learning more about the biology of tumor metastasis. Perhaps this will also lead to the discovery of new anticancer drugs.

Cancer Metastasis Genes

Cell fusion experiments, similar to those described earlier for the discovery of tumor suppressor genes, have shown that when metastatic tumor cells are fused with nonmalignant cells, the resulting hybrid cells that are tumorigenic are not metastatic,[74] suggesting the presence of metastasis suppressor genes. A putative gene of this type has now been found.

A metastasis suppressor gene, called *nm23*, was identified by mRNA "subtraction" experiments comparing the content of mRNA found in metastatic versus nonmetastatic murine melanoma cells.[75] The levels of *nm23* mRNA were ten-fold lower in melanoma cell lines of high metastatic potential compared to those with low potential. Subsequently, a similar gene has been found in human cells and low levels of its expression have been correlated with metastasis and poor patient prognoses in breast cancer.[76] However, in human colon tissue, *nm23* mRNA levels were increased in colon carcinoma cells compared to normal colonic mucosa,[77] suggesting that *nm23* gene expression is controlled differently in different tissues.

Through an intriguing bit of comparative genetic sleuthing, the function of the *nm23* gene has been found. There is a gene in the fruitfly Drosophila that, when mutated, causes morphologically deformed wing discs in the larval stage. This gene, called *awd* for abnormal wing discs gene, has been cloned and sequenced. After the *nm23* gene sequence was determined, a gene database search revealed that it was 78% homologous to the *awd* gene. A further clue came when the cDNA clones for nucleoside diphosphate kinase (NDP kinase) were isolated from the slime mold Dictyostelium and from a Myxococcus microorganism. These cDNA clones were found to be highly homologous to the *nm23/awd* gene, and the *awd* gene product was subsequently shown to be a NDP kinase.[78]

NDP kinases are an ubiquitous family of enzymes that catalyze the transfer of the terminal phosphate group of 5′-triphosphate nucleotide donors to diphosphate nucleotide acceptors—e.g., GDP to GTP via ATP. These kinases participate in functions that could affect tumor cell proliferation and metastasis by an action on G-protein–coupled signal transduction mechanisms that regulate microtubule assembly, since GTP is required for this function. The NDP kinase coded for by the *awd* gene is associated with microtubules in Drosophila larvae.[78] What role this might have in tumor metastasis is uncertain at this point, but since microtubules are important for cell locomotion and for response to external signals mediated by the ECM, loss of regulatory mechanisms mediated by NDP kinases could result in loss of normal matrix–cell interactions.

Inhibitors of Tumor-Cell Metastasis

Based on a search for compounds that could inhibit cell motility as a potential inhibitory mechanism of tumor metastasis, a Merck compound, L651582, was tested for its antitumor activity.[79] The rationale for this was that certain tumors secrete an autocrine motility factor that stimulates cell locomotion via G protein–coupled inositol trisphosphate (IP3) generation. L651582, originally developed to inhibit coccidiosis microorganisms, was shown to inhibit proliferation and clonogenic growth of human melanoma, breast and ovarian carcinomas, and *ras*-transformed rat fibroblasts.[79] The drug also significantly prolonged the survival time of nude mice transplanted intraperitoneally with a metastatic human ovarian carcinoma.

Inhibitors of the enzyme glucosylceramide synthase also may provide an approach to inhibit tumor metastasis. There is evidence that carbohydrate residues of cell surface glucosphingolipids (GSLs) play a role in metastasis by being involved in cell attachment. Moreover, GSL composition has been found to differ in cell lines with high versus low metastatic potential. An inhibitor of glucosylceramide synthase is D-threo-1-phenyl-2-decanoylamino-3-morpholino-l-propanol (D-PDMP). Treatment of murine Lewis lung carcinoma cells in culture with D-PDMP produced a time-dependent decrease in levels of all cellular GSLs, reduced the cells' invasive capacity for reconstituted basement membranes, and diminished the lung colonizing ability of treated cells compared to untreated cells after tail vein injection of cells into mice.[80]

The invasive capacity of human bladder carcinoma cells through an artificial basement membrane has been reported to be reduced by staurosporine, a microbial alkaloid isolated from a *Streptomyces* species and a potent inhibitor of protein kinase C. A rationale for this is that total PKC activity was found to be twofold higher in an invasive bladder carcinoma line than in a noninvasive one.[81] The drug, at concentrations producing minimal cell toxicity, inhibited the penetration of the invasive cell line in a dose-dependent manner by decreasing cell motility rather than tumor cell attachment.[81] Another approach to blocking tumor cell metastasis is to design and synthesize peptides that mimic the tumor cell-ECM attachment factors or block the tumor cell surface receptors involved in degradative enzymes being released.[82]

Drug Resistance

Drug resistance is one of the major problems in cancer chemotherapy today, as it has been since the onset of the systemic use of drugs to treat cancer in the 1940s. The advantage that oncologists have today is that many of the mechanisms of drug resistance are understood, and research is leading to new ways to circumvent or at least reduce the development of drug resistance. The mechanisms of drug resistance include: decreased drug uptake or increased drug efflux—e.g., overexpression of the P-glycoprotein product of the *mdr* genes; alterations in activating or deactivating enzymes—e.g., aldehyde dehydrogenase (cyclophosphamide), folylpolyglutamate synthetase (methotrexate), metallothionein (cisplatin); changes in target enzymes—e.g., dihydrofolate reductase (methotrexate), topoisomerase II (etoposide); changes in DNA repair enzymes—e.g., O^6-methylguanine alkyltransferase (alkylating agents); and alterations in glutathione S-transferases (alkylating agents).

The various mechanisms of drug resistance have been discussed in earlier chapters and some methods to alleviate drug resistance have been described. In the case of overexpression of the *mdr* genes, for example, calcium channel blockers have been shown to override some of the effects of elevated P-glycoprotein expression (see Chapter 4).

There is growing evidence for the role of glutathione-S-transferases (GSTs) in drug resistance (reviewed in ref. 83). This family of enzymes catalyzes the conjugation of electrophilic compounds to glutathione, a sulfhydryl-containing tripeptide present at high concentrations (5–10 mM) in mammalian cells. Glutathione helps maintain the redox potential inside cells and is a key player in oxidation and conjugation reactions in drug-metabolizing pathways. An end result of these reactions is to convert lipophilic compounds into more polar metabolites that are then excreted.

Many anticancer drugs are metabolized via such pathways, and alterations in GSTs and/or ratios of reduced to oxidized glutathione are found in cells resistant to anticancer drugs, particularly alkylating agents. Such alterations include increased reduced glutathione (GSH) levels and increased GST activity, sometimes involving a particular GST isozyme.[83] GSTs utilize GSH in a number of drug-metabolizing activities, including conjugation reactions and peroxidase activity that can inactivate anticancer drugs.

Several potential approaches to modulating drug resistance in cancer cells by altering GSH or GST activity have been thought of.[83] However, one must keep in mind that a lowering of GST or GSH in tumor cells could also lower these components in normal cells and render the normal cells more sensitive to drug toxicity. Furthermore, increasing these activities in normal cells to protect them from the onslaught of anticancer drugs could also elevate these protective factors in cancer cells and render them more drug resistant. Nevertheless, some potentially useful points of attack exist.

Cellular GSH levels can be reduced by buthione sulfoximine (BSO), an inhibitor of GSH biosynthesis. In cell culture studies and nude mouse experiments, BSO has been shown to enhance the toxic effects of the alkylating agent melphalan for human ovarian cancer cells but not for normal bone marrow cells.[84] The use of inhibitors of GST activity, if they could be made selective for tumor cell GST isoenzymes or delivered selectively to tumor cells, is another potential approach. Such inhibitors include peptide analogs of GSH such as γ-glutamylaspartylglycine, covalent inactivators of GSTs such as tetrachloro-1,4-benzoquinone that can bind to cysteine in the active site of the enzyme, and competitive inhibitors of GST that may compete with alkylating agents for GST binding. The diuretic agent ethacrynic acid and the prostaglandin I analog piriprost may be such competitive inhibitors.[83]

Chaperonins/Protein Folding

The formation of biologically functional proteins in cells is a highly organized and complex process (reviewed in refs. 85–87). The folding and assembly of proteins has been studied extensively *in vitro*, but it is clear that these processes *in vivo* are assisted by a variety of cellular folding "factors." Thus, more than just a thermodynamically driven process, dependent only upon primary amino acid composition, is involved inside cells. Such *in vivo* folding, often called "assisted folding," appears to involve both enzymatic activities and protein–protein interactions.

Key enzyme activities include protein disulfide isomerase (PDI), thioredoxinlike proteins, and peptidyl prolyl cis-trans isomerases. PDI is an endoplasmic reticulum-associated enzyme, with sequence homology to *E. coli* thioredoxin, that catalyzes the formation of native disulfide bonds during the folding of proteins in the ER to form their active functional conformation. Other thioredoxinlike proteins have been found in the ER, and these may also be involved in protein folding processes that involve disulfide bond formation or rearrangement.

The peptidyl prolyl isomerases (PPIases) are an ubiquitous family of proteins found in all organisms, from bacteria to humans. These proteins appear to catalyze the interconversion of *cis* and *trans* rotamers of proline during protein folding. Interestingly, it has been found that members of this family of proteins are receptors for the immunosuppressive drugs cyclosporin A and FK506. These receptors are called cyclophilin (or CsA) and FK-binding protein (FKBP), respectively, although the immunosuppressive activity of these drugs occurs at concentrations lower than those necessary to inhibit PPIase activity.[87] The actual function of PPIases in intact cells remains to be established, but they appear to act in catalyzing slow steps in the initial folding and/or rearrangement of proteins, as evidenced by the role of a cyclophilin-related protein in the folding of rhodopsins 1 and 2 in Drosophila and of type-I collagen in chick embryo fibroblasts.

A number of other cellular proteins, collectively called "chaperones" or "chaperonins," that are involved in protein folding, assembly, and translocation events have also been identified. In another example of how nature utilizes similar motifs to solve different problems, these proteins have been found to be identical with, or have a sequence homology similar to, what were originally identified as heat shock proteins (hsps) or stress-related proteins. Members of this family carry out such functions as stabilization of unfolded proteins so they don't aggregate before achieving a native conformation or assembling into biologically functional oligomers. They are also involved in receptor assembly and stabilization, protein translocations, targeting of malformed proteins for degradation, assembly of cell-matrix structures, protein secretion, and protection of proteins from heat- or stress-induced degradation.[87]

Some of the functions of the 70 kDa heat shock protein (hsp 70) family of chaperones is illustrated in Figure 14–6. The hsp 70 protein or its non-stress-induced cellular homolog, hsc 70, binds to nascent unfolded proteins in the ER as they are being synthesized, or shortly after they are synthesized, by recognizing a 7- to 9-amino acid structure with a particular aliphatic side chain hydrophobic "fingerprint" rather than a consensus amino acid sequence.[86] This could explain how these proteins recognize an unfolded or incompletely folded structure of several different proteins. Then hsp 70–bound unfolded proteins are translocated into the ER lumen where they can be stabilized by binding to another hsp 70–related protein known as BiP (named for its immunoglobulin-binding protein activity) until the folding and assembly process is completed. The final steps during which BiP is released require ATP hydrolysis. Similar events go on during translocation of proteins into the mitochondria and in protection of proteins from heat- or stress-induced degradation.

Now, one could imagine all sorts of ways that this intricate machinery could go awry during the initiation or progression events in cancer cells. And there is indirect evidence that this does occur. For example, as noted above, one of the ways in which cancer cells lose their ability to interact normally with their environment is by altering their cell–cell adhesion properties and their ability to interact with the extracellular matrix (ECM). The formation of adhesive protein complexes and of the ECM requires a carefully orchestrated assembly of multiple components. For example, assembly of a normal ECM requires the precise assembly of laminin, heparan sulfate proteoglycans (HSPG), type IV collagen, fibronectin, etc. Assembly of laminin and HSPG core protein occurs in the ER before translocation and secretion[88] and most likely requires the action of chaperones, since these are very large oligomeric glycoproteins. Furthermore, biosynthesis

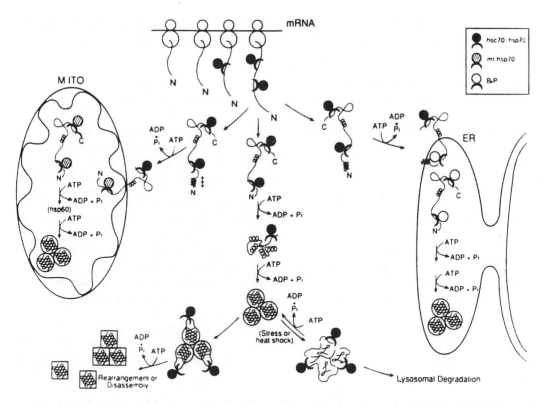

Figure 14–6 Illustration of the proposed roles of stress-70 proteins in eukaryotic cells during the folding and membrane translocation of nascent polypeptides, during molecular rearrangements or disassembly, in protection from stress and in protein turnover. (From Gething and Sambrook.[87])

of laminin chains and their assembly into 450 kDA laminin is altered in certain kinds of human cancer.[89]

Another example is the diminished assembly of the dimeric glycoprotein hormone human chorionic gonadotropin (hCG) in choriocarcinoma cells compared to normal placenta.[90] Since the rate-limiting event in the assembly of the α and β subunits of hCG is the folding of the β subunit,[91] and this appears to be a chaperone-assisted process, there may be a defect in the folding and assembly processes for hCG and other complex proteins in cancer cells.

Whether such defects in protein folding and assembly could be corrected by therapeutic intervention or, alternately, whether such processes could be selectively interfered with in cancer cells in a way that would block their proliferation or induce their demise isn't clear, but this presents a large and intriguing area for future research. It has been reported that the nitrosourea anticancer drug BCNU transcriptionally activates expression of the hsp 70 and hsp 90 genes by a process that requires protein synthesis.[92] This induction process is unlike that of heat shock or heavy metals, and implies that BCNU damages newly synthesized proteins as the trigger for activating a heat shock gene transcription factor.

Cellular Differentiation

It has been known for some time that malignant cells can be induced in cell culture, and in some instances *in vivo*, to differentiate into more normal, less malignant cells (reviewed in ref. 93). Examples include: (1) the implantation of mouse teratocarcinoma cells into a blastocyst derived from a normal pregnant mouse, with the subsequent normal differentiation of the teratocarcinoma cells into components of normal tissues; (2) the differentiation of murine and human myeloid leukemia cells by a variety of agents, including steroid hormones, anticancer drugs such as actinomycin D and cytosine arabinoside, dimethyl sulfoxide (DMSO), and various growth factors; (3) the induction of differentiation of erythroleukemia cells by a large variety of agents, including DMSO, anticancer drugs, and hexamethylene bisacetamide (HMBA); (4) the neural-like differentiation of neuroblastoma cells by a variety of agents that increase intracellular levels of cyclic AMP.

While a variety of such inducing agents can alter the malignant phenotype of animal and human cancer cells grown in culture or in experimental animals, until recently the value of such therapy for cancer patients had not been definitively recognized.[94] Recent studies have shown a decreased recurrence rate in patients with head and neck cancer who were receiving oral doses of the vitamin A analog trans-retinoic acid,[95] an agent known to induce differentiation of epithelial tissues. A further example occurred when some studies by Huang and colleagues at Shanghai Second Medical University became known. They reported complete remissions in 24 patients with acute promyelocytic leukemia who were treated with all-trans-retinoic acid (tretinoin).[96] Similar results have been reported from studies in France and the United States.[97,98]

The mechanism of action appears to involve a gene rearrangement process leading to the translocation of the retinoic acid receptor alpha (RARα) gene from chromosome 17 to chromosome 15 near the myl protooncogene locus,[99] producing a rearranged receptor. This rearranged receptor is somehow able to respond to exogenous retinoic acid, possibly by removing a dominant negative effect of the rearranged receptor and making the malignant cells more receptive to normal growth-modulating or differentiation-inducing cytokines. At any rate, the success of such therapy indicates a real potential for differentiation-inducing compounds, at least in the treatment of leukemia. It is possible, perhaps even probable, that such compounds will have to be used in combination with more classical chemotherapeutic agents to achieve maximum benefit. It is also likely that tretinoin represents a first generation of such therapeutically effective agents, with many more to come.

Chemoprevention

According to cancer epidemiologists, 70% to 80% of all human cancers are due to lifestyle and environmental factors. Thus, in theory at least, most human cancers should be preventable. It is estimated that about 30% of cancers in the Western world are caused or at least promoted by cigarette smoking. This includes, in addition to cancers of the lung, cancers of the oral cavity, esophagus, urinary bladder, kidney, and pancreas. Thus, cessation of cigarette smoking would reduce a major cause of cancers in the United States and in other industrialized countries of the world.

Diet is another major factor in cancer causation. High-fat diets have been associated with breast, colorectal, and prostate cancers. On the other side of the coin, some foods have been associated with reducing the risk of certain cancers. This includes foods rich in vitamin A and vitamin C, cruciferous vegetables containing aromatic isothiocyanates, and foods of high fiber content. These kinds of epidemiological data, as well as cell culture and experimental animal studies, have suggested that various chemicals could prevent the onset or progression of cancer—hence the term "chemoprevention."[100]

A number of potential chemopreventative agents have been identified, including the retinoic acid analogs discussed above, and they appear to act at different stages in the carcinogenic process (Fig. 14–7).[101] Some appear to block activation of chemical carcinogens and therefore prevent the initiation phase (e.g., vitamin C and isothiocyanates). Some may increase detoxification of carcinogens (e.g., glutathione and S_2O_3). Others appear to inhibit the promotion phase (e.g., β-carotene, retinoids, tamoxifen, dehydroepiandrosterone, and calcium). Some of these compounds may also act at more than one step in inhibiting carcinogenesis.

At any rate, sufficient interest has been generated by these data to initiate a number of

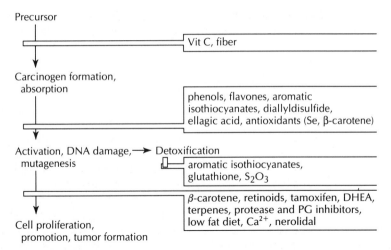

Figure 14–7 Cancer chemoprevention: strategies. Various agents that can be used in experimental systems to inhibit specific steps in the carcinogenic process. Certain agents appear to act at more than one step, and in several cases the precise mechanisms are not known. *Vit C,* vitamin C; *Se,* selenium; *DHEA,* dehydroepi-androsterone; *PG,* prostaglandin. (From Weinstein.[101])

clinical trials (reviewed in ref. 101). Among these are the chronic ingestion of β-carotene and retinoids in men at high risk for lung cancer from smoking or asbestos exposure, the use of the antioxidant vitamin E plus β-carotene to prevent lung cancer in women who smoke, and treatment with tamoxifen of women at risk for developing breast cancer.

By the very nature of the endpoints to be measured—e.g. the *lack* of getting cancer or a recurrence of cancer—these studies will have to be ongoing for a number of years. In the meantime, it would seem prudent to take several steps to stack the cards in one's favor by avoiding smoking and eating a diet rich in fruits and vegetables and other foods that contain β-carotene, vitamin C, aromatic isothiocyanates, fiber, and calcium.

REFERENCES

1. S. Linn: How many pols does it take to replicate nuclear DNA? *Cell 66:*185 (1991).

2. R. A. Bambara and C. B. Jessee: Properties of DNA polymerases δ and ε, and their roles in eukaryotic DNA replication. *Biochim. Biophys. Acta 1088:*11 (1991).

3. R. V. LaRocca, C. A. Stein, R. Danesi, M. R. Cooper, M. Uhrich, and C. E. Myers: A pilot study of suramin

in the treatment of metastatic renal cell carcinoma. *Cancer 67:*1509 (1991).

4. H. K. Jindal, C. W. Anderson, R. G. Davis, and J. K. Vishwanatha: Suramin affects DNA synthesis in HeLa cells by inhibition of DNA polymerases. *Cancer Res. 50:*7754 (1990).

5. M. A. Eisenberger, L. M. Reyno, D. I. Jodrell, V. J. Sinibaldi, K. H. Tkaczuk, R. Sridhara, E. G. Zuhowski, M. H. Lowitt, S. C. Jacobs, M. J. Egorin: Suramin, an active drug for prostate cancer: Interim observations in a phase I trial. *J. Natl. Cancer Inst. 85:*611 (1993).

6. A. Maxwell and M. Gellert: Mechanistic aspects of DNA topoisomerases. *Adv. Protein Chem. 38:*69 (1986).

7. C. S. Marrow and K. H. Cowan: Multidrug resistance associated with altered topoisomerase II activity—topoisomerases II as targets for rational drug design. *J. Natl. Cancer Inst. 82:*638 (1990).

8. A. M. Deffie, D. J. Bosman, and G. J. Goldenberg: Evidence for a mutant allele of the gene for DNA topoisomerase II in adriamycin-resistant P388 murine leukemia cells. *Cancer Res. 49:*6879 (1989).

9. J. P. Eder, B. A. Teicher, S. A. Holden, K. N. S. Cathcart, L. E. Schnipper, and E. Frei: Effect of novobiocin on the antitumor activity and tumor cell and bone marrow survivals of three alkylating agents. *Cancer Res. 49:*595 (1989).

10. G. J. Finlay, B. C. Baguley, and K. Snow: Multiple patterns of resistance of human leukemia cell sublines to amsacrine analogues. *J. Natl. Cancer Inst. 82:*662 (1990).

11. R. B. Mitchell, R. C. Moschel, and M. E. Dolan: Effect of O[6]-benzylguanine on the sensitivity of human tumor xenografts to bis(2-chloroethyl)-1-nitrosourea and on DNA interstrand cross-link formation. *Cancer Res. 52:*1171 (1992).

12. A. B. Pardee, R. Schlegel, and D. A. Boothman:

"Pharmacological interference with DNA repair," in *Anticarcinogenesis and Radiation Protection*, ed. by P. A. Cerutti, O. F. Nygaard, and M. G. Simic. New York: Plenum, 1987, pp. 431–436.

13. D. A. Boothman, D. K. Trask, and A. B. Pardee: Inhibition of potentially lethal DNA damage repair in human tumor cells by β-lapachone, an activator of topoisomerase I. *Cancer Res. 49*:605 (1989).

14. B. F. Pugh and R. Tjian: Mechanism of transcriptional activation by Sp1: Evidence for coactivators. *Cell 61*:1187 (1990).

15. J. W. Lillie and M. R. Green: Activator's target in sight. *Nature 341*:279 (1989).

16. T. Hai and T. Curran: Cross-family dimerization of transcription factors Fos/Jun and ATF/CREB alters DNA binding specificity. *Proc. Natl. Acad. Sci. USA 88*:3720 (1991).

17. H. R. Herschman: Extracellular signals, transcriptional responses and cellular specificity. *Trends Biochem. Sci. 14*:455 (1989).

18. T. Curran and J. I. Morgan: Barium modulates c-fos expression and post-translational modification. *Proc. Natl. Acad. Sci. USA 83*:8521 (1986).

19. J. T. Holt, T. V. Gopal, A. D. Moulton, and A. W. Nienhuis: Inducible production of c-fos antisense RNA inhibits 3T3 cell proliferation. *Proc. Natl. Acad. Sci. USA 83*:4794 (1986).

20. K. T. Riabowol, R. J. Vosatka, E. B. Ziff, N. J. Lamb, J. R. Feramisco: Microinjection of fos-specific antibodies block DNA synthesis in fibroblast cells. *Mol. Cell. Biol. 8*:1670 (1988).

21. E. L. Wickstrom, T. A. Bacon, A. Gonzales, D. L. Freedman, G. H. Lyman, and E. Wickstrom: Human promyelocytic leukemia HL-60 cells proliferation and c-myb protein expression are inhibited by an antisense pentadecadeoxynucleotide targeted against c-myc mRNA. *Proc. Natl. Acad. Sci. USA 85*:1028 (1988).

22. J. T. Holt, R. L. Redner, and A. W. Nienhuis: An oligomer complementary to c-myc messenger RNA inhibits proliferation of HL-60 promyelocytic cells and induces differentiation. *Mol. Cell. Biol. 8*:963 (1988).

23. J. Izant and H. Weintraub: Inhibition of thymidine kinase gene expression by antisense RNA: A molecular approach to genetic analysis. *Cell 36*:1007 (1984).

24. B. Calabretta: Inhibition of protooncogene expression by antisense oligodeoxynucleotides: Biological and therapeutic implications. *Cancer Res. 51*:4505 (1991).

25. C. Szczylik, T. Skorski, N. C. Nicolaides, L. Manzella, L. Malaguarnera, D. Venturelli, A. M. Gewirtz, and B. Calabretta: Selective inhibition of leukemia cell proliferation by BCR-ABL antisense oligodeoxynucleotides. *Science 253*:562 (1991).

26. P. H. Watson, R. T. Pon, and R. P. C. Shiu: Inhibition of c-myc expression by phosphorothioate antisense oligonucleotide identifies a critical role for c-myc in the growth of human breast cancer. *Cancer Res. 51*:3996 (1991).

27. C. Melani, L. Rivoltini, G. Parmiani, B. Calabretta, and M. P. Colombo: Inhibition of proliferation by c-myb antisense oligodeoxynucleotides in colon adenocarcinoma cell lines that express c-myb. *Cancer Res. 51*:2897 (1991).

28. T. Hunter and J. Pines: Cyclins and cancer. *Cell 66*:1071 (1991).

29. J. Pines: Cyclins: Wheels within wheels. *Cell Growth and Differentiation 2*:305 (1991).

30. B. C. Baguley: Cell cycling, cdc2, and cancer. *J. Natl. Cancer Inst. 83*:896 (1991).

31. L. Hartwell: Defects in a cell cycle checkpoint may be responsible for the genomic instability of cancer cells. *Cell 71*:543 (1992).

32. S. A. Aaronson: Growth factors and cancer: *Science 254*:1146 (1991).

33. P. Yaish, A. Gazit, C. Gilon, and A. Levitzki: Blocking of EGF-dependent cell proliferation by EGF receptor kinase inhibitors. *Science 242*:933 (1988).

34. T. Hunter: A thousand and one protein kinases. *Cell 50*:823 (1987).

35. T. Hunter: Protein-tyrosine phosphatases: The other side of the coin. *Cell 58*:1013 (1989).

36. E. H. Fischer, H. Charbonneau, and N. K. Tonks: Protein tyrosine phosphatases: A diverse family of intracellular and transmembrane enzymes. *Science 253*:401 (1991).

37. J. K. Klarlund: Transformation of cells by an inhibitor of phosphatases acting on phosphotyrosine in proteins. *Cell 41*:707 (1985).

38. P. Taylor and P. A. Insel: "Molecular basis of drug action," in *Principles of Drug Action*, ed. by W. B. Pratt and P. Taylor. New York: Churchill Livingston, 1990, pp. 103–200.

39. L. F. Allen, R. J. Lefkowitz, M. G. Caron, and S. Cotecchia: G-protein-coupled receptor genes as protooncogenes: Constitutively activating mutation of the α_{1b}-adrenergic receptor enhances mitogenesis and tumorigenicity. *Proc. Natl. Acad. Sci. USA 88*:11354 (1991).

40. S. Hermouet, J. J. Merendino, Jr., J. S. Gutkin, and A. M. Spiegel: Activating and inactivating mutations of the α subunit of G_{i2} protein have opposite effects on proliferation of NIH 3T3 cells. *Proc. Natl. Acad. Sci. USA 88*:10455 (1991).

41. K. Endo, Y. Igarashi, M. Nisar, Q. Zhou, and S. I. Hakomori: Cell membrane signaling as target in cancer therapy: Inhibitory effect of N,N-dimethyl and N,N,N-trimethyl sphingosine derivatives on in vitro and in vivo growth of human tumor cells in nude mice. *Cancer Res. 51*:1613 (1991).

42. T. Hunter: Cooperation between oncogenes. *Cell 64*:249 (1991).

43. J. M. Bishop: Molecular themes in oncogenesis. *Cell 64*:235 (1991).

44. J. B. Gibbs: Ras C-terminal processing enzymes— new drug targets? *Cell 65*:1 (1991).

45. R. Sager: Tumor suppressor genes: The puzzle and the promise. *Science 246*:1406 (1989).

46. H. Harris: The analysis of malignancy by cell fusion: The position in 1988. *Cancer Res. 48*:3302 (1988).

47. E. J. Stanbridge: Human tumor suppressor genes. *Annu. Rev. Genet. 24*:615 (1990).

48. A. G. Knudson, Jr.: Hereditary cancer, oncogenes, and antioncogenes. *Cancer Res. 45*:1437 (1985).

49. R. A. Weinberg: Tumor suppressor genes. *Science 254*:1138 (1991).

50. D. Malkin, F. P. Li, L. C. Strong, J. F. Fraumeni, Jr., C. E. Nelson, D. H. Kim, J. Kassel, M. A. Gryka, F. Z. Bischoff, M. A. Tainsky, and S. H. Friend: Germ line p53 mutations in a familial syndrome of breast cancer, sarcomas, and other neoplasms. *Science 250*:1233 (1990).

51. M. Hollstein, D. Sidransky, B. Vogelstein, and C. C. Harris: p53 mutations in human cancers. *Science 253*:49 (1991).

52. B. Vogelstein, E. R. Fearon, S. R. Hamilton, S. E. Kern, A. C. Preisinger, M. Leppert, Y. Nakamura, R. White, A. M. M. Smits, and J. L. Bos: Genetic alterations during colorectal tumor development. *New. Engl. J. Med. 319*:525 (1988).

53. S. J. Baker, A. C. Preisinger, J. M. Jessup, C. Paraskeva, S. Markowitz, J. K. V. Willson, S. Hamilton, and B. Vogelstein: p53 gene mutations occur in combination with 17p allelic deletions as late events in colorectal tumorigenesis. *Cancer Res. 50*:7717 (1990).

54. E. Bayever, K. M. Haines, P. L. Iversen, R. W. Ruddon, S. J. Pirruccello, C. P. Mountjoy, M. A. Arneson, and L. J. Smith: Selective cytotoxicity to human leukemic myeloblasts produced by oligodeoxyribonucleotide phosphorothioates complementary to p53 nucleotide sequences. Leukemia and Lymphoma, 1993 (in press).

55. P. Iversen: In vivo studies with phosphorothioate oligonucleotides: Pharmacokinetics prologue. *Anti-Cancer Drug Design 6*:531 (1991).

56. C. Hanski, J. Sheehan, M. Kiehntopf, B. Stolze, H. Stein, and E-O. Riecken: Increased number of accessible sugar epitopes defined with monoclonal antibody AM-3 on colonic mucins is associated with malignant transformation of colonic mucosa. *Cancer Res. 51*:5342 (1991).

57. E. W. Easton, J. G. M. Bolscher, and D. H. v. d. Eijnden: Enzymatic amplification involving glycosyltransferases forms the basis for the increased size of asparagine-linked glycans at the surface of NIH 3T3 cells expressing the N-ras proto-oncogene. *J. Biol. Chem. 266*:21674 (1991).

58. P. D. Yurchenco and J. C. Schittny: Molecular architecture of basement membranes. *FASEB J. 4*:1577 (1990).

59. R. P. Mecham: Receptors for laminin on mammalian cells. *FASEB J. 5*:2538 (1991).

60. V. Cioce, V. Castronovo, B. M. Shmookler, S. Garbisa, W. F. Grigioni, L. A. Liotta, and M. E. Sobel: Increased expression of the laminin receptor in human colon cancer. *J. Natl. Cancer Inst. 83*:29 (1991).

61. K. Vleminckx, L. Vakaet, Jr., M. Mareel, W. Fiers, and F. V. Roy: Genetic manipulation of E-Cadherin expression by epithelial tumor cells reveals an invasion suppressor role. *Cell 66*:107 (1991).

62. U. H. Frixen, J. Behrens, M. Sachs, G. Eberle, B. Voss, A. Warda, D. Lochner, and W. Birchmeier: E-Cadherin-mediated cell-cell adhesion prevents invasiveness of human carcinoma cells. *J. Cell Biol. 113*:173 (1991).

63. L. A. Liotta, P. S. Steeg, W. G. Stetler-Stevenson: Cancer metastasis and angiogenesis: An imbalance of positive and negative regulation. *Cell 64*:327 (1991).

64. I. J. Fidler: Critical factors in the biology of human cancer metastasis: Twenty-eighth G.H.A. Clowes Memorial Award Lecture. *Cancer Res. 50*:6130 (1990).

65. L. M. Matrisian: Metalloproteinases and their inhibitors in matrix remodeling. *Trends Genet. 6*:121 (1990).

66. J. F. Cajot, J. Bamat, G. E. Bergonzelli, E. K. O. Kruithof, R. L. Medcalf, J. Testuz, and B. Sordat: Plasminogen-activator inhibitor type 1 is a potent natural inhibitor of extracellular matrix degradation by fibrosarcoma and colon carcinoma cells. *Proc. Natl. Acad. Sci. USA 87*:6939 (1990).

67. M. Nakajima, D. Lotan, M. M. Baig, R. M. Carralero, W. R. Wood, M. J. C. Hendrix, and R. Lotan: Inhibition of retinoic acid of type IV collagenolysis and invasion through reconstituted basement membrane by metastatic rat mammary adenocarcinoma cells. *Cancer Res. 49*:1698 (1989).

68. J. Folkman, K. Watson, D. Ingber, and D. Hanahan: Induction of angiogenesis during the transition from hyperplasia to neoplasia. *Nature 339*:58 (1989).

69. P. Basset, J. P. Bellocq, C. Wolf, I. Stoll, P. Hutin, J. M. Limacher, O. L. Podhajcer, M. P. Chenard, M. C. Rio, and P. Chambon: A novel metalloproteinase gene specifically expressed in stromal cells of breast carcinomas. *Nature 348*:699 (1990).

70. A. Albini, A. Melchiori, L. Santi, L. A. Liotta, P. D. Brown, W. G. Stetler-Stevenson: Tumor cell invasion inhibited by TIMP-2. *J. Natl. Cancer Inst. 83*:775 (1991).

71. J. Rozhin, A. P. Gomez, G. H. Ziegler, K. K. Nelson, Y. S. Chang, D. Fong, J. M. Onoda, K. V. Honn, and B. F. Sloane: Cathepsin B to cysteine proteinase inhibitor balance in metastatic cell subpopulations isolated from murine tumors. *Cancer Res. 50*:6278 (1990).

72. S. S. Chauhan, L. J. Goldstein, and M. M. Gottesman: Expression of cathepsin L in human tumors. *Cancer Res. 51*:1478 (1991).

73. E. Koivunen, A. Ristimaki, O. Itkonen, S. Osman, M. Vuento, and U-H. Stenman: Tumor-associated trypsin participates in cancer cell-mediated degradation of extracellular matrix. *Cancer Res. 51*:2107 (1991).

74. E. Sidebottom and S. R. Clark: Cell fusion segregates progressive growth from metastasis. *Br. J. Cancer 47*:399 (1983).

75. P. S. Steeg, G. Bevilacqua, L. Kooper, U. P. Thorgeirsson, J. E. Talmadge, L. A. Liotta, and M. E. Sobel: Evidence for a novel gene associated with low tumor metastatic potential. *J. Natl. Cancer Inst. 80*:200 (1988).

76. C. Hennessy, J. A. Henry, F. E. B. May, B. R. Westley, B. Angus, and T. W. J. Lennard: Expression of the antimetastatic gene nm23 in human breast cancer: An association with good prognosis. *J. Natl. Cancer Inst. 83*:281 (1991).

77. M. Haut, P. S. Steeg, J. K. V. Willson, and S. D. Markowitz: Induction of nm23 gene expression in human colonic neoplasms and equal expression in colon tumors of high and low metastatic potential. *J. Natl. Cancer Inst. 83*:712 (1991).

78. J. Biggs, E. Hersperger, P. S. Steeg, L. A. Liotta, and A. Shearn: A Drosophila gene that is homologous to a mammalian gene associated with tumor metastasis codes for a nucleoside diphosphate kinase. *Cell 63*:933 (1990).

79. E. C. Kohn and L. A. Liotta: L651582: A novel antiproliferative and antimetastasis agent. *J. Natl. Cancer Inst. 82*:54 (1990).

80. J-I. Inokuchi, M. Jimbo, K. Momosaki, H. Shimeno, A. Nagamatsu, and N. S. Radin: Inhibition of experimental metastasis of murine Lewis lung carcinoma by an inhibitor of glucosylceramide synthase and its possible mechanism of action. *Cancer Res. 50*:6731 (1990).

81. G. K. Schwartz, S. M. Redwood, T. Ohnuma, J. F. Holland, M. J. Droller, B.C-S. Liu: Inhibition of invasion of invasive human bladder carcinoma cells by protein kinase C inhibitor staurosporine. *J. Natl. Cancer Inst. 82*:1753 (1990).

82. G. B. Fields: Synthetic peptides and tumor cell metastasis. *Peptide Res.* 6:115 (1993).

83. D. J. Waxman: Glutathione S-transferases: Role in alkylating agent resistance and possible target for modulation chemotherapy—a review. *Cancer Res.* 50:6449 (1990).

84. R. F. Ozols, K. G. Louie, J. Plowman, B. C. Behrens, R. L. Fine, D. Dykes, and T. C. Hamilton: Enhanced melphalan cytotoxicity in human ovarian cancer in vitro and in tumor-bearing nude mice by buthionine sulfoximine depletion of glutathione. *Biochem. Pharmacol.* 36:147 (1987).

85. L. E. Hightower: Heat shock, stress proteins, chaperones, and proteotoxicity. *Cell* 66:191 (1991).

86. G. C. Flynn, J. Pohl, M. T. Flocco, and J. E. Rothman: Peptide-binding specificity of the molecular chaperone BiP. *Nature* 353:726 (1991).

87. M. J. Gething and J. Sambrook: Protein folding in the cell. *Nature* 355:33 (1992).

88. G. P. Frenette, R. W. Ruddon, R. F. Krzesicki, J. A. Naser, and B. P. Peters: Biosynthesis and deposition of a noncovalent laminin-heparan sulfate proteoglycan complex and other basal lamina components by a human malignant cell line. *J. Biol. Chem.* 264:3078 (1989).

89. G. P. Frenette, T. E. Carey, J. Varani, D. R. Schwartz, S. E. G. Fligiel, R. W. Ruddon, and B. P. Peters: Biosynthesis and secretion of laminin and laminin-associated glycoproteins by nonmalignant and malignant human keratinocytes: Comparison of cell lines from primary and secondary tumors in the same patient. *Cancer Res.* 48:5193 (1988).

90. L. A. Cole, R. J. Hartle, J. J. Laferla, and R. W. Ruddon: Detection of the free beta subunit of human chorionic gonadotropin (HCG) in cultures of normal and malignant trophoblast cells, pregnancy sera, and sera of patients with choriocarcinoma. *Endocrinology* 113:1176 (1983).

91. J. S. Beebe, K. Mountjoy, R. F. Krzesicki, F. Perini, and R. W. Ruddon: Role of disulfide bond formation in the folding of human chorionic gonadotropin β subunit into an $\alpha\beta$ dimer assembly-competent form. *J. Biol. Chem.* 265:312 (1990).

92. R. A. Kroes, K. Abravaya, J. Seidenfeld, and R. I. Morimoto: Selective activation of human heat shock gene transcription by nitrosourea antitumor drugs mediated by isocyanate-induced damage and activation of heat shock transcription factor. *Proc. Natl. Acad. Sci. USA* 88:4825 (1991).

93. R. W. Ruddon: *Cancer Biology,* 2nd ed., ch. 4, New York: Oxford University Press, 1987. pp. 164–189.

94. L. M. DeLuca: Retinoids and their receptors in differentiation, embryogenesis, and neoplasia. *FASEB J.* 5:2924 (1991).

95. W. K. Hong, S. M. Lippman, L. M. Itri, D. D. Karp, J. S. Lee, R. M. Byers, S. P. Schantz, A. M. Kramer, R. Lotan, L. J. Peters, I. W. Dimery, B. W. Brown, and H. Goepert: Prevention of second primary tumors with isotretinoin in squamous-cell carcinoma of the head and neck. *New Engl. J. Med.* 323:795 (1990).

96. M. E. Huang, Y. C. Ye, S. R. Chen, J. R. Chai, J. X. Lu, L. Zhao, L. J. Gu, and Z. Y. Wang: Use of all-trans retinoic acid in the treatment of acute promyelocytic leukemia. *Hamatol. Bluttransfus.* 32:88 (1989).

97. S. Castaigne, C. Chomienne, M. T. Daniel, P. Ballerini, R. Berger, P. Fenaux, L. Degos: All-trans retinoic acid as a differentiation therapy for acute promyelocytic leukemia I. Clinical results. *Blood* 76:1704 (1990).

98. R. P. Warrell, Jr., S. R. Frankel, W. H. Miller, D. A. Scheinberg, L. M. Itri, W. N. Hittelman, R. Vyas, M. Andreeff, A. Tafuri, A. Jakubowski, J. Gabrilove, M. S. Gordon, and E. Dmitrovsky: Differentiation therapy of acute promyelocytic leukemia with tretinoin (all-trans-retinoic acid). *New Engl. J. Med.* 324:1385 (1991).

99. H. de The, C. Chomienne, M. Lanotte, L. Degos, and A. Dejean: The t(15;17) translocation of acute promyelocytic leukaemia fuses the retinoic acid receptor alpha gene to a novel transcribed locus. *Nature* 347:558 (1990).

100. M. B. Sporn and D. L. Newton: Chemoprevention of cancer and retinoids. *Fed. Proc.* 38:2528 (1979).

101. I. B. Weinstein: Cancer prevention: Recent progress and future opportunities. *Cancer Res. (Suppl.)* 51:5080s (1991).

Index